Quick Reference to Cardiovascular Diseases

Quick Reference to Cardiovascular Diseases

edited by

Edward K. Chung, M.D.,

F.A.C.P., F.A.C.C.

Professor of Medicine
Jefferson Medical College of
Thomas Jefferson University;
Director of the Heart Station
Thomas Jefferson University Hospital
Philadelphia, Pennsylvania

with 36 contributors

J. B. Lippincott Company
Philadelphia • Toronto

ISBN 0-397-50366-0

Library of Congress Catalog Card No. 76-50094

Printed in the United States of America

3   5   6   4

Library of Congress Cataloging in Publication Data

Main entry under title:

Quick reference to cardiovascular diseases.

    Bibliography: p.
    Includes index.
    1.   Cardiovascular system—Diseases—
Handbooks, manuals, etc.   I.   Chung, Edward K.
[DNLM: 1.   Cardiovascular diseases—
Handbooks.   WG100 Q6]
RC667.Q5   616.1'002'02   76-50094
ISBN 0-397-50366-0

To My Wife, Lisa
and
To Linda and Christopher

CONTRIBUTORS

David I. Abramson, M.D., F.A.C.P.
Professor Emeritus of Medicine, Physical
  Medicine and Rehabilitation
Abraham Lincoln School of Medicine
University of Illinois, College of Medicine,
Chicago, Illinois
Consultant, West Side Veterans
  Administration Hospital
Chicago, Illinois
Consultant, Veterans Administration
  Hospital
Hines, Illinois

Mark M. Applefeld, M.D.
Assistant Professor of Medicine
Division of Cardiology and
Attending Physician
University of Maryland School of Medicine
  and Hospital
Baltimore, Maryland

Donal M. Billig, M.D., F.A.C.S., F.A.C.C.
Professor of Surgery
Hahnemann Medical College and Hospital of
  Philadelphia
Philadelphia, Pennsylvania
Attending Thoracic and Cardiovascular
  Surgeon
Monmouth Medical Center
Long Branch, New Jersey

Edward K. Chung, M.D., F.A.C.P., F.A.C.C.
Professor of Medicine
Jefferson Medical College of
Thomas Jefferson University
Director of the Heart Station
Thomas Jefferson University Hospital
Philadelphia, Pennsylvania

Lisa S. Chung, M.D.
Chief Medical Officer and Medical Director
United States Public Health Service
Philadelphia, Pennsylvania

I. Sylvia Crawley, M.D.
Associate Professor of Medicine (Cardiology)
Emory University School of Medicine
Atlanta, Georgia
Chief, Cardiology Section
Atlanta Veterans Administration Hospital
Decatur, Georgia

Stuart M. Deglin, M.D.
Fellow in Cardiology
Waterbury Hospital
Waterbury, Connecticut

Formerly, Fellow in Cardiology
Thomas Jefferson University
Philadelphia, Pennsylvania

Martial A. Demany, M.D., F.A.C.C.
Clinical Instructor in Medicine
Case Western Reserve University School of
  Medicine
Associate Cardiologist of the Cardiovascular
  Laboratory
St. Vincent Charity Hospital
Cleveland, Ohio

Mary Allen Engle, M.D., F.A.A.P., F.A.C.C.
Professor of Pediatrics
Director of Pediatric Cardiology
The New York Hospital—Cornell Medical
  Center
New York, New York

**Edward D. Frohlich, M.D., F.A.C.P.,
  F.A.C.C.**
Vice President, Education and Research
Alton Ochsner Medical Foundation
Director, Division of Hypertensive Diseases
Ochsner Medical Institutions
New Orleans, Louisiana

Edward Genton, M.D., F.A.C.P., F.A.C.C.
Professor of Medicine
Associate Dean for Health Services
McMaster University
Faculty of Medicine
Hamilton, Ontario

**Frank Gerbode, M.D., F.A.C.S., F.R.C.S.
  Hon., F.R.C.S.E. Hon., F.A.C.C.**
Clinical Professor of Surgery, Emeritus
Stanford University School of Medicine
Palo Alto, California
Clinical Professor of Surgery, Emeritus
University of California, San Francisco
San Francisco, California
Chief, Department of Cardiovascular Surgery
Pacific Medical Center
San Francisco, California

John F. Goodwin, M.D., F.R.C.P., F.A.C.C.
Professor of Clinical Cardiology
Royal Postgraduate Medical School
Consultant Physician
Hammersmith Hospital
London, England

Ronald Gottlieb, M.D., F.A.C.P., F.A.C.C.
Assistant Professor of Medicine

Jefferson Medical College of
Thomas Jefferson University
Co-Director, Cardiac Catheterization
  Laboratory
Thomas Jefferson University Hospital
Philadelphia, Pennsylvania

Charles R. Hatcher, Jr., M.D., F.A.C.S.,
  F.A.C.C.
Professor of Surgery and
Chief, Thoracic and Cardiovascular Surgery
Emory University School of Medicine
Director, Emory University Clinic
Atlanta, Georgia

Richard B. Hornick, M.D., F.A.C.P.
Professor of Medicine and
Director, Division of Infectious Diseases
University of Maryland School of Medicine
Baltimore, Maryland

J. O'Neal Humphries, M.D., F.A.C.P.,
  F.A.C.C.
Professor of Medicine
Robert L. Levy Professor in Cardiology and
Associate Director for Clinical Cardiology
The Johns Hopkins University School of
  Medicine and Hospital
Baltimore, Maryland

J. Willis Hurst, M.D., F.A.C.P., F.A.C.C.
Professor and Chairman
Department of Medicine
Emory University School of Medicine
Atlanta, Georgia

Roland H. Ingram, Jr., M.D., F.A.C.P.
Associate Professor of Medicine
Harvard Medical School
Cambridge, Massachusetts
Director, Respiratory Division
Peter Bent Brigham Hospital
Boston, Massachusetts

Nicholas Johnson, M.D.
Fellow, Department of Cardiovascular
  Surgery
Heart Research Institute
Institutes of Medical Sciences, Pacific
  Medical Center,
San Francisco, California

Charles S. Kleinman, M.D.
Fellow in Pediatric Cardiology
Cardiovascular Research Institute
University of California San Francisco,
  School of Medicine
San Francisco, California

Stephen C. Manus, M.D.
Fellow in Cardiology
Thomas Jefferson University
Philadelphia, Pennsylvania

Dean T. Mason, M.D., F.A.C.P., F.A.C.C.
Professor of Medicine
Professor of Physiology
Chief, Section of Cardiovascular Medicine
University of California, Davis
School of Medicine
Davis, California

Richard R. Miller, M.D., F.A.C.C.
Associate Professor of Medicine
Director, Cardiac Catheterization
  Laboratory and
Director, Cardiology Clinics
Section of Cardiovascular Medicine
University of California, Davis
School of Medicine
Davis, California

James P. O'Neil, M.D.
Assistant in the Department of Internal
  Medicine
Section of Cardiology
Burlington County Memorial Hospital
Mount Holly, New Jersey
Consultant in Cardiology
Zurbrugg Memorial Hospital
Riverside, New Jersey
Formerly, Fellow in Cardiology
Thomas Jefferson University
Philadelphia, Pennsylvania

Charles E. Rackley, M.D., F.A.C.C.
Professor of Medicine and
Director, Specialized Center of Research for
  Ischemic Heart Disease
Department of Medicine
University of Alabama
School of Medicine
Birmingham, Alabama

Myles S. Schiller, M.D.
Fellow in Pediatric Cardiology
The New York Hospital—Cornell Medical
  Center
New York, New York

Ralph Shabetai, M.D., F.R.C.P.(Edin.),
  F.A.C.P., F.A.C.C.
Professor of Medicine
University of California, San Diego
School of Medicine
Chief, Cardiology Service

San Diego Veterans Administration Hospital
La Jolla, California

David H. Shapiro, M.D., F.A.C.S.
Clinical Assistant Professor of Surgery
University of South Florida
College of Medicine
Consultant Attending Physician
Tampa Veterans Administration Hospital
Tampa, Florida
Chief, Section of General and Peripheral
 Vascular Surgery
Diagnostic Clinic
Largo, Florida
Associate Staff Physician, Morton F. Plant
 Hospital
Clearwater, Florida
Staff Physician, University General Hospital
Seminole, Florida

Panagiotis N. Symbas, M.D., F.A.C.S.,
 F.A.C.C.
Professor of Surgery
Thoracic and Cardiovascular Division
Emory University School of Medicine
Director, Thoracic and Cardiovascular
 Surgery Department
Grady Memorial Hospital
Director, Daniel C. Elkin Surgical Research
 Laboratory
Emory University School of Medicine
Atlanta, Georgia

Angelo Taranta, M.D.
Associate Professor of Medicine
New York University School of Medicine
Director of Medicine
Cabrini Health Care Center
New York, New York

Paul Walter, M.D.
Associate Professor of Internal Medicine
 (Cardiology)

Emory University School of Medicine
Atlanta, Georgia
Director, Coronary Care Unit
Atlanta Veterans Administration Hospital
Decatur, Georgia

James J. Wellman, M.D.
Instructor in Medicine
Harvard Medical School
Cambridge, Massachusetts
Junior Associate in Medicine
Peter Bent Brigham Hospital
Boston, Massachusetts

Nanette K. Wenger, M.D., F.A.C.P.,
 F.A.C.C.
Professor of Medicine (Cardiology)
Emory University School of Medicine
Director, Cardiac Clinics
Grady Memorial Hospital
Atlanta, Georgia

Myron W. Wheat, Jr., M.D., F.A.C.S.,
 F.A.C.C.
Clinical Professor of Surgery
University of Louisville
School of Medicine
Louisville, Kentucky
Chairman, Department of Surgery
Chief, Thoracic and Cardiovascular Surgery
Diagnostic Clinic
Largo, Florida

Henry A. Zimmerman, M.D., F.A.C.P.,
 F.A.C.C.
Director, Marie L. Coakley, Cardiovascular
 Laboratory
Chief, Cardiovascular Service
Saint Vincent Charity Hospital
Cleveland, Ohio

PREFACE

The primary intention of this book is to describe common cardiovascular diseases that are frequently encountered in our daily practice. Therefore, the purpose of this publication is *not* to discuss in depth various subjects in medicine nor to describe in detail all cardiovascular diseases.

The contents are intended to be clinical, concise, and practical so that this book will provide all physicians with up-to-date materials that will assist them directly in the daily care of their patients with common cardiovascular problems. It is a common experience that we never have sufficient time to read in depth the standard textbooks and journals when presented with a clinical emergency with cardiovascular problems.

The format of each chapter is intended to be uniform, and the information is organized into an outline structure in order to provide a quick reference to cardiovascular problems, in diagnosis as well as management. Thus, most chapters include general considerations, definitions, etiology, pathophysiology, classifications, symptoms and signs, laboratory findings, diagnosis, differential diagnosis, complications, management, and prognosis.

The book will be particularly valuable to family physicians, emergency room physicians, practicing internists, cardiologists, house staff, and cardiology fellows, as well as coronary care unit nurses. In addition, medical students will also obtain from this book a general approach to various cardiovascular problems.

I am sincerely grateful to all the authors for their valuable contributions to this book. I also wish to thank my personal secretary, Miss Theresa McAnally for her devoted and cheerful secretarial assistance. She has been most valuable in handling correspondence to all contributors in addition to typing many chapters of mine for this book.

EDWARD K. CHUNG, M.D.

CONTENTS

Quick Reference to
Cardiovascular Diseases

1. HISTORY TAKING AND PHYSICAL DIAGNOSIS OF CARDIOVASCULAR SYSTEMS

Stuart M. Deglin, M.D., *and Edward K. Chung,* M.D.

GENERAL CONSIDERATIONS

Appropriate care for patients, whether or not they suffer primarily from cardiovascular disease, depends upon adequate collection of clinical information and definition of the problems.

The techniques by which information is gathered can be categorized as medical history, physical examination, and laboratory evaluations. Although some disorders are best diagnosed by a single modality, a full understanding of the patient's problem generally requires the use of multiple types of information. For example, the diagnosis of a typical angina pectoris is established by means of the medical history alone in many cases, but physical examination and laboratory parameters may be necessary to determine whether the etiology is coronary artery disease, aortic stenosis, thyrotoxicosis, or anemia. Special procedures, such as cardiac catheterization and exercise ECG (stress) testing, are frequently necessary for the diagnosis as well as the treatment.

In recognition of the importance of establishing a complete diagnosis, the New York Heart Association has suggested that the following factors be considered in evaluation of cardiovascular problems:[19]

1. Etiology: Congenital, rheumatic, atherosclerotic, hypertensive, endocrinologic, or other underlying causes may be responsible.

2. Anatomy: There may be valvular or coronary lesions, myocardial infarction, or chamber enlargement.

3. Physiology: Cardiac arrhythmias or heart failure may be present.

4. Functional ability: The amount of activity the patient can perform should be assessed.

The importance of assistance from nonphysician health care professionals should be recognized. Frequently, information obtained by nurses, pharmacists, dieticians, and social workers is of key importance in understanding and treating the patient's problems.

THE MEDICAL HISTORY IN CARDIOVASCULAR DISEASES

1. *Goals of history taking*
   A. Establish rapport with the patient.
   B. Obtain information about the patient.
   (1) Collect information that may lead to formation of a diagnosis.
   (2) Assess the severity of the problem.
   (3) Determine other sources of information, for example, the names of other physicians who have seen the patient and previous laboratory studies.
   (4) Assess the patient's personality traits.
   (5) Assess the patient's level of understanding.
   (6) Assess the patient's personal goals and requirements with regard to activity status.

2. *Symptoms*
   Patients with significant cardiac disease may be free of symptoms. On the

1

other hand, symptoms commonly associated with heart disease, such as dyspnea, chest pain, fainting episodes, or lightheadedness, may originate in another organ system or occur in the absence of any organic disease (See Chap. 31).

A. *Pain*

(1) Angina Pectoris

(a) Angina pectoris is chest discomfort that occurs intermittently when coronary blood flow is inadequate to meet the metabolic demands of the heart.

(b) It is usually characterized as being dull, aching, squeezing, or pressure-like. Patients may complain of "indigestion or burning in the chest" but deny the presence of chest pain per se.

(c) The discomfort typically occurs during physical activity, emotional excitement, or exposure to cold weather. It commonly occurs after meals.

(d) It usually begins in the middle of the chest (retrosternally). There are areas to which the discomfort commonly radiates, including the upper extremities, the jaw, the neck, the back, or the epigastric region. There may be no radiation at all or there may be no chest discomfort with the sensation occurring only in one of the areas mentioned above.

(e) The duration of angina is usually only a few minutes if the patient stops his activity. If the patient takes nitroglycerine sublingually, there is usually relief in 1 to 5 minutes.

(f) Angina pectoris that occurs with a changing pattern in a given patient, that is, with greater frequency, severity, or with less provocation or less reliable response to rest and nitroglycerine has been given various names including unstable angina, accelerated angina, crescendo angina, impending myocardial infarction, or the intermediate syndrome.[8]

(2) Myocardial infarction: The pain of myocardial infarction differs from that of angina pectoris in several ways.

(a) Severity: It is generally more severe.

(b) Duration: It is often more prolonged, lasting up to several hours or even days.

(c) Relationship to activity: It commonly occurs at rest.

(d) Response to nitroglycerine is less predictable.

(e) Distribution of pain is similar in myocardial infarction and angina pectoris.

(3) Pericarditis (See Chap. 8)

(a) The history of a preceding event that could cause pericarditis is an important clue in interpreting the chest pain (e.g., cardiac surgery, myocardial infarction [Chap. 31], a viral syndrome, or renal disease [Chap. 8]).

(b) The pain is sharp in nature.

(c) It is located precordially and may radiate into the shoulders and neck.

(d) It is exacerbated by respiratory movements and the supine position and may be relieved by sitting forward.

(4) Dissecting thoracic aortic aneurysm (see Chap. 14)

(a) The pain is sharp and severe.

(b) Its location is precordial or interscapular.

(c) It is not related to respiration.

(5) Intermittent claudication

(a) Pain in any part of the leg, most commonly the calf, may be due to arterial insufficiency.

(b) It occurs when the muscles of the leg are exercised and usually resolves with rest.

(c) It may be described as a cramp, a "pins-and-needles" sensation, or a sensation that the leg is "going to sleep."

(6) Shoulder-hand syndrome, Tietze's syndrome, hyperventilation syndrome (see Chap. 31).

B. *Palpitations*

(1) Palpitations may be defined as an uncomfortable awareness of the heartbeats.

(2) Patients may note that their heart is "beating fast," "pounding," or "skipping beats."

(3) If the palpitations represent premature beats or tachycardia, the patient will often be able to describe their frequency, rate, duration, precipitating factors, and whether they are regular or irregular. The patient may be better able to describe the cardiac rhythm associated with his palpitations by tapping his hand against his chest.

(4) Events other than arrhythmias may cause similar sensations, including vigorous ventricular contractions associated with exercise, anxiety, aortic stenosis, or the hyperkinetic heart syndrome. Heart murmurs or arterial bruits audible to the patient are sometimes interpreted as palpitations.

C. *Breathlessness* Dyspnea should be characterized with regard to:

(1) Relationship to activity. Intermittent dyspnea at rest is unusual in organic disease without a preceding history of exertional dyspnea.[24]

(2) Relationship to position. If dyspnea is worse in the supine than in the upright position, it is called orthopnea and is highly suggestive of congestive heart failure. The number of pillows the patient requires to breathe comfortably at night may be a helpful clue to the relative severity of the problem.

(3) Abruptness of onset. Abrupt shortness of breath may occur with pulmonary embolism (see Chap. 12), acute left heart failure (see Chap. 19) due to myocardial infarction or acute malfunction of the mitral valve apparatus.[13] Abrupt dyspnea that awakens the patient from sleep and is relieved by the upright position is termed paroxysmal nocturnal dyspnea. It implies congestive heart failure.

(4) Association with cough. If the production of purulent sputum accompanies dyspnea, a pulmonary infectious etiology should obviously be considered. The production of frothy, pink material is typical of acute pulmonary edema. Nonproductive cough is often associated with heart failure (see Chap. 19).

D. *Syncope*

Syncope is a transient loss of consciousness due to inadequate cerebral blood flow. The same pathophysiology may result in lightheadedness without actual loss of consciousness. Generally, syncope should be characterized according to its relationship to:

(1) Activity. The syncope of aortic stenosis, for example, is often exertional.

(2) Palpitations. Syncope preceded by palpitations may suggest an arrhythmic etiology.

(3) Position. Syncope occurring when the patient stands rapidly may represent orthostatic hypotension that may be due to carotid atherosclerosis, diabetes mellitus, or antihypertensive medications (see Chaps. 3 and 18). Syncope related to motion of the neck may be related to carotid atherosclerosis (see Chap. 28).

E. *Fatigue*

(1) Fatigue related to cardiovascular disease largely reflects a low cardiac output.

(2) If fatigue is present without dyspnea, pulmonary congestion is probably absent (e.g., in chronic mitral insufficiency).

(3) Fatigue may occur if volume depletion or potassium depletion occurs following treatment of heart failure.

3. *Signs*

A. *Hemoptysis*

Cardiovascular causes of hemoptysis include:

(1) Mitral stenosis (see Chap. 5)

(2) Rupture of a pulmonary arteriovenous fistula

(3) Rupture of an aortic aneurysm (usually luetic) into the trachea (see Chap. 14)

The differential diagnosis includes pulmonary infarction (see Chap. 12), pulmonary infections, and neoplasm.

B. *Cyanosis*

(1) Cyanosis may be present at birth due to a congenital right to left shunt (see Chap. 10).

(2) It may be acquired later in life in the presence of congenital heart disease with increases in right to left shunting or reversal of a left to right shunt (see Chap. 10).

(3) It may occur in the face of severe congestive heart failure (see Chap. 19).

C. *Fluid retention* (see Chap. 19)

The physician should always ask about swelling of the ankles, weight gain, and increasing abdominal girth.

(1) The development of edema is a late development when due to congestive heart failure.

(2) Edema may not be due to heart failure but rather to hypoproteinemia, obesity, or impaired venous drainage (see Chap. 16).

4. *Family history*

A. There are a number of genetically transmitted syndromes associated with heart disease,[11,21,25] examples of which include:

(1) Marfan's syndrome

(2) Mitral valve prolapse-click syndrome (Chap. 6)

(3) Progressive muscular dystrophy (Chap. 9)

(4) Myotonia dystrophica

(5) Q-T interval syndrome (Chap. 31)

(6) Down's syndrome (Chap. 10)

B. A positive family history is an important risk factor in coronary artery disease (see Chap. 2) and may be related to familial hyperlipidemias, diabetes mellitus, and hypertension.

5. *Social history*

A. Cigarette smoking is an important risk factor for coronary heart disease (see Chap. 2).

B. Alcohol abuse is a common cause of cardiomyopathy (see Chap. 9).

C. Crowded living conditions with less complete health care may be associated with a greater incidence of rheumatic heart disease.[2]

6. *Past medical history*

Previous medical problems have an obvious effect on the current cardiovascular status. A few examples include:

A. Previous coronary artery disease may help explain recurrences of chest pain or heart failure.

B. A history of syphyllis may point to the explanation of aortic insufficiency.

C. Previous trauma may account for a newly recognized A-V fistula, aortic insufficiency, or pericarditis.

PHYSICAL EXAMINATION

It is important to recognize that positive physical findings in the cardiovascular examination are often manifestations of pathophysiologic occurrences. In addition to the recognition of a given cardiovascular abnormality, these findings may provide valuable clues to the etiology and severity of a disease process and often provide valuable information regarding the efficacy of treatment. The physician should have a routine format for his approach to the physical examination to avoid omissions. The standard categories of inspection, palpation, percussion, and auscultation provide a useful guideline.

1. *Inspection*

A. *General appearance*

(1) Obesity may be a cause of a variety of symptoms and may be a risk factor for development of cardiovascular disease (see Chap. 31).

(2) Obvious cachexia points to severe debilitation that may be due to organic heart disease or other underlying disorders.

(3) The patient's affect and the amount of discomfort he appears to be experiencing, if any, may give important clues to the significance of his complaints.

(4) There are various facial and skeletal manifestations of congenital and systemic disorders, which are beyond the scope of this chapter.[11,21]

B. *Peripheral circulation*

Inspect the color of the lips, skin, and extremities.

(1) Generalized pallor or discoloration of the skin may imply impaired cardiac output.

(2) Localized pallor or trophic lesions suggest impairment of regional blood flow, either transient or constant[7] (see Chap. 16).

    (a) Occlusive arterial disease

    (b) Raynaud's phenomenon

    (c) Buerger's disease

(3) Generalized flushing of the skin occurs with peripheral vasodilatation. This may reflect a high cardiac output as in:

    (a) Pregnancy

    (b) Arteriovenous fistulae

    (c) Thyrotoxicosis

(4) Cyanosis

    (a) Peripheral cyanosis

        (i) Due to increased oxygen extraction in low output states

        (ii) Occurs in exposed parts of the body

        (iii) Associated with coldness of skin

        (iv) Disappears with warming

    (b) Central cyanosis[16]

        (i) Diffusely involves both skin and mucous membranes

        (ii) Skin temperature is normal

        (iii) Does not disappear with warming of the skin

        (iv) Is accompanied by a low arterial oxygen saturation

        (v) Occurs when at least 5 grams per cent of reduced hemoglobin is circulating and therefore may be absent in the presence of profound anemia.

        (vi) Occurs with right to left intracardiac shunting, pulmonary hypoventilation, or impaired oxygen diffusing capacity in the lungs.

        (vii) Reversal of flow at the level of a patent ductus arteriosus results in a normal color of the head and upper extremities and cyanosis of the lower extremities (differential cyanosis). This is because the right to left shunting occurs below the levels of the subclavian and carotid arteries[17] (see Chap. 10).

        (viii) Greater cyanosis in the upper extremities suggests complete transposition of the great vessels with a preductal coarctation or aortic interruption.[25]

C. *Clubbing of the digits*

(1) Obliteration of the angle between the nail and skin fold

(2) Exaggerated convexity of the nail itself

(3) Widening and thickening of the terminal phalanges of the fingers and toes

(4) May occur as a familial anomaly in otherwise normal individuals or with noncardiac diseases, such as hepatic cirrhosis

(5) It is most commonly associated with central cyanosis and a significant cardiorespiratory disorder.

D. *Jugular venous pulse*

(1) Technique of observation

    (a) The patient's trunk should be elevated to the point where venous pulsations are maximal—usually 15 to 30 degrees.

    (b) The head should not be turned enough to tense the tissues of the neck thus obscuring the pulse wave.

    (c) Venous pulsations may be best observed on either side of the neck just above the middle third of the clavicle, in the suprasternal notch and the supraclavicular fossae.

(d) The venous pulsations should be observed simultaneously with palpation of the opposite carotid pulse for timing purposes.

(2) Differentiation from arterial pulsations

(a) The venous pulse cannot be palpated.

(b) The venous pulse normally has three distinct waves rather than the single arterial pulse.

(c) Venous pulsations are easily obliterated by lightly placing a finger over the vein just above the clavicle.

(d) Venous pulsations and distention normally decrease when the patient sits up from the recumbent position.

(e) Inspiration decreases venous pulsations and distension by increasing the filling of the right side of the heart. ↓ intrathoracic pressure

(f) Valsalva maneuver has exactly the opposite effect.

(3) Normal jugular venous wave form

(a) The *A wave* is produced by right atrial contraction. It begins before the first heart sound.

(b) The *C wave* is recorded on pulse tracings, but often cannot be seen on physical examination.[16] It occurs simultaneously with the beginning of ventricular systole.

(c) The *V wave* is caused by right atrial filling just prior to tricuspid opening.

(d) The *X descent* follows the A wave as a result of atrial relaxation.

(e) The *Y descent* follows the V wave upon opening of the tricuspid valve.

(4) Abnormalities of the *a* wave

(a) The *a* wave is increased in amplitude whenever there is impaired right ventricular compliance or obstruc-

tion to right atrial emptying, as in the following conditions:

(i) Tricuspid stenosis
(ii) Pulmonic stenosis
(iii) Pulmonary hypertension
(if not associated with a septal defect, which would result in dissipation of pressure through the defect)

(b) Cannon waves are said to occur when the atria contract against a closed tricuspid valve.

(i) A-V junctional rhythms (where ventricular contraction and atrial contraction occur simultaneously) cause a cannon wave with each beat (see Chap. 21).

(ii) Irregularly occurring cannon waves may result from ectopic beats originating in any area or from A-V dissociation even if the atrial mechanism is sinus (see Chap. 21).

(c) The *a* wave is absent in atrial fibrillation

(d) In sinus tachycardia this wave may fuse with the preceding *v* wave and be difficult to define.

(5) Abnormalities of the X descent

(a) Tricuspid insufficiency results in a less negative descent because of regurgitation of blood from the right ventricle into the right atrium. If the regurgitation is severe, there may be complete loss of the negative deflection and fusion of the *c* and *v* waves. This is occasionally called a *giant V wave.*

(b) In the presence of active or constrictive pericarditis there may be exaggeration of the negative X descent.

(6) Abnormalities of the Y descent

(a) A rapid Y descent implies rapid right ventricular filling.

(b) In constrictive pericarditis the Y descent is followed by a rapid rise and then it levels off because diastolic filling is arrested by the rigid pericardium. This causes the characteristic diastolic dip and plateau (or square root sign) of constricting pericarditis.

(7) Abnormalities of the V wave

The V wave is exaggerated in significant tricuspid insufficiency because of systolic reflux into the right atrium.

E. *Venous pressure*

The commonest cause of elevated venous pressure is right heart failure (of any cause). Elevations of intrathoracic pressure, most strikingly caused by the Valsalva maneuver, may also cause elevation of the neck veins; the patient should be breathing quietly when examination of the venous pulse is taking place.

Venous pressure may be estimated by using the veins of the hand, or internal or external jugular veins.

(1) For examination of veins of the hand, the patient should lie at about a 30 degree angle. The hand should be held below the level of the heart until the veins fill and then gradually be elevated until they collapse. This normally occurs approximately at the level of the sternal angle.

(2) If the external jugular veins are used, the trunk should be elevated 30 to 60 degrees. The vein is lightly compressed by placing a finger just superior and parallel to the clavicle. After the vein has filled, the compression is withdrawn and the level of filling above the sternal angle is observed. This is generally less than 3 centimeters.

(3) The internal jugular vein may also be used to estimate venous pressure. The patient is positioned as described above for evaluation of jugular venous waves and the vertical distance above the sternal angle recorded. Again this is normally less than 3 centimeters.

(4) If no elevation of venous pressure is noted, the presence of hepatojugular reflux should be assessed.

(a) It is abnormal to note an elevation of the level of filling of the internal jugular vein after 30 to 60 seconds of firm pressure over the right upper quadrant of the abdomen.

(b) The presence of such elevation implies that the right ventricle cannot accept the increased returning volume caused by abdominal pressure.

F. *Skeletal deformities*

Skeletal deformities, such as pectus excavatum, which may cause apparently abnormal physical findings in a healthy patient, must be observed (see Chap. 31).

2. *Palpation*

A. Arterial pulses

(1) Purpose of examining the arterial pulse

(a) To determine the heart rate

(b) To determine the cardiac rhythm

(c) To determine the patency of the arteries

(d) To determine the characteristics of the pulse waves

(2) Technique of examination of the arterial pulse

(a) The patient should recline at approximately 30 degrees.

(b) The carotid pulse is palpated with the head turned just slightly toward the ipsilateral side.

(c) Apply just enough pressure to maximally appreciate the arterial wave form.

(d) Arterial pulse rate should be compared with the simultaneously auscultated heart rate.

(e) The amplitude of the carotid, radial, brachial, femoral, popliteal, dorsalis pedis, and posterior tibial pulses should be recorded and compared with the contralateral pulse.

(f) Radial and femoral pulses should be palpated simultaneously to determine their relative times of onset. Normally the femoral pulse arrives just before the radial. Bilateral delay of the femoral pulse indicates aortic obstruction below the origin of the left subclavian artery (as in coarctation of the aorta) or bilateral iliac artery disease.[18]

(3) The normal carotid pulse

(a) The upstroke, representing the beginning of left ventricular ejection, rises rapidly and terminates in a smooth rounded peak.

(b) The descending limb has a more gradual slope.

(c) The dicrotic notch is usually not clearly palpated although a slight change in the slope of the descent may be detected.

(4) Normal peripheral pulses

(a) Arrive later than the carotid pulse

(b) Have a steeper rise and fall than the carotid pulse

(c) Because of this deformation of the arterial pulse as it moves peripherally, peripheral pulses are generally less suitable than the carotid pulse for providing information about ventricular ejection.

(5) Categories of abnormalities of the arterial pulse

(a) The amplitude of the arterial pulse is determined by

(i) Left ventricular stroke volume

(ii) The rate of ejection

(iii) The pulse pressure (the difference between systolic and diastolic pressure)

(iv) Distensibility of the arterial bed

(v) Peripheral resistance

(vi) The distance from the heart to the vessel being palpated

(b) A low amplitude pulse is the result of diminished stroke volume, narrow pulse pressure, or increased peripheral resistance.

(i) Heart failure

(ii) Obstruction to flow as in valvular stenosis

(iii) Impairment of ventricular filling as in constrictive pericarditis

(c) Bounding or hyperkinetic pulses are the result of a large stroke volume, wide pulse pressure, and lowered peripheral resistance.

(i) Stress, exercise, or fever

(ii) Aortic regurgitation

(iii) Carotid atherosclerosis (elevated systolic pressure and thus widened pulse pressure)

(iv) Thyrotoxicosis

(v) Pregnancy (see Chap. 31)

(vi) Hyperkinetic heart syndrome (see Chap. 31).

(6) Specific abnormalities of the arterial pulse

(a) *Pulsus parvus et tardus* is the low amplitude pulse with a slowly rising upstroke characteristic of aortic stenosis. In addition, patients with this valve lesion may have a systolic thrill palpable in the carotid pulse ("carotid shudder").[26]

(b) Pulsus bisfiriens

(i) *Pulsus bisfiriens* consists of a rapid initial upstroke and two distinct peaks or palpable impulses in systole.

(ii) It is characteristic of aortic insufficiency and of muscular subaortic stenosis.

(iii) When present as a finding in aortic insufficiency, it implies that the lesion is hemodynamically significant.[26]

(iv) It may not be present at rest but can frequently be provoked by the Valsalva maneuver or inhalation of amyl nitrite.

(c) *Dicrotic pulse*

(i) This pulse form also has two palpable peaks, the second one following an exaggerated dicrotic notch.

(ii) Its presence usually implies severe functional impairment of myocardium.

(iii) It is most clearly differentiated from a bisfiriens pulse by simultaneous auscultation of the heart sounds. Both waves of a bisfiriens pulse occur in systole, that is, before the second heart sounds. The dicrotic wave follows the second heart sounds.

(d) *Pulsus alternans*

(i) This indicates a regular variation of the pulse ampltiude (i.e., alternating beats have noticeably lower amplitudes than the preceding beats).

(ii) It implies impaired ventricular function.

(iii) It is often present in pericardial tamponade.

(iv) It is often associated with electrical alternans.

(e) *Pulsus paradoxicus*

(i) This refers to a greater than normal decrease in systolic pressure and pulse wave amplitude during inspiration (greater than 10 mm. Hg decrease).

(ii) It classically occurs in conjunction with pericardial tamponade but may occur in many circumstances where respirations are labored.[18]

B. Palpation of the precordium

(1) Technique: the precordium is most accurately palpated with the patient in the supine position.

(2) The normal left ventricular apical impulse:

(a) Located in the fourth or fifth left intercostal space. No further lateral than the midclavicular line.

(b) It is a brief outward impulse no more than 2 or 3 cm. in diameter.

(3) The precordium in left ventricular hypertrophy

(a) Increased amplitude of the apical impulse

(b) Prolonged duration of the apical impulse

(c) Lateral displacement of the impulse if there is dilatation of the ventricle

(d) A more diffuse apical impulse is often present

(4) Other abnormalities of the apical impulse

(a) A prominent presystolic impulse has the same hemodynamic significance as the fourth heart sound (to be described in the discussion of cardiac auscultation below).

(i) Its presence usually implies impaired compliance of the left ventricle, which may be due to aortic stenosis or hypertensive or ischemic heart disease.[1]

(ii) Its presystolic timing is confirmed by its occurrence just before the first heart sound or the carotid upstroke.

(iii) Its presence is helpful in ruling out significant mitral stenosis.[26]

(b) A prominent, rapid diastolic filling impulse ("palpable S_3") may be found in left ventricular failure or mitral regurgitation.

(5) Palpation of the right ventricle

(a) The right ventricle cannot normally be palpated

(b) In the presence of right ventricular hypertrophy there may be a systolic lift along the lower left sternal border.

(c) Right ventricular enlargement is sometimes better appreciated by placing the examining finger tips just under the inferior margin of the sternum and feeling the descending impulse. This is particularly true in patients with chronic pulmonary disease[20] (see Chap. 13).

(6) Palpation of the pulmonary artery

When pulmonary arterial hypertension is present, a systolic pulmonary arterial impulse may be felt high up along the left sternal border.

(7) Thrills (see Chaps. 4, 5 and 10).

Thrills are low frequency vibrations associated with loud heart murmurs.

(a) The thrill of mitral stenosis is palpated at the apex in diastole.

(b) Mitral regurgitation is palpated in systole at the apex.

(c) Aortic stenosis is palpated in the second right intercostal space.

(d) Pulmonic stenosis is usually palpated in the second left intercostal space.

(e) Ventricular septal defects produce a thrill, palpable in the third or fourth left intercostal space, which radiates medially.

3. *Percussion*

A. Many authors feel that percussion makes only a limited contribution to the cardiovascular examination.[9]

B. The technique finds its greatest usefulness in demonstrating abnormally increased cardiac dullness to the right of the sternum as in:

(1) Dextrocardia

(2) Loss of volume of the right lung with mediastinal displacement

(3) Tension pneumothorax of the left lung

(4) Large pericardial effusions[26]

4. *Auscultation* (see Chaps. 4, 5 and 10)

A. *Technique of auscultation*

(1) Every attempt must be made to examine the patient in an environment free of extraneous noise.

(2) The patient may have to be positioned in a number of different ways during the examination in order to accentuate various findings.

(a) The murmur of aortic insufficiency may be heard only if the patient is leaning forward during full expiration.

(b) The diastolic rumble of mitral stenosis is best heard while the patient lies in the left lateral decubitus position. The murmur of mitral stenosis is often very localized in a small area.

(c) A click or systolic murmur may not be heard in the mitral valve click-prolapse syndrome unless the patient sits upright or stands[9] (see Chap. 6).

(d) Occasionally, the patient may have to stand "on all fours" to enable the physician to hear a pericardial rub.

(3) Use of stethoscope

(a) High pitched events are best heard with the diaphragm of the stethoscope:

(i) Valve closure sounds

(ii) Systolic ejection and nonejection clicks

(iii) Regurgitant murmurs

(iv) The murmur of ventricular septal defect

(b) When the diaphragm is used it should be applied to the chest with relatively heavy pressure

(c) Auscultation of low frequency events require use of the bell of the stethoscope:

(i) Gallop rhythm

(ii) The murmurs of mitral and tricuspid stenosis

(d) The bell should be applied lightly, with just enough pressure to form an air seal with the skin.

(4) Sequence of the auscultatory examination

(a) Determine heart rate and rhythm. Discrepancies between the apical heart rate and the peripheral pulse rate (pulse deficit) implies less effective peripheral perfusion with some beats. The pulse deficit is very common in atrial fibrillation with rapid ventricular response (see Chap. 21).

(b) The heart sounds should be evaluated at each auscultatory area (see below).

(c) Only one cardiac event should be examined at a time. In order to identify an event, it is often helpful to concentrate on a single part of the cardiac cycle.

B. *Auscultatory areas*

There are four classical auscultatory areas corresponding to points over the precordium at which events originating in each valve are best heard. These locations are not necessarily related to the anatomic position of the valve nor do all sounds heard at the area originate in the valve that names it.[14] Therefore, the auscultatory examination should not be limited to only these areas.

(1) The cardiac apex is the best location over which to listen for murmurs originating in the mitral valve, the opening snap of mitral stenosis, and nonejection clicks. In addition, gallop sounds, aortic valvular murmurs, and the aortic component of the second heart sound may be well heard at this area.

(2) The pulmonic area consists of the second and third interspaces just left of the sternum. Murmurs originating in the pulmonic valve as well as the components of the second heart sound and the murmur of a patent ductus arteriosus are well studied in this area.

(3) The second intercostal space to the right of the sternum is sometimes called the aortic area. The murmurs originating at the aortic valve, the components of the second heart sounds, and aortic ejection clicks are well heard at this area.

(4) The fourth and fifth interspaces to the right of the sternum have been called the tricuspid area. Murmurs of tricuspid stenosis and insufficiency, and ventricular septal defect are often well heard in this area. The murmur of aortic insufficiency, when due to disease of the aortic root, is well heard here as well.

C. *Valve closure sounds*

(1) The first heart sounds are produced by closure of the atrioventricular valves.

(a) Mitral closure normally precedes tricuspid closure by 0.02 to 0.03 second so that audible splitting of the first heart sound is a common normal occurrence.[12]

(b) Wide splitting of the first heart sounds at the apex may suggest right bundle branch block.

(c) The most important clinical significance of splitting of the first heart sounds is its differentiation from other systolic sounds that may be confused with splitting, such as systolic ejection sounds. The impression of a loud first heart sound at the pulmonic area may be a clue that an ejection sound is really present, since the first heart sound is usually relatively faint at the base of the heart.

(d) Unusually loud first heart sounds at the apex are heard in mitral stenosis, hyperkinetic states, and in the presence of a short P-R interval.[12]

(2) The second heart sounds are produced by closure of the semilunar valves.

(a) Splitting of the second heart sounds is caused by asynchronous closure of the pulmonic and aortic valves. Aortic closure occurs first.

(b) Due to increased venous return during inspiration right ventricular emptying is prolonged. This causes the widest splitting of the second heart sound to occur during inspiration. Conversely, the second sound is generally single or only narrowly split during expiration.

(c) Abnormally wide splitting of the second heart sound occurs in conditions causing delayed pulmonary closure or early aortic closure.

(i) Right bundle branch block, pulmonic stenosis, and left to right shunts (e.g., atrial septal defect) cause delayed pulmonic closure.

(ii) Mitral insufficiency causes early aortic closure because of abbreviated systolic ejection time.[26]

(d) Reversed splitting of the second heart sounds occurs when aortic closure is delayed to the extent that it is preceded by pulmonic closure.

(i) In this situation, the second heart sound is more widely split in expiration than during inspiration.

(ii) Conditions causing reversed splitting include left bundle branch block, aortic stenosis, and left ventricular dysfunction due to ischemia or cardiomyopathies.

(e) Fixed splitting of the second heart sounds (i.e., no respiratory variation) classically occurs in atrial septal defects because inspiratory increases in venous return are associated with reciprocal changes in the volume of left to right shunting.[21]

(f) The intensity of the aortic component of the second heart sounds is increased by systemic hypertension and decreased in aortic stenosis if mobility of the valve leaflets is impaired.

(g) The intensity of the pulmonic component is increased in pulmonary hypertension of any cause and decreased by pulmonic stenosis.

(h) If the pulmonic component exceeds the aortic component in intensity at the second left intercostal space, or if at the apex the pulmonic component is heard at all, it can be considered to be abnormally loud.[15]

D. *Gallop sounds*

Gallop rhythm describes the presence of a pathological third or fourth heart sound, or both, which may create a cadence resembling the gallop of a horse. These sounds are usually best heard at the apex, using the bell of the stethoscope and may be accentuated if the patient turns to the left lateral decubitus position.

(1) The atrial gallop is due to ventricular filling by the volume of blood expelled from the contracting atria. It occurs shortly before the first heart sound.

(2) In young people, a fourth heart sound with the same timing described above may be a normal finding.

(3) In adults, the atrial gallop usually implies impaired compliance of the ventricles (inability to accept volume without an abnormally high rise in end-diastolic pressure).[3]

(4) Clinical conditions in which the atrial gallop may be found include:

(a) Coronary heart disease. The atrial gallop may increase in intensity, or a new one may appear during episodes of acute ischemia, and this is evidence in favor of angina pectoris[4] (see Chap. 2).

(b) Cardiomyopathies (including idiopathic hypertrophic subaortic stenosis, see Chap. 9)

(c) Systemic or pulmonary hypertension may cause left- or right-sided gallops, respectively.

(d) Aortic stenosis. If the atrial gallop is due to aortic stenosis in a young patient in the absence of another cause (such as coronary artery disease), the outflow obstruction is likely to be significant.[3]

(5) The atrial gallop is more easily heard in the presence of varying degrees of A-V block (see Chap. 21).

(6) Ventricular gallops occur in early diastole during rapid ventricular filling approximately 0.15 second following the aortic component of the second heart sound.[4]

(7) Like the atrial gallop, it is a low-pitched sound.

(8) In timing and quality, it is identical to the physiologic third heart sound found in young people. It must be interpreted, therefore, in conjunction with all available clinical information.

(9) The ventricular gallop may occur in conditions causing volume overloading of the ventricle or myocardial damage, such as:

(a) Mitral or aortic insufficiency

(b) Left to right shunts

(c) Cardiomyopathies

(d) Coronary heart disease

(10) When a ventricular gallop is due to diseased myocardium, its presence implies myocardial decompensation.[20]

E. *Ejection sounds*

These are high-pitched sounds that occur at the onset of ventricular ejection.

They may be due to sudden distention of the vessel beyond the semilunar valve or they may originate at the valve leaflets.

(1) Pulmonic ejection sounds are best heard at the pulmonic area. It is heard with valvular pulmonic stenosis, pulmonary hypertension, and other causes of dilatation of the pulmonary artery.

(2) Aortic ejection sounds are well heard at the apex. They occur in valvular aortic stenosis (if the valve leaflets remain pliable) and in other conditions causing a dilated aorta, such as coarctation of the aorta and ascending aortic aneurysms.

F. *Systolic clicks* (see Chap. 6)

G. *Opening snaps of the atrioventricular valves*

Mitral and tricuspid opening snaps occur in most cases of stenosis of these valves. These sounds are sharp and high-pitched. In isolated mitral stenosis, increasing severity of the lesion causes higher atrial pressures and earlier opening of the valve. A relatively short interval between the aortic component of the second heart sound and the opening snap (A_2 - OS interval) implies severe mitral stenosis.

H. *Pericardial friction rubs* (see Chap. 8)

(1) Pericardial rubs are composed of brief, scratchy sounds.

(2) There may be one, two, or three components corresponding to atrial systole, ventricular systole, and ventricular diastole. It is difficult to be certain that the sound is a pericardial rub if only one component is present.

(3) Pericardial rubs may vary in intensity with respiration and may be present intermittently.

(4) They are best heard with the patient leaning forward or on all fours.

(5) They may be heard in spite of the presence of pericardial effusion.[10]

I. *Heart murmurs* (see Chaps. 4, 5 and 10)

(1) A heart murmur is a series of vibrations that occurs when blood velocity becomes critically high across an area of vascular narrowing or irregularity.[26]

(2) Heart murmurs must be characterized according to:

(a) Timing in the cardiac cycle

(i) Systolic murmurs begin with or after the first heart sound and end at or before the second heart sound

(ii) Diastolic murmurs begin at or after the second heart sound and end at or before the first heart sound

(iii) Continuous murmurs begin between the first and second heart sounds and continue into diastole

(b) Intensity: They are graded in order of increasing loudness.

(c) Pitch (e.g., high, low)

(d) Configuration (e.g., diamond shape)

(e) Quality (e.g., rumbling, blowing)

(f) Duration

(g) Radiation

(3) Further subdivision of murmurs by timing (see below) both is a convenient method by which to classify them and provides important information concerning their pathophysiology.

(4) Midsystolic ejection murmurs occur when blood is ejected across the semilunar valves. They may occur because of aortic or pulmonic stenosis, including supravalvular and subvalvular, increased ejection rate (as in pregnancy, anemia, or thyrotoxicosis), dilatation of the aortic or pulmonic valve, and sometimes in normal persons.

(a) They begin shortly after the first heart sounds, since it requires a certain time period to develop sufficient intraventricular pressure to open the valve.

(b) As ejection velocity increases, their intensity increases and then gradually decreases (crescendo-decrescendo configuration).

(c) In the presence of significant ventricular outflow obstruction, the murmur usually peaks after the first half of systole.[26]

(d) Aortic stenosis is the prototypic midsystolic murmur. It is loudest in the second right intercostal space and radiates into the neck.

(5) Holosystolic (pansystolic) murmurs are produced by flow from a high- to a low-pressure area throughout systole.

(a) The murmur of mitral regurgitation, for example, begins immediately after the first heart sounds, since ventricular pressure is greater than atrial pressure from the very onset of the systole. The murmur continues as long as the gradient exists. The murmur may last until or beyond the second heart sounds.[26]

(b) A mitral regurgitation murmur may radiate from the apex to either the left axilla or along the left sternal border toward the aortic area.

(c) The increased intensity of the murmur of tricuspid insufficiency accompanying inspiration is an important feature.

(d) Ventricular septal defects in the absence of pulmonary hypertension cause holosystolic murmurs.

(6) Early systolic murmurs begin with the first heart sounds and end before the second heart sounds. They may occur with:

(a) Ventricular septal defects with pulmonary hypertension or small ventricular septal defect in the absence of pulmonary hypertension

(b) Acute mitral insufficiency (because rapid pressure increase in the atrium causes a loss of the ventriculoatrial gradient during systole).

(7) Late systolic murmurs begin well after the beginning of ventricular ejection and continue to or through the second heart sounds.

(a) They are generally best heard at the apex.

(b) The usual causes are the mitral valve click-prolapse syndrome (see Chap. 6) and papillary muscle dysfunction.

(8) Early diastolic murmurs are due to aortic and pulmonic insufficiency.

(a) The murmur of aortic regurgitation begins with the aortic component of the second heart sounds, that is, as soon as ventricular pressure falls below aortic diastolic pressure.

(b) The murmur is generally decrescendo in configuration.

(c) It has a high pitch because of the high velocity of flow.

(d) The severity of regurgitation is often inversely related to the duration of the murmur. With severe regurgitation, aortic diastolic pressure falls rapidly and may equalize with ventricular pressure relatively early, causing cessation of the murmur.[22]

(e) It should be remembered that aortic insufficiency may also cause a diastolic rumble at the apex: the Austin-Flint murmur.

(f) There are two forms of murmurs of pulmonic insufficiency, one associated with pulmonary hypertension, and the other due to valvular disease.

(i) In pulmonic insufficiency due to pulmonary hypertension, there is a large diastolic gradient. The murmur is therefore high-pitched, follows the second heart sounds immediately, and continues throughout diastole.

(ii) In the absence of pulmonary hypertension there is usually a silent period between the pulmonic second heart sounds and an initiation of the murmur. The murmur is relatively low in frequency.[5]

(9) Mid-diastolic murmurs are most commonly due to mitral and tricuspid stenosis. Both are low-pitched "rumbles" and are initiated by an opening snap. They decrease in intensity during diastole and may become louder

again with atrial contraction (so-called presystolic accentuation) during sinus rhythm.

(10) Functional diastolic murmurs may occur due to increased volume of flow across the A-V valves in the absence of stenosis. Examples include:

(a) Mitral or tricuspid insufficiency

(b) Patent ductus arteriosus

(c) Left to right shunts

(11) Continuous murmurs imply the presence of a high to low pressure gradient that maintains blood flow without interruption from systole into diastole. They are generally due to one of four hemodynamic mechanisms:[22]

(a) Aortopulmonary connections (most commonly patent ductus arteriosus)

(b) Arteriovenous communications, which may be congenital or acquired

(c) Persistent gradients across stenotic vessels, as in severe carotid arterial obstructive lesions

(d) Rapid flow through non-stenotic vessels, such as bronchial arterial collaterals in pulmonary atresia or venous hums.[22]

J. *Useful maneuvers in cardiac auscultation*

A variety of pharmacological and physiological manipulations can be used to alter ascultatory findings, and aid in their evaluation for the assessment of the clinical diagnosis.[6]

(1) Respiration

(a) Inspiration causes increased venous return. This results in increased intensity of various heart murmurs due to right-sided lesions, such as tricuspid stenosis and tricuspid regurgitation.

(b) Right-sided gallop sounds are increased in intensity during inspiration.

(2) Posture

Sudden standing after the patient has been in the sitting position results in a decrease in venous return. This may cause a decrease in the murmurs of pulmonic and aortic stenosis but an increase in the murmur of idiopathic hypertrophic subaortic stenosis (by decreasing ventricular size and therefore increasing the obstruction).

(3) Valsalva maneuver

By increasing intrathoracic pressure and thereby decreasing venous return, performance of the Valsalva maneuver has the same effect on the murmurs mentioned above as sudden standing.

(4) Amyl nitrite

This drug is a potent vasodilator. It causes a marked decrease in systemic peripheral resistance and reflex increase in cardiac output.

(a) It causes an increase in intensity of the majority of "forward flowing" murmurs

(b) It causes a decrease in intensity of the regurgitant murmurs of aortic, mitral, and pulmonic regurgitation.

(c) It is particularly helpful in differentiating organic mitral stenosis (which increases after amyl nitrite) from the Austin-Flint murmur (which decreases in intensity).

REFERENCES

1. Benchimol, A. and Diamond, E. G.: The normal and abnormal apexcardiogram. Am. J. Cardiol., *12*:368, 1963.
2. Besterman, E.: The changing face of acute rheumatic fever. Br. Heart J., *32*:599, 1970.
3. Caulfield, W. H. et al.: The clinical significance of the fourth heart sound in aortic stenosis. Am. J. Cardiol., *28*:179, 1971.
4. Craige, E.: Gallop rhythm. *In* Friedberg, C. K. (ed.): Physical Diagnosis in Cardiovascular Disease. New York, Grune & Stratton, 1969.
5. Craige, E. and Castle, R. F.: Heart sounds and murmurs. In Conn, H. L. and Horowitz, O. (eds.): Cardiac and Vascular Diseases. Philadelphia, Lea & Febiger, 1971.
6. Dohan, M. C. and Criscitiello, M. G.: Physiological and pharmacological manipula-

tions of heart sounds and murmurs. Mod. Concepts Cardiovasc. Dis., *39*:121, 1970.

7. Fairbairn, J. F., Juergens, J. L., and Spittell, J. A.: Peripheral Vascular Diseases, ed. 4. Philadelphia, W. B. Saunders, 1972.

8. Fischl, S. J., Herman, M. V. and Gorlin, R.: The intermediate coronary syndrome. N. Engl. J. Med., *288*:1193, 1973.

9. Fontana, M. E. et al.: The varying clinical spectrum of the systolic click-late systolic murmur syndrome. Circulation, *43*:807, 1970.

10. Fowler, N. O.: Pericardial disease. *In* Hurst, J. W. (ed.): The Heart, Arteries and Veins. New York, McGraw-Hill, 1974.

11. Harris, W. S.: The cardiovascular system. *In* Goodman, R. M. (ed.): Genetic Disorders of Man. Boston, Little Brown & Co., 1970.

12. Harvey, W. P., and Perloff, J. K.: Some recent advances in clinical auscultation of the heart. *In* Friedberg, C. K. (ed.): Physical Diagnosis in Cardiovascular Diseases. New York, Grune & Stratton, 1969.

13. Hurst, J. W.: Symptoms due to heart disease. *In* Hurst, J. W. (ed.): The Heart, Arteries and Veins, ed. 3. New York, McGraw-Hill, 1974.

14. Hurst, J. W. and Schlant, R. C.: Principles of ascultation. *In* Hurst, J. W. (ed.): The Heart, Arteries and Veins, ed. 3. New York, McGraw-Hill, 1974.

15. Leatham, A.: The first and second heart sounds. *In* Hurst, J. W. (ed.): The Heart, Arteries, and Veins, ed. 3. New York, McGraw-Hill, 1974.

16. Likoff, W.: Examination of the cardiovascular systems. *In* Chung, E. K. (ed.): Non-Invasive Cardiac Diagnosis. Philadelphia, Lea & Febiger, 1976.

17. Luisada, A. A.: Examination of the Cardiac Patient. New York, McGraw-Hill, 1965.

18. Marx, H. J. and Yu, P. N.: Clinical examination of the arterial pulse. *In* Friedberg, C. K. (ed.): Physical Diagnosis in Cardiovascular Disease. New York, Grune & Stratton, 1969.

19. New York Heart Association: Nomenclature and Criteria for Diagnosis of Diseases of the Heart and Great Vessels, ed. 7. Boston, Little, Brown & Co., 1973.

20. O'Rourke, R. A. and Braunwald, E.: Physical examination of the heart. *In* Wintrobe, M. W. (ed.): Principles of Internal Medicine, ed. 7. New York, McGraw-Hill, 1974.

21. Perloff, J. K.: The Clinical Recognition of Congential Heart Disease. Philadelphia, W. B. Saunders, 1970.

22. ———: Systolic, diastolic and continuous murmurs. *In* Hurst, J. W. (ed.): The Heart, Arteries and Veins, ed. 3. New York, McGraw-Hill, 1974.

23. Shah, P. M. and Yu, P. N.: Gallop rhythm. Am. Heart J., *78*:823, 1969.

24. Silber, E. N. and Katz, L. N.: Heart Disease. New York, Macmillan, 1975.

25. Silverman, M. E. and Hurst, J. W.: Inspection of the Patient. *In* Hurst, J. W. (ed.): The Heart, Arteries and Veins, ed. 3. New York, McGraw-Hill, 1974.

26. Tavel, M. E.: Clinical Phonocardiography and External Pulse Recording, ed. 2. Chicago, Yearbook Medical Publishers, 1972.

2. CORONARY HEART DISEASE

I. Sylvia Crawley, M.D., *Paul Walter*, M.D., *and J. Willis Hurst*, M.D.

DEFINITIONS

Any pathological process involving the coronary arteries may result in myocardial ischemia, which may produce certain symptoms, physical findings, or laboratory abnormalities. This chapter will deal almost exclusively with coronary atherosclerotic heart disease, but the reader is reminded that many forms of heart and arterial disease can produce angina pectoris or myocardial infarction. Also, there are other forms of heart disease that can mimic myocardial infarction. Some of these situations are associated with a different prognosis and require different management.

1. *Coronary arteriosclerosis* is a nonspecific term that includes several conditions producing hardening of the coronary arteries.

2. *Coronary atherosclerosis* is a specific disease that predominantly involves the intima and is the most common cause of coronary artery disease in the United States.

3. *Coronary atherosclerotic heart disease* is said to be present when coronary atherosclerosis has become severe enough to produce myocardial ischemia.

4. *Ischemic heart disease* is a general term for any type of heart disease resulting from inadequate myocardial oxygenation. It may result from any form of coronary artery disease as well as severe aortic valvular disease, obstructive cardiomyopathy, coronary emboli, and other causes.

5. *Angina pectoris* is a subjective manifestation of myocardial ischemia (ischemic heart disease). The term does not imply etiology and should never be used without further qualification.

6. *Myocardial infarction* is a pathological term that the clinician uses only in the context of certain subjective and objective data. Again, the term does not suggest etiology.

GENERAL CONSIDERATIONS

Coronary heart disease is the leading cause of death in this country. Unlike most congenital and rheumatic forms of heart disease, it may be severe and life-threatening, even though the physical examination, electrocardiogram, and chest roentgenogram may be normal. The major symptom is chest pain, and expertise in its analysis is an important clinical skill. Since death is not infrequently the first manifestation of coronary heart disease, one should learn to recognize early or warning symptoms and signs as well as risk factors contributing to the development and progression of coronary atherosclerosis.

ETIOLOGY OF CORONARY ATHEROSCLEROTIC HEART DISEASE

1. Coronary atherosclerosis is a pathologic condition of the coronary arteries characterized by a combination of changes of the intima of the arteries.[30] The earliest lesions of atherosclerosis are fatty streaks. Fatty streaks may progress to fibrous plaques and eventually to lesions complicated by ulceration, hemorrhage, calcification, and thrombosis.

2. Although knowledge of the etiologic events is incomplete, it is clear that no single factor is responsible for the development of atherosclerosis.

3. Epidemiologic studies have established the association between certain factors and coronary atherosclerosis. The most important of these are elevated serum lipids (cholesterol and triglyceride), hypertension, cigarette smoking, and abnormal glucose tolerance.

4. Obesity, sedentary living, and psychosocial tensions may enhance development of atherosclerosis, but the evidence for these factors is less certain.

5. Some family groups have a greater risk of developing coronary atherosclerosis at a younger age. The roles of genetic and environmental factors in such unfortunate families are not known. Many such families, however, have major risk factors that can be favorably altered.

6. Although the relation between risk factors and the development of coronary atherosclerotic heart disease is accepted, the benefits of modifying the major risk factors need further clarification. There is evidence that the cessation of smoking leads to a lower risk of developing coronary atherosclerotic heart disease. In the high-risk human subject there is some evidence that preventive dietary measures may partially prevent coronary events and reduce the mortality from coronary atherosclerotic heart disease. The beneficial effects of a prudent diet for patients who have sustained a myocardial infarction is less apparent than in patients who have not had evidence of coronary atherosclerotic heart disease.

7. The presence of risk factors in an individual patient does not offer a great deal of help to the effort to diagnose the cause of chest pain, and the absence of such factors does not exclude coronary atherosclerotic heart disease.

PATHOPHYSIOLOGY[2]

The basic pathophysiology of coronary atherosclerotic heart disease is an imbalance of myocardial oxygen supply and demand. Oxygen supply may decrease, or demand may increase beyond the limits of coronary perfusion reserve, resulting in ischemia.

1. *Myocardial oxygen supply*

A. Myocardial metabolism is predominantly aerobic. Since myocardial oxygen extraction is 70 to 80 percent, increased myocardial oxygen needs must be met by increased blood flow.

B. Blood flow to the left ventricle occurs primarily in diastole and is influenced by cardiac output, diastolic arterial pressure, intramyocardial pressure, and coronary arteriolar resistance.

C. Increased coronary blood flow can occur by increasing cardiac output and diastolic arterial pressure, by decreasing coronary arteriolar resistance and intramyocardial pressure, and by developing collateral vascular channels.

D. Intramyocardial pressure, influenced by ventricular diastolic pressure and volume, is greatest in the subendocardial region. The subendocardium is therefore more prone to the adverse effects of decreased coronary blood flow.

2. *Myocardial oxygen demand*

A. The major determinants of myocardial oxygen consumption are heart rate, myocardial tension developed during contraction (influenced by ventricular volume and systolic pressure), and the contractile state.

B. Heart rate and systolic blood pressure, and to a lesser extent heart size, are simple observations that can aid in determination of myocardial oxygen needs.

C. The adverse influences of heart rate and systolic blood pressure can be decreased by clinical interventions.

3. *Myocardial ischemia*

A. Myocardial ischemia is the physiologic consequence of impaired myocardial perfusion, whether it be diffuse as in severe aortic stenosis or segmental as in coronary atherosclerotic heart disease.

B. The sequence of events in the production of myocardial ischemia as well as the spectrum of clinical manifestations is variable and not completely understood.

C. A significant degree of narrowing of the lumen of a coronary artery may be well tolerated as long as myocardial needs are minimized. If the same degree of narrowing is associated with increased myocardial needs or decreased coronary flow, myocardial ischemia can result.

D. Myocardial ischemia may be transient or prolonged, depending on the effectiveness of physiologic compensatory mechanisms or medical interventions.

E. The subjective manifestation of myocardial ischemia is pain in the chest or its equivalent. The exact mechanisms of pain production by myocardial ischemia are unclear. Other symptoms are the result of secondary effects produced by impaired cardiac performance. Their severity and duration are determined by the extent and reversibility of ischemia.

CLASSIFICATION

Implicit in the definition of coronary atherosclerotic heart disease are the subjective and objective manifestations of the disease. A clinical classification of these findings is appropriate and provides a practical approach to the care of patients. The clinical taxonomy of the spectrum of coronary atherosclerotic heart disease (Fig. 2-1) previously proposed will be used.

SYMPTOMS AND SIGNS OF CORONARY ATHEROSCLEROTIC HEART DISEASE[15]

1. *Symptoms*

A. *Angina pectoris,* "brief pain" attributed to myocardial ischemia, is typically a retrosternal discomfort brought on by exertion or emotion and relieved by rest. It usually lasts at least 3 to 5 minutes, and rarely more than 20 minutes. Nitroglycerin usually relieves angina pectoris in 1 to 3 minutes. The discomfort is not necessarily described as a pain but rather as a fullness, ache, pressure, tightness, or burning. The discomfort may occur in the jaw, neck, throat, interscapular area, or arm; it may be on the left more often than the right, and may occur with or without simultaneous chest discomfort. The intensity of the discomfort frequently increases following its onset. It may be precipitated by sudden exposure to a cold environment. Seemingly nonstrenuous activities such as shaving, hair combing, or putting dishes in a cabinet may bring on angina. Angina pectoris may occur at rest, soon after assuming the recumbent position, or it may awaken the patient from sleep.

B. *Prolonged pain* of myocardial ischemia has the same pain characteristics as brief pain, but the duration is longer (30 minutes to several hours). The pain may be more severe and may be associated with nausea and diaphoresis. It may occur at rest or during exertion. Myocardial necrosis may be associated with "prolonged pain."

C. *Other cardiovascular symptoms* may be associated with "brief pain" or "prolonged pain." During angina pectoris patients may notice dyspnea or weakness that resolves promptly with relief of the angina. There may be palpitation, dizziness, or near syncope. During prolonged pain these symptoms may be more prominent and may persist. Other

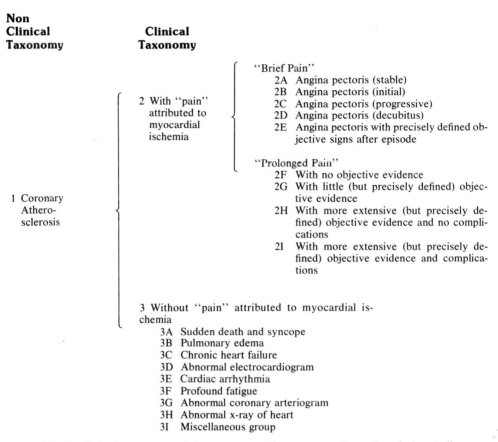

Non Clinical Taxonomy

Clinical Taxonomy

1 Coronary Atherosclerosis

2 With "pain" attributed to myocardial ischemia

"Brief Pain"
2A Angina pectoris (stable)
2B Angina pectoris (initial)
2C Angina pectoris (progressive)
2D Angina pectoris (decubitus)
2E Angina pectoris with precisely defined objective signs after episode

"Prolonged Pain"
2F With no objective evidence
2G With little (but precisely defined) objective evidence
2H With more extensive (but precisely defined) objective evidence and no complications
2I With more extensive (but precisely defined) objective evidence and complications

3 Without "pain" attributed to myocardial ischemia
3A Sudden death and syncope
3B Pulmonary edema
3C Chronic heart failure
3D Abnormal electrocardiogram
3E Cardiac arrhythmia
3F Profound fatigue
3G Abnormal coronary arteriogram
3H Abnormal x-ray of heart
3I Miscellaneous group

Fig. 2-1. A clinical taxonomy of the spectrum of coronary atherosclerotic heart disease used in this discussion. (From Hurst, J. W. [ed.]: The Heart, Arteries, and Veins, p. 1039. New York, McGraw-Hill, 1974).

cardiovascular symptoms in the absence of chest pain may result from coronary atherosclerotic heart disease but are less specific. Palpitations, syncope, dyspnea, orthopnea, and paroxysmal nocturnal dyspnea can occur.

D. Symptoms of coronary atherosclerotic heart disease should be sought in all patients, even though the problem for which they seek medical advice is not referable to the heart. It is sometimes difficult to elicit a history of angina pectoris. When chest discomfort is present, it is important to obtain as precise a history as possible to aid in classification and management. The following are a series of open-ended questions that may aid the physician in this endeavor:

(1) Do you have any sort of uncomfortable feeling in your chest, neck, or arms?

(2) What does it feel like?

(3) When did you first notice the trouble?

(4) When is it most severe (when you first noticed it or moments later)?

(5) What are you usually doing when it occurs?

(6) Give some examples of activities that bring it on.

(7) How long does it last?

(8) What do you do when it comes on?

(9) Does anything else bother you at the time?

(10) Do you have it when sitting and relaxed?

(11) Do you ever awaken from sleep?

(12) What awakens you?

(13) Do you have the pain (or discomfort) while shaving or taking a bath?

(14) What things does it keep you from doing that you would like to do?

(15) How frequently does it occur—daily, several times a week, etc.?

(16) Is the discomfort worse now than last week or last month?

(17) Has the frequency, duration, or severity changed in recent weeks?

(18) Do you take nitroglycerin for each attack?

(19) How long does the discomfort last after you place the nitroglycerin under the tongue?

(20) How many nitroglycerin tablets do you use per week or month?

2. *Signs*

A. During brief pain (angina pectoris) transient abnormalities, including an ectopic precordial bulge, atrial and ventricular gallops, or an apical systolic murmur of papillary muscle dysfunction, may be found. The transient occurrence of these findings during an episode of chest discomfort is helpful in attributing the pain to myocardial ischemia.

B. Similar physical findings may be present in patients with acute myocardial infarction and may persist.

C. Complications of prolonged myocardial ischemia may produce other findings, including pulmonary rales, jugular venous distension, hypotension, and shock.

D. The development of a systolic murmur during acute myocardial infarc-tion may be due to mitral regurgitation as a result of papillary muscle dysfunction, rupture of papillary muscle, or ventricular septal rupture.

LABORATORY ABNORMALITIES ASSOCIATED WITH CORONARY ATHEROSCLEROTIC HEART DISEASE

The electrocardiogram and chest roentgenogram are part of the data base collected on every patient. Cardiac enzymes, exercise electrocardiograms, blood lipids, and cardiac catheterization are obtained on patients with certain clinical syndromes.

1. *Electrocardiogram*

A. The electrocardiogram is of value in the identification of myocardial ischemia and myocardial infarction.

B. Horizontal or down-sloping S-T segment depression of 1 mm. or more beyond the J point is characteristic, although not pathognomonic of myocardial ischemia.

C. 50 to 70 per cent of patients with stable angina pectoris have normal electrocardiograms during pain-free periods.

D. Electrocardiograms recorded during a bout of angina show characteristic S-T segment depression in some, but not all, patients.

E. Other electrocardiographic abnormalities, including nonspecific ST-T wave changes, atrioventricular and intraventricular conduction delays and arrhythmias, are nonspecific for coronary atherosclerotic heart disease.

F. In the syndromes of "variant" angina pectoris, electrocardiograms reveal S-T segment elevation indicative of an epicardial "injury current" (Printzmetal syndrome). Serious ventricular arrhythmias and atrioventricular block are common complications of this type of angina pectoris.

2. *Exercise electrocardiography*

A. Exercise electrocardiography is

used for early detection of latent ischemic heart disease and for evaluation of treatment.

B. The usefulness of this test is limited by false-positive and false-negative results.[17] Among the common causes of a false-positive exercise test are: recent digitalis administration, hypokalemia, hyperventilation, hypertensive heart disease, and the Wolff-Parkinson-White syndrome.

C. Exercise testing may be hazardous in persons with myocardial infarction or a recent change in stable angina pectoris. To insure patient safety, resuscitative equipment (including defibrillator) must be available during the test.

D. A marked displacement of the S-T segment as a result of Stage I and II exercise is a clue to more serious obstruction of the coronary arteries, such as left main coronary artery obstruction or its equivalent.[4]

3. *Electrocardiographic abnormalities associated with myocardial infarction*[14,27]

A. The electrocardiogram may be normal or may show only nonspecific abnormalities in the presence of infarction.

B. A single normal electrocardiogram does not exclude acute myocardial infarction, because the electrocardiographic changes may not occur or may be delayed hours to several days.

C. The electrocardiographic abnormalities resulting from acute transmural myocardial infarction include Q waves combined with typical S-T segment elevation and T-wave alterations.

D. Many infarcts, however, are subendocardial or intramural and do not produce abnormal Q waves.

E. Diagnostic Q waves may never appear if a transmural infarction is small or located in an electrically silent area of the heart.

F. Left bundle branch block and left ventricular hypertrophy are common electrocardiographic abnormalities that may prevent the appearance of new Q waves.

G. A QRS complex deformed by several prior infarctions will rarely be significantly changed by a subsequent infarction.

H. The QRS complex abnormalities associated with the Wolff-Parkinson-White syndrome, pulmonary emphysema, left ventricular hypertrophy, cardiomyopathy, pulmonary embolus, and the cardiomyopathy of neuromuscular disease can mimic myocardial infarction.

I. Hyperventilation may produce S-T segment depression that is indistinguishable from the electrocardiographic changes of subendocardial ischemia.

J. Pericarditis, eletrolyte disturbances, use of digitalis, and subarachnoid hemorrhage are among the many other conditions that may alter the S-T segment and T waves of the electrocardiogram.

4. *Chest roentgenogram*

A. A roentgenogram of the chest should be obtained on every patient with coronary atherosclerotic heart disease.

B. The heart size as shown on the chest roentgenogram is usually normal in patients with angina pectoris and with a first myocardial infarction.

C. Cardiac enlargement may be seen in the patient with chronic heart failure.

D. The chest roentgenogram may reveal signs of pulmonary congestion due to left ventricular dysfunction in patients with acute myocardial infarction, even when other clinical signs of heart failure are absent.

E. A ventricular aneurysm may be suggested by the chest roentgenogram.

5. *Cardiac enzymes*

A. When heart muscle cells are irreversibly injured, enzymes may be liberated into the bloodstream via the coronary lymphatic drainage. Commonly, following a myocardial infarction, the activity of certain enzymes in the serum is elevated.

B. The serum glutamic oxaloacetic transaminase (SGOT), lactic dehydrogenase (LDH) and creatine phosphokinase (CPK) determinations are the enzymes most commonly used in the laboratory diagnosis of acute myocardial infarction in man.

C. Since these enzymes are found in organs of the body other than the heart, disease processes in other organs may produce elevations of any one or all of these enzymes.

D. Because of poor specificity, it is hazardous to make the diagnosis of myocardial infarction on the basis of an isolated elevation of the SGOT, total LDH, or total CPK in the absence of other evidence.

E. The enzyme determinations of greatest value are the isoenzymes of CPK and LDH. If a patient is seen within 48 hours of the time of chest pain, the determination of the total CPK or of the CPK isoenzymes offers the greatest specificity. If the patient with myocardial ischemia is seen after 48 hours of chest pain, the LDH isoenzymes, because of their prolonged elevation (10 to 12 days) are the enzyme determinations of choice.

F. The total CPK is commonly elevated following an intramuscular injection of any substance. Recognition of this important fact may prevent a false-positive diagnosis of myocardial infarction in a patient with noncardiac chest pain.

G. When the symptoms of myocardial ischemia are classic and the electrocardiographic abnormalities are definite, serum enzymes are not needed for diagnostic purposes.

H. Serum enzyme determinations should be obtained and may offer further objective evidence of myocardial necrosis in the patient with chest pain typical of myocardial ischemia, but whose electrocardiogram is normal or shows only nonspecific changes.

I. The finding of normal serum enzymes does not eliminate the possibility of a coronary event.

6. *Blood lipids*

It is well established that hyperlipidemia is an important factor in the development of coronary atherosclerosis. The reader is referred to Fredrickson for a discussion of hyperlipidemia.[10]

7. *Coronary arteriography and left ventriculography*

A. With refined techniques, the risk of coronary arteriography and left ventriculography have been decreased to a low figure in skilled hands. For example, the mortality is 0.1 per cent at Emory University Hospital.

B. The procedure is performed for diagnostic purposes or prior to coronary artery surgery. Coronary arteriography and left ventriculography are performed to determine: the location and extent of the obstructive disease, the status of the distal vessels beyond the obstructive lesions, the contractile state of the myocardium (generalized and localized), the left ventricular ejection fraction, and the presence of disease other than coronary atherosclerosis.

C. A coronary arteriogram and left ventriculogram are indicated in patients with: stable angina pectoris that interferes with an acceptable life-style; initial angina pectoris with recurrent episodes of angina at rest, despite medical treatment; progressive angina pectoris; angina decubitus, Printzmetal angina; repeated bouts of prolonged myocardial ischemia with no objective signs, or with ST and T changes; mild angina pectoris with one or two episodes of prolonged myocardial ischemia having 2 mm or greater S-T segment displacement in the electrocardiogram produced by Stage I or II treadmill exercise; and angina pectoris with objective signs in the electrocardiogram (such as Q waves) if the angina is disabling.

D. In general, patients who have large hearts and congestive heart failure should not be studied because they are not ideal candidates for coronary artery surgery, unless a ventricular aneurysm is being sought.

E. Patients who have myocardial infarction and are pain-free are not studied.

DIAGNOSIS

Criteria for recognition of the clinical syndromes outlined in Fig. 2-1 are as follows.[15]

1. *"Brief pain"* attributed to myocardial ischemia

A. In *stable angina pectoris* (2A in Fig. 2-1), the pain is predictably brought on by specific forms of effort. The amount of effort required to produce an episode varies from patient to patient and determines the degree of incapacity. Assuming no change in physical activity, the number of attacks and their duration is a fairly predictable pattern. The physical examination, electrocardiogram, and chest roentgenogram are frequently normal.

B. With *initial onset of angina pectoris* (2B), the pattern can be quite variable. Within days to a few weeks (up to one month) prior to seeing a physician, the patient may experience infrequent attacks with moderate exertion or may have frequent daily attacks with mild exertion or during rest. On initial evaluation there may be no objective evidence by physical exam or electrocardiogram.

C. *Progressive angina pectoris* (2C) implies a change in a previously stable pattern. There may be an increase in frequency of attacks with less effort, a recent onset of rest or nocturnal pain, or more severe attacks requiring more nitroglycerin for relief. Progressive angina pectoris may be overlooked if the patient is not questioned regarding any recent change in activity, because the patient may actually have decreased activities to maintain a stable pattern.

D. *Decubitus angina pectoris* (2D) is that which occurs at rest without any obvious precipitating factor. It may occur during the day or at night.

E. At the time of initial evaluation of *angina pectoris* there may be certain *objective signs* (2E), the significance of which can only be determined by subsequent events. Q waves may be present initially or S-T and T-wave changes may be present that may either remain unchanged or may, within days to weeks, be associated with additional electrocardiographic findings and enzyme changes of myocardial infarction. (See p. 22)

2. *"Prolonged pain"* attributed to myocardial ischemia

A. Prolonged pain of myocardial ischemia (2F, 2G, 2H, 2I) is that which lasts for 30 minutes or longer and may occur at rest, during exertion, or nocturnally. There may be no objective abnormalities.

B. A spectrum of electrocardiographic abnormalities may be present initially or may develop later.

C. The determination of the levels of cardiac enzymes in the blood may or may not be useful, and they are not available when the patient is first seen.

D. Complications including left ventricular dysfunction or cardiac arrhythmias may be present initially or may develop later.

E. Patient management must be instituted without the advantage of all objective data that can ultimately be collected. These subgroups may be defined on a day-to-day basis and allow the physician to react appropriately.

F. The specific subset is characterized by labeling the condition as prolonged myocardial ischemia and stating the objective data.

DIFFERENTIAL DIAGNOSIS

"Brief Pain" Attributed to Myocardial Ischemia

A variety of conditions associated with chest discomfort are sometimes confused with angina pectoris. In many cases, a careful analysis of the symptoms related by the patient will enable the physician to differentiate angina pectoris from other causes of chest discomfort.

1. *Anxiety*

A. Patients with anxiety may have several types of discomfort that may be confused with angina pectoris: lancinating or stabbing precordial pain, precordial aching pain that last hours or days, substernal tightness associated with hyperventilation, or a choking sensation in the throat due to globus hystericus. This discomfort is not precipitated by physical exertion and is not relieved promptly by rest.

B. The occurrence of pain with emotional upset is common in patients with anxiety, but is also a feature of angina pectoris.

C. Patients with anxiety may complain of palpitation, claustrophobia, fatigue, and fear of crowds.

D. Forced hyperventilation for 2 minutes may reproduce the patient's symptoms and clarify the nature of the complaints.

E. Classic "ischemic" S-T segment depression of 1 mm. or more during hyperventilation and exercise or T-wave inversion are common electrocardiographic findings in patients with anxiety and the hyperventilation syndrome. An electrocardiogram recorded during and following hyperventilation helps to identify the anxious patient with a false-positive electrocardiogram.

2. *Disorders involving the bony skeleton, joints, and skeletal muscle*

A. Pain in the chest and arms can be produced by a variety of disorders involving the bony skeleton, joints, and skeletal muscle.

B. The discomfort is precipitated by movement of a local area rather than by a total bodily effort, and may last for seconds or for hours.

C. Careful palpation and active or passive movement of the involved structures may reproduce the patient's symptoms.

D. Tenderness of the muscles of the chest wall, and painful swelling of the anterior costochondral joints (Tietze's syndrome) are two common problems that may be detected by the physical examination.

3. *Esophageal disorders*

A. The discomfort associated with reflux esophagitis also simulates angina pectoris. The pain is usually located in the lower substernal area. Recumbency and the ingestion of highly seasoned foods and alcohol may aggravate the discomfort.

B. Esophageal spasm may closely mimic the pain of myocardial ischemia. A positive Bernstein test or elevated pressure in the esophagus suggests this diagnosis. A hiatal hernia may or may not be present.

"Prolonged Pain" Attributed to Myocardial Ischemia

1. *Acute pericarditis*

A. With the combination of chest pain, fever, and a pericardial friction rub, there may be difficulty in distinguishing between acute pericarditis and prolonged myocardial ischemia with secondary pericarditis.

B. The pain of pericarditis is characteristically aggravated by deep inspiration, change of body position, and coughing.

C. The rapid appearance of fever and a pericardial friction rub suggest pericarditis rather than myocardial infarction with pericarditis. These signs are usually, but not always, delayed for several days following myocardial infarction.

D. The electrocardiographic abnormalities in acute pericarditis are confined to the S-T segment and T waves. The QRS complex is not altered except for occasional decreases in amplitude due to pericardial effusion. The S-T segment and T-wave changes due to diffuse epicardial injury are found most commonly in patients with pericarditis, but may be produced by apical epicardial injury associated with infarction.

2. *Dissecting aortic aneurysm*

A. Although many of the symptoms of dissecting aortic aneurysm resemble those of prolonged myocardial ischemia, a careful history of the onset and development of symptoms and a detailed examination usually permit a distinction to be made.

B. In both conditions there is severe chest pain, but the pain of dissecting aortic aneurysm often has its peak at the onset, and may have more widespread radiation to the posterior thorax, the lumbar region, the epigastrium, or the lower extremities.

C. Aortic regurgitation, not previously present, wide differences in blood pressures or in pulses between legs, arms, or carotid arteries, and pulsation of the sternoclavicular joint favor dissecting aneurysm.

D. Roentgenologic examination sometimes discloses a progressive widening of the aorta.

3. *Pulmonary embolism*

A. Marked dyspnea, tachypnea, or cyanosis accompanying the onset of chest pain suggests the diagnosis of pulmonary embolism.

B. Syncope may be the major complaint when the embolism is massive.

C. Helpful physical findings include: signs of acute tricuspid regurgitation, wide splitting of the second heart sound with an increased intensity of the pulmonic component, and right ventricular gallop sounds.

D. Sinus tachycardia, atrial fibrillation, and atrial flutter may occur in patients with pulmonary embolism.

E. Alterations of the QRS complex may suggest inferior or anterior myocardial infarction in some patients.

F. The serum enzymes, SGOT, total LDH, and total CPK, may be elevated following either myocardial infarction or pulmonary infarction and are of little differential value; however, a determination of isoenzymes of CPK and LDH are useful in identifying the heart or the lung as the source of enzyme elevation.

4. *Acute abdominal disorders*

A. A perforated peptic ulcer, cholelithiasis, and acute cholecystitis, acute pancreatitis, and acute intestinal obstruction can produce a clinical picture that may be mistaken for myocardial ischemia.

B. If the patient is in shock, depression of the S-T segment in the electrocardiogram may cause confusion.

5. *Cafe Coronary*

A. The signs and symptoms of a "cafe coronary" may mimic an episode of myocardial ischemia.

B. The typical setting is that of a man at a restaurant having a few drinks of alcohol and eating meat. He suddenly aspirates a large bolus of poorly chewed meat and then clutches his chest, becomes cyanotic, and collapses. Such patients cannot talk because of total airway obstruction.

C. Cafe coronary is cured by alleviation of the tracheal obstruction.

COMPLICATIONS

Pericarditis, pulmonary embolism, cardiogenic shock, acute pulmonary edema, cardiac arrhythmias, and cardiac rupture (including septal rupture, papillary muscle rupture, and external rupture of the heart) are important complications of myocardial infarction. Recent studies have shown that these serious complications can occur as a result of myocardial ischemia in the absence of objective evidence of myocardial infarction (serum enzyme elevation or diagnostic electrocardiographic changes). Many patients in the "brief pain" groups should be monitored for arrhythmias and other complications, just as the patients in the "prolonged pain" groups are monitored.

1. *Atrial arrhythmias*[7]

A. The major mechanisms responsible for the atrial arrhythmias appear to be left ventricular dysfunction and atrial ischemia or infarction.

B. Premature atrial contractions are not of consequence, except that they sometimes precipitate atrial tachyarrhythmias or give warning of the likelihood of developing atrial fibrillation.

C. Atrial tachycardia is uncommon in patients with myocardial infarction.

D. Atrial tachycardia with block may result from digitalis toxicity.

E. Atrial fibrillation is commonly initiated by a premature atrial contraction occurring early in the cardiac cycle. In atrial fibrillation, the loss of an effective synchronized atrial contraction and the presence of a rapid irregular ventricular rate combine to decrease the cardiac output.

F. Atrial flutter is less common than atrial fibrillation in the setting of myocardial infarction. Most frequently, a 2:1 AV conduction ratio results in a ventricular rate in the vicinity of 150 beats per minute. This rapid ventricular rate may cause serious hemodynamic deterioration.

G. The persistence of rapid sinus tachycardia is a serious complication that is not generally appreciated. Persistent sinus tachycardia is commonly a sign of severe left ventricular dysfunction.

2. *Junctional arrhythmias*

A. Myocardial ischemia may produce an accelerated junctional pacemaker focus with rates greater than 60 beats per minute.

B. Accelerated junctional rhythms associated with inferior infarction are usually benign.

C. Patients with anterior infarction and AV junctional tachycardia have a poor prognosis.

3. *Ventricular arrhythmias*

A. The most common arrhythmia associated with myocardial infarction is premature ventricular contraction (PVC). PVCs occur in approximately 80 per cent of patients constantly monitored during acute myocardial infarction. Their significance lies in their proclivity to precipitate ventricular tachycardia or ventricular fibrillation, although these potentially lethal arrhythmias can arise without any preceding PVCs.

B. Much emphasis has been placed on PVCs that occur in the vulnerable phase of the cardiac cycle (on the T wave of the previous beat). Although this type of PVC is more likely to initiate a serious ventricular tachyarrhythmia, repetitive ventricular beating may be precipitated by PVCs that originate outside the vulnerable phase.

C. Accelerated idioventricular rhythm has been recognized with increasing frequency in myocardial infarction. It is more common than rapid ventricular tachycardia and is less serious.

4. *Bradycardia*[25]

A. Sinus bradycardia may be seen as a transient or persistent slow rate, with or without hypotension. The combination of sinus bradycardia and hypotension frequently represents a vagovagal reaction, the hemodynamic consequences of which include a decrease in cardiac output and in peripheral vascular resistance.

B. The bradycardia associated with myocardial infarction may be due to second degree or complete heart block. As a rule, heart block associated with anterior myocardial infarction is more serious than block related to inferior infarction.

C. With inferior infarction, AV block usually occurs in the AV node. Complete heart block follows a period of Type I second-degree block and the escape pacemaker is located above the bifurcation of the bundle of His. As a result, the QRS complex is usually of normal duration. The rate of this pacemaker is between 45 and 60 beats per minute.

D. In anterior infarction, AV block usually results from extensive disease in the bundle branches. Progression to complete heart block is sudden, and is only occasionally preceded by Type II second-degree AV block. The QRS duration is 0.12 seconds or greater, and the idioventricular escape rhythm is 40 beats per minute or less. The escape pacemaker may suddenly stop, producing asystole.

E. Bradycardia due to any mechanism may increase ventricular ectopy.

5. *Ventricular dysfunction*[22]

A. A varying degree of impaired left ventricular function occurs in most patients with acute myocardial infarction.

B. Patients with mild infarctions frequently demonstrate abnormal elevations of the left ventricular filling pressure during the first few days after infarction. Symptoms of congestive heart failure are absent, and the only abnormal physical finding may be an atrial gallop.

C. With congestive heart failure, the left ventricular end-diastolic pressure tends to be substantially elevated. Dyspnea and orthopnea are frequently absent, but the following physical findings suggest the presence of heart failure: ventricular diastolic gallop, persistent sinus tachycardia, pulsus alternans, inspiratory rales, and abnormal neck vein distention.

D. Even when the physical examination is normal, the chest roentgenogram may show interstitial pulmonary edema.

E. Cardiogenic shock is associated with extensive loss of left ventricular myocardium due to recent myocardial infarction. At times, the problem occurs because a new infarction is added to an old infarction. The state of shock further reduces coronary perfusion pressure, resulting in continuing focal myocardial ischemia and necrosis.

F. The hemodynamic changes accompanying shock due to myocardial infarction are variable. In general, the left ventricular end-diastolic pressure is elevated, the cardiac output is markedly decreased, and the peripheral vascular resistance is elevated.

G. In a few patients, hypovolemia may contribute to the shock state. The first clue to occult hypovolemia may be the recording of a normal or low pulmonary artery wedge pressure.

6. *Pericarditis*

A. Pericarditis is often unrecognized because of the absence of a pericardial friction rub or characteristic S-T segment elevation.

B. Chest pain occurring a few days after infarction that is aggravated by inspiration, a change of position, coughing, or swallowing should suggest pericarditis.

C. Atrial arrhythmias or recurrent fever developing a few days to a week following myocardial infarction are other clues to the presence of this condition.

7. *Pulmonary embolism*

Pulmonary embolism may cause episodes of dyspnea, atrial arrhythmias, or sudden death. Deep venous thrombosis is more common in patients with severe congestive heart failure, shock, preexisting venous disease, and in patients over the age of 70.

8. *Systemic arterial emboli*

A. Systemic arterial emboli originate in left ventricular mural thrombi.

B. Arterial emboli may produce infarction of the brain, kidney, spleen, and intestinal tract.

C. Peripheral embolism in an extremity is characterized by acute pain, loss of sensation, coldness of the extremity, loss of arterial pulsation, and (later) loss of motion of the affected muscles.

9. *Cardiac rupture*

A. External rupture of the heart following myocardial infarction leads to hemopericardium, cardiac tamponade, and sudden death. Death may occur within a few minutes after rupture, but occasionally there is a survival period of several hours.

B. Rupture of a papillary muscle may be suspected when a holosystolic murmur and acute pulmonary edema and shock develop suddenly in a patient with recent myocardial infarction. Severe mitral regurgitation due to papillary rupture may not be associated with a heart murmur and should be considered in any patient with shock and heart failure.

C. Rupture of the ventricular septum produces a systolic murmur near the lower sternal border and pronounced signs of acute heart failure. At times, the murmur may be located at the apex. The discovery of a new systolic murmur in a patient with acute infarction is not diagnostic of rupture of the ventricular septum or papillary muscle because a systolic murmur may be caused by papillary muscle dysfunction. The cause of such a murmur should be clarified by cardiac catheterization if the patient is not doing well.

10. *Ventricular aneurysm*

A. A ventricular aneurysm is a late complication of myocardial infarction that is suggested by: an abnormal precordial pulsation located medially or superiorly to the cardiac apex, persistent S-T segment elevation of the electrocardiogram, and an abnormal contour of the left cardiac border in the roentgenogram of the chest.

B. Refractory heart failure, recurrent arterial emboli, and recurrent ventricular tachycardia are major complications of ventricular aneurysm.

11. *Sudden death*

The most common cause of sudden death in adults is coronary atherosclerotic heart disease. In many patients, sudden death is the first and only clinically recognizable manifestation of the disease.

MANAGEMENT[15]

"Brief Pain" Attributed to Myocardial Ischemia

1. *Stable angina pectoris* (2A in Fig. 2-1)

A. *Nitroglycerin* is probably the most important drug in the therapy of angina pectoris. Its administration results in prompt relief of pain within 1 to 3 minutes. It is preferable to begin with a small dosage of 0.32 mg. (1/200 g.) or 0.16 mg. (1/400 g.) in order to minimize side effects, especially headache. Some patients may require 0.64 mg. (1/100 g.) to obtain optimum effect. The patient should be instructed to carry nitroglycerin at all times and to take it promptly at the onset of pain. Nitroglycerin may be repeated every 5 minutes for three doses. The patient should seek medical attention if this fails to relieve pain. Nitroglycerin should be used before an event that is known to precipitate angina pectoris. The medication is not addictive. It will deteriorate with exposure to light and moisture (failure to experience a slight burning of the tongue or a throbbing sensation in the neck, throat, or head are signs that the medication has deteriorated).

B. *Long acting nitrites* are useful for patients with stable angina pectoris who are more than minimally incapacitated. Isosorbide dinitrite sublingually is recommended at an initial dosage of 2.5

to 5 mg. every 6 hours with a gradual increase to 5 to 10 mg. every 2 to 4 hours. Symptomatic orthostatic hypotension should be avoided. Severe headaches when therapy is first begun can discourage patient compliance. Thus, initial therapy with a low dosage and patient reassurance are helpful.

C. *Nitrol ointment*[23] (2%) is especially helpful for nocturnal angina. An initial dose of ½ to 1 inch is applied at bedtime, and may be gradually increased to 2 inches. It can be used throughout the day by using similar amounts applied every 4 to 6 hours. This preparation is especially helpful if propranolol must be stopped for any reason.

D. *Propranolol*[21] is one of the great pharmaceutical advances in the treatment of angina pectoris. The drug is indicated in the treatment of mild angina pectoris; its use should not be reserved for severe angina pectoris, as was formerly suggested. Propranolol is a beta-adrenergic blocking agent that decreases myocardial contractility and heart rate, resulting in a decrease in myocardial oxygen requirement. The initial dosage is 10 mg. every 6 hours, which may be gradually increased by 10 mg. increments to doses as great as 80 to 100 mg. every 6 hours. The dosage can be increased, provided the resting heart rate is 55 beats per minute or greater, there is no symptomatic orthostatic hypotension, and there are no signs or symptoms of heart failure or bronchospasm. Other side effects (headache, fatigue, nausea, or diarrhea) may require a reduction of dose. Propranolol should not be used in patients with severe bronchospasm, heart block, or severe congestive heart failure. It should be used with caution if sinus bradycardia is already present, if there is evidence of moderate left ventricular failure, or if the patient takes insulin for diabetes mellitus.

E. *Digitalis* can be useful in the treatment of angina pectoris. It is indicated in those patients with nocturnal angina and may be useful if rest angina is present. A trial of digitalis in all patients with incapacitating angina after maximum therapy with other drugs is reasonable. Frequently, the left ventricular hemodynamics and left ventricular angiogram are abnormal in the absence of clinical signs of heart failure. Therapy can be instituted simply with a daily dose of 0.25 mg.

F. *Diuretics* are indicated if there is evidence of congestive heart failure and may be helpful if nocturnal angina is prominent.

G. The correction of *factors known to aggravate angina pectoris* is important. Obesity, smoking, hypertension, and anemia are frequent offenders. Thyrotoxicosis should be treated if present.

2. *Angina Pectoris, Initial* (2B), *Angina Pectoris, Progressive* (2C), *Angina Pectoris, Decubitus* (2D).

These are categories of unstable angina and imply that a patient's status has changed within days or weeks. *Since their course is unpredictable at the time of initial assessment, these patients should be managed as though a myocardial infarction had occurred.* Patients in Category 2E "brief pain" with objective signs have actually had an infarction.

A. *Hospitalization* is indicated for patients with: previously stable angina that was infrequent, which is now occurring several times daily; previously stable angina pectoris precipitated by moderate exertion, which is now occurring at rest or nocturnally; progressive angina with new electrocardiographic abnormalities; or those with the initial onset of angina occurring daily.

B. *Drug therapy* in these groups is similar to that outlined under stable angina pectoris. Drug dosages should be increased in increments, as long as the patient continues to have pain. Nitroglycerin may be used for episodes of pain, as long as they are brief. Long-acting nitrites may be increased on a daily basis as long as hypotension is not significant. Propranolol dosage, after an initial 10 mg. dose to observe blood pressure and heart rate response may be increased by 10 mg. increments every 12 to 24 hours, until a dosage of 40 to 60 mg. every 6 hours is reached. Careful patient monitoring for side effects is imperative. Nitroglycerin, long-acting nitrites, and propranolol may be instituted initially. Digitalis can be added at any point, keeping in mind the general indications discussed in the management of stable angina pectoris.

C. *Electrocardiographic monitoring* in a coronary care unit for 48 hours or longer is important if arrhythmias develop or if pain continues. Physical activity should be restricted as long as the pain pattern is not resolving.

D. *Coronary arteriography* and *coronary artery surgery* are often indicated when the symptoms of myocardial ischemia continue for 3 or 4 days (see p. 32).

E. *Diagnostically,* additional objective data should be collected during hospitalization. An electrocardiogram should be obtained daily for the first few days or longer if there is recurrence of pain. An electrocardiogram just prior to discharge should be obtained to detect any late changes and to serve as a baseline during subsequent evaluations. Serial determinations of cardiac enzymes my be helpful. Both the cardiac examination and an electrocardiogram during pain may provide useful information.

F. The *day-to-day evaluation* of response to therapy and additional objective data will determine the duration of hospitalization and treatment. The point is, these patients may be placed in one of two groups. One group of such patients may be managed medically because they have no more difficulty, and another group may be moved on to coronary surgery. The indications for surgery are changing monthly, and more and more

patients are being placed in this group. (See p. 33)

"Prolonged Pain" Attributed to Myocardial Ischemia

Each of these subgroups (2F, 2G, 2H, and 2I) should be managed initially as though myocardial infarction had occurred. The same is true for brief pain with objective signs (2E). The clinical course and additional objective data may modify subsequent assessment and management.

1. The patient should be *admitted to the coronary care unit.* Relief of pain should be accomplished as promptly as possible. If there is dyspnea or persistent pain, oxygen should be administered. Blood pressure, cardiac rhythm, and urine output should be monitored.

2. *Relief of pain* is best accomplished with intravenous administration of opiates. Morphine sulfate in 1- to 2-mg. increments every 2 to 4 minutes (total dose 5 to 10 mg.) or meperidine hydrochloride (Demerol) in 25 mg. increments (total dose 75 to 100 mg.) are frequently used. Respiratory depression, manifested as a decreased amplitude or rate of respiratory excursions, should be avoided. Smaller doses should be used in patients with lung disease, pulmonary edema, hypotension, or myxedema. Since morphine sulfate has a vagotonic effect, meperidine hydrochloride is preferable in the presence of bradycardia.

3. *Digitalis* should be used if there is evidence of left ventricular dysfunction. A ventricular gallop, rales, neck vein distention, interstitial edema on x-ray examination or sinus tachycardia are indications for its use. Significant left ventricular dysfunction may be present with a normal heart size on x-ray.

4. *Diuretics* are useful in the management of left ventricular failure. They must be used cautiously in acute myocardial infarction to avoid hypovolemia. A small initial dose is recommended.

5. For a discussion on the treatment of *cardiac arrhythmias,* see Chapter 21.

6. Patients in subsets 2F, 2G, or 2H *without complications* are allowed out of bed to use the bedside commode on the day after admission They may sit in a chair at the bedside as long as this does not produce hypotension, arrhythmias, or fatigue. They are transferred from the coronary care unit about the third day, are walking about the room on the fifth day and in the hallway by the ninth day, and can anticipate discharge after a total of 12 to 14 days' hospitalization.

7. Patients with *mild complications* (subset 2I) require slightly longer hospitalization, approximately 3 weeks, and ambulation is permitted slightly later in the hospital course. The presence of heart failure, recurrent chest pain, or arrhythmias does not necessarily preclude ambulation, as long as these problems are not worsened by such activities. An ambulation program should begin early and should be progressive.[16]

8. While the patient is in the coronary care unit he should be given a soft diet, a stool softener, and a mild sedative. Visits by family and friends should be brief.

9. *Anticoagulants* are given for patients with QRS changes associated with S-T, T changes in the electrocardiogram, or with only S-T, T changes.[18,19]

10. The measurement of *cardiac enzymes* in the blood is indicated when the electrocardiogram is not specific, but such measures are not indicated in patients with definite electrocardiographic changes of severe ischemia or infarction.

11. *Vasodilator therapy* with sodium nitroprusside or phentolomine[3] or nitroglycerin[1] improves hemodynamics in patients with *left ventricular failure* complicating acute myocardial infarction. It has also been demonstrated that these agents may decrease S-T segment elevation (implying decreased ischemic injury) during acute myocardial infarction.[9] Further work in this area is needed

to clarify the value of vasodilator therapy.

12. The patient with prolonged pain due to myocardial ischemia with a normal electrocardiogram or with S-T, T changes should have *coronary arteriography* and *coronary artery surgery* if the pain recurs for several days despite treatment. An electrocardiogram made during pain may reveal the Printzmetal phenomenon of S-T segment elevation, which should hasten the performance of coronary arteriography. Bypass surgery is indicated if obstruction is present, but not when coronary artery spasm alone is present (see below). As a rule, coronary arteriography with coronary surgery is not performed in patients with overt myocardial infarction.

13. *Intraaortic balloon pumping* may be useful in the management of complications of acute myocardial infarction. *Cardiogenic shock* may be temporarily alleviated by this intervention.[2] This will allow further evaluation of the cause of shock by cardiac catheterization and angiographic studies.

Rupture of the ventricular septum, papillary muscle rupture, and ventricular aneurysm may be present. With current surgical expertise, these lesions may be approached with encouraging results.[20] Rupture of the ventricular septum and ventricular aneurysm may result in severe heart failure without cardiogenic shock. If the response to medical therapy is acceptable, surgical repair is best postponed for 4 to 6 weeks.[8] Surgery performed earlier may be successful if all problems of cardiac anatomy can be repaired simultaneously.[6]

Coronary Bypass Surgery

The use of a saphenous vein or internal mammary artery bypass graft for the treatment of obstructive coronary disease has increased rapidly during the last 5 years.[24] This procedure has now earned a definite and major place in the treatment of certain patients with symptomatic coronary atherosclerotic heart disease.

1. The perfection of low-risk coronary arteriography, left ventriculography, and coronary artery surgery are responsible for the wide use of these procedures. The overall risk of coronary artery surgery at Emory University Hospital is 3.5 per cent. The operative mortality in certain clinical subsets is less than 2 per cent.

2. We do not recommend coronary bypass surgery for asymptomatic patients; for patients with cardiac enlargement and heart failure; for patients over 70 years of age, although there are exceptions; or for patients with other disabling diseases.

3. Coronary artery surgery should be used for the following conditions:

A. Stable angina pectoris that is severe enough to interfere significantly with the patient's life-style. As a rule, the patient is on nitroglycerin, isosorbide, and propranolol, but every possible dosage schedule should not be tried before moving on to surgery because valuable time can be wasted.

B. Initial angina pectoris with recurrent episodes of angina at rest despite medical treatment, progressive angina pectoris, and angina decubitus (see earlier definitions).

C. Recurrent prolonged myocardial ischemia with or with out S-T and T-wave changes in the electrocardiogram.

D. Stable angina pectoris associated with a markedly positive exercise electrocardiogram (2 mm. S-T segment displacement produced by Stage I or II exercise on the treadmill) and left main coronary artery obstruction or left main equivalent (proximal anterior descending and proximal circumflex obstruction) on coronary arteriography.

E. Angina pectoris that continues after a myocardial infarction when a period of time has elapsed after the acute infarction.

4. There is increasing evidence that life is prolonged by coronary bypass surgery more than by medical management.[29] Our own work at Emory University Hospital supports this view. We do not at this time recommend surgery for this reason. We recommend surgery for symptoms and promise the patient that there is an 80 per cent chance of relieving the symptoms and that 80 per cent of the vein grafts remain patent.[13] Having counseled the patient that surgery is to be performed in an effort to relieve symptoms, we then add that the evidence is now accumulating that life may be prolonged.

5. The preceding suggestions represent our current view. The field is changing and the watchword should be to collect data carefully, analyze it in a meticulous manner, and keep an open mind. Regretably, coronary bypass surgery will not solve all the problems because surgery cannot be performed in all patients (e.g., those with poor distal vessels) and the atherosclerotic process continues after bypass has been successfully performed.

PROGNOSIS

It is difficult to determine the prognosis of coronary atherosclerosis and coronary atherosclerotic heart disease. There is no other common disorder in medicine in which an individual is so likely to die suddenly. Sudden death accounts for at least 50 per cent of the deaths due to coronary atherosclerotic heart disease. The appearance of any of the many clinical events related to coronary atherosclerotic heart disease is unpredictable and the prognosis varies with the event.

1. Most patients with angina pectoris

live at least 5 to 10 years after the onset of this symptom.

2. Patients with unstable angina pectoris (groups 2B, 2C, 2D, 2F, and 2G shown in Fig. 2-1) have a worse prognosis. A recent report showed that 14 per cent of patients with unstable angina developed an acute myocardial infarction within three months of the onset of the symptoms.[11]

3. Associated complications of coronary atherosclerotic heart disease such as congestive heart failure, cardiac enlargement, and hypertension, adversely influence the long-range prognosis.

4. Acute myocardial infarction complicated by shock lasting one hour or longer, or by acute pulmonary edema is associated with a mortality rate approaching 80 per cent.

5. The resting electrocardiogram provides useful prognostic information in patients who survive a myocardial infarction. Electrocardiographic manifestations of myocardial ischemia, myocardial necrosis, conduction defects, atrial fibrillation, and frequent ventricular premature beats are associated with an increased mortality.

6. An elevation of enzymes of 4 to 8 times normal generally indicates that the area of infarction is large and that complications are likely to develop.[28]

7. The severity of coronary atherosclerosis[12,24] and the degree of left ventricular dysfunction are important predictors of survival. Patients with one-vessel coronary disease have a mortality rate of 2 per cent per year after the disease is diagnosed. If two or three major coronary arteries are stenosed, the mortality rate is 10 per cent per year or about 50 per cent in 5 years. These data apply to patients in the stable phase of their disease and should not be applied to patients with one of the unstable syndromes. Obstruction of the main left coronary artery is associated with a particularly unfavorable prognosis.[5]

REFERENCES

1. Armstrong, P. W. et al.: Vasodilator therapy in acute myocardial infarction. A comparison of sodium nitroprusside and nitroglycerin. Circulation, *52*:1118, 1975.
2. Bregman, D. et al.: Intraoperative unidirectional intra-aortic balloon pumping in the management of left ventricular power failure. J. Thoracic Cardiovasc. Surg., *70*:1010, 1975.
3. Chatterjee, K. et al.: Hemodynamic and metabolic response to vasodilator therapy in acute myocardial infarction. Circulation, *48*:1183, 1973.
4. Cheitlin, M. D. et al.: Correlation of "critical" left coronary artery lesions with positive submaximal exercise tests in patients with chest pain. Am. Heart J., *89*:305, 1975.
5. Cohen, M. V. and Gorlin, R.: Main left coronary disease. Circulation, *52*:275, 1975.
6. Crosby, I. K. et al.: Resection of acute posterior ventricular aneurysm with repair of ventricular septal defect after acute myocardial infarction. J. Thoracic Cardiovasc. Surg., *70*:57, 1975.
7. DeSanctis, R. W., Block, P., and Hutter A. M.: Tachyarrhythmias in myocardial infarction. Circulation, *45*:681, 1972.
8. Donahoo, J. S. et al.: Factors influencing survival following post infarction ventricular septal defects. Ann. Thoracic Surg., *19*:648, 1975.
9. Flaherty, J. F. et al.: Intravenous nitroglycerin in acute myocardial infarction. Circulation, *51*:132, 1975.
10. Fredrickson, D. S.: A physician's guide to hyperlipidemia. Mod. Concepts Cardiovasc. Dis., *41*:31, 1972.
11. Fulton, M. et al.: Natural history of unstable angina. Lancet, *1*:860, 1972.
12. Gurggnof, G. W., and Parker, J. O.: Prognosis in coronary artery disease. Circulation, *51*:146, 1975.
13. Hatcher, C. R. et al.: The surgical treatment of unstable angina pectoris. Ann. Surg., *181*:754, 1975.
14. Hurst, J. W., (ed.): The Heart, Arteries, and Veins. ed. 3. New York, McGraw Hill, 1974.
15. Hurst, J. W.: Editorial: Ambulation after myocardial infarction. N. Engl. J. Med., *292*:746, 1975.
16. Hurst, J. W., and Myerburg, R. J.: Introduction to Electrocardiography. ed. 2. New York, McGraw Hill, 1973.
17. Kattus, A. A.: Exercise electrocardiography: recognition of the ischemic response, false positive and negative patterns. Am. J. Cardiol., *33*:721, 1974.
18. Lonascia, J., Gordis, L., and Schmerler, H.: Retrospective evidence favoring use of an-

ticoagulants for myocardial infarctions. N. Engl. J. Med., *292*:1362, 1975.

19. Modan, B. et al.: Reduction of mortality in myocardial infarction by anticoagulant therapy. N. Engl. J. Med., *292*:1359, 1975.
20. Mundth, E. D., and Austen, W. E.: Surgical measures for coronary heart disease. N. Engl. J. Med., *293*:124, 1975.
21. Nies, A. S. and Shand, D. G.: Clinical pharmacology of propranolol. Circulation, *52*:6, 1975.
22. Rackley, C. E. and Russell, R. O.: Left ventricular function in acute myocardial infarction and its clinical significance. Circulation, *45*:231, 1972.
23. Reichek, N. et al.: Sustained effects of nitroglycerin ointment in patients with angina pectoris. Circulation, *50*:348, 1974.
24. Ross, R. S.: Ischemic heart disease: An overview. Am. J. Cardiol., *36*:946, 1975.
25. Rotman, M. and Wanger, A. G.: Bradyarrhythmias in acute myocardial infarction. Circulation, *45*:703, 1972.
26. Rubio, R. and Berne, R. M.: Regulation of coronary blood flow. Progr. Cardiovasc. Dis., *18*(2):105, 1975.
27. Schlant, R. C. and Hurst, J. W. (eds.): Advances in Electrocardiography. New York, Grune & Stratton, 1972.
28. Sobel, B. E. et al.: Estimation of infarct size in man and its relation to prognosis. Circulation, *46*:640, 1972.
29. Spencer, F. C. et al.: The long-term influence of coronary by-pass grafts on myocardial infarction and survival. Ann. Surg., *180*:439, 1974.
30. Wissler, R. W. and Geer, J. C., (eds.): The Pathogenesis of Atherosclerosis. Baltimore, Williams & Wilkins, 1972.

3. HYPERTENSION AND HYPERTENSIVE HEART DISEASE

Edward D. Frohlich, M.D.

DEFINITION

1. Because we know that the higher the arterial pressure—systolic or diastolic—the greater the cardiovascular morbidity or mortality, a corollary may be stated that the higher the systolic or diastolic pressure, the greater will be the cardiovascular risk.

2. Because we, as physicians, deal best with "normal ranges," we have now accepted that an elevated systolic pressure is considered to be one in excess of 140 mm. Hg on several repeated observations; likewise, a diastolic pressure is considered to be elevated if it is repeatedly in excess of 90 mm. Hg. It should be remembered, however, that these arbitrary levels are already considerably elevated in the pediatric age group.

3. In recent years, the level of diastolic pressure above which practicing physicians have been urged to treat patients with arterial hypertension is 104 mm. Hg (High Blood Pressure Education Program). This is because the results of the Veterans Administration Cooperative Study demonstrated efficacy of antihypertensive therapy in male patients whose diastolic pressures were 105 mm. Hg and more. Nevertheless, there is a tremendous weight of evidence provided through life insurance actuarial data and major epidemiological prospective studies (e.g., Framingham Study) that indicates that patients whose diastolic pressure levels fall between 90 and 105 mm. Hg have a greater risk of cardiovascular morbidity than individuals whose diastolic pressures are less than 90 mm. Hg.

GENERAL CONSIDERATIONS

Systemic arterial hypertension afflicts approximately 20 per cent of the adult population in the United States. It is the prime cause of congestive heart failure and is a major risk factor of atherosclerotic coronary arterial disease. Therefore, its recognition, evaluation, and treatment are serious medical and public health problems. Since cardiovascular disease is responsible in the United States for more deaths than the sum of all other causes, it is obvious that proper management ought to significantly reduce its devastating complications. This is the challenge of modern-day preventive cardiology.

By itself, arterial hypertension is merely a clinical sign. Its evaluation should be approached with the same consideration as an abnormal heart rate or body temperature. Good medicine requires identification of the causes or mechanisms of abnormalities. Then, with the mechanism having been found, the appropriate therapy can be initiated.

Data from public health, insurance, and epidemiological services have demonstrated that no matter whether systolic or diastolic levels are considered, the higher the blood pressure, the greater the morbidity and mortality rate. Thus, a 35-year-old man with a pressure of 130/90 mm. Hg has a life span 4 years less than his normotensive counterpart. This same individual has a 9-year reduction in life expectancy if his pressure is 140/90 mm. Hg, and a 17-year reduction if his pressure is 150/100 mm. Hg.

Recent information indicates that no matter what the cause of the hypertension, control of arterial pressure with antihypertensive drugs is associated with significantly reduced morbidity and mortality.

CLASSIFICATIONS

Etiological Classification of Hypertension

Primary (hypertension of undetermined cause)
  Labile (borderline)
  Systolic
  "Benign" essential
  Malignant essential
Secondary (related to a cause)
  Renal
    Parenchymal (pyelonephritis,
      glomerulonephritis, cystic disease, etc.)
    Renal arterial
      Atherosclerotic
      Nonatherosclerotic (fibrosing)
      Other (embolic, perinephric hematoma,
        etc.)
    Renoprival
  Endocrine
    Thyrotoxicosis
    Hyperparathyroidism
    Pheochromocytoma
    Acromegaly
    Adrenal cortical (Cushing's syndrome and
      disease, licorice, primary aldosteronism,
      biosynthetic enzymatic defects)
    Oral contraceptives
  Aortic coarctation
  Neural (porphyria, poliomyelitis, increased
    intracranial pressure, diencephalic syndrome,
    lead encephalitis, cord transection)

1. *Etiological* (see list above)
  A. *Primary hypertension*

We know of no specific cause for the elevated arterial pressure in most patients with systemic hypertension. At first thought, this might seem frustrating (if not inexcusable) when one considers the amount of time, effort, energy, and resources expended to understand this enormous clinical problem.

However, the physician must realize that with advancing understanding of the hypertension problem, most authorities are arriving at the conclusion that this problem is one of "disregulation." Thus, rather than thinking of hypertension as a single homogeneous disease, we now consider the problem as a complex and heterogeneous grouping of clinical conditions characterized by an elevated arterial pressure and brought about through a loss of regulation of the pressor mechanisms involved in maintaining arterial pressure at normal levels.

About 80 to 90 per cent of the cases of hypertension seem to have no specific identifiable etiology. These individuals with hypertension of undetermined cause are said to have "essential hypertension," a term that now refers to "hypertension of idiopathic cause." However, the term "essential" did not always reflect this meaning; the early German literature indicated that the elevated arterial pressure was essential for life.

We know now that this term *essential* is what has been behind the erroneous clinical thinking that if one reduces arterial pressure in the patient with *essentialle hypertonie,* poor tissue perfusion of the brain, heart, and kidneys will result.

  B. *Secondary hypertension*

Of the remaining 10 to 20 per cent of patients with arterial hypertension, an identifiable cause or known disease can be identified. These persons, then, are said to have secondary forms of hypertension (see list on this page), in contrast with those patients with so-called essential hypertension.

The physician should not be misled into thinking that just because a cause of hypertension is identified, the hypertension is "curable."

It is true that patients with aortic coarctation and pheochromocytoma generally have a normal blood pressure with correction or removal of the lesions. However, this is not so with

hypertension associated with parenchymal disease of the kidney; and only a
certain percentage of patients with renal
arterial disease or with adrenal tumors
have a normal pressure after correction
of the problem.

It is for this reason that we prefer to
view patients with systemic arterial
hypertension in terms of the pressor
mechanisms involved. As this concept
has become more widely considered,
and as we use antihypertensive drugs
with more specific actions, we believe a
mechanistic approach to hypertension
will become more popular.

2. *Pathophysiological* (see Table 3-1
and 3-2)

We have therefore found it extremely
useful to classify hypertension according
to pressor mechanisms (Table 3-1). Even
when there is a single cause, several
pressor mechanisms are usually operative.

For example, in the patient with renal
arterial disease, in whom the renopres-
sor mechanism is predominant (increased plasma renin activity or an-
giotensin), other mechanisms, including
hormonal (secondary hyperaldosteronism), volume (contracted in-

***Table 3-1.* Classification of Known Hypertensive Diseases According to Pressor Mechanisms**

Primary Pressor Mechanisms	Clinical Diagnosis	Other Implicated Mechanisms	Specific Tests
Mechanical	Coarctation of aorta	Renopressor	Chest x-ray, angiography
Catecholamines	Pheochromocytoma	Volume, renopressor, neural	Urine assay (VMA, cate-cholamines, meta- and normetanephrines)
Renopressor	Renal arterial disease	Aldosterone, volume, neural	Renal arteriography, renin or angiotensin
Hormonal	Thyrotoxicosis	Thyroid, sympathetic	Thyroid function studies
	Hyperparathyroidism	Calcium on vascular smooth muscle	
	Hypertension induced by oral contraceptives	Renopressor	Renin, withdrawal
	Acromegaly, gigantism	?	HGH
	Cushing's syndrome or disease	Compounds D, F	17-OH steroids
	Primary hyper-aldosteronism	Volume, electrolytic	Aldosterone, renin
	Adrenal virilism	Volume, electrolytic	Ketosteroids
	Hydroxylase deficiencies	Volume, electrolytic	Corticosteroids
	DOC-tumors	Volume, electrolytic	17-OH steroids
Volume	Renal parenchymal disease	Electrolytes, renopressor	IVP, culture, biopsy, renal function studies
Neural	? Essential hypertension; labile hypertension	Volume, ? renopressor	Hemodynamics
	Beta-adrenergic hyper-circulatory state	? Adenylate cyclase, cAMP	Hemodynamics, isoproterenol
	Porphyria	? Renopressor	Porphobilinogen
	Diencephalic syndrome		

Table 3-2. **Pressor Mechanisms in Essential Hypertension**

Type of Hypertension	Main Mechanism	To Evaluate Mechanisms
? Labile, mild essential	Catecholamines Adenylate cyclase system	Hemodynamic studies
Malignant	Renopressor ? Renal depressor	Plasma volume Aldosterone
Volume dependent	Hormonal (steroids)	Fluid volumes Electrolytes Hormonal assays
"Low renin"	Volume, electrolytes	Aldosterone, 18-OH, DOC, etc.
Neurocirculatory asthenia	Neural	Heart rate
Hyperdynamic beta-adrenergic circulatory state	Neural	Hemodynamics
Diencephalic syndrome	Neural	Postural studies

travascular volume), and neural factors (increased adrenergic activity), may participate in maintaining his hypertension.

The patient with aortic coarctation, with a simple mechanical obstruction to flow causing elevated proximal pressure, may also demonstrate increased plasma renin activity and hyperkinetic circulation.

The patient with pheochromocytoma exhibits, in addition to increased circulating and excreted catecholamines, increased plasma renin activity and contracted intravascular volume.

This mechanistic approach to the "secondary" forms of hypertension is even more useful when evaluating the mechanisms involved in maintaining the elevated pressure in the run-of-the-mill essential hypertensive patient.

Thus, if one explores the role of each secondary mechanism, he will be able to treat more specifically the patient with "volume-dependent" essential hypertension, mild essential hypertension with a hyperkinetic circulation, more severe "vasoconstricted" essential hypertension with markedly elevated arterial pressure, contracted intravascular volume, exudate retinopathy with hyperreninemia and secondary hyperaldosteronism, the patient with low-, normal-, or high-renin essential hypertension, and so forth (Table 3-2).

These considerations are extremely important, for identification of new "causes" for patients having essential hypertension will only come about through the identification of operative pressor mechanisms. It is for this reason that the search goes on for another adrenal steroid hormone that will expand intravascular volume and reduce plasma renin activity. The logical source of hypertensive patients for this group is those with so-called low-renin or volume-dependent essential hypertension.

SYMPTOMS AND SIGNS

1. *No symptoms*

The general statement made over and again is true: there are no specific signs and symptoms attributable to the hypertensive diseases *except for the determi-*

nation of arterial pressure by the examining physician.

This point should be kept in mind by every physician: arterial hypertension will never be diagnosed if the arterial pressure is not measured.

A second corollary can be made: if we are to prevent the target organ complications of systemic arterial hypertension, the patient with the earliest stage of the disease must be recognized—*and treated.*

2. *Common symptoms*

There are many statements that the most common symptoms associated with hypertension are:

Headache
Fatigue
Epistaxis

The physician must remember that these are, in fact, the most common symptoms that affect most patients. However, the patient with early morning headache (the one that may awaken the patient) may have associated hypertension; and a sudden onset of severe vertical headache should bring to mind the rupture of a Berry aneurysm with subarachnoid hemorrhage.

3. *Important physical signs*

A. A most important physical sign is the recognition of the absent femoral arterial pulsations associated with coarctation of the aorta.

B. Another physical examination technique necessary in the periodic examination of all hypertensive patients is the careful study of the progressive vascular and exudative changes in the optic fundi.

C. In general, the physician can detect advancing vascular disease associated with hypertension by the progression of the degree of focal and generalized constriction of the retinal arterioles and the development of exudates and hemorrhages in the fundi as the hypertensive disease becomes accelerated.

D. Papilledema is the hallmark of malignant hypertension.

4. *Hormonally dependent hypertension*

A. Hormonally dependent hypertension is generally not associated with edema.

B. The patient with primary aldosteronism has no evidence of edema, and the symptoms are primarily associated with the accompanying hypokalemia: muscle weakness and easy fatigability.

C. Patients with Cushing's disease or syndrome demonstrate truncal obesity, "buffalo hump," purple striae, etc., but no edema (with these latter patients, previous photographs of the patient are always helpful).

D. The patient with pheochromocytoma can be almost always detected by his symptoms of pressure elevations associated with flushing, palpitations, sweating, sensations of skipped heart beats, and so forth.

5. *Renal hypertension*

A. Signs of anemia, weakness, and peripheral edema are all signs of renal failure; these may occur in the patient with long-standing systemic hypertension or hypertension associated with chronic parenchymal disease of the kidney.

B. The patient with essential hypertension and early renal functional impairment will, however, first complain of nocturia.

C. Always worth repeating is the finding of the abdominal bruits that should strongly suggest renal arterial disease—especially if the bruits are well localized and of both systolic and diastolic timing. These bruits may also be heard over the flank areas.

6. *Heart failure*

Symptoms of tiredness, easy fatigue, diminished exercise tolerance, and shortness of breath should of course bring to mind long-standing hypertension associated with left ventricular failure.

The most common cause of heart failure today is hypertension. However, even before left ventricular failure occurs, there are specific signs and symptoms that should permit the physician to determine whether the heart is involved by systemic arterial hypertension.

First, the patient with labile (borderline) or mild hypertension may complain of palpitations and rapid heart action. These symptoms of cardiac awareness may be the manifestations of increased adrenergic participation in the development of the hypertensive process; and treatment may be directed not only to produce remission of these symptoms but also reversal of the hypertensive disease.

As hypertensive heart disease becomes more involved, and as vascular resistance progressively increases, the myocardium adapts to the increased afterload and pressure work; ventricular hypertrophy occurs.

This may be detected by the evidence of reduced left ventricular compliance even before overt left ventricular hypertrophy is seen by chest roentgenogram and electrocardiogram; the electrocardiogram demonstrates left atrial abnormality; a fourth heart sound may become audible, and these may be confirmed by echocardiographic techniques.

When the left ventricular hypertrophy is evident by chest roentgenogram or electrocardiogram (or echocardiogram), the patient may have the symptoms of palpitations, feelings of "skipped beats," and inability to sleep because of his "pounding heart."

On physical examination, a loud second aortic sound, left ventricular lift, palpable (and audible) fourth heart sound may be present, and possibly findings of left ventricular failure may also develop.

The physician should remember that as myocardial oxygen demand increases with the level of arterial pressure and size of the heart, symptoms of coronary insufficiency may develop; these can remit with reduction of arterial pressure.

DIAGNOSIS AND LABORATORY FINDINGS

1. *General features*

Having considered the pressor mechanisms in classifying the hypertensive patient, diagnostic and differential diagnostic considerations are obvious. Thus, even the *routine blood count* becomes a physiological clinical tool. Does the high hemoglobin or hematocrit so frequently observed in hypertension reflect a healthy, plethoric man, or is it a physiological expression of contracted plasma volume in a patient having "stress polycythemia" or the Gaisbock syndrome? Measurement of plasma volume (using radioiodinated human serum albumin) becomes a sophisticated diagnostic tool that differentiates this possibility. In carefully controlled clinical studies, plasma volume has been found to vary inversely with the height of diastolic pressure in patients with essential hypertension, renal arterial disease with hypertension, or pheochromocytoma. In contrast, plasma volume was *directly* related to the height of diastolic pressure in hypertensive patients with renal parenchymal disease, aldosterone-producing tumors, and volume-dependent essential hypertension.

2. *The 24-hour urine collection*

A. The 24-hour urine collection need not be utilized only in those patients suspected of having severe renal disease, endocrine disorders, or pheochromocytoma.

B. Urine that is collected from any untreated hypertensive outpatient on a liberal dietary sodium intake (in excess of 100 mEq of sodium in 24 hours) can be measured wisely for sodium, potassium, creatinine, and protein.

C. The excretion of more than 50

mEq of potassium per 24 hours suggests the variety of diseases associated with potassium wastage (including primary aldosteronism, Cushing's syndrome or disease, renal disease), provided the causes of secondary aldosteronism are included (e.g., vomiting, diarrhea, chronic laxative ingestion, and oral contraceptive therapy).

D. Oral contraceptive therapy also invalidates plasma volume determinations.

E. The quantitative protein excretion value should help with differential diagnosis of renal disease.

F. Thus, the normal kidney should not excrete more than 0.2 g. of protein in 24 hours, while excretion between 0.2 and 0.4 g. is compatible with any type or severity of hypertension.

G. Protein excretion in excess of 0.4 to 0.5 g. indicates renal parenchymal disease; if protein excretion exceeds 2.0 to 3.0 g., chronic pyelonephritis should be considered as secondary to an additional renal disease since, in this form of renal disease, massive proteinuria per se is highly unusual.

H. Of course, if arterial pressure is extremely high, excessive proteinuria will result from an increased "sieving" effect; this should diminish markedly once pressure is reduced, provided the patient does not have renal parenchymal disease.

3. *Routine urinalysis*

In addition to the 24-hour urine collection, routine urinalysis and urine culture are important in the initial evaluation of the hypertensive patient. Too often, the randomly collected urine specimen is not studied by the physician.

Many reports have shown, particularly in premenopausal women, that asymptomatic bacteriuria is exceedingly common.

The presence of casts and red cells and white cells found in the fresh specimen are critically important.

The pH and specific gravity, simple as they are, may provide the first clues of primary aldosteronism. Thus, in order to substantiate a diagnosis of primary aldosteronism, the search begins for:

A. A repeatedly alkaline urine specimen

B. A lower than expected specific gravity

C. An inappropriately normal or expanded plasma volume for the level of diastolic pressure

D. Carbohydrate intolerance

E. Mild hypokalemic alkalosis

4. *Serum electrolytes determinations*

In order to evaluate electrolytic balance, one should obtain not only a random serum potassium concentration, but also potassium should be considered in association with the other major ions, including sodium, chloride, bicarbonate, calcium, and phosphate.

It is noteworthy that there is a greater prevalence of hypertension among patients having hypercalcemia from any cause. This is believed to result from the elevated serum calcium concentration per se, rather than the underlying disease process or from nephrocalcinosis. In this regard, 70 per cent of patients having primary hyperparathyroidism are hypertensive, and with the removal of the adenoma, arterial pressure becomes reduced even when nephrocalcinosis is present. Moreover, calcium infusion into normotensive subjects may elevate arterial pressure and increase vascular resistance.

5. *Serum uric acid concentration and carbohydrate tolerance*

A. Since diuretic therapy with any of the many thiazide congeners is commonly associated with hyperglycemia, occasional glycosuria, and hyperuricemia, it is wise to obtain a baseline serum uric acid concentration and carbohydrate tolerance prior to initiation of therapy.

B. We have yet to find insulin-dependent diabetes mellitus developing de novo during thiazide therapy.

C. Even when the fasting blood sugar was normal, an abnormality of carbohydrate tolerance (2- to 4-hour glucose tolerance test) was demonstrated in all patients who later developed thiazide "diabetes."

6. *Radiographic tests*

Perhaps no specialized area of clinical evaluation has been so exploited in the hypertensive patient as the variety of radiographic tests developed for diagnosing the "curable" forms of renal hypertension.

The best screening test for renal arterial disease is the intravenous pyelogram, which has developed a variety of modifications including mannitol or urea washout, with or without rapid films at the outset.

The major diagnostic criteria (no matter what technique is employed) include:

A. Delayed appearance

B. Renal asymmetry (the right kidney is normally 0.5 cm. shorter than the left)

C. Hyperconcentration of contrast material on the affected side

The presence of calyceal clubbing, contour irregularity, or scarring should suggest chronic pyelonephritis.

Asymmetry, delayed appearance, and pelvic hyperconcentration of contrast material should suggest main or branch stenosis of the renal artery.

Nevertheless, the old adage holds true, "If one wants to see renal arterial disease, he must look at the renal arteries." The sophistication, practicality, and soundness of the techniques of selective renal arteriography have provided an outstanding opportunity for preoperative diagnosis of the renal arterial diseases. Moreover, this technique has provided the means for understanding the natural history of these diseases.

Selective renal arterial and venous catheterization permits specific identification of different pathological types of arterial lesions and an estimation of differential concentrations of renal venous renin, respectively, thereby providing excellent criteria for selecting appropriate therapy.

Thus, the patient with a renal arterial plaque, associated with atherosclerotic coronary or cerebral disease, may not be considered for corrective surgery until renal function becomes compromised or medical antihypertensive therapy is ineffective.

The patient with medial fibroplasia ("string of beads" lesion), a fibrosing disease of the renal arteries that does not progress rapidly, may be treated first with drugs. This provides an observation period to determine whether the stenosis is stable or progressive.

If an arterial lesion is identified, and if renin is secreted in a concentration equal to or greater than 1.5 times that of the unaffected kidney, corrective surgery may be considered.

These techniques have relegated other differential renal function studies by ureteral catheterization techniques to a position of historical interest.

7. *Comments on renal artery disease*

Additional comment concerning the clinical characteristics of renal arterial disease is necessary. Classically, the patient has been described as being young, a known hypertensive with sudden or increased severity of disease, unresponsive to medical therapy, or associated with accelerated or malignant hypertension. These points may be true; frequently, however, the disease runs a more benign course. A young woman is often hospitalized for evaluation of hypertension (including renal arteriography) only to have the pressure fall to normotensive levels on the following day. Consequently, she is discharged without a diagnosis having been established. Thus, while unresponsiveness to antihypertensive therapy or development of malignant hypertension may suggest "renovascular" hypertension, they are not the typical or exclusive features.

COMPLICATIONS

1. *Hypertensive heart disease*
   A. The electrocardiogram and the chest roentgenogram are exceedingly important diagnostic tools for determining the progression of hypertensive heart disease.
   B. *Left atrial abnormality*
      (1) The earliest sign of cardiac involvement in hypertension is the electrocardiographic finding of left atrial abnormality (see Abnormal Diagnostic Cardiac Criteria below).

Abnormal Diagnostic Cardiac Criteria

Left atrial abnormality (ECG)—two of four
   P wave in Lead II $\geq$ 0.3 mv. and $\geq$0.12 sec.
   Bipeak interval in notched P wave $\geq$0.04 sec.
   Ratio of P wave duration to PR segment $\geq$ 1.6
      (Lead II)
   Terminal atrial forces (in V_1) $\geq$ 0.04 sec.
Left ventricular hypertrophy
   Ungerleider Index $\geq$+ 15% (chest x-ray alone)
   Ungerleider Index $\geq$ + 10% (chest x-ray + 2 of
      following ECG criteria)
   Sum of tallest R and deepest S waves $\geq$ 4.5
      mv. (precordial)
   LV "strain" i.e., QRS and T wave vectors
      180° apart
   QRS frontal axis $\leq$ 0°
All 3 ECG criteria (above)

      (2) These left atrial changes may be present without evidence of left ventricular enlargement.
      (3) They do not reflect atrial disease per se but, rather, the response of a dynamic atrium to the less compliant ventricle as hypertrophy is developing (but prior to becoming clinically evident).
      (4) Not infrequently, this electrocardiographic abnormality coexists with the auscultatory finding of a fourth heart sound, or presystolic atrial gallop.
   C. *Ventricular hypertrophy*
   Then, as clinical ventricular hypertrophy becomes obvious, it may be identified by a variety of electrocardiographic or roentgenographic criteria (see Abnormal Diagnostic Cardiac Criteria above).
   D. *Left ventricular failure*
   Eventually, if the hypertension remains untreated, left ventricular failure and its associated clinical findings supervene.
   E. Not infrequently, because of the very high association of atherosclerosis and hypertension, the complications of *coronary insufficiency, myocardial infarction,* and *ventricular aneurysm* appear during the course of chronic hypertensive heart disease.
2. *Coronary arterial disease*
   A. Hypertension is generally acknowledged as a major risk factor in coronary arterial disease, together with diabetes mellitus, hyperlipidemia, and cigarette smoking.
   B. Since atherosclerosis is so commonly found in hypertension, it is logical to screen the hypertensive population for these three factors and expect a very high yield.
   C. Hence, a lipid "profile," serum uric acid, and carbohydrate tolerance are important factors to evaluate in an individual hypertensive patient.
   D. Moreover, knowledge of one abnormality can provide deeper insight into another (e.g., hyperlipidemia and carbohydrate intolerance).
3. *Angina pectoris*
   A. Chest pain may develop in a patient with hypertension as a result of:
      (1) Coronary arterial disease
      (2) The increased demand for oxygen by a hypertrophying myocardium subjected to a progressively increasing pressure and afterload
      (3) Both (1) and (2)
   B. Control of arterial pressure in itself may be enough to produce a remission of chest pain.
4. *Aortic dissection*
   A. Hypertension is a not-infrequent finding in a patient with a dissecting aortic aneurysm.

B. Control of arterial pressure in these patients may be associated not only with remission of pain but with arrest of the dissecting process.

C. This will permit further evaluation of the condition, and, in some patients, may be the major therapy used.

5. *Renal failure*

A. With progression of hypertension, thickening of the small arterial and arteriolar walls progresses.

B. This results in the changes of nephrosclerosis when the renal vessels are involved.

C. Clinically, this may be expressed by:

(1) Nocturia

(2) Reduced renal concentrating ability

(3) Proteinuria (usually less than 0.4 g. daily).

6. *Accelerated and malignant hypertension*

A. The patient with accelerated hypertension has an elevated diastolic arterial pressure (not infrequently in excess of 130 mm. Hg, but the magnitude is irrelevant) associated with exudative retinopathy, hemorrhages, and exudates.

B. In malignant hypertension, the disease has progressed still further.

C. The optic fundi reveal papilledema.

D. When tissue (e.g., kidney) is studied microscopically, necrotizing arteriolitis is found.

E. Not infrequently, this disease is associated with severe proteinuria, which usually diminishes markedly with reduction of pressure. However, if malignant hypertension is associated with severe renal parenchymal disease (e.g., chronic glomerulonephritis), the proteinuria may not diminish.

Prior to the time when antihypertensive therapy was available, malignant hypertension was uniformly fatal, 97 per cent of the patients dying within 3 months. At present, if diagnosed and treated early enough (this is not unusual today), remarkable prolongation of life will result. Indeed, information on intrarenal pathology is available as long as 15 years after diagnosis of malignant hypertension in which the kidney shows a characteristic onion-skin appearance of "healed arteriolitis."

7. *Hypertensive encephalopathy*

This is a condition of severely elevated arterial pressure associated with nausea, vomiting, and headache that progresses to coma and is accompanied by clinical signs of neurological deficit.

B. With intravenous infusion of nitroprusside or trimethaphan, or with injection of diazoxide, arterial pressure falls and the patient promptly awakens from coma, with disappearance of the nausea, vomiting, headache, and neurological deficits.

C. Where treatment has not been made available early enough, the syndrome proceeds to stroke, "chronic encephalopathy," or malignant hypertension. Reversibility then is much slower and much more in doubt.

MANAGEMENT

1. *Secondary hypertension*

A. While any drug therapy that reduces arterial pressure may be of value in treating hypertensive diseases, common sense dictates that the more specific the therapy, the better one may expect the control of pressure to be (see Pressor Mechanisms and Antihypertensive Therapy below).

B. In certain "secondary" types of hypertension, the specific therapy might well be surgical. For example:

(1) Excision of the aortic coarctation

(2) Repair of the renal arterial lesion or nephrectomy

(3) Removal of the cortical or

Pressor Mechanisms and Antihypertensive Therapy

Mechanism	Therapy
Mechanical	Correction of obstruction; reserpine
Renopressor	Surgical correction
	Methyldopa or propranolol (plus diuretic if necessary)
	Angiotensin II receptor inhibitors (e.g., saralasin)
	Converting enzyme inhibitors
Catecholamines	Surgical correction (removal of pheochromocytoma)
	Alpha- and/or beta-adrenergic receptor blockade
Hormonal	Surgical removal of tumor
	Adrenal steroid biosynthetic inhibitors
	Hormonal antagonists
	Diuretics; adrenergic inhibitors
Volume	Diuretics (thiazide "loop" diuretics)
	Dialysis (blood or peritoneal)
	(May also require vasodilators)
Neural	Ganglion blockade (acute)
	Sympatholytics (methyldopa, clonidine, guanethidine, reserpine, etc.)
	Adrenergic receptor blockade

medullary adrenal tumor most likely will restore normotension.

C. Even in these forms of hypertension (not infrequently following repair of coarctation) there may be a paradoxical, post-operative hypertensive episode. This may develop through lack of an immediate neural readaptation, and "stopgap" reserpine therapy provides remission of the elevation in pressure.

D. Certain patients with *renal arterial disease* may have extensive bilateral or branch involvement that precludes surgery. In these instances, medical therapy is indicated with specific agents.

E. Certain antihypertensive drugs (e.g., methyldopa and propranolol) can inhibit renin release and normalize the pressure and the hyperkinetic circulation, either alone or in conjunction with diuretics. In these patients, careful follow-up of renal function and renal size is necessary.

F. Even patients with *adrenal medullary or cortical tumors* may be treated medically if surgery is contraindicated or impossible.

G. *Pheochromocytomas* have been treated for as long as 17 years with alpha-adrenergic receptor blocking drugs.

H. *Aldosterone-producing tumors* may be treated with spironolactone alone or with sodium restriction and/or more potent diuretics.

I. Spironolactone is a mild diuretic that specifically antagonizes the hormone at the renal tubule level and possibly within the adrenal gland. Its main value in this instance is as a potassium-sparing diuretic.

2. *Primary hypertension*

A. Although a standardized treatment program has been demonstrated to be successful (Table 3-3), it is acknowledged that patients with "essential" hypertension may also be treated specifically. Thus, mildly hypertensive patients (i.e., those with a hyperkinetic circulation, or with "high renin" activity) may be treated with *propranolol*.

B. Recent reports also indicate that beta-blockade in conjunction with *peripheral vasodilating drugs* (i.e., hy-

Table 3-3.* Standard "Stepped Care" Treatment Approach

Therapy Stage	Drug	Daily Dose Range
One	Thiazide congeners (e.g., hydrochlorothiazide)	50–100 mg.
	plus	
Two	Rauwolfia derivatives (e.g., reserpine)	0.25–0.50 mg.
	or	
	Methyldopa	500–3000 mg.
	or	
	Propranolol	60–320 mg.
	plus	
Three	Hydralazine	75–200 mg.
	or plus	
Four	Methyldopa or Guanethidine or Clonidine	500–3000 mg. 10–200 mg. 0.4–3.6 mg.

*The physician adds additional antihypertensive therapy to the maximal dose of previous level of therapy when arterial pressure fails to become reduced to normotensive levels (less than 140/90 mm. Hg).

dralazine) may be effective in established essential hypertension, even in those patients without evidence of a hyperkinetic circulation. And, as with any antihypertensive agent, treatment is enhanced with *diuretic therapy.* This latter effect has been explained by three possible mechanisms:

(1) The diuretic further contracts intravascular and extracellular fluid volumes.

(2) It reduces vascular responsiveness to circulating pressor substances, possibly through a membrane effect on vascular smooth muscle.

(3) It has a possible direct effect on baroreceptors.

C. At any rate, the potentiative effect of diuretic agents (and by dietary sodium deprivation as well) upon all antihypertensive drugs is well established.

D. A listing of the major available antihypertensive agents with their respective doses is presented in Table 3-4.

E. *Low sodium diet therapy*

Unlike its value in edematous states (e.g., cardiac, renal, or hepatic failure), sodium restriction by itself is of no practical value in uncomplicated hypertension unless the dietary sodium intake is less than a range of 200 to 500 mg. daily. If sodium intake is greater than this, there will be only minimal antihypertensive value.

More important, moderate sodium re-

***Table 3-4.* The Major Antihypertensive Drugs and Doses**

Agent	Usual Initiating Dose	Maximum Daily Dose
Diuretics (these agents are compiled in equivalent forms so that one agent is the same as another)		
Chlorothiazide	500 mg. b.i.d.	1000 mg.
Hydrochlorothiazide	50 mg. b.i.d.	100 mg.
Furosemide	40 mg. b.i.d.	As high as 2.0 g.
Spironolactone	25 mg. q.i.d.	100 mg.
Smooth muscle relaxants		
Hydralazine	10 mg. q.i.d.	200 mg.
Nitroprusside	60 μg./ml.	
Rauwolfia derivatives		
Reserpine (typical of this group)	0.25 mg. q.d. (oral)	0.25 mg.
Reserpine (parenteral)	0.5 mg. (to see if unusual response)	2.5 to 5.0 mg. q. 6 H
Adrenergic inhibitors		
Methyldopa	250 mg. t.i.d. or q.i.d.	4.0 g.
Guanethidine	10 mg. q.d.	150–250 mg.
Clonidine	0.1 mg. b.i.d.	2.4 mg.
Trimethaphan	1 mg./ml., IV	
Receptor antagonist		
Alpha-		
Phenotolamine	5 mg., IV	10 mg. or by infusion
Dibenzylene	5 mg. b.i.d.	As necessary; see text
Beta-		
Propranolol	10 mg. q.i.d.	160 mg. q.i.d. (see text for precautions and contraindications)

striction complicates the evaluation of hypertension because it promotes secondary hyperaldosteronism. Thus, diuretic agents are far more effective than dietary sodium restriction.

F. *Volume-dependent hypertension*

(1) For those essential hypertensive subjects with volume-dependent hypertension, diuretic therapy should be the first therapeutic consideration. This may be accomplished with spironolactone (25 to 100 mg. four times daily) if hyperaldosteronism seems at all possible.

(2) Addition of thiazide therapy should also be considered if the spironolactone, by itself, is ineffective.

G. *Loop diuretics*

"Loop" diuretics (i.e., furosemide or ethacrynic acid) should not be used in hypertensive patients with normal renal function because these agents demonstrate a shorter duration of action, a re-

bound effect, more potassium wastage, and are no more effective than the thiazide diuretics.

However, in patients with chronic renal disease and renal insufficiency, loop diuretics may be more efficacious since, unlike hydrochlorothiazide (with the dose limited to 50 mg., twice daily), they can be increased until an effect is ultimately achieved. Thus, if furosemide (40 mg., four times daily) is ineffective in an azotemic patient, the dosage may be increased to 80, 120, 160, or even 200 mg. four times daily.

When a diuretic is indicated, the thiazides should be considered first. If these are ineffective in promoting the desired diuresis, the "loop" diuretics may be employed—but not with thiazides.

H. *Adrenolytic therapy*

For those patients having high diastolic pressures that require potent adrenolytic therapy, the agents to be considered should be methyldopa, clonidine, or guanethidine.

(1) Methyldopa acts on the peripheral adrenergic nerve ending as a false neurotransmitter (alpha-methyl-norepinephrine on the norepinephrine receptor sites) and possibly also inhibits renin release from the kidney.

(2) Clonidine acts in the brain, stimulating alpha-adrenergic receptor sites centrally and thereby inhibiting sympathetic outflow from the brain.

(3) Guanethidine is a more long-acting sympatholytic agent, acting at the peripheral nerve ending, but it depletes norepinephrine stores and thereby provides less neurotransmitter to be bound at the receptors. This agent should be administered only once daily, at noontime, to lessen the early morning postural hypotension. More frequent administration is unnecessary because it has a duration of action for as long as 1 month when the patient has been on long-term therapy.

(4) As with other agents, diuretics enhance the effectiveness of these drugs and thereby reduce the required dosage.

3. *Hypertensive emergencies*

A hypertensive emergency should not be defined solely in terms of the height of arterial pressure. Indeed, the physician should repeatedly measure pressure to confirm sustained hypertension and to obtain baseline records.

In the absence of neurological symptoms, cardiac failure, or papilledema, dramatic intravenous therapy should be avoided. In any event, baseline chest roentgenogram, electrocardiogram, electrolytes studies, renal function studies, and a hemogram should be obtained prior to initiating therapy.

If immediate pressure reduction is indicated (e.g., with hypertensive encephalopathy, coma, or malignant hypertension associated with cardiac failure or neurological changes), intravenous hydralazine (10 to 20 mg.), alpha-methyldopa (250 to 500 mg.), or infusion of the ganglion-blocking agent, trimethaphan (1 mg./ml.) may be used.

Hydralazine should be used with extreme caution in patients with left ventricular decompensation or coronary insufficiency, because use of this agent will be associated with reflex tachycardia and possibly with increased myocardial work.

Reserpine (parenteral) should be avoided, since in azotemic or comatose patients it can produce changes in sensorium that confuse the clinical assessment.

Once any parenteral therapy program is begun, oral antihypertensive therapy should be studied so the patient may be weaned from intravenous drugs as soon as possible.

SUGGESTED READINGS

Bhatia, S. and Frohlich, E. D.: The "hypertensive" evaluation. Am. Family Physician, *5*:83, 1972.

Chrysant, S. and Frohlich, E. D.: Side effects of antihypertensive drugs. Am. Family Physician, *9*:94, 1974.

Cohn, J. N. (ed.): Hypertension 1974. Arch. Intern. Med., *133*:911, 1974.

Dustan, H. P., et al.: Arterial pressure responses to discontinuing antihypertensive drug treatment. Circulation, *37*:370, 1968.

Dustan, H. P., Tarazi, R. C., and Hinshaw, L. B.: Mechanisms controlling arterial pressure. In Frohlich, E. D. (ed.): Pathophysiology: Altered Regulatory Mechanisms in Disease, ed. 2. pp. 49–82. Philadelphia, J. B. Lippincott, 1976.

Frohlich, E. D.: Clinical-physiological classification of hypertensive heart disease in essential hypertension. In Onesti, G., Kim, K. E., and Moyer, J. H., (eds.): Hypertension: Mechanisms and Management pp. 181–190. New York, Grune & Stratton, 1973.

———: Hypertension 1973: Treatment—why and how. Ann. Intern. Med., *78*:717, 1973.

———: Hypertension. In Conn, H. F., (ed.): Current Therapy 1976, pp. 208–224. Philadelphia, W. B. Saunders, 1976.

———: Pathophysiology of hypertension. In

Kurtzman, N. A., (ed.): Renal Hypertension Springfield, Charles C Thomas, (in press).

Frohlich, E. D. et al.: Physiological comparison of labile and essential hypertension. Circ. Res., *27*(I):55, 1970.

Frohlich, E. D., Tarazi, R. C., and Dustan, H. P.: Clinical-physiological correlations in the development of hypertensive heart disease. Circulation, *44*:446, 1971.

————: Re-examination of the hemodynamics of hypertension. Am. J. Med. Sci., *257*:9, 1969.

Genest, J., Koiw, E., and Kuchel, O. (eds.): International Textbook on Hypertension. New York, Blakiston, Publications/McGraw-Hill (in press).

Kaplan, N. M.: Clinical Hypertension. New York, Medcom, 1973.

Laragh, J. H. (ed.): Hypertension Manual. New York, Yorke Medical Books, 1974.

National High Blood Pressure Education Program, National Heart and Lung Institute: Performance Characteristics, Learning Objectives and Evaluation Approaches for the Education of Physicians in High Blood Pressure. Report of the Working Group on the Training and Evaluation of Physicians in High Blood Pressure. Circulation, *51*:10, 1975.

Onesti, G., Kim, K. E., and Moyer, J. H. (eds.): Hypertension: Mechanisms and Management. New York, Grune & Stratton, 1973.

Tarazi, R. C. et al.: Plasma volume and chronic hypertension. Relationship to arterial pressure levels in different hypertensive diseases. Arch. Intern. Med., *125*:835, 1970.

Veterans Administration Cooperative Study Group on Antihypertensive Agents: Effects of treatment on morbidity in hypertension. II. Results in patients with diastolic blood pressure averaging 90 through 114 mm Hg. J.A.M.A., *213*:1143, 1970.

Veterans Administration Study Group on Antihypertensive Agents: Effects of treatment on morbidity in hypertension. III. Influence of age, diastolic pressure, and prior cardiovascular disease; further analysis of side effects. Circulation, *45*:991, 1972.

4. RHEUMATIC FEVER

Angelo Taranta, M.D.

DEFINITION

Rheumatic fever is an inflammatory disease that occurs as a sequel to group A beta-hemolytic streptococcal infection of the throat. It consists clinically of a number of manifestations that tend to occur in the same patients, simultaneously or in close succession: polyarthritis, carditis, Sydenham's chorea, erythema marginatum, and subcutaneous nodules.

GENERAL CONSIDERATIONS

1. Relationship to connective tissue diseases and to autoimmune diseases

Rheumatic fever is often grouped with rheumatoid arthritis, systemic lupus erythematosus, dermatomyositis, etc., under the general heading of "connective tissue diseases" and with Hashimoto's thyroiditis, Goodpasture's syndrome, etc., under the label of "autoimmune diseases." Although rheumatic fever shares features with both of these overlapping sets of disorders, it also differs from them—not only because of its distinctive clinical and histopathologic features, but also because its specific eliciting factor is known. Moreover, patients with connective tissue diseases often have manifestations of more than one disease (e.g., "sclerodermatomyositis," "mixed connective tissue disease"), while this is exceptional in patients with rheumatic fever.

2. Regional decline of rheumatic fever incidence: consequent complacency and disinterest

Starting in the 1920s the incidence of rheumatic fever has been decreasing in the more affluent countries. Some poor countries, in which the disease was thought to be rare, are now recognized as having a comparatively high incidence, especially where overcrowding prevails. However, even in the more affluent countries the disease still occurs in pockets of poverty, and, less frequently, elsewhere. The decrease of incidence has engendered complacency and lack of interest, which is unfortunate since rheumatic fever is one of the most preventable among the serious diseases of man, and even one case of it is one too many.[7]

ETIOLOGY

1. *Streptococcal etiology*

The streptococcal etiology of rheumatic fever is generally accepted on the basis of five main lines of evidence:

A. A recent streptococcal infection can be demonstrated by serologic means in most patients with rheumatic fever of recent onset.[11]

B. Adequate treatment of streptococcal infections reduces by 90 percent the attack rate of rheumatic fever.[17]

C. The 10 per cent of attacks that do occur follow treatment failures (i.e., failures to eradicate streptococci from the throat).

D. Continual administration of antistreptococcal medications largely prevents recurrences of the disease—which are frequent otherwise.[14]

E. Recurrences of rheumatic fever in patients receiving continual antistreptococcal prophylaxis occur only after "streptococcal breakthroughs" (i.e., after streptococcal infections that occur despite prophylaxis).[14]

2. *Viral etiology*

The viral etiology of rheumatic fever, in vogue many years ago, has been recently resurrected.[2] Lesions similar to those of rheumatic fever have been produced in the hearts of monkeys with Coxsackie virus infections. Nevertheless, the lines of evidence listed above militate against viral infection as the cause of rheumatic fever.

EPIDEMIOLOGY

1. *Relationship of the epidemiology of rheumatic fever to that of streptococcal infections*

A. Rheumatic fever is extremely rare before the age of 3 years, and is observed most frequently between the ages of 5 and 15 years, when streptococcal infections are most frequent.

B. Similarly, the geographic distribution, incidence, and severity of rheumatic fever reflect the frequency and severity of streptococcal infections.

C. In epidemics of streptococcal pharyngitis (characterized by exudative pharyngitis accompanied by antibody response, and followed by prolonged carriage of group A streptococci), the incidence of rheumatic fever is about 3 per cent.

D. In endemic situations, the infections are usually milder, and the attack rate of rheumatic fever is much lower (about 0.3%).

2. *Epidemiology of recurrences*

A. Patients who have had previous attacks of rheumatic fever show a greatly increased attack rate of rheumatic fever following streptococcal infections (10–50%).

B. The attack rate is related to the severity of the streptococcal infection in these patients.

C. In addition, the attack rate is related to the time of the previous attack of rheumatic fever, and is higher in patients with rheumatic heart disease.[9]

3. *Genetic factors*

A. Rheumatic fever tends to "run in families," but whether this is due to

common environment, to common genes, or to both, has remained unclear.

B. The concordance rate for rheumatic fever is considerably higher in monozygotic than in dizygotic twins.

C. The kind of rheumatic manifestations tends to be similar in monozygotic twins, and is similar, to a lesser extent, in other siblings.

D. However, even in monozygotic twins, the concordance rate is only 20 per cent indicating a limited penetrance of the genetic predisposition, despite the ubiquity of the eliciting environmental factor—streptococcal infections.[10]

4. *Ethnic minorities and overcrowding*

A. Rheumatic fever in the United States is more common in certain ethnic minorities—Blacks, Puerto Ricans, Chicanos, and American Indians—but no intrinsic genetic predisposition has been demonstrated.

B. Rather, environmental factors, particularly crowding in the home, appear to account for the increased incidence, most likely because crowding facilitates the spread of streptococcal infections.[5]

PATHOPHYSIOLOGY

Little is known about the chain of events that links streptococcal infection to rheumatic fever.

1. *Hypersensitivity or allergy*

A. Some similarities between rheumatic fever and serum sickness ("latent period" between inciting event and sequel, sterile and transient arthritis) led, years ago, to the hypothesis that an immune reaction is responsible for rheumatic fever.

B. However, the similarity of rheumatic fever and serum sickness is superficial: serum complement is decreased in serum sickness, but, is increased in rheumatic fever, and the latent period characteristically shortens with repeated attacks in serum sickness, but not in rheumatic fever.

2. *Autoimmunity*

A. More recently, autoantibodies to heart muscle have been demonstrated in the serum of most patients with rheumatic fever, and a variety of immunologic cross-reactions have been discovered between streptococci and mammalian tissues.

B. Moreover, gammaglobulins and complement have been identified in the myocardium of children dying of acute rheumatic carditis.

C. These observations led to the hypothesis that streptococci cause rheumatic fever by eliciting the formation of heart-reactive antibodies.[6]

D. It is not clear, however, whether these antibodies are capable of fixing to their respective antigens in the healthy human heart in vivo (similar antibodies elicited in the rabbit circulate in the blood stream, but do not fix to the heart).

E. A point that is even less clear is whether these antibodies, once fixed, can cause rheumatic carditis.

F. An experimental model of rheumatic fever would be handy, but of those proposed, none has been generally accepted.

3. *Toxins*

A. In the face of this uncertainty, it is pertinent to remember that streptococci produce a number of powerful toxins, some of which may cause inflammation by lysosome disruption or lymphocyte activation.

B. One of these, streptolysin O, is acutely cardiotoxic in intact animals and in tissue culture.

C. Another, streptolysin S, is non-antigenic, an interesting property in a disease with a tendency to recur (since antigenicity would interfere with toxin action on repeated exposure).

D. In addition, some of the constituents of the streptococcal cell itself are toxic.

These toxic factors, singly or in combination, may well play a role in the elicitation of one or more manifestations of rheumatic fever.[16] For a detailed discussion of pathogenic mechanisms, see reference 12.

4. *Mechanisms of specific manifestations*

A. *Heart Failure*

(1) When heart failure occurs during the acute stage of rheumatic fever, it is usually due to myocarditis rather than to valvular damage.

(2) Conversely, when heart failure occurs years after an acute attack, it is usually due to progessive valvular deformities, initiated during the acute attack.

B. *Pericarditis*

Pericarditis may occasionally cause circulatory embarrassment by cardiac tamponade.

C. *Prolongation of the P-R interval*

(1) The P-R interval in the electrocardiogram is often prolonged in acute rheumatic fever, but this conduction disturbance is just as frequent in patients with clinically detectable carditis as in those without it.

(2) Moreover, patients with prolonged P-R interval have no worse cardiac prognosis than those without it.

(3) Hence, the mechanism responsible for P-R prolongation, whatever it may be, must be different from that responsible for clinically-detectable carditis.

D. *Extracardiac manifestations*

(1) Among the extracardiac manifestations, chorea, because of its symptoms, may be inferred to specifically involve the basal ganglia, but the few pathologic observations have revealed, instead, a diffuse involvement of the brain.

(2) Biopsies of the skin in cases of erythema marginatum have failed to show any alteration whatsoever.

(3) The subcutaneous nodules of

rheumatic fever (which are histologically indistinguishable from those of rheumatoid arthritis, unless the latter are biopsied later) seem to require a mechanical cofactor, appearing as they do in sites where the subcutaneous tissues rest directly on bony plates (extensor surface of the ulna, skull, and in proximity to joints).

CLASSIFICATION

1. *Rheumatic fever: acute, chronic, active, and inactive*
A. Most attacks of rheumatic fever are of relatively short duration.
B. The terms "rheumatic fever" and "acute rheumatic fever" are often used interchangeably.
C. A minority of attacks are of long duration or "chronic."
D. A special, very rare type of chronic rheumatic fever (or of rheumatic fever sequel) is Jaccoud arthritis, a fibrositis of the hand causing mild deformities that has been reported to follow repeated attacks of acute rheumatic fever.
E. Both acute and chronic rheumatic fever are considered active forms of the disease.
F. "Inactive" rheumatic fever denotes, instead, the status which follows acute (or chronic) rheumatic fever.

2. *Importance of specific manifestations in classification and diagnosis*
Whenever the diagnosis of rheumatic fever is made, it is important to ascertain which manifestations are present and to specify them in the diagnosis. This is particularly true of carditis, since its presence and severity greatly affect prognosis. Instead of simply stating, as is so often done in medical summaries, "the patient had an attack of rheumatic fever," with no further diagnostic details, the reader is urged to be more specific, as in the following diagnosis:
A. "Rheumatic fever with carditis, cardiomegaly, and failure"

B. "Residual lesions: aortic and mitral regurgitation with mild cardiomegaly but no heart failure"

SYMPTOMS AND SIGNS

1. *Arthritis* (see list below)
A. Arthritis is the most common manifestation of rheumatic fever.
B. Its incidence in first attacks increases with age.
C. It affects mostly large joints, especially knees and ankles.
D. Each joint is inflamed only for a week or two at the most, even in the absence of therapy.
E. In typical, untreated cases, new joints become affected as the attack progresses; the joints first affected tend to get better first ("migratory polyarthritis").
F. The total duration of the arthritis attack, including all the joints affected in succession, rarely exceeds 1 month, even in the absence of therapy.
G. Pain and tenderness are usually acute.
H. Characteristically, roentgenograms of the involved joints fail to show abnormal findings and the arthritis heals without residue (for a very rare exception, see Jaccoud arthritis, above).

2. *Carditis*
A. *General features*
(1) Carditis is the most serious manifestation of rheumatic fever.
(2) Its incidence in first attacks decreases with increasing age.
(3) It is often diagnosed by physical signs only in a patient who comes to medical attention because of noncardiac symptoms: joint pains or, rarely, the involuntary movements of Sydenham's chorea.
(4) Less frequently, carditis is diagnosed in a patient coming to medical attention because of cardiac symptoms: shortness of breath, dependent edema, right upper quadrant pain (caused by acute distention of the liver).

Jones Criteria (Revised) for Diagnosis of Rheumatic Fever*

Major Manifestations
  Carditis
  Polyarthritis
  Chorea
  Erythema marginatum
  Subcutaneous nodules
Minor manifestations
  Clinical
    Previous rheumatic fever or rheumatic heart disease
    Arthralgia
    Fever
  Laboratory
    Acute phase reactions
      Erythrocyte sedimentation rate
      C-reactive protein
      Prolonged P-R interval
      Leukocytosis
  Supporting evidence of streptococcal infection
    Increased titer of streptococcal antibodies
      ASO (antistreptolysin O)
      Other antibodies
    Positive throat culture for group A streptococcus
    Recent scarlet fever

*The presence of two major criteria, or of one major and two minor criteria, indicates a high probability of the presence of rheumatic fever. Evidence of a preceding streptococcal infection greatly strengthens the possibility of acute rheumatic fever. Its absence should make the diagnosis doubtful (except in Sydenham's chorea or long-standing carditis). (The Jones Criteria, revised, for Guidance in the Diagnosis of Rheumatic Fever. © 1967 American Heart Association.) Reprinted with permission. This pamphlet is available from local Heart Associations.

(5) In either case, the physical signs are mostly auscultatory—organic heart murmurs and sometimes pericardial friction rubs.
  B. *Specific findings*
    (1) Apical systolic murmur
      (a) The most commonly heard murmur during acute rheumatic fever is an organic apical systolic murmur indicative of mitral regurgitation.
      (b) It is long, usually occupying the whole of systole (holosystolic).
      (c) Its loudness is at least two, but usually three or more, on a scale of six.
      (d) Its pitch tends to be high, its character blowing.
      (e) A corollary of its loudness is that the murmur can be heard also in the axilla and that it is not obliterated by inspiration or by changes in posture.
    (2) Apical mid-diastolic murmur
      (a) Often associated with the murmur just described is an apical mid-diastolic murmur (Carey Coombs murmur), which starts with the third heart sound and ends distinctly before the first heart sound.
      (b) It should be differentiated from the murmur of established mitral stenosis, which is rumbling in character, is often preceded by the opening "snap" of the mitral valve, and, in the presence of sinus rhythm, is accentuated in presystole (due to the accelerated blood flow engendered by the "atrial kick").
      (c) While the murmur of established mitral stenosis is due to actual narrowing of the valve orifice, the Carey Coombs murmur appears to be due to "relative" stenosis of the mitral valve in relation to the dilated ventricular chamber, often combined with increased flow due to fever.
    (3) Basal Diastolic Murmur
      (a) Less frequent than the apical murmur is a basal diastolic murmur, indicative of aortic regurgitation.
      (b) This is a high-pitched, blowing murmur of "decrescendo" intensity, usually heard best along the left sternal border on the third or second interspace.
      (c) It may be short and faint and therefore difficult to hear.
    (4) Pericardial friction rubs
      (a) Pericardial friction rubs are scratchy, crunchy, crackling, or leathery sounds that can sometimes be altered by varying the pressure of the stethoscope against the chest wall.
      (b) They are usually not limited to a single phase of the cardiac cycle (systole or diastole), and may sometimes vary with the phase of respiration (pleuropericardial rubs).
    (5) Other auscultatory findings
      (a) Tachycardia: present even

during sleep—unlike emotional tachycardia—and often persists even after the temperature has returned to normal.

(b) Gallop rhythm

(i) Gallop rhythm, usually a protodiastolic gallop resulting from accentuation of the third heart sound;

(ii) Less frequently, a presystolic gallop resulting from accentuation of the usually inaudible fourth heart sound

(iii) A combination of (i) and (ii)—"summation" gallop

(c) Decrease of intensity of the first heart sound: this may become indistinct, "impure," or "mushy" due to a first degree A-V block, which, by delaying ventricular contraction, allows the mitral leaflets to float back towards the atria before systole.

3. Chorea

Chorea (Sydenham's chorea, chorea minor) is characterized by involuntary, abrupt, purposeless movements, muscular weakness, and emotional lability. The movements may involve all muscles, but especially those of the face and upper limbs.

A. Bizarre grimaces and inappropriate grins are common (Fig. 4-1).

B. Handwriting becomes clumsy or even impossible.

C. Speech is often halting, jerky, or slurred.

D. Muscular weakness is best revealed by asking the patient to squeeze the examiner's hands, which results in variations of pressure ("relapsing grip," "milkmaid's grip").

E. The emotional lability is manifested by crying, restlessness, giddy, inappropriate behavior, and litigiousness.

F. The knee-jerk may have a "hung-up" or pendular quality (the leg remains elevated longer than normal or may start to come down only to go up again—Gordon's sign).

G. The hands, when projected forward, tend to become flexed at the wrist and hyperextended at the metacarpophalangeal joints, with straightening of the fingers and abduction of the thumb ("spooning" or "dishing" of the hands).

H. It is interesting to note that chorea tends to appear later than other rheumatic manifestations in any given attack of rheumatic fever, and sometimes appears alone ("pure chorea").

4. *Subcutaneous nodules*

A. The subcutaneous nodules of rheumatic fever are seldom seen at present.

B. They are firm and painless, round or ovoid, with a diameter of up to 2 cm.

C. The skin overlying them is not inflamed and can be moved over them.

D. They occur on bony surfaces or near tendons.

5. *Erythema marginatum*

A. Erythema marginatum, another rare manifestation of rheumatic fever, is an evanescent, nonpruritic pink rash, which appears usually on the trunk and proximal parts of the limbs.

B. It extends centrifugally with a sharp outer margin, while the center returns gradually to normal—hence the name, "erythema marginatum."

C. The margin of the lesion is usually continuous, making a ring—hence its other name, "erythema annulare."

The five manifestations described above (see p. 54) are called "major" not because they are severe (certainly the last two are not) but because they are more specific for rheumatic fever than temperature elevation or arthralgia. Fever, however, is almost always present at the onset of rheumatic polyarthritis; it is often present in isolated carditis, but seldom in isolated chorea.

6. *Recurrences of rheumatic fever*

A. There is a similarity of clinical manifestations of recurrences to those of the preceding attack.

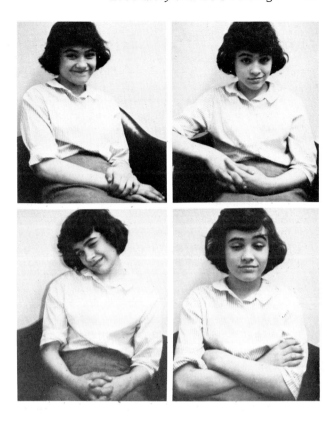

Fig. 4-1. Characteristic grimaces of a patient with Sydenham's chorea (Hollander, J. L. and McCarty, D. J., Jr. (eds.): Arthritis and Allied Conditions, ed. 8. Philadelphia, Lea and Febiger, 1972).

B. The pattern of rheumatic fever manifestations tends to repeat itself in successive attacks.

C. This is particularly important in the case of carditis; patients who escape it in the first attack have a generally good prognosis even in the event of recurrences, either because they escape carditis altogether, or because their carditis is mild and leaves no residual heart disease.[3]

LABORATORY AND ECG FINDINGS

Laboratory findings in rheumatic fever fall under three general headings: evidence of a recent streptococcal infection, manifestations of a systemic inflammatory state, and autoantibodies to heart antigens. Only the first two have general applicability so far; both strengthen the diagnostic suspicion; the absence of either throws doubt on the diagnosis (with the exception of chorea and long-standing carditis). In addition, the ECG often shows a prolongation of the P-R interval.

1. *Evidence of recent streptococcal infections*

A. *ASO titers*

(1) Eighty per cent of patients with acute rheumatic fever observed early in their course have elevated antistreptolysin O (ASO) titers.

(2) The remaining 20 per cent have elevation of one or more of the other streptococcal antibody tests (antistreptokinase, antihyaluronidase, antideoxyribonuclease, antidiphosphopiridinenucleotidase).[11,14]

(3) All of these antibody tests are based on the inhibition of a specific toxic

or enzymatic activity of streptococcal culture filtrate.

(4) Unfortunately, only the ASO test is generally available, and all the tests are time-consuming.

B. *Streptozyme*

(1) Recently, a simple, rapid test based on a different principle (the agglutination of sheep red cells coated with a mixture of streptococcal antigens) has become commercially available (Streptozyme).

(2) It is more sensitive than any other single streptococcal antibody test and, in small series, has been reported to be positive in 100 per cent of cases of rheumatic fever.[1]

C. *Throat culture*

A positive throat culture for group A streptococci may provide presumptive evidence of streptococcal infection which should, however, be confirmed by antibody determinations.

2. *Laboratory manifestations of a systemic inflammatory state*

A. Laboratory manifestations of a systemic inflammatory state in rheumatic fever include an elevated erythrocyte sedimentation rate, a positive test for C-reactive protein, and leukocytosis.

B. Usually, changes in the C-reactive protein tests precede those in the erythrocyte sedimentation rate.

C. With the exception of "pure" or isolated chorea, untreated rheumatic fever is consistently accompanied by elevation of the ESR, positivity of the CRP, or, more commonly, by both.

3. *Antiheart antibodies*

A. Antiheart antibodies are demonstrable by a variety of techniques in the serum of patients with rheumatic fever.

B. They are also found, however, in the serum of patients with uncomplicated streptococcal infections or with acute glomerulonephritis, though usually at a lower titer.[6]

C. Because of this overlap, as well as because of technical difficulties, these tests have not entered general use as yet.

4. *Cardiac arrhythmias*

A. Prolongation of the P-R interval occurs in 25 to 40 per cent of the patients.

B. Other arrhythmias may include: Wenckebach A-V block, A-V dissociation, and even complete A-V block.

DIAGNOSIS

Since none of the clinical or laboratory manifestations of rheumatic fever is characteristic enough to be diagnostic, the diagnosis must be based on appropriate combinations of them.

1. *Jones criteria*

A. T. D. Jones divided the manifestations of rheumatic fever into "major" and "minor" according to their diagnostic usefulness (see p. 55). These criteria have been widely accepted and have proved useful especially in avoiding overdiagnosis.

B. He proposed that the presence of two major or of one major and two minor manifestations indicates a high probability of the presence of rheumatic fever.

2. *The role of history*

A. If the physician sees the patient early in the attack, he should be able to observe directly the various manifestations or to note their absence. In such cases, the role of history-taking will be limited to ascertaining whether the patient has had rheumatic fever earlier, and whether he had scarlet fever 2 to 4 weeks previously.

B. A positive answer to either of these questions makes rheumatic fever more likely.

C. In the absence of scarlet fever, a history of recent sore throat is consistent with the diagnosis of rheumatic fever, but is too nonspecific to be taken as evidence of recent streptococcal infection.

D. Many sore throats are viral; many streptococcal infections are subclinical; hence the diagnosis of recent streptococcal infection should be made serologically.

E. If the physician first sees the patient after the acute manifestations have subsided, the history is of great importance and is often critical.

3. *Arthritis*

Arthritis is a term that should be restricted to cases with objective evidence of joint inflammation, such as swelling, heat, and redness, or at least tenderness or limitation of motion.

A. It is important to distinguish polyarthritis (a major manifestation) from arthralgia (a minor manifestation), and arthralgia from myalgia (not a manifestation of rheumatic fever).

B. Although the typical joint manifestation of rheumatic fever is migratory polyarthritis, arthritis is sometimes so short-lived that it has no time to migrate.

C. To facilitate diagnosis, anti-inflammatory treatment should be withheld until the character of the arthritis has declared itself.

D. Any arthritis that persists in the same joint for more than 1 week should make one think of another diagnosis, especially in children.

E. Arthritis is more severe, and more frequent in adults; it also lasts longer.

F. The arthritis of rheumatic fever responds readily to aspirin, while that of many other arthritides does not.

4. *Carditis*

Rheumatic carditis is always associated with one or more of the three murmurs described earlier: organic apical systolic murmur, mid-diastolic apical murmur, aortic diastolic murmur. Hence, the paramount importance of careful auscultation.

A. *Apical systolic murmur*

(1) Functional systolic murmurs may be mistaken for the organic systolic murmur of mitral regurgitation, especially when their loudness is increased by fever or anemia.

(2) Unlike the murmur of mitral regurgitation, however, most functional systolic murmurs are heard best along the left sternal border, in the third or second interspace (Still's murmur, innocent ejection-type murmurs).

(3) The functional systolic murmurs are limited to the first two-thirds of systole, and tend to have a mid-systolic accentuation.

(4) The functional systolic murmurs have generally low pitch and they lack the "blowing" or "steam-jet" quality of mitral regurgitation murmurs.

(5) Some functional murmurs have a "groaning" or "twanging-string" quality; they are often heard best along the lower left sternal margin or between it and the apex.

B. *Mid-diastolic murmur*

At the apex, physiologic third heart sounds may be mistaken for mid-diastolic murmurs. Differentiation of the two rests mainly on the perceptible duration of the latter.

C. *Basal diastolic murmur*

(1) The aortic diastolic murmur is notoriously easy to miss, and good training of the ear (under supervision) is essential to learn to detect it.

(2) Overdiagnosis of aortic regurgitation, less commonly a problem, will be avoided if one remembers that this high-pitched, decrescendo murmur starts right at the end of the second sound and has a definite duration.

D. *Pericardial friction rub*

One must be wary not to confuse a pericardial rub with the sounds made by chest hair rubbing against the stethoscope.

5. *Chorea*

Chorea must be differentiated from "tics" (repetitive, stereotyped, localized movements).

6. *Subcutaneous   nodules   and erythema marginatum*

A. Subcutaneous nodules must sometimes be differentiated from enlarged lymph nodes (especially in rubella).

B. Erythema marginatum must sometimes be differentiated from cutis marmorata, a fixed, reticular bluish discoloration of the skin.

7. *Laboratory findings*

A. The role of the laboratory is mainly confirmatory when it reveals the existence of a recent streptococcal infection and of a systemic inflammatory state.

B. The lack of either throws doubt on the diagnosis (with the exception of isolated chorea and of long-standing carditis).

DIFFERENTIAL DIAGNOSIS

1. *Rheumatoid arthritis*

A. The fever of juvenile rheumatoid arthritis may have wide swings reminiscent of a "septic" or "hectic" temperature curve; the fever of rheumatic fever is steadier.

B. A period of high fever without any localizing sign and persisting for weeks or even more than a month may occur in juvenile rheumatoid arthritis (Still's type), but not in rheumatic fever.

C. The onset of arthritis is almost always rapid in rheumatic fever; it is often gradual in rheumatoid arthritis.

D. An arthritis limited to the small joints of the hands or feet, and especially an arthritis involving the cervical spine or the temporomandibular joints should make one think of rheumatoid arthritis rather than of rheumatic fever.

E. Morning stiffness is not a feature of rheumatic fever.

F. At any given level of objective involvement, the arthritis of rheumatic fever is distinctly more painful and tender than that of rheumatoid arthritis.

G. Low ASO and streptozyme titers will be against rheumatic fever.

H. Rheumatoid factor tests are of limited usefulness because they are often negative in the initial phase of adult rheumatoid arthritis and are persistently negative in juvenile rheumatoid arthritis.

I. The differential diagnosis between rheumatic fever and rheumatoid arthritis is often difficult early in the attack; later it becomes easier, because the arthritis of rheumatic fever is of shorter duration.

2. *Systemic lupus erythematosus (SLE)*

A. Kidney involvement, onset of the disease after exposure to sunlight, and hyperkeratotic rash with follicular plugging and central atrophy favor SLE.

B. Organic heart murmurs and a history of a recent sore throat favor rheumatic fever.

C. Antinuclear antibodies are almost always present in SLE, and serum complement is often decreased.

3. *Subacute bacterial endocarditis (SBE)*

A. SBE must be considered whenever a patient with rheumatic heart disease develops an unexplained fever of more than a few days' duration.

B. Arthralgia and arthritis of one or more joints occur frequently in SBE, especially in children, and may lead to an erroneous diagnosis of rheumatic fever.

4. *Sickle-cell anemia*

A. Sickle-cell anemia may cause diagnostic confusion because of joint pains, fever, and heart murmurs.

B. The erythrocyte sedimentation rate is usually elevated in rheumatic fever, but not in sickle-cell anemia.

C. A sickle-cell preparation will dispel the confusion—unless both diseases coexist.

MANAGEMENT

1. *General measures and bed rest*

A. All patients with rheumatic fever should be examined daily for the first 2 or 3 weeks of the illness, primarily to find out whether carditis is developing and to start treatment promptly should heart failure appear.

B. Discussions at the bedside concerning heart murmurs or cardiomegaly are better avoided; often the patient misunderstands and worries needlessly.

C. All patients should be in bed for the first 3 weeks of illness because carditis is immediately present in some, and may appear later in others.

D. Strict bed rest, however, should be limited to patients with arthritis of the lower limbs (to decrease their pain) and to those with carditis and cardiomegaly (not to overtax their inflamed hearts).

E. After this initial period of observation, the bed rest regimes should be tailored to the manifestations of the disease that are present in the particular patient.

2. *Management for specific manifestations*

A. *Patients with polyarthritis and no carditis* are usually asymptomatic by the second or third week of aspirin treatment. In the third or fourth week they may be gradually ambulated, while continuing the aspirin.

B. *Patients with carditis manifested by significant murmurs, but with no definite cardiomegaly or heart failure* (with or without polyarthritis) should be kept in bed for 1 month. The bed rest need not be strict, and in the last week may be broken by periods of supervised ambulation of a few hours per day.

C. *Patients with carditis and cardiomegaly, but no congestive heart failure* (with or without polyarthritis) should be kept on bed rest for 6 weeks; this should be strict for the first 2 weeks. For the last 2 weeks, the patient can be allowed out of bed for a few hours daily.

D. *Patients with carditis and congestive heart failure* (with or without polyarthritis) should be kept on strict bed rest until failure is controlled. It is wise to maintain a modified bed rest until

a month after anti-inflammatory treatment is stopped (if no rebound ensues), or until 2 weeks after the spontaneous subsidence of a rebound.

3. *Analgesic or anti-inflammatory treatment*

A. *In cases with arthralgia only, or with mild arthritis and no carditis,* the patient may be given analgesics only. This is particularly wise when the diagnosis is not beyond doubt; it also has the advantage of not engendering rebounds.

B. *Patients with moderate or severe arthritis but no carditis, or with carditis but no cardiomegaly or fever* will be treated with aspirin: two-thirds to three-fourths grains per pound per day for the first 2 weeks, and one-half grain per pound per day for the following 6 weeks. Sometimes slightly larger doses may be necessary to control arthritis.

C. *Patients with carditis and cardiomegaly, but no congestive heart failure* (with or without polyarthritis) should be started on aspirin (see above). In patients with marked cardiomegaly, however, aspirin is often insufficient to control fever, discomfort and tachycardia, or does so only at toxic or near-toxic doses. These patients may then be switched to steroids (see below).

D. *Patients with carditis and heart failure* (with or without polyarthritis)

(1) All patients should receive prednisone, starting with a dose of 40 to 60 mg. per day, to be increased if control of heart failure is not achieved.

(2) In cases of extreme acuteness and severity, therapy should be started by intravenous administration of methylprednisone (Solu-Medrol, 10 to 40 mg.) followed by oral prednisone.

(3) After 2 or 3 weeks, prednisone may be slowly withdrawn, decreasing the daily dose at the rate of 5 mg. every 2 or 3 days. When tapering is started, aspirin at standard doses should be added and continued for 3 or 4 weeks after prednisone is stopped. This "over-

lap" therapy reduces the incidence of post-therapeutic clinical rebounds.

(4) The termination of anti-inflammatory treatment may be followed in all rheumatic fever patients by the reappearance within 2 or 3 weeks of laboratory abnormalities (laboratory rebounds), or of clinical abnormalities as well (clinical rebounds).

(5) All the laboratory rebounds and most of the clinical rebounds are best left untreated or should be treated symptomatically with analgesics or small doses of aspirin, lest the full treatment be followed by another rebound and the duration of the attack lengthened.

(6) Only the most severe clinical rebounds necessitate reinstitution of the full original treatment.

(7) Unfortunately, most well-controlled studies have failed to prove that treatment with steroids decreases the incidence of residual rheumatic heart disease.[15] Nevertheless, such treatment is indicated in patients with severe carditis and failure because of the distinct impression that death during the acute attack may be averted thereby.

(8) In about 5 to 10 per cent of all patients with rheumatic fever, a persistently elevated erythrocyte sedimentation rate is observed for months after termination of therapy. This is a benign, unexplained phenomenon that should not alter the medical management.

(9) However, a persistently-elevated C-reactive protein level often heralds a protracted course with subsequent flare-ups; these patients should be supervised closely.

4. *Diuretics and cardiotonic medication*

The heart failure of rheumatic carditis is often controlled with bed rest and steroids only. If it is not:

A. Diuretics may be added first, followed by digitalis if needed.

B. Digitalis should be used with caution because its therapeutic range may be decreased in rheumatic carditis.

C. The need for digitalis should be reevaluated at the end of the rheumatic attack, and periodically thereafter. In assessing the effect of digitalis, one should distinguish "cardiac" tachycardia, which is also present during sleep ("sleeping tachycardia") from emotional tachycardia, that subsides during sleep.

D. As in congestive failure from other causes, oxygen is indicated in the presence of dyspnea or cyanosis.

E. Morphine and rotating tourniquets are indicated in pulmonary edema.

5. *Sedation or tranquilization*

A. Patients with chorea may benefit from administration of barbiturates or tranquilizers.

B. Since chorea often occurs as an isolated manifestation or a few months after arthritis or carditis, anti-inflammatory medication is not usually needed.

C. Although steroids in large doses have been reported to control choreic movements, it is difficult to be sure, because the course of chorea is unpredictable and well-controlled studies are lacking. Since steroids (especially at large doses) are not harmless, it would be unwise to use them in any but the most severe cases of chorea.

PREVENTION OF RHEUMATIC FEVER RECURRENCES

Patients who have had an attack of rheumatic fever are prone to develop it again. Since recurrences may follow asymptomatic as well as symptomatic streptococcal sore throat, the physician cannot rely on diagnosis and treatment of streptococcal pharyngitis for prevention of rheumatic recurrences, but must institute *continual* prophylaxis.

1. *Initial "eradicating" treatment* As soon as the diagnosis of rheumatic fever is made—not sooner, lest other possible diagnoses be obscured—the patient should be started on antistreptococcal prophylaxis with an initial therapeutic (streptococcal-eradicating) dose or

course of antibiotics (as outlined under "appropriate treatment" below). Thanks to this "eradicating" treatment, one can then start continual prophylaxis with a "clear slate," and clearly identify new infections, should they occur.

2. *Continual parenteral prophylaxis*

A. Best results are obtained with the injection of 1.2 million units of benzathine penicillin G every four weeks (Fig. 4-2).

B. This treatment is particularly recommended in high-risk patients:

(1) Those with rheumatic heart disease

(2) Those whose previous attack of rheumatic fever was recent (3 years or less)

(3) Those with multiple attacks

C. Additional risk factors are:

(1) Young age (childhood and adolescence)

(2) Exposure to young people

(3) Crowding in the home

3. *Continual Oral Prophylaxis*

A. In patients intolerant of benzathine penicillin prophylaxis because of pain at the site of injection, continual oral medication may be prescribed.

B. Its success, of course, depends on the compliance of the patient, which may be poor even when the patient seems to be cooperative.

C. Sulfadiazine (0.5 g. once daily in children weighing less than 60 pounds and 1 g. in the others), and oral penicillin (200,000 to 250,000 units twice a day) are about equally effective.

D. Patients on sulfadiazine should have a blood count after 2 weeks, and also whenever they develop a rash in association with fever or sore throat. The drug should be stopped if the white count falls below 4000 and the neutrophil level falls below 35 per cent.

E. For the exceptional patient who may be sensitive to both penicillin and sulfa, erythromycin may be prescribed (100 to 250 mg., twice daily).

F. It should be remembered that an-

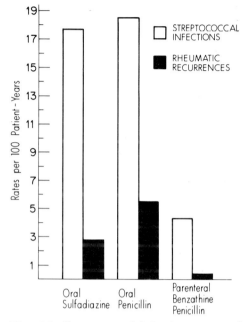

Fig. 4-2. Streptococcal infection rates and rheumatic recurrence rates per 100 patient-yr. in children and adolescents with previous rheumatic fever. The three prophylactic regimes were tested concurrently: sulfadiazine, 1 g./day, orally in a single dose (675 patient yr.); penicillin G, 0.2 million units/day orally in a single dose, ½ hr. before breakfast (545 patient-yr.); and benzathine penicillin G, 1.2 million units i.m. every 4 wks. (560 patient-yr.). (Taranta, A. and Gordis, L.: The prevention of rheumatic fever: opportunities, frustrations, and challenges. Cardiovasc. Clin. *4*:1, 1972.)

tistreptococcal prophylaxis is not 100 per cent effective—particularly oral prophylaxis.

G. The occurrence of sore throat in patients on prophylaxis requires an immediate throat culture and appropriate treatment.

4. *Duration of continual prophylaxis*

For maximum protection, continual prophylaxis may be maintained for the lifetime of the patient. This is particularly important for patients with rheumatic heart disease. The risk factors mentioned above may serve as a guide to the physician, so that he may apply pressure and persuasion in accordance with the need for protection of the particular patient.[8]

PREVENTION OF INITIAL ATTACK OF RHEUMATIC FEVER ("PRIMARY PREVENTION")

1. *General approach*

A. While the prevention of recurrences of rheumatic fever is very important for the protection of individual patients, the eradication of rheumatic fever can only be accomplished by prevention of first attacks.

B. Moreover, the hearts of many patients are irreparably damaged by a first attack; for them, the triumphs of secondary prophylaxis are no consolation.

C. Although highly effective, prophylaxis of first attacks is hampered by the sheer size of the population at risk, and by the imperfect methods of diagnosing streptococcal pharyngitis.

D. Streptococcal infections of the skin, which can cause glomerulonephritis, have not been associated with rheumatic fever, and will not be considered further here.

2. *Throat culture*

Patients with fever, fiery red throat with exudate, and tender anterior cervical lymph nodes are more likely than others to have a streptococcal pharyngitis, but even this "classic" picture may be caused by viruses. Conversely, some mild sore throats may be streptococcal and may be followed by rheumatic fever or glomerulonephritis. Therefore, it is considered prudent to take a throat culture in all patients with acute pharyngitis, and to treat all those with a positive culture. Hoarseness, conjunctivitis, cough and simple coryza are usually *not* associated with streptococcal infections; therefore, patients with these symptoms need not be cultured.

A. The throat culture should be taken *before* antibiotic therapy.

B. The tongue should be depressed, the throat should be clearly visualized and well lit, and the swab must be rubbed vigorously over each tonsillar area without touching the tongue or the lips.

C. One may then send the swab to a laboratory, following the laboratory's instructions, or one may streak the swab directly on a blood agar plate and then incubate and read the plate.[13]

D. The cost of the throat culture, which is often excessive, can be reduced by using state laboratories (whenever available) or by doing the culture in one's own office. Alternatively, one may ask commercial or hospital laboratories to omit the unnecessary garnishes of identification of all bacterial species (usually, the only important organisms to identify are group A beta-hemolytic streptococci), and of antibiotic sensitivity (all group A beta-hemolytic streptococci are sensitive to pencillin).[7]

3. *Onset of treatment*

This depends on how sick the patient is, on the one hand, and on how compliant he is considered to be, on the other.

A. *Patients in advanced state*

(1) Treatment may be started at once in a febrile, toxic patient with exudative pharyngitis, especially during the winter and spring months.

(2) This is particularly true for those patients who may not be expected to return for treatment.

(3) Often, in emergency room practice and other kinds of episodic medical care, the doctor perceives that the patient is not likely to come back and that treatment will be given "either now or never;" he should then act accordingly.

B. *Patients in mild state*

(1) On the other hand, the milder the symptoms and signs, and the closer

the patient-doctor relationship, the safer it is to delay treatment until an etiologic diagnosis is made.

(2) One should remember that a few days' delay in initiating treatment has not been shown to be harmful in terms of rheumatic fever prevention.

(3) Although many parents of patients are anxious to obtain "instant treatment," experience has shown that they can be educated to accept a less empirical approach.

(4) In many middle-class communities, the use of a throat culture as a basis for treatment is becoming recognized as a trademark of good care.

C. *Patients treated before obtaining culture result*

If treatment is started with an oral agent before the culture results are known, these options remain open:

(1) To discontinue medication the morning after, if the throat culture is negative for beta-hemolytic streptococci

(2) To discontinue medication one day later, if they are not of group A

4. *Appropriate treatment*

Given the present state of knowledge, eradication of streptococci from the throat is the aim of treatment, not only to prevent rheumatic fever, but to interrupt the chain of contagion. Eradication depends upon the choice of drug and the length of time effective blood levels are maintained.

A. *Penicillin*

(1) Penicillin is the drug on which the largest amount of favorable data has been accumulated.

(2) It can be administered by the oral route (200,000 to 250,000 units 3 to 4 times per day), at least ½ hour before or 1 hour after meals for 10 days, even though symptoms will abate earlier.

(3) Advantages of the oral route are: a lower incidence of severe allergic reactions, and the option to discontinue the drug if the diagnosis is not confirmed by culture or if allergy develops.

(4) The chief drawback is failure to complete the prescribed course. Such failure is surprisingly common, especially in clinic or emergency-room patients, because the patient, his parents, and at times the doctor, do not understand the importance of treating a sore throat that is no longer sore.

(5) In fact, the main reason for treatment is prevention of sequelae—rheumatic fever and glomerulonephritis—not the amelioration of symptoms.

(6) The most reliable way to guarantee adequate therapy is by a single injection of benzathine penicillin G, 0.6 million units in children weighing less than 60 pounds, or 1.2 million units in the others.

(7) If a combination of procaine penicillin and benzathine pencillin is used, the latter should still be given in the amounts just noted.

(8) Buffered penicillin G, the least expensive preparation, seems to be just as effective in the treatment of streptococcal pharyngitis as penicillin V or phenethicillin.

(9) Penicillin allergy is a cause of genuine concern, especially when dealing with adults.

(10) Care should be taken to obtain a good history and to keep epinephrine (adrenalin) at hand.

B. *Erythromycin*

For patients with a history of penicillin allergy, erythromycin should be prescribed, 20 mg. per pound per day (not to exceed 1 g. per day) for 10 days.

C. *Sulfonamides*

Sulfonamides, which are effective agents in continual prophylaxis, should not be used for therapy because they suppress, but do not eradicate, group A streptococci.

D. *Tetracyclines*

Tetracyclines should not be used because 40 per cent of group A streptococcal strains are resistant to them.

E. *Treatment for family members*

(1) Family members of a patient with symptomatic streptococcal pharyngitis are at high risk of being infected.

(2) It seems prudent, therefore, to culture all family contacts with recent upper respiratory symptoms and to treat those with positive cultures.

(3) Some physicians elect to culture all family contacts.

5. *Follow-up*

A. *Reasons for follow-up visits*

(1) To ascertain whether the infection has cleared or is relapsing

(2) To stimulate compliance

(3) To find out whether streptococcal sequelae have resulted

B. *Timing of follow-up visits*

(1) In the case of oral medication, the follow-up visit should be set at 2 to 10 days after the end of the medication

(2) In the case of repository medication, follow-up should be at 2 to 10 days after the estimated end of a bactericidal concentration (14 to 16 days for 600,000 units and 21 to 28 days for 1.2 million units of benzathine penicillin).

6. *Recurrences*

A. Clinical and bacteriologic (sore throat with positive throat culture)

B. Bacteriologic only (positive throat culture without sore throat)

Current recommended practice is to treat both kinds of recurrences with a second course of penicillin (preferably benzathine penicillin, by injection) or erythromycin by mouth.

PROGNOSIS

1. Sequelae of rheumatic fever are essentially limited to the heart, and depend on the presence and severity of carditis.

2. Among large recent series of patients followed from their acute attack onwards, rheumatic heart disease has not developed in those who had no clinical evidence of carditis during the acute attack.

3. An exception may be noted in patients whose first attack of rheumatic fever took the form of "pure" chorea, who may develop rheumatic heart disease (usually mitral stenosis) gradually and insidiously over the years.

4. Among patients with clinical evidence of carditis during the acute attack, the incidence of residual rheumatic heart disease increases with increasing severity of the initial carditis.

5. Thus, in one study (Table 4-1) the incidence of residual heart disease was higher in patients who, at the time of the initial carditis, had systolic and mid-diastolic apical murmurs, than in those who had systolic murmurs only, and among the latter it was higher in those who had loud murmurs.

6. The incidence of residual heart disease was highest in patients who had congestive heart failure, pericarditis, or both during the acute attack.[15]

7. In another study, the incidence of residual heart disease (8 years after the attack) among patients with initial carditis was maximum in patients with marked enlargement of the heart during the acute attack, and minimum in patients with organic murmurs, but without cardiomegaly during the acute attack.[4]

8. In both series, the incidence of residual heart disease was higher after recurrences than after first attacks.

9. It is of interest that mitral stenosis which, after 5 years, was present only in approximately 1.4 per cent of patients, increased to approximately 5 per cent by the end of 10 years, and that mitral stenosis was usually preceded by a severe attack of rheumatic carditis in males (6 of 8 cases had had failure, pericarditis, or both) but not in females (only 5 of 16 cases had had the manifestations mentioned).[15]

10. For unknown reasons, natives of India develop mitral stenosis at a much

Table 4-1. **Prognosis in Relation to Cardiac Status at Start of Treatment***

Cardiac Status at Start of Treatment	No. of Cases Observed for 5 Years	Per Cent With No Murmur After 5 Years	No. of Deaths in 5 Years
No carditis	71	96	0
Questionable carditis	32	84	0
Apical systolic murmur, grade I only†	39	82	0
Apical systolic murmur, grade II or III only	60	68	2
Apical systolic and apical mid-diastolic murmurs	44	48	1††
Basal diastolic with or without other murmurs	45(15)§	53(27)§	1
Failure and/or pericarditis	33	30	1
Preexisting heart disease without failure and/or pericarditis	80	30	5‡
Preexisting heart disease with failure and/or pericarditis	22	0	6

*The combined results of all three treatment groups. Modified from U.K. and U.S. Joint Report. Circulation 32:457, 1965.
†Grades I, II and III are increasingly loud, but all refer to murmurs considered organic in this classification.
††Death from acute nephritis and uremia.
§Excluding one U.K. center which had exceedingly high incidence of basal diastolic murmurs.
‡Includes one death from acute intestinal obstruction.

earlier age than Westerners; up to one-third of all mitral commissurotomies are performed in patients below the age of 20 years.

REFERENCES

1. Bisno, A. L. and Ofek, I.: Serologic diagnosis of streptococcal infection: Comparison of a rapid hemagglutination technique with conventional antibody tests. Am. J. Dis. Child., 127:676, 1974.
2. Burch, G. E., Giles, T. D., and Colcolough, H. L.: Pathogenesis of "rheumatic" heart disease: Critique and theory. Amer. Heart J., 80:556, 1970.
3. Feinstein, A. R. and Spaguolo, M.: Mimetic features of rheumatic fever recurrences. N. Engl. J. Med., 262:533, 1960.
4. Feinstein, A. R. et al.: Rheumatic fever in children and adolescents: a long-term epidemiologic study of subsequent prophylaxis, streptococcal infections, and clinical sequelae. VII. Cardiac changes and sequelae. Ann. Intern. Med., 60 (Feb. Supp):87, 1964.
5. Gordis, L., Lilienfeld, A., and Rodriguez, R.: Studies in the epidemiology and preventability of rheumatic fever: II. Socioeconomic factors and the incidence of acute attacks. J. Chronic Dis., 21:655, 1969.
6. Kaplan, M. H. and Svec, K. H.: Immunologic relation of streptococcal and tissue antigens: III: Presence in human sera of streptococcal antibody cross-reactive with heart tissue; as-

sociation with streptococcal infections, rheumatic fever, and glomerulonephritis. J. Exp. Med., 119:651, 1964.
7. Rheumatic Fever and Rheumatic Heart Disease Study Group, Inter-Society Commission for Heart Disease Resources (A. Taranta, chairman; members: J. Fiedler, C. Frank, B. S. Gilson, L. Gordis, C. Hufnagel, M. Markowitz, L. W. Wannamaker): Prevention of rheumatic fever and rheumatic heart diseases. Circulation, 41:A-1, 1970.
8. Rheumatic Fever and Rheumatic Heart Disease Study Group, Inter-Society Commission for Heart Disease Resources (A. Taranta, Chairman; members: J. Fiedler, B. S. Gilson, L. Gordis, C. Hufnagel, H. Kloth, M. Markowitz, L. W. Wannamaker): Community resources for the management of patients with rheumatic heart disease. Circulation, 44:A-273, 1971.
9. Spagnuolo, M., Pasternack, B., and Taranta, A.: The risk of rheumatic recurrences after streptococcal infections: a statistically-controlled prospective study of clinical and social factors. N. Engl. J. Med., 285:641, 1971.
10. Spagnuolo, M. and Taranta, A.: Rheumatic fever in siblings: similarity of its clinical manifestations. N. Engl. J. Med., 278:183, 1968.
11. Stollerman, G. H. et al.: Relationship of immune response to group A streptococci to the course of acute, chronic and recurrent rheumatic fever. Am. J. Med., 20:170, 1956.
12. Taranta, A.: Rheumatic fever made difficult. Paediatrician, 5:74, 1976.
13. Taranta, A. and Moody, M.: Diagnosis of streptococcal pharyngitis and rheumatic fever:

symposium on laboratory diagnosis. Pediatr. Clin. North Am., *18*:125, 1971.

14. Taranta, A. et al.: Rheumatic fever in children and adolescents: a long-term epidemiologic study of subsequent prophylaxis, streptococcal infections, and clinical sequelae. IV. Relation of the rheumatic fever recurrence rate per streptococcal infection to the titers of streptococcal antibodies. Ann. Intern. Med., *60* (Feb. Supp.): 47, 1964.

15. U.K. and U.S. Joint Report: The natural history of rheumatic fever and rheumatic heart disease: Cooperative clinical trial of ACTH, cortisone and aspirin. Circulation, *32*:457, 1965.

16. Wannamaker, L. W.: The chain that links the heart to the throat. Circulation, *48*:9, 1973.

17. Wannamaker, L. W. et al.: Prophylaxis of acute rheumatic fever by treatment of the preceding streptococcal infection with various amounts of depot penicillin. Amer. J. Med., *10*:673, 1951.

SUGGESTED READINGS

Markowitz, M. and Gordis, L.: Rheumatic Fever *In* Schaffer, A. J. (ed): Major Problems in Clinical Pediatrics, vol. II. Philadelphia, W. B. Saunders, 1972.

Stollerman, G.: Rheumatic Fever and Streptococcal Infection. New York, Grune & Stratton, 1975.

5. VALVULAR HEART DISEASE

J. O'Neal Humphries, M.D

GENERAL CONSIDERATIONS

Obstruction to forward flow (stenosis) or regurgitation of flow at any of the four heart valves is considered to be valvular heart disease. Clinically, a broad range of severity of stenosis or regurgitation is encountered. Isolated stenosis or regurgitation of a single valve or combinations of stenosis and regurgitation of one or more valves are all possible, although the left heart valves are more often involved.

The efficiency of a pump of any variety depends on two things: (1) the power of the pump, and (2) the proper function of the inflow and outflow valves. Diminished power or malfunction of the valves leads to inefficiency of the pump and, if either one or both are severe enough, will lead to reduced effectiveness of the pump. This results in a decreased volume that can be handled and an increase in volume and pressure proximal to the pump. When the effectiveness of the heart pump is diminished, this results in a reduced cardiac output and an increased volume and pressure in the filling chambers (and vessels leading to filling chambers). This combination is referred to as *heart failure* (see Chap. 19).

For simplicity's sake, it is desirable to consider the right and left side of the heart as separate pumps. Malfunction of the valves is much more common on the left side of the heart than on the right side. Inadequate performance of the left pump results in a reduced cardiac output and increased volume and pressure in the left atrium and pulmonary vasculature (pulmonary congestion), whereas inadequate performance of the right pump leads to a reduced cardiac output and increased volume and pressure in the right atrium and systemic venous system (systemic congestion).

To a certain degree, compensatory adjustments of the heart muscle can maintain the overall performance of the pump even when one or more valves are malfunctioning. However, this causes hypertrophy, dilatation, and even damage to the heart muscle so that eventually the compensatory mechanisms are exhausted. Peripheral compensatory processes also occur to insure adequate nutrient supply to tissues. Increased extraction of oxygen by peripheral organs attempts to adjust for the decrease in oxygen delivery associated with the reduced cardiac output and may be detected by measuring wide oxygen concentration differences between arterial and venous blood samples.

Auscultation remains the most powerful screening technique for valvular heart disease in the symptomatic and asymptomatic patient (see Chap. 1). It is simple, safe, and reasonably accurate when done by experienced physicians. Other aspects of the cardiac examination play a major role in establishing the severity and consequences of the valvular disease, as do selected laboratory studies.

Less common and clinically insignificant valvular lesions are purposely omitted in this chapter because they are beyond the scope of this book.

AORTIC STENOSIS

1. *Definition*

   A. Reduction in the valve orifice size is considered to be aortic stenosis.

   B. Reduction of the valve ring itself as part of underdevelopment of the entire left heart may cause serious difficulty in infancy.

C. In the adult, however, stenosis is always associated with abnormalities of the leaflet.

2. *General features*

A. Obstruction to outflow of the left ventricle is most commonly due to disease at the level of the aortic valve leaflets, but occasionally may be due to a constriction of the ascending aorta (supravalvular stenosis) or a fibrous ring or tunnel within the left ventricle just below the aortic leaflets (subvalvular stenosis).

B. The severity of obstruction varies immensely and determines the extent of compensatory responses, symptoms, and therapy.

C. The clinical presentation, laboratory studies, and management will be arbitrarily divided into three categories: (a) mild, (b) moderate, and (c) severe; although the disorder is actually a continuous spectrum.

3. *Etiology*

A. Congenital bicuspid valve

(1) The most common cause of aortic stenosis is a congenital bicuspid formation of the valve leaflets.

(2) This may be severe at birth and cause serious difficulty during infancy or childhood, but more commonly the stenosis is mild in infancy and childhood.

(3) With the passage of time, however, the obstruction tends to increase so that moderate stenosis is present during the third and fourth decade of life and severe stenosis develops during the fifth decade or later.

(4) This slow increase in severity of stenosis is due to progressive sclerosis, thickening, and eventually calcification of the valve, so that there is a progressive reduction in the orifice.

(5) This disorder is seen about twice as frequently in men as in women.

B. Aortic stenosis in the aged

(1) Occasionally even the leaflets

of a normal tricuspid aortic valve may become rigid and cause stenosis.

(2) This develops in the eighth and ninth decades of life and is only rarely severe.

C. Rheumatic fever:

(1) Practically the only other cause of aortic stenosis is rheumatic fever.

(2) With this process, the severity of the stenosis also tends to progress slowly.

(3) Eventually the obstructed valve is indistinguishable from the end-stage of the congenitally abnormal valve.

4. *Pathophysiology*

Obstruction to left ventricular outflow requires the development of higher left ventricular pressure in order to maintain a normal systemic arterial pressure. The difference between the left ventricular and aortic systolic pressure is referred to as the aortic valve gradient. High left ventricular pressures are accompanied by hypertrophy of the left ventricular mass. In order to generate the higher left ventricular systolic pressures, the end-diastolic pressure is elevated.

A. If unrelieved, severe aortic stenosis may lead to eventual ventricular decompensation with ventricular dilatation and markedly elevated diastolic pressures.

B. Such a state is associated with elevated left atrial and pulmonary venous pressures and the development of pulmonary congestion.

C. The high pressures developed by the left ventricle are associated with increased needs of oxygen by the heart muscle cells themselves.

D. This increased need may play a role in the angina pectoris syndrome, which may develop with or without associated coronary artery disease.

E. The scarring and calcification of the aortic leaflets will eventually extend to the valve ring and even into the surrounding heart tissue.

F. Involvement of the adjacent portions of the cardiac conducting system is of particular importance.

5. *Symptoms*

A. There are no symptoms during most of the years when aortic stenosis is mild or moderate, and the patient may be totally unaware that he has a cardiac disorder.

B. When the obstruction becomes severe, however, the patient may develop (1) syncope; (2) angina pectoris of effort; (3) congestive heart failure; or (4) a combination of any or all of these.

C. There is nothing specific about any of these presentations, and it is necessary to consider aortic stenosis whenever any of these symptoms develop.

D. It is also necessary to consider other possible causes of these symptoms in the patient with the signs of aortic stenosis. For instance, coronary heart disease may be the cause of the symptoms and the aortic stenosis is only mild and incidental.

E. A-V block is frequently seen with calcific aortic stenosis and may be the cause of syncope in these patients.

6. *Signs*

The signs of aortic stenosis vary according to the severity of obstruction.

A. Mild aortic stenosis

(1) With mild aortic stenosis, as in childhood and adolescence, the only finding may be a loud ejection click heard at the apex and a short, early systolic murmur.

(2) The aortic second sound is usually loud and is best heard in the aortic area.

B. Moderate aortic stenosis

(1) As moderate obstruction develops, the murmur becomes louder and longer.

(2) It is loudest at the aortic area, but may be transmitted to the supraclavicular fossa, carotid vessels, and apex of the heart.

(3) The murmur is harsh but ends well before the aortic second sound, which is well maintained.

(4) The ejection click is also maintained.

(5) By this time the obstruction is beginning to significantly alter the character of the arterial pulse.

(6) There is usually a shudder on the upstroke and the upstroke is slightly prolonged.

(7) The apex impulse may still be normal but more often is slightly sustained and a presystolic shoulder (''a'' wave) may be felt before the major systolic impulse.

C. Severe aortic stenosis

(1) With the passage of time, the stenosis becomes severe and the valve is thickened and heavily calcified.

(2) The ejection sound is no longer present and the aortic second sound is markedly diminished or absent.

(3) The murmur may be faint to very loud but will always be long and occupy almost all of systole.

(4) At the aortic area the murmur is usually harsh but may contain some musical components.

(5) The murmur may be faint in a patient with an increased anterior-posterior chest diameter and/or a reduced cardiac output.

(6) In older men with a barrel chest and severe distress due to heart failure, the murmur may be faint and even overlooked.

(7) In these patients, it is important to listen for an aortic murmur in the suprasternal notch and also to look for the other signs of aortic stenosis outlined below.

(8) The murmur of aortic stenosis is usually well transmitted to the apex of the heart, where it may have a pure or musical quality.

(9) Since the murmur sounds so different at the base and the apex, it is not surprising that the patient is often

mistakenly felt to have both aortic stenosis and mitral regurgitation.

(10) A fourth heart sound is heard preceding the first heart sound at the apex, but a gallop cadence may be difficult to discern.

(11) It is not unusual to hear a decrescendo diastolic blow of aortic regurgitation along the left sternal border in the patient with severe aortic stenosis. This does not represent significant regurgitation.

(12) With severe aortic stenosis the carotid pulse is strikingly abnormal, and this is one of the most important clinical findings, since very few other things cause the abnormality.

(13) The abnormal quality is characterized by a very slow and long upstroke, with or without a faint shudder, and by an overall small quality to the pulse. This pulse character is best appreciated over the carotid vessels and may not be present in the brachial, radial, or femoral pulses.

(14) The apical impulse is also quite characteristic in severe aortic stenosis. It is strong and sustained for all of systole and has a prominent presystolic component ("a" wave). This type of apex is not specific for aortic stenosis, but the demonstration of a normal apical impulse would be strong evidence against severe aortic stenosis.

7. *Laboratory findings*
    A. *Electrocardiography*
    (1) The electrocardiogram (ECG) may be normal at any stage in the course of aortic stenosis.

(2) With severe aortic stenosis, the ECG is usually abnormal and may show varying signs of left ventricular hypertrophy from mere reduction in amplitude of the T waves in leads I, aVL, V_5 and V_6 to the full-blown picture of left ventricular hypertrophy.

(3) Left anterior hemiblock and left bundle branch block are commonly seen.

(4) Complete A-V block may develop in calcific aortic stenosis.
    B. *Chest x-ray*
    (1) The cardiac thoracic ratio on the chest roentgenogram is often normal, even in severe aortic stenosis.

(2) The apical contour, however, is abnormal.

(3) There is often prominence of the ascending aorta and calcium in the area of the aortic valve.

(4) Calcium in the area of the aortic valve can practically always be seen when the stenosis is severe, if looked for with screen-intensified fluoroscopy.
    C. *Phonocardiography*
    Phonocardiography can confirm the auscultatory features outlined above, and graphic recordings dramatically display the abnormalities of the carotid pulse and apex impulse.
    D. *Echocardiography*
    (1) Echocardiography is most useful in the evaluation of the patient with a basal systolic murmur in whom aortic stenosis is being considered and/or in whom the severity of the disease is uncertain.

(2) When a good recording can be obtained, clear distinction can be made between all stages of the disorder: namely, a normal valve appears different from a bicuspid, mildly obstructed valve, and that appears different from a thickened, sclerotic, moderately obstructed valve, and finally that appears different from a heavily calcified, severely obstructed valve.
    E. *Cardiac catheterization and angiography*
    (1) In the adult it is usually possible to establish with reasonable certainty the degree of stenosis by clinical and noninvasive laboratory studies; heart catheterization is not usually needed.

(2) If the stenosis is felt to be severe, and the patient is being considered for surgery, however, it may be important to study the patient with heart

catheterization and angiography to establish the severity of the obstruction and to estimate possible associated disease, such as obstructed coronary arteries, primary disease of the myocardium, and other valve disease.

(3) Pressures recorded in the left ventricle are usually 50 to 100 mm. Hg higher than in the aorta during systolic (systolic gradient) in severe stenosis.

(4) Also during end-diastole there is abnormal elevation of pressures in the left ventricle.

(5) In the child or young adult, mild aortic stenosis can usually be identified, but it may be difficult to distinguish moderate from severe aortic stenosis by any method other than heart catheterization.

8. *Differential diagnosis*

A. *Supravalvular aortic stenosis*

(1) This is rare and associated with mental retardation and abnormal facies.

(2) The stenosis is due to a constriction at the beginning of the aorta just above the sinuses of Valsalva.

B. *Membranous subvalvular aortic stenosis*

(1) It is uncommon, usually severe, and thus usually causes difficulty in childhood.

(2) An ejection click is not present despite a young age.

(3) Heart catheterization and angiography are needed to distinguish this lesion from moderate or severe aortic valve stenosis in the child or young adult.

C. *Hypertrophic cardiomyopathy (often referred to as idiopathic hypertrophic subaortic stenosis)*

(1) This is a commonly inherited disorder of left ventricular muscle of unknown etiology, which may have symptoms similar to those of valvular aortic stenosis.

(2) Though the disorders share some clinical signs, there are easy ways to distinguish the two.

(a) In hypertrophic cardiomyopathy, ejection from the left ventricle is rapid and results in a sharp rising, often bifid carotid pulse that is quite distinct from the small, slow rising pulse of valvular aortic stenosis.

(b) The murmur of hypertrophic cardiomyopathy is loudest along the left sternal edge or apex and poorly heard in the aortic area and carotid vessels.

(c) Though the ECG and chest roentgenogram may be similar in the two disorders, the echocardiogram is quite different and is helpful in distinguishing the two. For more detailed discussion of this disorder, see Chapter 9.

D. *Mitral regurgitation*

(1) Occasionally the murmur of mitral regurgitation can be referred to the base of the heart and even be louder there than at the apex.

(2) For some reason, this murmur may increase in intensity in mid-systole and truly simulate the murmur of aortic stenosis.

(3) With severe mitral regurgitation, the cardiac output may be low and the carotid pulse small, and thus the difficulty continues.

(4) Since this peculiar transmission of a mitral regurgitant murmur is seen when this disorder develops abruptly (ruptured chordae tendineae or head of a papillary muscle) then it is not uncommon for the left atrium to be of normal size on ECG, chest roentgenogram, and echocardiography, and for sinus rhythm to be maintained.

9. *Treatment*

A. *Medical management*

(1) An isolated bicuspid aortic valve or stenosis due to rheumatic fever with little obstruction requires no specific treatment.

(2) However, these patients are at increased risk of developing bacterial endocarditis and should be carefully instructed in the appropriate use of an-

tibiotics before any dental procedures, certain operations, or manipulation of infected skin lesions. (See Chap. 7 for presently recommended antibiotic programs.)

B. *Surgical management*

(1) Symptomatic and severe aortic stenosis

(a) When the severity of the aortic stenosis increases so that symptoms develop, then surgical replacement of the diseased valve with a prosthesis is indicated.

(b) Though not a true emergency, there is some urgency about completing the evaluation and surgery, since the frequency with which further difficulty, or sudden death, develops in the next 1 to 36 months is high.

(c) Until the evaluation and surgery can be completed, the patient may need to restrict his activities.

(d) Digitalis and diuretics as well as salt restriction are indicated in those patients with congestive heart failure.

(2) Asymptomatic patients with severe aortic stenosis

(a) There are asymptomatic patients with severe aortic stenosis in whom elective surgery is appropriate.

(b) In the older age group with calcific aortic stenosis, those patients with large pressure gradients between the left ventricle and aorta should undergo surgical replacement of the valve.

(c) Presumably the cardiac output is normal in these patients, in which case a gradient of 80 mm. Hg or greater should be considered an indication for surgery.

(d) The rate at which difficulty will develop in these patients is sufficient to justify surgical intervention.

(e) In those asymptomatic patients with a normal cardiac output and with gradients between 50 and 80 mm. Hg, the decision is more controversial.

(f) When a gradient below 50 mm. Hg is found, a conservative program should be followed. This should include periodic re-evaluation with the appropriate clinical and noninvasive studies.

(g) The asymptomatic child or young adult with severe stenosis may obtain adequate relief of the stenosis by commissurotomy of the valve. This is especially important to complete if there are signs of left ventricular hypertrophy with S-T segment and T wave changes on the ECG (systolic overloading pattern).

10. *Prognosis*

A. With mild aortic stenosis, the prognosis is good because the severity of the stenosis progresses slowly.

B. The patient may remain active and free of symptoms for 10 to 50 years.

C. The rate of progression is quite variable, and periodic re-evaluation is a most important part of the care.

D. As already indicated, the prognosis is quite poor once symptoms have developed.

E. Almost all patients will continue to have symptoms and most will die within three years.

The prognosis after successful valve replacement is discussed in Chapter 30.

AORTIC REGURGITATION

1. *Definition*

Regurgitation of blood from the aorta to the left ventricle does not occur in the normal situation. Regurgitation occurs most commonly from damage to the valve leaflets but also may result from dilatation of the aortic valve ring, damage to the ascending aorta, and, rarely, by communications between the aorta and left ventricle.

2. *General features*

In contrast to aortic stenosis, there are many causes of aortic regurgitation (the previously most common etiologies, rheumatic fever and syphilis, are now overshadowed by the many other causes). The clinical signs, prognosis, and management of aortic regurgitation vary enormously in the different degrees of severity: mild, moderate, or severe. This must be kept in mind in all of the following discussions.

3. *Etiology*

There are many causes of regurgitation of blood from the aorta to the left ventricle.

A. Syphilitic aortitis used to be common but now is rare.

B. Rheumatic involvement of the aortic valve is also less commonly seen.

C. A congenital bicuspid valve may occasionally present with severe regurgitation.

D. Cystic medial necrosis of the aorta may be seen in patients with other features of the Marfan syndrome, but more commonly it is the only apparent feature of the syndrome. Cystic medial necrosis is one of the causes of sudden severe aortic regurgitation.

E. Other causes include:

(1) Bacterial endocarditis

(2) Dissecting hematoma or aneurysm of the aorta

(3) Ruptured sinus of Valsalva

(4) Relapsing polychondritis

(5) Ankylosing spondylitis

F. Minor degrees of aortic regurgitation are seen in patients with:

(1) Calcific aortic stenosis

(2) Chronic systemic hypertension

(3) A variety of systemic inflammatory diseases.

4. *Pathophysiology*

A. In order to maintain adequate peripheral organ perfusion, it is necessary for the left ventricle to eject the usual stroke volume plus the volume that regurgitates from the aorta into the left ventricle.

B. The ventricular stroke volume can be more than 2 times greater than normal.

C. This results in dilatation and hypertrophy of the left ventricle which maintains the circulatory state until the left ventricle fails.

D. Because of the combination of peripheral vasodilatation and the leak into the ventricle in diastole, the diastolic blood pressure is low and the systolic pressure is high.

5. *Symptoms and signs*

A. *Severe aortic regurgitation*

(1) The most common symptomatic presentation of severe aortic regurgitation is pulmonary congestion.

(2) While this may be gradual in onset, it could be abrupt and may result in great distress. This distress is due to left ventricular failure and results in not only pulmonary edema but also inadequate cerebral and other peripheral organ perfusion.

(3) The patient may be stuporous, confused, or even combative.

(4) In these circumstances, aortic regurgitation may be difficult to recognize.

(5) The murmur of aortic regurgitation may be soft and short.

(6) The peripheral signs of aortic regurgitation may be absent. The loss of the peripheral signs is due to the reduction in the speed of left ventricular ejection, replacement of the usual peripheral vasodilation by vasoconstriction, and a high left ventricular diastolic pressure.

(7) This patient may have a blood pressure of 100/40, or even 90/50, a small volume peripheral pulse, and a short aortic diastolic murmur that is very difficult to hear.

(8) Recognition of this clinical presentation is crucial, since valve surgery is needed urgently.

B. *Mild aortic regurgitation*

(1) In mild aortic regurgitation, the patient is asymptomatic and the cardiovascular examination normal except

for the decrescendo diastolic murmur, which is loudest along the left sternal border (Erb's point).

(2) With mild or moderate aortic regurgitation, the patient may remain asymptomatic for many years.

C. *Moderate to severe aortic regurgitation*

(1) More severe regurgitation may cause the patient to have symptoms of effort dyspnea and excessive sweating.

(2) These patients present the "classical" signs of aortic regurgitation.

(3) The skin is warm, flushed, and damp with visible arterial pulsations striking in the neck.

(4) To palpation, the pulse is bounding with a rapid rise and fall and may have a double or bisferiens quality.

(5) There may be head bobbing, capillary pulsations, pistol shots over the arteries, to-and-fro murmurs over peripheral arteries when the stethoscope is applied with pressure (Duroziez' sign).

(6) The arterial pulse pressure is wide with elevation of the systolic and reduction of the diastolic pressures.

D. *Apical impulse*

(1) The character of the apical impulse is most important in quantitating the severity of aortic regurgitation.

(2) With mild regurgitation, the apical impulse is normal but, as the severity increases, the impulses become forceful and more sustained, larger, and displaced downward and outward.

(3) With the development of left ventricular failure, a diastolic filling impulse may be felt.

E. *Heart murmurs*

(1) The typical decrescendo diastolic blow of aortic regurgitation is quite characteristic and almost diagnostic of the disorder.

(2) The aortic murmur is usually heard best along the left lower sternal border.

(3) The murmur may be louder along the right lower sternal border than

the left in disorders associated with marked dilatation of the root of the aorta, such as cystic medial necrosis or syphilis, whereas the murmur is practically always louder to the left in rheumatic disease of the aortic valve.

(4) With very mild regurgitation, the murmur may be short but this may also be true with gross regurgitation and severe left ventricular failure.

(5) With moderate or severe regurgitation, the murmur is long and extends throughout diastole.

(6) Whenever there is significant regurgitation, an aortic systolic murmur will be present.

(7) This murmur occupies only the early part of systole but may be harsh and loud.

(8) A diastolic rumble with or without a presystolic murmur (Austin Flint murmur) may be heard at the apex in a patient with severe aortic regurgitation, especially when ventricular failure develops.

F. *Other auscultatory findings*

(1) The first sound may be followed by a prominent ejection click.

(2) Diminished intensity of the first sound occurs with the development of left ventricular failure.

(3) A fourth heart sound gallop is unusual in the absence of other disease.

(4) But, a third sound gallop is common even in the absence of congestive heart failure.

6. *Laboratory studies*

A. *Chest x-ray*

(1) The chest roentgenograph may show enlargement of the left ventricle.

(2) A cardiothoracic ratio of greater than 60 per cent is seen with severe or gross aortic regurgitation.

(3) Dilatation of the ascending aorta is seen in syphilis, cystic medial necrosis, Marfan syndrome, relapsing polychondritis, but usually not with rheumatic disease.

(4) Huge dilatation of the aortic

root and aortic ring can be hidden within the cardiac silhouette in patients with cystic medial necrosis.

B. *Electrocardiography*

(1) Left ventricular hypertrophy of diastolic overloading pattern and P wave abnormalities are seen on the electrocardiogram when the regurgitation is severe.

(2) Atrial fibrillation is very rare in the absence of associated mitral disease.

C. *Echocardiography*

(1) The echocardiogram may be helpful in some patients by demonstrating enlargement of the aortic root, calcification or vegetation on the aortic leaflets, or bicuspid valve configuration.

(2) The echocardiogram is useful in the examination of left ventricular function and evaluation of the presence or absence of associated mitral stenosis.

D. *Cardiac catheterization and angiography*

(1) Cardiac catheterization and angiography are not needed to establish the diagnosis of aortic regurgitation, since the clinical examination and noninvasive studies are specific enough.

(2) However, when considering surgical intervention, contrast aortography is valuable in delineating the various pathological processes of the aortic root.

7. *Differential diagnosis*

A. The decrescendo diastolic murmur of aortic regurgitation may be simulated by pulmonary regurgitation in a patient with pulmonary hypertension, but associated findings are quite different in the two situations.

B. Rupture of a sinus of Valsalva aneurysm into the right side of the heart may simulate aortic regurgitation. However, the management of the two is not dissimilar, and aortography is important in establishing the correct diagnosis.

C. Peripheral signs of the arterial system similar to aortic regurgitation may be seen in a variety of disorders with a very low peripheral arterial resistance, such as:

(1) Traumatic arteriovenous fistulae

(2) Patent ductus arteriosus

(3) Thyrotoxicosis

(4) High fevers

8. *Complications*

A. With profound heart failure, there is inadequate systemic circulation and impairment of the function of end organs, especially the brain and kidneys.

B. Even the patient with mild aortic regurgitation is at increased risk of developing infective endocarditis.

9. *Management*

A. *Asymptomatic aortic regurgitation*

(1) The patient with mild or even moderate aortic regurgitation should be advised to lead an entirely normal life, but also should be urged to assume the responsibility of obtaining prophylactic antibiotics before dental and operative procedures and to arrange for periodic cardiac reevaluation.

(2) When there is evidence of cardiac enlargement and moderately severe or severe aortic regurgitation but no symptoms, many authorities would recommend the introduction of a digitalis preparation daily.

(3) These patients should be instructed to avoid heavy or exhausting physical activities.

(4) They should not participate in such activities as tennis or basketball; nor should their occupations require heavy exertion.

B. *Symptomatic aortic regurgitation*

(1) With the development of symptoms that are related to left ventricular failure, serious consideration for surgical replacement of the aortic valve is indicated.

(2) If the aortic regurgitation and heart failure have developed abruptly, it may be important to consider surgery on an emergency basis.

(3) These patients can be difficult to identify but astute observations can identify those who require immediate surgery.

C. *Asymptomatic but severe aortic regurgitation*

(1) Studies have shown that there are patients who are asymptomatic with severe aortic regurgitation who can be predicted to develop symptoms or to die within a short period of time.

(2) Thus, it is reasonable to consider the surgical management of these patients, once identified, even in the absence of symptoms.

(3) The combination of a pulse pressure of greater than 100 mm. Hg, left ventricular hypertrophy with S-T segment and T wave abnormalities on the electrocardiogram, and cardiomegaly on a chest roentgenograph (CT ratio rapidly increasing or greater than 60%) has been reported to identify such a group of patients with rheumatic aortic regurgitation and possibly can be applied to the general group.

(4) In those patients with disease of the ascending aorta, it may be necessary to replace that structure as well as the valve.

10. *Prognosis*

A. The long period of stability of the patient with mild or moderate aortic regurgitation should be emphasized.

B. Intervention at this stage is ill-advised unless it is dictated by the underlying disorder, such as dissecting hematoma of the aorta or incurable infective endocarditis.

C. Once severe aortic regurgitation develops and left ventricular hypertrophy is present on physical examination, chest x-ray, and electrocardiography, it is probable that symptoms of left ventricular failure will develop in the near future.

D. If surgery is to be deferred, it is wise to follow that patient with frequent reviews.

E. The prognosis with medical management once symptoms have developed is poor; progressive impairment of left ventricular failure can be expected and sudden death is not rare.

F. The prognosis after surgery is dependent on the degree and length of previous ventricular damage.

G. The ventricle may return to normal if the regurgitation developed abruptly and surgery was performed early, but this is unlikely if cardiomegaly has been present for a long period.

MITRAL STENOSIS

1. *Definition*

Obstruction to flow across the mitral orifice may be caused by adhesions between the two mitral leaflets, loss of mobility of the leaflets, and possibly fibrosis and rigidity of the chordae tendineae and papillary muscles.

2. *Etiology*

A. Valvulitis associated with one of the rheumatic fever syndromes is thought to be the cause of mitral stenosis in essentially all patients with this disorder.

B. A history of rheumatic fever is obtained in only about half of the patients with mitral stenosis.

C. The interval between the acute rheumatic fever and detection of mitral stenosis is variable; it may be as short as three years, but more commonly is 15 to 25 years.

D. Women are affected twice as commonly as men.

E. Congenital stenosis of the mitral valve is extremely rare.

3. *Pathophysiology*

A. Acute valvulitis causes little or no hemodynamic abnormalities.

B. However, with the passage of time the acute inflammatory process heals by scarring and eventually calcification. This results in fusion of the commissures, rigidity of the valve leaflets, and thickening and matting of the chordae tendineae. This process leads to obstruction of flow from the left atrium to the left ventricle.

C. Obstruction to flow across the mitral valve results in an elevation of the left atrial pressure, which is transmitted to the pulmonary veins and capillaries. This causes transudation of fluid into the perivascular and perialveolar area, making the lungs stiff. Further pressure rises may result in fluid accumulation in the alveoli or pulmonary edema. By necessity, elevation of the pulmonary venous pressure is associated with a rise in the pressure in the pulmonary artery and right ventricle. Sometimes spasm develops in the pulmonary arterioles and there is an inappropriate rise in the pulmonary artery and right ventricular pressures. This is especially likely to occur in the young female with significant mitral stenosis.

D. In addition to the pressure changes, mitral valve obstruction limits the forward flow of blood. This causes reduced exercise tolerance and stamina, but usually this occurs so slowly that the patient reduces his pace over the years and may not recognize his or her limitations.

E. The elevation of the pulmonary vascular resistance may be followed by right ventricular failure. Right ventricular failure leads to right atrial hypertension, which in combination with fluid retention due to reduced renal perfusion leads to systemic congestion.

4. *Symptoms*

A. Easy fatigue and decreased exercise tolerance may be present for many years without the patient's recognizing that he is disabled.

B. Dyspnea may be the first symptom noticed by the patient, but even this may be ignored until episodes of nocturnal dyspnea and orthopnea develop.

C. Occasionally the effort dyspnea may become less troublesome and the patient finally presents with the signs and symptoms of right ventricular failure.

5. *Signs*

A. Precordial palpation: the precordial examination is distinctive.

(1) The apical impulse is of very short duration and tapping in quality.

(2) A sustained apical impulse would negate the possibility of pure mitral stenosis and would suggest associated aortic valve or left ventricular muscle disease.

(3) Sometimes the opening snap and diastolic rumble can be palpated.

(4) When the pulmonary artery pressure is elevated, a tap at the end of systole may be felt high on the left sternal border and a parasternal heave along the lower sternal border.

B. Auscultation remains the principal method of detecting mitral stenosis.

(1) The diastolic rumble at the apex is almost diagnostic in itself.

(2) This is especially true if there is presystolic increase in pitch and intensity of the rumble and if the first sound is loud and an opening snap detected.

(3) The murmurs are increased in intensity during the first several cardiac cycles after the patient rolls onto his left side or after mild exercise.

(4) The auscultatory features may be atypical and difficult to hear.

(5) When the diseased mitral valves are very thickened, rigid, and partially calcified the first sound diminishes and may be soft. In this setting, the opening snap is also reduced or absent. Also, in this setting, the murmurs may be diminished in intensity and very difficult to hear.

6. *Laboratory studies*

A. *Electrocardiography*

(1) The electrocardiogram may be normal.

(2) It may show notched and broad P waves in leads I, II, III and aVF, and a biphasic P wave with a prominent negative component in lead V_1.

(3) With pulmonary hypertension, there may be signs of right ventricular hypertrophy.

(4) Atrial fibrillation (often coarse fibrillation waves) is common.

B. *Chest x-ray*

The chest roentgenograph has the following features:

(1) Prominence of the upper lobe vasculature

(2) Straightening of the left heart border due to enlargement of the left atrial appendage

(3) A double density of an enlarged left atrium

(4) Subtle enlargement of the left atrium can be best detected in the lateral or right anterior oblique view with barium in the esophagus.

(5) Right ventricular enlargement

(6) Potentially all the signs of pulmonary congestion and edema

C. *Echocardiography* is extremely valuable in the evaluation of the stenotic mitral valve.

(1) First, in a desperately ill patient, echocardiographic demonstration of normal mitral motion excludes mitral stenosis as a cause for the patient's distress.

(2) Second, when mitral stenosis is present, the echocardiogram can demonstrate enlargement of the left atrium, indicate rigidity and calcification of the valve, and grossly estimate the severity of the obstruction.

D. *Cardiac catheterization and angiography*

Cardiac catheterization and angiography is needed only in confusing cases and to evaluate other valvular function and ventricular function.

7. *Diagnosis*

A. In pure mitral stenosis, the diagnosis is not difficult and is made by auscultation.

B. When there is multiple valve disease, the severity of the mitral stenosis may be more difficult to determine.

C. The echocardiogram provides a good estimation of degree of obstruction.

D. Cardiac catheterization may be necessary in some complex cases.

E. In any patient with pulmonary hypertension, mitral stenosis should be carefully considered and either excluded or established.

F. Most cases of pulmonary hypertension are not correctable, but relief of mitral stenosis can dramatically reduce the pulmonary artery pressure.

8. *Differential diagnosis*

A. *Left atrial myxoma (see also Chap. 11)*

(1) A left atrial myxoma may cause symptoms very similar to mitral stenosis and also have similar clinical signs so that even the best observer may be fooled.

(2) The apical diastolic rumble is similar in nature and the "tumor plop," an early diastolic sound, can be easily mistaken for an opening snap.

(3) Carefully performed echocardiography can usually distinguish the two, but angiography may be necessary.

(4) If a left atrial myxoma is suspected, transseptal catheterization should not be performed and the left atrium must be visualized on films taken late after injection of the contrast material into the pulmonary artery.

(5) If a myxoma is demonstrated, surgical removal should be completed promptly.

B. *Aortic regurgitation*

(1) The Austin Flint murmur of severe aortic regurgitation may simulate the murmur of associated mitral stenosis.

(2) Marked left ventricular hypertrophy, a diminished first sound, and absent opening snap favor the Austin Flint mechanism as a cause of the murmur.

(3) Echocardiography is helpful in distinguishing these two possibilities.

C. *Atrial septal defect*

(1) A diastolic rumble may be heard in the mid precordium in a patient with a large left to right shunt through an

atrial septal defect, due to torrential flow across the tricuspid valve.

(2) The features on the chest roentgenogram and echocardiogram allow distinction of these two disorders.

9. *Complications*

A. *Atrial fibrillation*

(1) Atrial fibrillation develops in many patients with significant mitral stenosis.

(2) The onset of atrial fibrillation with a rapid ventricular rate may precipitate symptoms for the first time.

(3) These symptoms may disappear after the rate is slowed by digitalis.

B. *Hemoptysis* is not uncommon and occasionally can be large in quantity.

C. *Systemic emboli*

(1) Systemic emboli may occur in any patient with mitral stenosis but is especially likely if atrial fibrillation is also present.

(2) The clinical presentation of the systemic embolus depends entirely upon the end organ involved.

(3) The most common sites are the bifurcation of the aorta and the femoral, cerebral, renal, and mesenteric arteries.

10. *Management*

A. *Digitalization*

Though digitalis does not help in the care of the patient with isolated mitral stenosis and sinus rhythm, this drug is the mainstay of management once atrial fibrillation develops.

B. *Surgical approach*

(1) The development of symptoms due to mitral stenosis signifies the need for consideration of surgical relief of the stenosis.

(2) Mitral commissurotomy continues to provide excellent relief of symptoms for a period of many years in properly selected patients.

(3) The final decision of whether a commissurotomy will adequately relieve the stenosis without producing severe regurgitation, will have to be made at the time of surgery.

(4) The clues that a commissurotomy may be adequate include a loud, sharp first heart sound and opening snap, absence of calcium on fluoroscopy, and demonstration of a thin, mobile valve on the echocardiogram and angiogram.

(5) If it is estimated that the diseased mitral valve will have to be replaced, it is wise to maintain medical management as long as the patient is only minimally limited. This includes control of the ventricular rate in the patient with atrial fibrillation, anticoagulation in the patient who has had a systemic embolus, and periodic reexamination.

(6) Replacement of the valve with a prosthesis does relieve the stenosis but life-long anticoagulation is required, and there are other late postoperative complications of any prosthetic valve.

C. *Conversion of atrial fibrillation*

(1) Conversion of atrial fibrillation to normal sinus rhythm can sometimes be maintained, especially if the patient can be treated with quinidine.

(2) Also the patient is usually maintained on digitalis to provide some atrioventricular block in case atrial fibrillation recurs.

(3) To reduce the risk of systemic embolization, the patient should be given anticoagulants for several weeks prior to the attempted conversion.

(4) If valve surgery is planned for the patient, it is wise to postpone the conversion attempt until after surgery.

D. *Anticoagulation*

(1) When a systemic embolus complicates the course of mitral stenosis, there is good reason to maintain the patient on anticoagulation chronically to reduce the risk of recurrence.

(2) Some authorities recommend chronic anticoagulation in all patients with mitral valve disease and persistent atrial fibrillation.

11. *Prognosis*

A. Under most circumstances, the degree of stenosis and the disability are very slowly progressive over a period of years.

B. The exceptions to this may go in either direction.

C. The course may be absolutely stable for years and years with the patient remaining asymptomatic into the sixth and seventh decades.

D. On the other hand, the process may progress rapidly and cause severe disability in young adulthood, especially in the female.

E. The slow appearance of symptoms may be abruptly altered by the development of atrial fibrillation.

F. Following a successful commissurotomy, the patient can usually return to a fully active life.

G. Because of the possibility of restenosis, the patient must be reevaluated periodically. This reevaluation might include only a history and physical examination, but chest roentgenographs, electrocardiographs, and echocardiograph may be obtained as indicated.

The care of the patient with a prosthesis in the mitral area is discussed in Chapter 30.

MITRAL REGURGITATION

1. *Definition*

To understand the multiple etiologies of mitral regurgitation, it is important to be familiar with the complex anatomy of the mitral apparatus.

A. Competence depends on the following:

(1) Integrity of the valve leaflets

(2) Proper size and function of the annulus

(3) Integrity of all of the chordae tendineae

(4) Integrity and proper contraction of the papillary muscles

(5) Proper function of the left ventricular muscle

B. Damage to any of these structures may lead to regurgitation of blood from the left ventricle to the left atrium.

2. *Etiology*

A. *Rheumatic fever*

(1) Rheumatic fever causes an acute valvulitis, which may lead to scarring and retraction of the leaflets, although stenosis is more common.

(2) Infective endocarditis may damage the leaflets, causing scarring, clefts, and perforations.

(3) Congenital clefts of the leaflets occur with or without other associated congenital cardiac disorders.

B. *Mitral valve prolapse syndrome (see Chap. 6)*

(1) One of the most common causes of mitral regurgitation is prolapse of the mitral leaflets into the left atrium during systole.

(2) The primary abnormality that allows this prolapse remains uncertain.

(3) Proposed causes of such prolapse include

(a) Dilatation of the mitral valve annulus

(b) Primary mucoid degeneration of the mitral valve

(c) Excessive length of the chordae tendineae

(d) Impaired contraction of the papillary muscles or the portion of the left ventricle from which the papillary muscles arise.

(4) The severity of the mitral regurgitation due to mitral valve prolapse varies from minimal to gross.

C. *Chordae tendineae rupture and papillary muscle dysfunction or rupture*

(1) Chordae tendineae may rupture spontaneously or secondary to infective endocarditis or nonpenetrating chest trauma.

(2) When an entire papillary muscle ruptures, usually due to acute infarction, severe pulmonary congestion and

shock develop abruptly and lead to death shortly.

(3) On the other hand, rupture of one portion of a papillary muscle causes severe mitral regurgitation, but the patient may survive if adequate ventricular function remains.

(4) Mitral regurgitation due to ischemia or scarring of the papillary muscle is most commonly mild and related to slight misfit of the leaflets.

(5) On the other hand, occasionally a patient develops severe mitral regurgitation during episodes of angina pectoris presumably due to ischemia of a papillary muscle.

D. *Left ventricular dilatation*

(1) When the left ventricle is dilated due to any cause, the unique relationship of the papillary muscles, chordae tendineae, and mitral leaflets is distorted, and mitral regurgitation develops.

(2) If the ventricular dilatation can be reversed, then the mitral regurgitation of this cause can be eliminated.

(3) Dilatation of the mitral valve annulus out of proportion to overall enlargement of the left ventricle does not occur in the absence of structural disorder of the annular tissue as seen in the Marfan syndrome or prolapsed mitral valve syndrome.

3. *Pathophysiology*

A. The abrupt development of severe mitral regurgitation results in marked elevation of left atrial and pulmonary venous pressure and thus pulmonary congestion. The "v" wave in the left atrium may be as high as 60 to 70 mm. Hg.

B. Abrupt, severe mitral regurgitation may be intermittent when it is due to papillary muscle ischemia producing a dramatic clinical picture of episodes of great distress separated by periods of a relatively normal circulatory status and few or no signs of significant mitral regurgitation.

C. Chronic mitral regurgitation, especially of rheumatic origin, leads to marked dilatation of the left atrium. This allows a dampening of the pressure effects so that significant regurgitation can be present for years with only mild elevation of the left atrial and pulmonary venous pressures. However, steady progression can be expected when the regurgitation is significant, since ventricular enlargement occurs and this in turn tends to increase the mitral regurgitation.

D. Minimal or mild mitral regurgitation can be, and usually is, a remarkably stable state and can be present for a lifetime with no progression unless complicated by rupture of chordae tendineae or infective endocarditis.

4. *Symptoms*

A. The symptoms of mitral regurgitation are due to pulmonary congestion and low cardiac output.

B. Palpitation due to premature contractions or atrial fibrillation may develop.

C. Systemic emboli, though less common than in mitral stenosis, do occur, especially with atrial fibrillation and heart failure, and complicate the clinical picture.

D. Peculiar left inframammary pain may plague patients with prolapse of the mitral valve.

5. *Signs*

A. Palpation

(1) When mitral regurgitation is mild to moderate, the apical impulse is normal.

(2) With more severe regurgitation, the impulse is rather large, laterally placed, and sustained.

(3) With gross regurgitation, there may be a late systolic accentuation of the impulse and an early diastolic impulse coinciding with the third heart sound.

(4) The presence of pulmonary hypertension is associated with a para-

sternal heave, though such a heave may be felt with only moderate elevation of pulmonary artery pressure due to systolic expansion of the small left atrium pushing the right ventricle forward.

B. *Auscultation*

(1) Apical systolic murmur

(a) The classical sign of mitral regurgitation is the systolic murmur at the apex of the heart.

(b) The typical systolic murmur is holosystolic, plateau in intensity and pitch, and blowing in quality.

(c) This murmur is usually transmitted loudly to the left axilla and left back.

(d) Occasionally, the murmur may be transmitted to the upper sternal areas and even the neck vessels, which may cause confusion about the origin of the murmur.

(2) In rheumatic disease, the first heart sound is usually diminished, but may be normal or even increased in regurgitation of other etiologies.

(3) A third heart sound is characteristic of significant regurgitation and may be followed by a low pitched mid-diastolic murmur.

(4) A fourth heart sound is unusual unless the regurgitation is abrupt in development.

(5) An opening snap is occasionally heard even in the absence of mitral stenosis.

(6) Mitral valve prolapse syndrome

(a) The signs of mitral valve prolapse are quite variable from individual to individual and even from time to time in the same individual.

(b) A very high-pitched click, sounding like the diaphragm of the stethoscope crackling on the skin, may be the only auscultatory finding.

(c) There may be one or more of these clicks and the timing may extend from just after the first sound to just before the second sound.

(d) Sometimes a crescendo late systolic murmur follows the click or the murmur may be present without clicks.

(e) This late systolic murmur may also assume a whooping quality at times.

(f) The murmur of more severe regurgitation associated with mitral valve prolapse may be pansystolic, but is usually not plateau in intensity or pitch, peaking either in mid or late systole.

(7) Rarely, a patient with very gross mitral regurgitation will have no apical murmur or only an unimpressive soft murmur. This is most frequently seen in patients with gross regurgitation around a prosthetic mitral valve.

6. *Laboratory findings*

A. *Electrocardiography*

(1) The ECG may be normal.

(2) The ECG may show:

(a) Nonspecific S-T and T wave abnormalities

(b) Left ventricular hypertrophy

(c) P wave abnormalities

(d) Premature contractions

(e) Atrial fibrillation

(3) Even when there is rather marked cardiomegaly, it is common for the ECG not to have increased QRS voltage.

B. *Chest x-ray*

(1) The chest roentgenograph varies from normal to enormous dilatation of all cardiac chambers, especially the left atrium.

(2) The first chamber to enlarge is the left atrium, and in borderline cases this can best be detected with barium in the esophagus (lateral and right anterior oblique views).

(3) Elevation of the left atrial pressure may cause the redistribution of pulmonary blood flow with distension of the upper lobe vessels, pulmonary edema.

(4) Calcification of the mitral annulus may be seen in patients with pro-

lapse of the mitral valve, and calcification of the valve tissue is not uncommon in rheumatic mitral regurgitation.

C. *Echocardiography* can be of great value by demonstrating:

(1) Left ventricular size and contraction

(2) Left atrial size

(3) Clots and tumors

(4) Mitral valve excursion

(5) Specific changes of mitral valve prolapse (see Chap. 6)

D. *Cardiac catheterization*

(1) Findings of cardiac catheterization may be normal with mild to moderate mitral regurgitation.

(2) With severe regurgitation, there is elevation of right-sided pressures and elevation of the pulmonary capillary wedge or left atrial pressures, especially of the "v" waves. With abrupt, severe regurgitation, the "v" waves may be as high as 60 to 70 mm. Hg and may be reflected as specific waves in the pulmonary artery.

(3) Left ventriculography "semiquantitates" the severity of the mitral regurgitation and also provides information about ventricular function, valve anatomy, and tumors or clots in the left atrium.

7. *Diagnosis*

A. Auscultation of an apical holosystolic murmur and of the various auscultatory findings of prolapse of the mitral valve in an asymptomatic individual without other abnormal cardiac findings is all that is necessary to make the diagnosis of mitral regurgitation but an electrocardiograph and chest roentgenograph are usually obtained for comparison with later examinations.

B. More severe mitral regurgitation or puzzling clinical presentations can be classified by echocardiography, cardiac catheterization, and angiography.

8. *Differential diagnosis*

A. *Hypertrophic cardiomyopathy*

(1) Hypertrophic cardiomyop-

athy may present with a systolic murmur that may simulate mitral regurgitation.

(2) Indeed, the murmur of hypertrophic cardiomyopathy may be due in part or wholly to mitral regurgitation.

(3) The clinical features of hypertrophic cardiomyopathy (see Chap. 9) and the rather typical echocardiographic and radionuclide studies of this disorder usually provide quick distinction once the diagnosis is considered.

B. *Aortic stenosis*

(1) The murmur of aortic stenosis may be transmitted to the apex where it may be of an entirely different quality than the harsh murmur at the base, but the apical murmur of aortic stenosis maintains its diamond shape and is usually musical in quality rather than blowing and holosystolic.

(2) The murmur of aortic stenosis increases after a premature beat or after inhalation of amyl nitrate, whereas the murmur of mitral regurgitation remains the same or decreases in these circumstances.

C. The murmur of *ventricular septal defect* is maximal in intensity along the left sternal border, as is the murmur of *tricuspid regurgitation*. The latter murmur may increase in intensity with inspiration and is associated with signs of right ventricular hypertrophy and the peripheral signs of the tricuspid regurgitation.

9. *Complications*

A. The most hazardous complication encountered with mild or moderate mitral regurgitation is infective endocarditis.

B. Spontaneous rupture of chordae tendineae may also cause abrupt worsening of the degree of mitral regurgitation.

C. Atrial fibrillation and systemic emboli are complications of more severe mitral regurgitation.

D. Premature contractions, both atrial and ventricular, are common in patients with prolapse of the mitral valve.

10. *Management*

A. Patients with mild or moderate regurgitation without cardiac enlargement should be examined periodically and carefully instructed in the use of prophylactic antibiotics before dental, instrumentation, and operative procedures. No restriction of activities is necessary.

B. With more severe regurgitation and cardiomegaly, it may be wise to maintain the patient on digitalis and advise that he or she avoid exhausting physical exertion.

C. The development of symptoms of pulmonary congestion or inadequate cardiac output is an indication for consideration for valvular surgery. Some cardiologists would prefer to attempt to eliminate symptoms with digitalis and diuretics and recommend surgery only if significant symptoms developed after the use of these agents.

D. The abrupt development of severe mitral regurgitation is associated with serious symptoms that are relieved by prompt surgery.

11. *Prognosis*

A. The extremely good prognosis of mild or even moderate mitral regurgitation is well documented.

B. Many patients can lead perfectly normal lives without any restrictions.

C. Mild or moderate regurgitation may progress to severe regurgitation slowly or abruptly; the latter is usually related to infective endocarditis or rupture of chordae tendineae.

D. Severe mitral regurgitation is usually a slowly progressive disorder that leads to incapacitation and reduced life expectancy.

SUGGESTED READINGS

Bacon, A. P. C. and Matthews, M. B.: Congenital bicuspid aortic valves and the etiology of isolated aortic valvular stenosis. Q. J. Med., 28:545, 1959.

Barlow, J. B. et al: The significance of late systolic murmurs. Am. Heart J., 66:443, 1963.

Braunwald, E. and Awe, W. C.: The syndrome of severe mitral regurgitation with normal left atrial pressure. Circulation, 27:29, 1963.

Burch, G. E., DePasquale, N. P., and Phillips, J. H.: The syndrome of papillary muscle dysfunction. Am. Heart J., 75:399, 1968.

Cohen, L. S., Friedman, W. F., and Braunwald, E.: Natural history of mild congenital aortic stenosis elucidated by serial hemodynamic studies. Am. J. Cardiol., 30:1, 1972.

Frank, S., Johnson, A., and Ross, J., Jr.: Natural history of aortic valvular stenosis. Br. Heart J., 35:41, 1973.

Goldschlager, N. et al.: The natural history of aortic regurgitation: a clinical and hemodynamic study. Am. J. Med., 54:577, 1973.

Harvey, W. P., Corrado, M. A., and Perloff, J. K.: "Right-sided" murmurs of aortic insufficiency (diastolic murmurs better heard to the right of the sternum than to the left). Am. J. Med. Sci., 245:533, 1963.

Kirklin, J. W., and Pacifico, A. D.: Surgery for acquired valvular heart disease. N. Eng. J. Med., 288:133, 1973.

Olesen, K. H.: The natural history of 271 patients with mitral stenosis under medical treatment. Br. Heart J., 24:349, 1962.

Roberts, W. C.: Anatomically isolated aortic valvular disease: the case against its being of rheumatic etiology. Am. J. Med., 49:151, 1970.

Roberts, W. C.: The congenitally bicuspid aortic valve: study of 85 autopsy cases. Am. J. Cardiol., 26:72, 1970.

Roberts, W. C., Braunwald, E., and Morrow, A. G.: Acute severe mitral regurgitation secondary to ruptured chordae tendineae: clinical, hemodynamic, and pathologic considerations. Circulation, 33:58, 1966.

Ross, J., Jr. and Braunwald, E.: Aortic stenosis. Circulation, 38[Supp. V]:61, 1968.

6. MITRAL VALVE PROLAPSE-CLICK SYNDROME

Ronald Gottlieb, M.D., and Edward K. Chung, M.D.

DEFINITION

1. Mitral valve prolapse exists when one, or both, of the leaflets of the valve abnormally protrude into the left atrium during systole.

2. Mitral regurgitation, nonspecific abnormality of S-T, T waves on the electrocardiogram, nonejection systolic click (or clicks), a systolic murmur, chest pain, and cardiac arrhythmias may be present.

3. Other names for the syndrome include:

    A. Barlow's syndrome *Myx. PVC MR*

    B. Floppy mitral valve syndrome

    C. Late mitral insufficiency

    D. Mitral click-murmur syndrome

    E. Mid-systolic click-late systolic murmur syndrome

    F. Billowing mitral leaflet syndrome

    G. Ballooning mitral valve leaflets

    H. Blue valve syndrome

    I. Myxomatous degeneration of the mitral valve

    J. Mucoid degeneration of the mitral valve

    K. A combination of the above.

4. Tricuspid valve prolapse has been shown to be associated with mitral valve prolapse in as many as 20 per cent of patients.

GENERAL CONSIDERATIONS

In less than two decades, since mitral valve prolapse was described by Barlow, the syndrome has gone from a curiosity to the most frequently diagnosed valvular abnormality in cardiovascular disease. The diagnostic hallmark on physical examination, the non-ejection systolic click, was originally thought to be an extracardiac event. Recently, it has been shown that the systolic click is secondary to redundancy of the mitral valve with resulting systolic protrusion into the left atrium. Mitral regurgitation may, or may not, be present in this syndrome.

As long as examination and angiography remained the only methods for establishing the diagnosis, the syndrome was often unrecognized by many physicians on casual examination. Because of a ready availability of echocardiography, 10 to 15 per cent of the population was found to have mitral valve prolapse by ultrasonic criteria. Many of these individuals, however, had neither clinical nor angiographic evidence of the syndrome. At present, therefore, a significant controversy exists as to what constitutes the diagnostic "gold standard" by which other methods may be judged.

Clinical manifestations may vary from a complete lack of symptoms to free mitral regurgitation that may require surgical intervention. Most cases have mild symptomatology consisting of either atypical chest pain and/or palpitations due to cardiac arrhythmias. Follow-up study suggests that only a few patients progress to the more severe form. Initial reports indicated that sudden death was a definite risk, but the fact now appears to have been overstated.

No treatment is indicated as long as the individual with this syndrome is asymptomatic. Prophylactic antibiotics should be administered, however, prior to dental or other surgical procedures as endocarditis is a distinct possibility. If chest pain is a problem, propranolol (Inderal) may be tried with variable responses. For cardiac arrhythmias, again propranolol is found to be the agent of choice in most cases. The prognosis is, in general, good although a long follow-up is not yet available for the determination of long-term prognosis.

ETIOLOGY

1. *Myxomatous degeneration of the mitral valve*
The usual pathologic finding has been myxomatous degeneration of the mitral valve.

   A. This refers to a process in which the collagenous supporting structure of the valve is replaced by loose metachromatically staining myxomatous tissue.

   B. There is increased intracellular accumulation of acid mucopolysaccharides composed of hyaluronic and/or chondroitin sulfates.

   C. Loss of fibrous tissue permits stretching of valve leaflets, and, hence, prolapse into the left atrium during systole.

2. *Marfan's syndrome*
   A. Similar pathology has been noted in Marfan's syndrome.

   B. Mitral valve prolapse may represent a *forme fruste* of that disease.

3. *Chemical compounds*
   A. Ingestion of certain compounds may be etiologically related to the disease.

   B. Beta-amino-proprionitrite ingestion (lathyrism) has caused changes similar to myxomatous degeneration.

4. *Ischemia*
   A. Ischemia has been suggested as playing a role in the chest pain and cardiac arrhythmia aspects of the syndrome.

   B. Traction on the papillary muscles is the postulated mechanism but convincing evidence is lacking.

   C. Coronary artery disease has not been etiologically linked to myxomatous degeneration.

5. *Rheumatic heart disease*
Rheumatic heart disease has not been shown to be etiologically related to myxomatous degeneration.

6. *Atrial septal defect*
   A. It has been shown that atrial septal defect often coexists with mitral valve prolapse.

   B. There is no clear etiologic connection between these entities, however.

7. *Familial incidence*
There has been some familial incidence.

PATHOPHYSIOLOGY

1. Redundancy of the valve leaflets permits varying degrees of *systolic prolapse into the left atrium*.

2. *A high pitched click (or clicks)* is produced as each prolapsing "segment" reaches its maximal posterior displacement.

3. *Mitral regurgitation*
Coaptation of the leaflets may be disrupted with resulting mitral regurgitation. Advanced cases may develop:

   A. Left ventricular and left atrial enlargement

   B. Pulmonary hypertension

   C. Atrial tachyarrhythmias

   D. Left- and right-sided congestive heart failure

4. *Ventricular function*
   A. Some investigators have found that the left ventricle may be angiographically abnormal.

   B. This would imply that the syndrome may be a form of cardiomyopathy.

5. *Cardiac arrhythmias*
   A. Both atrial and ventricular arrhythmias may occur.

   B. The etiology is unknown, but there is some evidence for either localized ischemia or cardiomyopathy.

6. *Chest pain*

Chest pain may be secondary to ischemia, perhaps of a papillary muscle placed under increased tension because of a prolapsing valve leaflet.

CLASSIFICATION

1. No useful classification has been developed, because the etiology of the syndrome remains in doubt.

2. Patients have been divided into the following categories:

    A. Those with posterior leaflet prolapse

    B. Those with anterior leaflet prolapse

    C. Those with both anterior and posterior leaflet prolapse

3. Others have divided cases into secondary and primary forms.

    A. *Secondary form*

The syndrome associated with:

    (1) Marfan's syndrome

    (2) Ischemic heart disease

    (3) Idiopathic hypertrophic subaortic stenosis

    (4) Atrial septal defect

    B. *Primary form*

Those found unassociated with any other abnormality. Wisdom of the former classification is dubious at best; it offers nothing of use clinically and may actually be in error, since the so-called primary form may simply be a less overt expression of the same disease as the secondary forms.

SYMPTOMS AND SIGNS

1. *Symptoms*

There are two major symptoms, including atypical chest pain and various complaints due to cardiac arrhythmias.

    A. *Chest pain*

    (1) Usually atypical in nature (i.e., not necessarily related to exertion or relieved by rest or nitroglycerin).

    (2) Often sharp and localized to the left chest.

    B. *Cardiac arrhythmias*

    (1) Relatively common. They may be atrial or ventricular arrhythmias with the latter predominating.

    (2) Ventricular premature contractions are most common and they may occur in isolated form, bigeminy or trigeminy, or occasionally, ventricular tachycardia.

    (3) Vectorcardiographic studies have indicated that ventricular premature beats frequently originate from the base of the left ventricle. From this observation, diastolic tactile stimulation may be a possible cause to provoke the ventricular ectopic beats.

    (4) Sudden death has been reported but recent recognition of the extent of the entity would seem to indicate that it must be extremely rare.

    (5) Recent reports indicate that Mobitz Type II A-V block or complete A-V block may occur in this syndrome but are also very rare.

    C. *Other findings*

Many patients with this syndrome are emotionally unstable and anxious young to middle-aged women.

2. *Physical findings*

The characteristic physical finding is the presence of one or more nonejection high-pitched systolic clicks frequently followed by a systolic murmur.

    A. The systolic murmur and the systolic click may not be present at rest or even after postural and pharmacological interventions.

    B. The systolic click (or clicks) may be heard only intermittently.

    C. The clicks and murmur are usually best heard along the lower left sternal border and at the apex.

    D. Systolic ejection click is a common source of diagnostic error.

    (1) May be followed by ejection murmur, adding to difficulty of diagnosis

    (2) May be generated across either aortic or pulmonic valve

    (3) Occur early in systole, are fol-

lowed by crescendo-decrescendo murmurs that end before the second heart sound and are best heard at the base of the heart rather than along the lower left sternal border or at the apex.

E. In general, physical and pharmacologic maneuvers that decrease left ventricular size or afterload (standing, Valsalva maneuver, isoproterenol and amyl nitrate) cause the click to move toward the first heart sound and the murmur to become longer and louder.

F. Maneuvers that increase left ventricular size or raise afterload (e.g., squatting, handgrip, and methoxamine) cause the click to move toward the second heart sound and the murmur to become shorter and softer.

G. The murmur is commonly a late systolic murmur, but it may be a pansystolic murmur due to mitral regurgitation.

H. Irregular cardiac rhythm or tachycardia can be detected when any cardiac arrhythmia is present.

I. In advanced and severe cases, the signs of left ventricular hypertrophy and congestive heart failure may be present.

LABORATORY FINDINGS

1. *Hematologic, serum chemistry and x-ray studies*
No diagnostic value.
2. *Carotid pulse tracings and apex-cardiography*
Very little use.
3. *Phonocardiography*
A. Valuable only for confirmation of the presence and timing of the click (or clicks) and the systolic murmur.

B. Mobility of both components can also be demonstrated in response to physical and pharmacologic maneuvers.
4. *The electrocardiogram*
A. The ECG may be normal or it may exhibit a variety of nonspecific changes.

B. S-T segment depression and T wave inversion that closely resemble myocardial ischemia are the most common ECG abnormalities.

C. These ECG findings are most often observed in leads II, III, aVF and V_5 and V_6, but they may be widespread. Recently, several patients with this syndrome showing ECG abnormalities compatible with diaphragmatic (inferior) myocardial infarction have been reported.

D. Pseudoanterior (or anteroseptal) myocardial infarction also occurs rarely in this syndrome.

F. The Q-T interval may be prolonged.

G. Rhythm disturbances, including atrial and ventricular premature contractions and paroxysmal atrial tachyarrhythmias, are common.

H. Mobitz Type II A-V block and complete A-V block also have been encountered.
5. *Echocardiography*
A. At present, echocardiography is the most valuable noninvasive laboratory study to diagnose the mitral valve prolapse-click syndrome.

B. One or both leaflets may be observed moving in a posterior direction during systole.

C. The diagnostic feature of echocardiogram in this syndrome is a posterior excursion of the leaflets during systole.

D. Its motion may occur at some time during systole or may be present throughout systole.

E. When phonocardiograms are recorded during echocardiography, the click coincides with the completion of the posterior excursion of the leaflet(s), or maximal degree of prolapse.

F. Nevertheless, there are some differences of opinion as to the technical aspects of obtaining the echocardiogram and its interpretation.

G. Thus, this technique may not

lead to a clear and unequivocal diagnosis in all cases.

6. *Cardiac catheterization and angiography*

A. Cardiac catheterization and angiography have the disadvantage of being invasive.

B. The question of whether angiography or echocardiography is more definitive is, for the present, as yet unresolved.

C. The ventriculogram is the useful aspect of the angiographic study.

(1) Both the right and left anterior oblique projections are helpful, but the former is usually more so than the latter.

(2) Which leaflet or leaflets are involved can usually be discerned.

(3) A problem occurs in differentiating very small degrees of prolapse from a normal variant, since the mitral valve commonly is minimally displaced posteriorly during systole. No absolute criteria yet exists for defining the limits of normal in this regard.

DIAGNOSIS

1. *Suspicion should be raised by any of the following:*

A. Atypical chest pain

B. Unexplained cardiac arrhythmias

C. Nonejection systolic click (or clicks) followed by a systolic murmur.

2. *Sex ratio*

Female over male predominates 2:1

3. *Establishing diagnosis*

A. Typical auscultatory findings, made by an experienced observer, are usually sufficient in many cases.

B. Electrocardiogram:

(1) S-T, T wave abnormalities described as above

(2) Cardiac arrhythmias described as above

C. Chest roentgenogram is usually normal.

D. More definitive confirmation

must be made from echocardiography and/or cardiac catheterization, but there is no complete agreement at present as to which is the more definite study.

(1) Echocardiography

(a) Should probably be study of first choice

(b) Simpler

(c) Safer

(d) Cheaper

(e) Limitations:

(i) Scans limited portion of valve, and prolapse could go undetected.

(ii) Differences of opinion as to interpretation exist

(iii) Therefore, cannot be used to rule out prolapse.

(2) Catheterization

Diagnostic pitfalls are as follows:

(a) Valve leaflets overlie themselves, and left ventricular shadow in right anterior oblique projection makes diagnosis difficult in some cases.

(b) The grey zone between very small prolapse and normal mitral valve has not yet been eliminated.

(c) In a great many cases, however, the diagnosis is apparent.

DIFFERENTIAL DIAGNOSIS

1. *Mitral regurgitation of other etiology*

A. It may be impossible to differentiate from mitral regurgitation of other etiology clinically when prolapse has progressed to holosystolic murmur, and click is no longer present.

B. If there is no associated rheumatic aortic valvular disease or mitral stenosis, pathologic examination may be only way to establish the diagnosis.

2. *Idiopathic hypertrophic subaortic stenosis (IHSS)*

A. IHSS may resemble mitral-valve-prolapse-click syndrome because of presence of systolic murmur that becomes louder with Valsalva maneuver.

B. Mitral regurgitation may also be

present in approximately 50 per cent of such patients.

    C. IHSS can be differentiated by:

        (1) Absence of click

        (2) Bisferiens carotid pulse

        (3) Triple apical impulse

        (4) Deep but narrow Q waves and/or left ventricular hypertrophy on the electrocardiogram.

    3. *Atrial septal defect*

    A. Atrial septal defect rarely causes the diagnostic difficulty.

    B. When it does, it is because of systolic ejection murmur.

    C. Atrial septal defect can be differentiated by:

        (1) Murmur loudest at the base with crescendo decrescendo in quality

        (2) Usual presence of widely split and fixed second heart sound

        (3) Hyperdynamic precordium to palpation

        (4) Increased pulmonary vasculature on chest x-ray

        (5) Common finding of incomplete right bundle branch block pattern on electrocardiogram.

    4. *Mitral stenosis*

Mitral stenosis causes difficulty only when the heart rate is rapid and the opening snap and murmur are erroneously felt to be in systole and misinterpreted as a click followed by a murmur.

COMPLICATIONS

    1. *Bacterial endocarditis*

    A. Bacterial endocarditis has been clearly documented to occur.

    B. Secondary complications of endocarditis may include

        (1) Destruction of mitral valve

        (2) Septic emboli (e.g., to brain, kidneys, lower extremities)

        (3) Anemia

        (4) Splenomegaly

    2. *Cardiac arrhythmias*

    A. *Atrial tachyarrhythmias*

        (1) Atrial tachyarrhythmias may include atrial premature beats, paroxysmal atrial tachycardia, atrial flutter, and fibrillation.

        (2) Atrial tachyarrhythmias may cause palpitations and minor symptoms, but they are rarely serious.

    B. *Ventricular tachyarrhythmias*

        (1) Ventricular premature contractions are the most common arrhythmia in this syndrome.

        (2) Ventricular tachycardia is occasionally observed.

        (3) Ventricular arrhythmias have the potential to create serious problems including sudden death.

    C. *A-V block*

On rare occasions, second degree or complete A-V block may occur.

    3. *Progression to severe mitral regurgitation*

    A. Severe mitral regurgitation occurs only occasionally.

    B. It may require mitral valve replacement with prosthesis.

MANAGEMENT

    1. *Antibiotic prophylaxis for bacterial endocarditis*

    A. Antibiotics should be prescribed for all dental or other surgical procedures.

    B. They should be given the day before, the day of, and 2 days after the procedure.

    C. Some suggested regimens:

        (1) Procaine penicillin G 300,000 units and aqueous penicillin 300,000 units intravenously one hour before procedure, followed by procaine penicillin G 300,000 units every 6 hours for 3 days.

        (2) Above regimen with intramuscular streptomycin 1 g. added to the first dose and 0.5 g. added to subsequent doses.

        (3) Ampicillin 0.5 g. intramuscular injection and gentamycin (1

mg./kg./dose if normal renal function) intramuscular injection one hour before the procedure and every 6 hours for 3 days.

D. Daily prophylaxis against recurrent streptococcal infection is *not* necessary.

2. *Treatment of cardiac arrhythmias* (see Chap. 24)

A. *Atrial arrhythmias*

(1) The treatment is required only when recurrent and troublesome.

(2) When the treatment is considered to be indicated, the drug of choice is propranolol (Inderal).

(3) If propranolol can not be used or the drug is ineffective, quinidine, procainamide or diphenylhydantoin may be used.

B. *Ventricular arrhythmias*

(1) Indications for therapy are not completely clear.

(2) Generally, the treatment is considered to be indicated in the following situations:

(a) Symptomatic ventricular arrhythmias

(b) Multifocal ventricular premature beats

(c) Ventricular group beats

(d) Frequent (5–6 or more per minute) ventricular premature beats

(e) R-on-T phenomenon

(f) Ventricular tachycardia

(3) The drug of choice:

(a) Propranolol (Inderal) seems to be most effective

(b) The second choice of drugs include lidocaine (Xylocaine), diphenylhydantoin (Dilantin), quinidine and procainamide (Pronestyl).

C. *A-V block*

On rare occasions, some patients with this syndrome may require artificial pacemaker for complete A-V block.

3. *Treatment of chest pain*

A. Chest pain may be poorly responsive to any therapy.

B. The most effective drug has been propanolol (Inderal).

4. *Treatment of severe mitral regurgitation*

A. Should be managed similar to mitral regurgitation of any other etiology.

B. Avoid surgery until patient has reached "moderately compromised" category of the New York Heart Association classification.

C. Treat atrial fibrillation, if present, with digitalis.

D. Valve replacement should be recommended when there are increasing symptoms with increasing heart size and the development of pulmonary hypertension.

E. Prosthetic valve function may be slightly less satisfactory in these patients because of involvement of the valve ring in the disease process leading to postoperative mitral regurgitation.

PROGNOSIS

1. *Typical case*

Average life span differs very little from normal individual.

2. *Factors that may lead to decreased life expectancy*

A. Progression of mitral regurgitation, which may require valve replacement; and the prognosis then becomes that of patient with prosthetic mitral valve.

B. Bacterial endocarditis

C. Cardiac arrhythmias may cause sudden death, but this is very rare indeed.

D. A long-term prognosis of this syndrome requires a further investigation.

SUGGESTED READINGS

Barlow, J. B. et al.: Late systolic murmurs and non-ejection ("mid-late") systolic clicks: An analysis of 90 patients. Br. Heart J., *30*:203, 1968.

Criley, J. M. et al.: Prolapse of the mitral valve: clinical and cine-angiocardiographic findings. Br. Heart J., *28*:488, 1966.

DelRio, C. et al.: Chest pain and post-exercise ECGs with normal coronary arteriograms in patients with click-late systolic murmur syndrome. Chest, *60*:292, 1971.

Dillon, J. C. et al.: Use of echocardiography in patients with prolapsed mitral valve. Circulation, *43*:505, 1971.

Edwards, J. E.: Clinicopathologic correlations: mitral insufficiency resulting from "overshooting" of leaflets. Circulation, *43*:606, 1971.

Fontana, M. E. et al.: The varying clinical spectrum of the systolic click-late systolic murmur syndrome. Circulation, *41*:807, 1970.

Fontana, M. E. et al.: Postural changes in left ventricular and mitral valvular dynamics in the systolic click-late systolic murmur syndrome. Am. J. Cardiol., *29*:262, 1972.

Gooch, A. S. et al.: Arrhythmias and left ventricular asynergy in the prolapsing mitral leaflet syndrome. Am. J. Cardiol., *29*:611, 1972.

Gulotta, S., Ewing, K., and Radmamabnan, V.: Mitral valve prolapse and left ventricular dysfunction. Circulation, *43* & *44*(Supp. II):173, 1971.

Jeresaty, R. M.: Mitral valve prolapse-click syndrome. In Sonnenblick, E. and Lesch, M. (ed.): Valvular Heart Disease.New York, Grune & Stratton, 1974.

Linhart, J. W. and Taylor, W. J.: The late apical systolic murmur: clinical hemodynamic and angiographic observations. Am. J. Cardiol., *18*:164, 1966.

McDonald, A. et al.: Association of prolapse of posterior cusp of mitral valve and atrial septal defect. Br. Heart J., *32*:554, 1970.

Pocock, W. A. and Barlow, J. B.: Etiology and electrocardiographic features of the billowing posterior mitral leaflet syndrome: analysis of a further 130 patients with a late systolic murmur or nonejection systolic click. Am. J. Med., *51*:731, 1971.

Ronan, J. A., Perloff, J. K., and Harvey, W. P.: Systolic clicks and the late systolic murmur. Intracardiac phonocardiographic evidence of their mitral valve origin. Am. Heart J., *70*:319, 1965.

Ronan, J. A., Waters, T. J., and Escorcia, E.: Effect of simple bedside maneuvers in the isolated systolic click. Circulation, Vol. *43* and *44*(Suppl. II):31, 1971.

Shankar, K. R. et al.: Lethal tricuspid and mitral regurgitation in Marfan's syndrome. Am. J. Cardiol., *20*:122, 1967.

7. ENDOCARDITIS AND MYOCARDITIS

Richard B. Hornick, M.D., *and Mark M. Applefeld,* M.D.

Part 1   Endocarditis

DEFINITION

1. *Endocarditis* is the term describing the clinical signs and symptoms occurring in patients with infection of the intact or damaged endothelium or prosthetic valves of the heart.

2. Infection can also arise inside cardiac chambers (i.e., left ventricle where jet of regurgitant blood through incompetent aortic valve impinges on the wall; in the right ventricle around the edges of a ventricular septal defect) or it can be associated with a patent ductus arteriosus, with coarctation of the aorta, or with arteriovenous fistulae. Thus, *endocarditis* is a restrictive term that needs further categorization (see Classification below) to be descriptive.

3. Because the infection is located on an endothelial surface, with organisms proliferating in a lesion that allows ready access to the circulation, most patients have a continuous bacteremia.

4. The infection itself provokes little inflammation in the amorphous material that layers on and around the bacterial colonies (these lesions are called *vegetations*). The presence of the bacteremia stimulates the production of fever, the most common sign in patients with endocarditis.

5. Infection can spread from the vegetations to cause abscess formation in the valve ring or annulus, especially in patients with infected prosthetic valves. Metastatic evidence of infection can be seen in the brain, heart, spleen, kidneys, and elsewhere.

GENERAL CONSIDERATIONS

Bacterial endocarditis is a unique infectious process involving normal or damaged heart valves as well as homografts and prosthetic valves. The number of microorganisms that have been implicated in this infection is large and includes common and exotic, virulent and low-virulence bacteria, as well as fungi, viruses, and rickettsia. Despite the wide range of known pathogens, there remain a few strains that are predominantly involved in infections of normal valves (e.g., staphylococcus, gonococcus), damaged valves (e.g., streptococcal species), and prosthetic valves (early onset: *Staphylococcus epidermiditis,* late onset: other streptococcal species). Prior to the availability of antibiotics, bacterial endocarditis was almost invariably fatal, with death occurring after a prolonged, relentless, debilitating illness. Appropriate antibiotic utilization has reduced the overall mortality, but sequelae persist and may be crippling. Many of the manifestations of endocarditis are not directly infectious in origin but rather are a consequence of immunological reactions. The diagnosis remains a significant problem, since endocarditis often is not suspected in patients who are ill for many weeks before a definite diagnosis is established. One of the major unanswered questions about endocarditis relates to the factors involved in the establishment of the infection on the heart valves. With the ample opportunities for infection to occur during acknowledged

95

frequent, transient bacteremias, why don't more infections ensue? The complex interaction of host defenses balanced by the number and virulence of the microorganisms requires further elucidation.

ETIOLOGY

1. The endothelium has the propensity to be infected, under the proper circumstances, by virtually all microorganisms.

2. Bacteria and other organisms can gain entrance to the circulation by many means; the skin, genitourinary and gastrointestinal tracts, and respiratory system are frequent sources. Ordinarily, bacteria, particularly less virulent pathogens, are cleared from the blood stream by the reticuloendothelial system. However, when large numbers of organisms are introduced (e.g., following dental extraction, particulary in the presence of a damaged heart valve or a foreign body), the clearing mechanisms are compromised and infection may occur.

3. Infection occurs most commonly on the mitral valve, then on the aortic, tricuspid, and pulmonary valves. Rarely, two or more valves may be infected. Patients with acute endocarditis, whether occurring on a normal or a prosthetic valve, are likely to be infected with *Staphylococcus aureus* or *Staphylococcus epidermiditis*. These two species cause over half the cases of early onset prosthetic valve endocarditis (PVE). Patients who are drug abusers are prone to develop infection with *S. aureus,* particularly on the tricuspid valve. The less virulent *S. epidermiditis* attacks the implanted foreign bodies in the heart.

Streptococcus pneumoniae, group A, beta hemolytic streptococci, *N. gonorrhoeae* and *Pseudomonas aeruginosa* are other bacterial species that infect normal heart valves. The pneumococcus causes disease of the aortic valve that often results in perforation of a cusp (e.g., ulcerative valvulitis). Formerly, the pulmonary valve was selectively infected by the gonococcus, but despite continued involvement of this pathogen in the etiology of endocarditis, it no longer demonstrates this predilection. While these organisms are the likely causes of infection in acute endocarditis, others usually associated with subacute infections may also initiate a rapid, fulminating type of infection.

4. Subacute bacterial endocarditis is a disease caused most commonly (in about 80 per cent of cases) by streptococci. These are the alpha hemolytic gram-positive cocci formerly known as *Streptococcus viridans* and they are a part of the normal oropharyngeal flora. Bacteremia with these organisms occurs after brushing the teeth vigorously, dental manipulation, and especially extractions. These organisms have a low virulence and are associated with endocarditis involving congenitally deformed valves, acquired damage to a valve, or the late-onset form of PVE. Aortic and mitral valves are most commonly involved.

Other streptococci, the enterococci, Lancefield group D, cause a more severe form of endocarditis. These organisms (the species *Streptococcus fecalis* is the standard-bearer of the group) are found in the gastrointestinal and genitourinary tracts. Following instrumentation of the genitourinary tract or delivery, they may gain entrance to the bloodstream and initiate either an acute or indolent form of endocarditis. In recent years *Streptococcus bovis,* a nonenteric enterococcus, has been isolated with increasing frequency. It is differentiated from *S. fecalis* by its increased susceptibility to penicillin.

5. Fungi causing endocarditis are usually histoplasma and various candida species. The latter are associated with disease in drug addicts who skin pop or

mainline, in diabetic patients, and in those patients with prosthetic valves.

6. Anaerobic bacteria have been recognized infrequently as causative agents, perhaps because the arterial blood oxidation-reduction potential inhibits their growth and thus is an unfavorable environment to initiate an infection. However, with vegetations present, the situation may be changed and microaerophilic or anaerobes may infect.

7. *Coxiella burnetii,* the rickettsia responsible for Q fever, produces a distinctive form of endocarditis. The vegetations are large, and the disease requires long term antibiotic therapy and/or surgical intervention.

8. Cell wall defective organisms can be isolated in hypertonic media from patients with endocarditis. They may represent streptococci or other bacteria that have had their normal cell wall synthesis interfered with by antibiotics, antibodies, or lysozymes. It has been suggested that these organisms are responsible for persistence or relapse of endocarditis.

9. About 15 per cent of patients with clinical manifestations of subacute endocarditis have persistently sterile blood cultures. The reasons for the absence of detectable bacteremia are unknown, but the fastidious nature of the organisms, cell-wall defective bacteria, the intracellular location and compromised status of bacteria in phagocytes may contribute. Previous antibiotic therapy increases the difficulty in isolation of bacteria.

PATHOPHYSIOLOGY

1. Damage to endothelium can occur at the edge of valves (i.e., point of closure), in regions of high pressure gradients across narrow orifices (i.e., aortic and mitral valves), and near arteriovenous fistulae. Colonization of these traumatized areas occurs from bacteria

in the bloodstream. The resulting vegetations form at the downstream side of these pressure gradients or on the margin of valve leaflet.

2. The bacteria become enmeshed in platelet and fibrin thrombi, which provide an environment that is both protective from host defense and also conducive to bacterial multiplication.

3. Bacteria most commonly associated with subacute endocarditis have surface antigens that allow them to adhere preferentially to endothelial cells. This may help to explain the unique ability of *S. viridans* to cause endocarditis but no other infectious process.

4. Bacterial colonies in the amorphous fibrin vegetation are protected from phagocytes and direct delivery of antibiotics because no vascular channels are present.

5. Multiplication of bacteria and enlargement of the vegetations by platelet and fibrin aggregation can lead to poor closure of valve leaflets. Scarring may occur, and causes retraction and valvular insufficiency. The infectious process may erode through a leaflet, resulting in a perforation. Infection may spread to the annulus and create abscesses in the myocardium. Rupture of chorda tendineae may occur. Mycotic emboli may cause aneurysms in the aorta or smaller vessels. The development of pericarditis arises from coronary artery embolization, myocardial abscess, or extension from valve ring.

6. Peripheral manifestations of endocarditis arise from sterile or mycotic emboli or from immunological reactions initiated by the chronic infection. Involvement of the right side of the heart is associated with frequent bouts of pneumonitis and pulmonary infarction. Left-sided disease produces emboli that can cause abscesses in the brain, kidneys, spleen, and other organs.

7. Patients with endocarditis may develop congestive failure because of

myocarditis or altered hemodynamics due to poorly functioning valves.

8. The usual prolonged duration of infection in SBE leads to increased reticuloendothelial function with enlargement of the spleen. It is usually palpable after 4 to 6 weeks of disease.

9. Rheumatoid factor can be detected in about 66 per cent of patients with SBE. This IgM antibody directed against the host's IgG is thought to be derived by the alteration that occurs in the proliferating IgG antibodies (detected as foreign by the host) directed against the microbes. Thus, the IgG-IgM (and perhaps microbe antigens or intact organisms) circulating immune complex can act to initiate vasculitis.

10. The immune complexes can react with complement, especially C_3 and C_4, so these levels are decreased in patients with endocarditis. Glomerulonephritis is one manifestation of endocarditis infection that appears to be mediated by this immunological reaction.

11. These deposits of IgM-IgG can also be found in small blood vessels and account for splinter hemorrhages, Osler's nodes, Janeway lesions, and Roth spots—each a consequence of vasculitis.

CLASSIFICATION

1. Endocarditis involving infections of previously normal heart valves frequently results in a fulminating infectious process. Duration of illness is less than 6 weeks. In such circumstances it is appropriate to use the term *acute bacterial endocarditis*. Blood cultures are positive in 95 per cent of patients.

2. Infections of valves damaged by rheumatic fever or congenitally altered valves usually results in an indolent but progressive infectious process. This is the most common form of endocarditis and frequently referred to as *subacute bacterial endocarditis*. Blood cultures are positive in 85 to 90 per cent of patients.

3. Infections of heart valves caused by fungi, rickettsia, or viruses are less common and are classified as to etiological agent (e.g., Q fever endocarditis, *Candida albicans* endocarditis).

4. Classification of endocarditis involving surgically repaired implanted prosthetic valves (PVE, prosthetic valve endocarditis) is predicated on time of onset of disease. Those infections arising in the first 60 postoperative days are entitled "early onset"; "late onset" disease includes those infections diagnosed after that period. This separation is useful because it establishes those etiologies that had origins in the pre- , post- , or intraoperative periods and thus suggests means of prevention or predicting the causative organisms

SYMPTOMS AND SIGNS

1. Disease incited by highly virulent pathogens, such as staphylococcus, enterococcus, or pneumococcus, usually presents with an abrupt onset of high fever, signs of toxicity, and often evidence of cardiac decompensation; while an insidious course is caused by low-virulence organisms (e.g., *Streptococcus viridans* or *Staphylococcus albus*). Under the latter circumstances, night sweats calling attention to late afternoon temperature elevation, anorexia, arthralgias, or worsening of chronic congestive failure may be found.

2. An apparent "stroke," cerebral vascular accident, is the initial manifestation in many patients. The presence of fever and murmur should signal the likelihood of endocarditis.

3. Endocarditis in narcotic addicts, representing 10 per cent of some series, often presents as pneumonitis or as a pulmonary embolus. Vegetations due to fungi frequently embolize to a major

arterial vessel, causing acute vascular insufficiency.

4. Fever, found in 90 to 100 per cent of patients, remains a sine qua non of disease. Low-grade elevations are common; a truly afebrile course is rare, though occurring in the setting of uremia, congestive failure, central nervous system hemorrhage, or prior antibiotic usage.

5. Murmurs are heard in 85 per cent of the cases. Daily variation in intensity probably relates to fluctuating temperature or progression of anemia. More significant and suggesting active infection is the appearance of new murmurs of aortic, mitral, or tricuspid regurgitation or a pericardial friction rub.

6. Acute tricuspid regurgitation may be manifested only by an atrial gallop. In the absence of a murmur, the gallop indicates a severe low pressure hemodynamic leak into a small, noncompliant atrium.

7. Splenomegaly is present in 25 to 60 per cent of instances and relates both to the duration of disease and the intent with which it is sought.

8. Osler's nodes, petechiae, and Roth's spots are recorded in 15, 30, and less than 5 per cent of cases, respectively. It is important to re-emphasize that older patients do not present in different fashion from their younger counterparts. Only 3 of 29 such individuals over age 60 studied by us had neither fever nor leukocytosis.

LABORATORY FINDINGS

1. Blood cultures are positive in 95 per cent of patients with acute endocarditis and 85 to 90 per cent in patients with subacute endocarditis.

2. The peripheral white count is usually slightly elevated. In SBE the chronic infection depresses bone marrow activity and anemia is present. The sedimentation rate is elevated.

3. Rheumatoid factor (latex agglutination titer) is elevated in about two-thirds of patients with SBE.

4. Serum cholesterol levels are usually reduced during the prolonged illness.

5. Microscopic hematuria occurs as a manifestation of the glomerulonephritis associated with SBE. In these patients, serum complement activity is decreased. In addition, BUN and creatinine levels are increased.

6. An echocardiogram may reveal vegetations on infected valves. ECG is of little diagnostic help. Nonspecific ST-T wave changes may be present. Evidence of a significant new arrhythmia may suggest myocardial abscess.

DIAGNOSIS

1. In a patient who presents with fever, anemia, leukocytosis, cardiac murmurs, and signs of peripheral emboli, diagnosis is obvious.

2. Four to six blood cultures will reveal the infecting organisms in 85 to 95 per cent of all cases. Repeatedly sterile blood cultures should raise suspicion of anaerobes, fungi, brucella, *Hemophilus influenzae*, mycoplasma, coxsackie virus, and *Coxiella burnetii*.

DIFFERENTIAL DIAGNOSIS

1. Presentation may be that of a primary neurologic, collagen vascular, pulmonary, or renal disorder, depending upon the nature of the infecting organism and the site of the vegetation.

2. Embolism to a coronary artery may simulate a myocardial infarction; to a peripheral artery, an acute vascular syndrome.

3. Endocarditis, particularly the subacute form, may mimic almost any systemic disease. Diagnosis rests upon this entity's being considered and excluded by appropriate laboratory studies.

4. Patients with fever and positive blood cultures following open heart surgery may not have endocarditis. Sande et al., have described prolonged gram-negative rod bacteremia without infection of the prosthetic valve. As yet there is no discriminating procedure that allows for differentiation of endocarditis from bacteremia and patients should receive adequate antibiotic therapy.

5. Splinter hemorrhages occur in normal individuals (e.g., in 25 per cent of freshman medical students). They and conjunctival petechial hemorrhages also appear following open heart surgery and do not necessarily indicate endocarditis.

COMPLICATIONS

1. The most frequent cause of mortality (50–60% of instances) is congestive heart failure due to valvular dysfunction. Valvular insufficiency may be caused by perforation of a leaflet, destruction of a cusp, or rupture of chordae tendineae. Less well appreciated is that large vegetations (particularly those due to fungi or *C. burnetii*) may obstruct flow of blood into or out of the ventricle.

2. Emboli to the brain, spleen, kidney, and coronary vessels are the next most common complication, occurring in 15 to 35 per cent of cases. Splenic and renal emboli are an infrequent cause of morbidity and mortality. Major cerebral emboli, reported in up to 30 per cent of patients, are most often found in the distribution of the middle cerebral artery. Occurring usually during active infection, they have been reported up to 2 years following completion of therapy. It should be stressed that 3 per cent of all cerebral emboli arise from valvular infection. Coronary arterial emboli may produce a myocardial infarction, abscess, or pericarditis. Septic mycotic aneurysms frequently cause acute intracranial or intra-abdominal hemorrhage.

MANAGEMENT

1. Appropriate antibiotic therapy depends upon identification of the infecting organism. Endocarditis is an infection that responds best to bactericidal, as opposed to bacteriostatic, antibiotics. As noted above (see Pathophysiology), antibiotics must diffuse into the vegetation to inhibit the bacteria rather than having a more direct access through inflamed tissue. When clinical evidence is overwhelming, the patient should have blood drawn for culture (5 cultures are sufficient over a 12–24 hour period) and antibiotics instituted. The delay in treating suspected acute endocarditis should be no longer than 2 to 4 hours.

2. Patients with acute endocarditis caused by staphylococci should receive intravenously a penicillinase-resistant drug, such as the penicillin-derived drugs: methicillin (16–20 grams daily), naficillin or oxacillin (4–8 grams daily), or cephalothin or cefazolin (10–14 grams daily). These antibiotics must be continued for 6 to 8 weeks in high doses to prevent relapses and to enhance chances for recovery. If the staph is sensitive to penicillin G, this drug remains the drug of choice. A daily dose of 16 to 20 million units for 6 to 8 weeks is needed.

Vancomycin (4-8 g. I.V. daily) or clindamycin phosphate (1.5-2.5 g. I.V. daily) can be given to patients with history of severe penicillin and cephalosporin hypersensitivities.

3. For treating patients with streptococcal infections, viridans group, penicillin is the drug of choice, as most strains are susceptible. Usual daily dose I.V. is 6 to 10 million units for an adult, with therapy continued for 4 to 6 weeks. Some authors have had good results with shorter courses by combining an aminoglycoside with penicillin for 2 or 3 weeks. Others have achieved good results with oral penicillin, 7.2 g. per day plus streptomycin, 0.5 g. b.i.d. for 3 to 4

weeks. In the latter regimen, care must be taken to insure that the organism is very sensitive to penicillin, that adequate blood levels are achieved, and that the patient is reliable. In allergic patients, cephalothin or vancomycin may be substituted.

4. The enterococcus is a more difficult pathogen to eradicate. Two drugs are mandatory. Penicillin, despite in vitro resistance, will be effective if given with aminoglycoside. These two drugs are synergistic for enterococci. Penicillin, 20 million units daily at least, plus 1 to 1.5 g. streptomycin has been the traditional combination. Ampicillin and kanamycin or gentamicin may be used. Therapy should be continued for 6 weeks. In patients allergic to penicillin, consideration should be given to attempts to control hypersensitivity reactions with corticosteroids and antihistamine drugs. Virtually no other antibiotic regimen is as effective as penicillin and aminoglycoside in treatment of enterococcal disease. If attempts to use these drugs fail despite antiallergic treatment, then vancomycin and streptomycin may be used.

5. Relapses occur in about 10 to 20 per cent of patients treated for endocarditis. Follow up cultures should be obtained at weekly intervals for 4 to 6 weeks following treatment, the period of highest incidence of relapse. Retreatment with higher doses of the same drug(s) and longer duration should be accomplished, provided the antibiotic sensitivity remains the same.

6. Supportive therapy for renal or cardiac failure should be prescribed as clinically indicated. Oxygen therapy may be useful to alleviate the tissue demands created by the increased host metabolism secondary to the fever and anemia.

7. Surgical removal of diseased valves and implantation of artificial valves may be life-saving. Criteria for intervention are controversial. Intractable heart failure is a definite indication. These patients, however, are poor surgical risks and a decision to operate should be reached promptly. Other reasons for surgery are presence of a large vegetation, overt embolic episodes, evidence of myocardial or ring abscess, and infection of a foreign body. The latter two are definite, whereas the former two are questionable.

8. Prophylaxis. All patients with damaged or prosthetic valves should receive antibiotic coverage following those procedures likely to cause bacteremia (e.g., dental work, instrumentation of the GU or GI tract, delivery of an infant, or surgical procedures involving contaminated fields). The drugs selected should be aimed at the organism likely to be encountered and given several hours prior to procedure and continued for that day and 2 days following. Penicillin should be part of any treatment and an aminoglycoside added for gastrointestinal or genitourinary tract manipulation.

A. Dental Work. Penicillin, 600,000 units I.M., one hour prior and penicillin P.O., 250 mg. q.i.d. for 3 days thereafter. Erythromycin, 250 mg. q.i.d. starting 2 hours prior and continuing for 3 days thereafter, can be used in penicillin-allergic patients.

B. Urologic or Gynecologic Procedures. Penicillin 600,000 units P.O. plus 200,000 units crystalin penicillin 1 hr. prior and q.d. for two days, or ampicillin 25–50 mg./kg. P.O. 1 hour prior then 25 mg./kg. q. 6 hours for remainder of day and 2 days thereafter. Both regimens add streptomycin 1–2 g. on day of and 2 days thereafter.

C. Cardiac Surgery. Methicillin, oxacillin, or cephalothin may be used along with gentamicin, each started one hour before surgery and maintained for 3 to 5 days afer surgery. During surgery special attention should be paid to drug administration, since the prolonged operative time and blood dilution with the heart pump contribute to inadequate levels of circulating antibiotic.

PROGNOSIS

Disease caused by susceptible organisms is associated with a 70 to 80 per cent survival rate if treated appropriately. Adverse factors affecting mortality are delay in diagnosis, presence of organisms not susceptible to available antibiotics, certain infecting organisms (i.e., staphylococci, enterococci, gram-negative rods), congestive heart failure, repeatedly sterile blood cultures, and infection on prosthetic heart valves. Relapses are seen in up to 10 per cent of cases and are most frequent within the first month of cessation of antibiotic therapy.

Part 2 Myocarditis

DEFINITION

1. Myocarditis is a direct infiltration of myocardial cells or their interstitium by bacteria, rickettsiae, viruses, or helminths, and by the inflammatory cells generated as a response to these agents.

2. Myocarditis may also be the consequence of myocardial cell damage due to toxins, physical and chemical agents, or hypersensitivity reactions.

3. It may occur either as a primary event (e.g., neonatal Coxsackie myocarditis) or secondary infection (e.g., subsequent to infective endocarditis or pneumonitis).

GENERAL CONSIDERATIONS

The myocardium is a unique and complex organ system. Any infectious or toxic process that damages myocardial cells directly by cytotoxicity or indirectly by the inflammatory response can seriously disturb the function of this system. Clinical myocarditis is relatively uncommon but by no means rare. Bacterial, viral, rickettsial, protozoal, and helminthetic agents have all been implicated as etiologies. Most patients with myocarditis have transient electrocardiographic changes during the course of their infectious disease. A few individuals develop overt signs and symptoms of cardiac dysfunction. Resolution of an inflammatory process in the myocardium is variable, although most often complete. Uncommonly, a persistent myocarditis with chronic congestive failure or a conduction abnormality may result. There is no specific therapy for patients with viral- or toxin-induced myocarditis.

ETIOLOGY

1. Virtually any microbe—bacteria, virus, rickettsia, or helminth—is capable of causing myocarditis.

2. Common agents include Coxsackie, group B, ECHO, influenza, polio, mumps, measles, and varicella viruses; *C. diphtheriae; S. pneumoniae;* and *R. rickettsiae.*

3. Although rare in the United States, *Trypanosoma cruzi* is a major cause of myocarditis (Chaga's Disease) in South America.

PATHOPHYSIOLOGY

1. Pyogenic bacteria seed the myocardium via hematogenous routes localizing in the interstitium with subsequent microabscess formation. Alternatively, infection may involve the myocardium contiguously from an infected heart valve or foreign body.

2. Rickettsial myocarditis is a consequence of a generalized vasculitis. Viral agents either may have a direct toxic effect on myocardial cells, causing necrosis and a subsequent inflammatory response, or may stimulate disease by the release of products from damaged cells.

3. Some microbial agents, notably *C. diphtheriae,* cause myocardial damage by the release of a toxin. Others (i.e., protozoan or helminthetic agents) incite an allergic reaction or parasitize a myocardial fiber causing eventual rupture and intense inflammation.

4. Myocarditis may be pathologically extensive and overwhelming or focal and microscopic. Some patients may demonstrate marked clinical evidence of myocardial dysfunction and yet have relatively scant histologic changes. This clinicopathologic dissociation is most typical of rickettsial diseases but is not confined to these agents. The extensive pathological involvement of other patients correlates well with their marked clinical signs.

5. When infecting agents localize in or near the conducting system (i.e., SA node, AV node, or Purkinje fibers), they may cause disturbance in both rhythm and conduction.

6. It is important to remember that the myocardium is intimately related to the pericardium. Individuals who experience episodes of pericarditis of any etiology invariably have a concomitant myocarditis.

SYMPTOMS AND SIGNS

1. Myocardial involvement during the course of an acute infectious illness may be obvious or incidental. Constitutional symptoms of fever, malaise, and arthralgia are often present and are construed by the physician as being consistent with the primary infectious process.

2. The not infrequent complaint of precordial discomfort typical of pericar-

ditis should direct the physician's attention towards the heart. Uncommonly, pain may resemble that of angina pectoris or a myocardial infarction. Such episodes have been ascribed to "relative" coronary insufficiency from reduced cardiac output or obliterative coronary arteritis.

3. The presence of tachycardia disproportionate to the degree of fever, unexplained hypotension, symptoms of congestive failure, or disturbance in rhythm or conduction should heighten the clinical suspicion of myocarditis, particularly when these abnormalities occur during the course of an otherwise uncomplicated infectious illness. Alternatively, physiological stresses from the infectious process itself, a toxic state, or hypoxia from pulmonary involvement may produce similar abnormalities when superimposed upon clinical or subclinical coronary artery or valvular heart disease.

4. Sudden death, presumably dysrhythmic, may be the initial manifestation of myocarditis. In one series this presentation was found in approximately 10 per cent of young patients.

5. Persistent fatigue is common during convalescence from an acute infectious illness, particularly if the episode has been prolonged. However, unrecognized myocarditis may also cause similar symptoms and should be considered as a possible etiology.

6. Most often, specific symptoms directing attention towards the myocardium are absent. Under these circumstances, diagnosis usually rests upon obtaining an abnormal electrocardiogram during the course of an acute infectious illness (see below).

7. Auscultatory clues to the diagnosis include softening of the first heart sound, increased intensity of pulmonic closure, the appearance of a gallop rhythm (particularly ventricular) or a systolic murmur. The latter is most often of short to

moderate duration, ejection in shape, grade I–II/VI, localized to the cardiac apex, and caused by ventricular dilatation with consequent misalignment of the papillary muscles. This spatial distortion causes the mitral leaflets to remain open during systole and permits mitral regurgitation. At rapid heart rates, embryocardia or first and second sounds that are indistinguishable in intensity, as well as loud summation gallops, are found. Pericardial friction rubs are not infrequent.

8. Emphasis needs to be placed upon proper positioning of the patient in the left lateral decubitus position and listening in a quiet room to detect these subtle auscultatory changes.

9. The appearance of congestive heart failure in the absence of underlying coronary artery or valvular heart disease is a significant diagnostic clue. On the other hand, for reasons mentioned above (see Pathophysiology), an infectious illness in a patient with valvular or coronary insufficiency may cause an increase in the amount of existing congestive failure in the absence of myocarditis.

10. Myocarditis should be considered in patients with normal serum potassium who have increased susceptibility to rhythm disturbances with relatively small doses of digitalis.

LABORATORY FINDINGS

1. An abnormal electrocardiogram is the most useful laboratory aid in establishing the diagnosis. Changes, usually present during the first week or two of disease, are found in up to 40 per cent of patients.

2. Decreased QRS voltage, ectopic atrial or ventricular beats, tachyarrhythmias (sinus, atrial fibrillation, or paroxysmal ventricular tachycardia), conduction disturbances (1st or 2nd degree AV block or right or left bundle branch block), axis shifts (especially left anterior hemiblock), and repolarization abnormalities have all been reported with variable frequency.

3. Repolarization abnormalities seen especially in the lateral precordial leads are usually interpreted as being nonspecific. They consist of slight ST segment shifts and T wave flattening or inversion. When specifically sought, these changes have been noted in up to 75 per cent of patients.

4. There are no distinctive radiographic changes of acute myocarditis. Characteristic findings include mild to moderate cardiomegaly with or without evidence of pulmonary vascular congestion. A globular cardiac silhouette suggesting pericardial effusion should be confirmed with echocardiography.

5. Elevation in the levels of GOT, LDH, and CPK is occasionally helpful. With recent interest in isoenzymes of LDH and CPK, separation of cardiac from noncardiac enzyme elevation may be easier.

6. Viral isolation from nasopharyngeal swabs, throat washings, and/or stool should be attempted. In addition, serial serum samples obtained at 2-week intervals should be frozen and saved. Paired sera should be tested simultaneously for a fourfold titer change.

DIAGNOSIS

1. As has been mentioned above, diagnosis most often rests upon obtaining an abnormal electrocardiogram during an otherwise uncomplicated illness.

2. Signs and symptoms directing the physician's attention towards the heart have been discussed. Otherwise unexplained congestive heart failure, a gallop rhythm, or appearance of rhythm or conduction disturbances deserve reemphasis as possibly indicating myocarditis.

DIFFERENTIAL DIAGNOSIS

The differential diagnosis includes coronary artery and valvular heart disease, neurocirculatory asthenia, and pericardial disease.

1. Patients with coronary artery disease and valvular heart disease usually give a long history of cardiac decompensation. However, an acute infectious illness may potentiate subclinical disease.

2. Familiarity with a symptomatic patient's personality and a lack of ECG changes usually permits a differentiation of neurocirculatory asthenia from myocarditis.

3. Idiopathic pericarditis causes the greatest problem in differential diagnosis.

COMPLICATIONS

1. Ectopic beats are the most frequent complication. Intractable arrhythmias and complete heart block are uncommonly reported. Permanent pacing has been required because of the latter.

2. Mild to moderate cardiac decompensation is not infrequent. Less often myocarditis may be fulminant and cause death from arrhythmia or cardiac failure.

3. Confirmed persistence of acute myocarditis with the development of a chronic myocardiopathy is seemingly unusual.

MANAGEMENT

1. Congestive heart failure should be managed by the use of digitalis and diuretics, with judicious sodium and fluid restriction.

2. When necessary, antiarrhythmic agents must be used cautiously because of occasional increased drug sensitivity.

3. Bed rest is indicated in the acute stages until the quality of the heart sounds improves, signs and symptoms of congestive failure decrease, and the electrocardiogram stabilizes. Resumption of activities should be gradual, extending over a period of weeks to months, and must be individualized for each patient.

4. Corticosteroids have been shown experimentally to be harmful if administered during the early stages of disease. Their use should be reserved only for intractable cases not responding to conventional measures.

PROGNOSIS

1. In general, prognosis is good, excluding only those patients who develop conduction disturbances or persistent, smoldering myocarditis.

2. Infrequently, patients complain of continued precordial chest discomfort or experience cardiac awareness.

3. Resting electrocardiographic abnormalities often revert to normal during the first year after resolution of acute disease. In some patients, these changes may persist. Approximately 45 per cent of patients manifest T wave flattening or inversion with standing or exercise testing during follow-up. Under these circumstances, care must be taken to avoid confusion with coronary artery disease.

4. Measurements of functional work capacity and heart volume tend to remain normal during the follow-up period.

SUGGESTED READINGS

Applefeld, M. M. and Hornick, R. B.: Infective endocarditis in patients over age 60. Am. Heart J., *88*:90, 1974.

Black, S., O'Rourke, R. A. and Karliner, J. S.: Role of surgery in the treatment of primary infective endocarditis. Am. J. Med., *56*:357, 1974.

Buchbinder, N. A. and Roberts, W. C.: Left-sided valvular active infective endocarditis—a study of forty-five necropsy patients. Am. J. Med., *53*:20, 1972.

Buddington, R. S. et al.: Exercise and sudden cardiac death. Circulation, *4*:93, 1973.

Cherubin, C. E. and Neu, H. C.: Infective endocarditis at the Presbyterian Hospital in New York City from 1938–1967. Am. J. Med., *51*:83, 1971.

Dismukes, W. E. et al.: Prosthetic valve endocarditis: analysis of 38 cases. Circulation, *48*:365, 1973.

Finland, M. and Barnes, M. W.: Changing etiology of bacterial endocarditis in the antibacterial era—experiences at Boston City Hospital, 1933–1965. Ann. Int. Med., *72*:341, 1970.

Gerzen, P. et al.: Acute myocarditis—a follow up study. Br. Heart J., *34*:575, 1972.

Harvey, W. P. et al.: Symposium: Clinical Recognition and Treatment of Primary Myocardial Disease. Circulation, *32*:828, 1965.

Kilbourne, E. D., Wilson, C. B., and Perrier, D.: The induction of gross myocardial lesions by a Coxsackie virus and cortisone. J. Clin. Invest., *35*:362, 1956.

Kluge, R. M. et al.: Sources of contamination in open heart surgery. J.A.M.A., *230*:1415, 1974.

Roberts, W. C. and Buchbinder, N. A.: Right-sided valvular infective endocarditis—a clinicopathologic study of twelve necropsy patients. Am. J. Med., *53*:7, 1972.

Sande, M. A. et al.: Sustained bacteremia in patients with prosthetic cardiac valve. N. Engl. J. Med., *286*:1067, 1972.

Saphir, O.: Myocarditis. Arch. Path., *32*:1000, 1941.

Woodward, T. E. et al.: Specific microbial infections of the myocardium and pericardium. Arch. Int. Med., *120*:270, 1967.

8. DISEASES OF THE PERICARDIUM

Ralph Shabetai, M.D.

DEFINITION

Pericarditis is the term applied to any alteration of the pericardium, whether or not inflammatory; whether or not infectious. Thus, in addition to the infectious pericarditis, we have for example, myxedematous, uremic, malignant, and cholesterol pericarditis. The term *pericardiopathy* may be preferable but is not in general use.

GENERAL CONSIDERATIONS

Pericarditis may be primary, when all the clinical findings are caused by the pericarditis, dominant, when the findings of pericardial disease dominate the clinical picture of a generalized disorder, or subordinate, when the clinical findings of pericarditis are overshadowed by those of the causative illness.[15] Pericardial involvement is much more frequently recognized at autopsy than at the bedside, where it is often silent; for example, the pericardium is involved in half of all cases of rheumatoid arthritis[5] but pericardial friction rub, tamponade, or constriction—while important in individual cases—are uncommon. Pericardial effusion is found by the pathologist in most cases with congestive heart failure but its clinical recognition is the exception and not the rule.

In almost all cases of pericarditis, anticoagulants should either not be administered or should be given with great circumspection. Acute hemorrhagic pericarditis may, under the influence of anticoagulants, cause bleeding into the pericardial sac and cause cardiac tamponade. Caution is advised regarding administration of anticoagulants to patients with pericardial effusion, at least until it has been ascertained that the fluid is not sanguinious. Administration of anticoagulants to patients with cardiac tamponade secondary to rupture of the left ventricle or dissecting hematoma of the aorta mistakenly diagnosed as cardiogenic shock may well prove to be a fatal error. On the other hand, anticoagulants are not contraindicated in patients with acute myocardial infarction who develop a pericardial friction rub on the second or third day.

Uncommon pericardial diseases are not included in this chapter because of limited space. Tumors involving pericardium are discussed in Chapter 11, whereas various traumas to the pericardium are discussed in Chapter 15.

ETIOLOGY

Pericarditis may be a feature of virtually any disease: in a recent article, Spodick lists no less than 75 causes.[15]

CLASSIFICATION

Several syndromes (with a degree of overlap), listed below, may occur:

Acute pericarditis
  Without clinically significant fluid
  With fluid: tamponade
  Rapidly constricting pericarditis
Subacute pericarditis
  Effusive-constrictive pericarditis
Chronic pericarditis
  Chronic constrictive
  Chronic pericardial effusion
Relapsing or recurrent pericarditis
  With pain, rub, and fever
  With fluid: sometimes tamponade

ACUTE PERICARDITIS WITHOUT SIGNIFICANT FLUID

1. *Etiology*

The most frequent causes are infectious (viral, bacterial tuberculosis), metabolic (uremia), and drug-related (hydralazine, procainamide); pericarditis can also be idiopathic.[4]

In clinical practice, pericardial infection by a virus or the tubercle bacillus is often difficult, tedious, or impossible to prove. Thus, overlap occurs with idiopathic pericarditis.

2. *Symptoms and signs*

Symptoms of the causative disease may be absent, obscure, or dominant. Fever is usually present.

A. *Pericardial pain*

(1) Pain accompanies most cases and may vary from mild to excruciating.

(2) The pain may imitate ischemic heart pain or pleurisy, and commonly has features reminiscent of both.

(3) Thus it may be precordial and yet be aggravated by inspiration and relieved by sitting up.

(4) Characteristically, it is referred to the trapezius ridge.

(5) The nature may range from knife-like and pleuritic to squeezing anginal.

B. *Pericardial friction rub*[13]

(1) Rub may be evanescent, as in pericarditis occurring in the first few days after myocardial infarction, or may persist for many days, as in uremic pericarditis.

(2) It may be very loud and coarse, even palpable, or soft.

(3) It is a scratchy superficial sound, best appreciated with the diaphragm of the stethoscope pushed firmly against the precordium, commonly at the lower left sternal edge.

(4) It usually has three components,[14] one before the first sound, one in systole, and one in diastole, but the presystolic and/or the diastolic components may be absent.

3. *Laboratory findings*

A. Most abnormalities reflect the underlying disease.

B. The ECG shows S-T segment elevation. This is frequently present in all 3 standard limb leads and several precordial leads.

C. This distribution as well as the subsequent evolution without Q waves helps differentiate the ECG of acute pericarditis from that of early acute myocardial infarction.

D. Reciprocal S-T segment depression is usually confined to leads aVR and V_1.[16]

E. The cardiac enzymes either remain normal or increase only moderately and the time course of recovery is slower than in acute myocardial infarction.

4. *Diagnosis*

A. Chest pain should always alert the physician to the possibility of pericarditis.

B. If the typical ECG and pericardial friction rub are present, the diagnosis is assured.

C. The physician must remember that beyond the pericarditis a potentially lethal but treatable condition may be lurking.

5. *Differential diagnosis*

A. Acute myocardial infarction

B. Dissecting hematoma (aneurysm) of the aorta

C. Massive pulmonary embolism

The above are the major diseases that must be considered in the differential diagnosis of those patients who present with the sudden onset of severe chest pain. In more obscure cases, especially when the pericardial rub, or some of its components, or the classical serial ECG changes have been missed, the physician must carefully consider all the known causes of chest pain.

6. *Complications*

Any patient with acute pericarditis may suffer:

    A. Relapses

    B. Tamponade

    C. Constriction

7. *Management*

    A. Pain is managed by appropriate analgesic.

    B. The wise physician tries to control pain with the simplest effective remedy available.

    C. Some patients respond quickly to anti-inflammatory agents (e.g., indomethacin).

    D. Some patients, e.g., those with Dressler's syndrome (pericarditis in the late recovery period of myocardial infarction) and those with frequent recurrences, require steroid therapy: 60 mg. per day of prednisone or its equivalent are given initially and the dose is then rapidly tapered to the lowest that controls symptoms.

    E. Patients with frequent relapses characterized by pain, fever, and pericardial friction rub in spite of several courses of indomethacin or steroids should be considered for elective pericardiectomy.

    F. Treatment of the underlying disorder (e.g., uremia) may of itself suffice to treat pericarditis.

    G. Anticoagulants are contraindicated, as they may precipitate bleeding into the pericardial space.

8. *Prognosis*

The prognosis is that of the causative disease or, when present, the complication of constriction or tamponade.

CARDIAC TAMPONADE

1. *Definition*

    A. Pericardial fluid, including blood, exerting increased pressure around the heart and thereby impeding cardiac filling.

    B. Severe tamponade occurs when a small volume of fluid rapidly enters the pericardial sac.

    C. Much larger volumes of fluid are needed to produce tamponade when the fluid accumulates slowly.

2. *Etiology*

The common causes include:

    A. Any cause of acute pericarditis

    B. Trauma: blunt or sharp

    C. Radiation

    D. Neoplastic disease

    E. Rupture of heart or great vessel

    F. Perforation (e.g., by catheters, pacing probes)

3. *Pathophysiology* [13]

    A. The pericardial space is normally a potential one with only a few drops of fluid. Normal intrapericardial pressure is approximately the same as intrapleural pressure (minus 2–5 mm. Hg).

    B. When fluid accumulates rapidly, the pericardium fails to stretch adequately and therefore intrapericardial pressure increases often to 20 or more mm. Hg.

    C. The filling of the heart is decreased, and by Starling's Law its stroke volume falls.

    D. Thus, raised venous pressure, decreased blood pressure, and tachycardia appear.

    E. Inspiration pools a significant portion of the already reduced stroke volume in the right heart and lungs, and increases intrapericardial pressure, thus during inspiration there is a dramatic fall in blood pressure and pulse volume (pulsus paradoxus). [10]

4. *Symptoms*

    A. Depending upon the rapidity and severity, the patient's state may vary from asymptomatic to moribund.

    B. When circulatory embarrassment is severe and sudden, as after massive trauma or rupture, consciousness is decreased or lost.

    C. When the cerebral status permits, the patient may complain of dyspnea, fullness in the chest, or chest pain.

D. When there is a slow leak of blood or the gradual accumulation of pericardial effusion, considerable tamponade may develop without the patient's being aware of it.

5. *Signs*

The major physical signs are (1) raised venous pressure; (2) decreased arterial pressure; (3) pulsus paradoxus; and (4) quiet precordium.

A. *Raised venous pressure*

(1) The venous pressure may be too high to permit pulsation of the jugular veins.

(2) The raised venous pressure can best be appreciated by examining the patient in the sitting posture.

(3) When in doubt, measure the central venous pressure.

(4) In traumatic cases with copious recent blood loss, venous pressure elevation may be much less severe.

(5) Similarly in patients with chronic disease, who have received prolonged intensive diuretic therapy, the venous pressure may be considerably lowered.

B. *Decreased blood pressure*

(1) Hypotension is common in advanced cases.

(2) The blood pressure may be normal in milder cases.

C. *Pulsus paradoxus*

(1) This physical finding can be detected at the bedside. The pulse is examined while the observer notes the phase of the patient's respiration.

(2) During inspiration there is a pronounced decrease in the amplitude of the pulse.

(3) In mild cases it may be necessary to request the patient to breathe deeply and slowly in order to enhance this physical finding.

(4) In very severe cases with hypotension, the radial pulse may be

difficult to feel, and under these circumstances it is difficult to appreciate pulsus paradoxus. In such cases the sign should be sought in larger vessels (e.g., the carotid and femoral arteries).

(5) An estimate of the degree of pulsus paradoxus can be obtained with the use of an ordinary clinical sphygmomanometer. The cuff is inflated in the standard manner. Deflation must proceed slowly and evenly. The Karatkoff sounds are auscultated and the physician simultaneously observes the sphygmomanometer reading and the phase of respiration. When the Karatkoff sounds first become audible, they are heard only during inspiration. As the cuff is slowly deflated, a point is reached at which the sounds are audible throughout the respiratory cycle. The difference in sphygmomanometer readings between these two points is an estimate of pulsus paradoxus, and is expressed in mm. Hg. This estimate should be made during normal respiration because deep breathing exaggerates pulsus paradoxus.

(6) Pulsus paradoxus may be accurately measured via a needle or small catheter placed in a systemic artery and connected to a transducer recorder system.

(7) Clinical observation of the pulses to detect pulsus paradoxus and serial measurement of the blood pressure to estimate its severity; along with observations of the jugular venous pulse or measurements of the central venous pressure are the most important tools available to the clinician who is following a patient with pericardial disease for the onset of tamponade or changes in its severity.

6. *Laboratory findings*

The principal laboratory tests include: electrocardiography, chest x-ray, and echocardiography.

A. *Echocardiography*

(1) Serial echocardiography[3] de-

tects increased pericardial fluid or indirect evidence of increased intrapericardial pressure.

(2) The latter is betrayed by a pendular motion of the heart within the pericardial fluid.

B. *Electrocardiography*

(1) Serial ECG to detect decreases in QRS voltages and, more important, the development of electrical alternans.

(2) Monitor leads are inadequate for the latter purpose, as alternans may not be obvious in the monitor lead.

(3) The ECG usually shows reduced voltage.

(4) In severe cases, the patient develops electrical alternans, in which each alternate complex varies between two configurations. This phenomenon may affect P, QRS and T and may be obvious in some leads and subtle in others.[16]

C. *Chest x-ray*

(1) Serial chest roentgenograms detect changes in heart size and in the appearance of the lung fields.

(2) This method, however, suffers the severe limitations inherent in portable chest roentgenography.

(3) Chest x-ray will show slight enlargement in very acute cases and considerable enlargement when time has allowed a larger effusion of blood or fluid.

(4) The lung fields are clear. This is helpful in distinguishing tamponade from heart failure.

7. *Diagnosis*[10]

A. Cardiac tamponade should be suspected in any patient with the triad of raised jugular or central venous pressure, hypotension, or pulsus paradoxus and a quiet precordium.

B. Suspicion is heightened when there is a cause of pericardial effusion or bleeding (e.g., pericarditis, recent cardiac operation or instrumentation) and

recent myocardial infarction and when there is other evidence of pericarditis: rub, pain, or ST segment elevation.

C. Except in the most dire emergencies, the presence of pericardial fluid must be established before an attempt is made to aspirate the pericardial space.

D. Diagnosis is best accomplished by echocardiography and second best by a radioactive cardiac blood pool scan.

E. Failing the availability of these reliable noninvasive methods, the presence of pericardial fluid can be established by the injection of carbon dioxide or radio-opaque contrast material into the right atrium.

8. *Differential diagnosis*

A. True pulsus paradoxus with an inspiratory fall of systolic arterial pressure greater than 10 mm. Hg pressure and a reduced pulse pressure is almost always caused by cardiac tamponade.

B. Pulsus paradoxus may be found in constrictive pericarditis, but this is usually in subacute cases in which some pericardial fluid is present.

C. An exaggerated respiratory variation in the pulse and in systolic blood pressure is found in most patients with labored respiration due to severe airway obstruction. This phenomenon does not include an inspiratory fall in pulse pressure and, strictly speaking, is not true pulsus paradoxus.

D. Nevertheless, increased respiratory effort is the commonest cause of inspiratory drop in systolic pressure[9] and this must be ruled out before a diagnosis of pulsus paradoxus and cardiac tamponade is made.

9. *Management by pericardiocentesis*

The only treatment of cardiac tamponade is removal of the pericardial fluid with consequent reduction of the intrapericardial pressure. Fluid may be removed via a needle, cannula, or catheter, or by open drainage.

Whenever possible the procedure must be carried out by, or in the presence of, a physician experienced in the technique; otherwise fluid may not be obtained and/or complications or even death may ensue.

A. Emergency pericardiocentesis

(1) When the physician encounters a moribund patient in clinical circumstances and with physical signs compatible with cardiac tamponade, it is his duty to pass a needle into the pericardium to attempt to withdraw a portion of the blood or fluid.

(2) A long number 17 gauge needle is suitable.

(3) The pericardial sac is most safely entered from the xiphisternal area.

(4) Not all of the fluid need be removed, because following the removal of 100 or 200 ml., a dramatic improvement usually follows, which allows time for more definitive management.

B. Elective pericardiocentesis

(1) Under all other circumstances the procedure is done in a planned elective manner, perferably in the cardiac catheterization, coronary care, or operating area.

(2) The presence of pericardial fluid is unequivocally established before the procedure is begun.

(3) Full facilities for cardiopulmonary resuscitation must be on hand (see Chap. 27).

(4) Tubes and containers suitable for diagnostic specimens as well as the means to measure intrapericardial pressure must be available.

(5) A central venous catheter or a cardiac catheter, such as the Swan-Ganz, should be in place in the right atrium or pulmonary artery.

(6) Isoproterenol infusion may be given (1–4 μg./min.) to improve hemodynamics while pericardiocentesis is being prepared.

(7) Using full aseptic technique, the pericardium is punctured. The operating table should be tilted head up or the patient can be propped up on pillows. If the procedure is carried out in a properly wired and grounded room, the tapping needle is attached to an electrocardiographic monitor.[1] If the needle tip touches the epicardium, the S-T segment is elevated several millimeters above the base line, indeed the QRS-T complex may become virtually monophasic. If the S-T segment elevation appears, the needle is withdrawn until the S-T segment returns to the isolelectric line. If there is any doubt about the adequacy of the electrical wiring of the room, the operator relies on S-T segment elevation in a conventional monitor lead and on the appearance of ventricular extrasystoles to warn himself that his needle has contacted the epicardium. This is because faulty grounding can cause ventricular fibrillation when a needle attached to an electrocardiograph touches the heart. In these circumstances, no direct connection between the needle and any electrical apparatus is permissible.

(8) The xiphisternal route is preferred because it avoids accidental puncture of the coronary vessel or the pleura.

(9) The skin is anesthetized 0.5 mm. below and to one side of the tip of the xiphoid process. A skin puncture is made with a number 11 blade.

(10) Pericardiocentesis is accomplished with a needle 3 or 4 inches long, number 17 or 18T gauge. Longer needles may be required in the obese, and wider ones if pus is suspected. The needle is first directed posteriorly until it is passed posterior to the xiphoid and the costal margin, the angle is then changed to cephalad with a 15 to 30° posterior tilt.

(11) The needle is slowly but steadily advanced and simultaneously gentle aspiration is maintained on a

syringe attached to the needle and the ECG is monitored until one or more of the following occur:

(a) Blood or fluid appears in the aspirating syringe

(b) S-T segment elevation or ventricular extrasystoles occur

(c) The needle is felt to touch the beating ventricle

(12) A sensation of the thickness and character of the pericardium is usually imparted to the operator when the needle is pushed through the pericardium.

(13) Tamponade is confirmed by the forceful flow of blood or fluid from the needle.

(14) Intrapericardial pressure should be measured before an appreciable volume of fluid has been aspirated. In tamponade, the pressure is always higher than atmospheric and may be over 20 mm. Hg. In the absence of cardiac disease, intrapericardial pressure is equal to central venous or pulmonary wedge pressure. When pressure transducers and an electronic recording device are not available, intrapericardial pressure is measured with a spinal manometer attached with plastic or rubber tubing to the needle with zero at the midchest level.

(15) Pericardiocentesis can be completed via the tapping needle or cannula. Many physicians prefer to exchange the needle for a catheter. This is easily accomplished by passing a guide wire into the pericardial space through the needle, removing the needle, and passing a thin-walled catheter with multiple side holes over the guide wire into the pericardium. The pericardium is then aspirated as completely as possible, and the tube may then be left in place for a few hours to several days for completion of drainage, insufflation of air or carbon dioxide into the pericardium for negative contrast studies, or for the administra-

tion of drugs directly into the pericardial space. Strict precautions to prevent the aspiration of small volumes of air into the pericardium are not necessary, but scrupulous asepsis should be practiced, and the tube should be removed as soon as it has accomplished its purpose or as soon as it ceases to function well.

(16) Recurrence of cardiac tamponade after successful pericardiocentesis is almost always an indication for prompt surgical drainage. Pericardiocentesis may need to be repeated while preparations for the operation are being made.

PERICARDIAL FLUID WITHOUT TAMPONADE

A considerable volume of fluid can accumulate slowly in the pericardium with minimal disturbance of hemodynamics and change in intrapericardial pressure. In chronic cases, well over a liter of fluid may be present and yet the pericardial pressure may remain zero, or 2 or 3 mm. Hg.

1. *Etiology*

Almost any pericarditis may cause effusion. The commonest causes are:

A. Tuberculosis

B. Active viral or idiopathic pericarditis

C. Chronic idiopathic effusive pericarditis

D. Malignancy

2. *Diagnosis of pericardial effusion*

A. *Clinical approach*

The clinical approach to pericardial effusion pursues the following logical steps:

(1) Diagnosis of the presence and quantity of fluid

(2) Evaluation of the pathophysiological effects of the fluid

(3) Examination of the fluid

(4) Treatment

B. *Physical findings*

(1) Cardiac dullness may be percussed lateral to the apex beat.

(2) Several conditions must be met before this sign can be applied:

(a) The cardiac impulse must be palpable, and it must be possible to localize the apex beat. In many patients with pericardial effusion, the apex beat becomes impalpable.

(b) The left lung must be free of disease that could impair the percussion note, and left pleural effusion and thickening must be absent. Pulmonary infiltrates and pleural effusions are frequent in pericardial effusion of several different etiologies.

(3) A pericardial friction rub may be present in acute and subacute cases.

C. *Laboratory findings*

(1) Chest x-ray

(a) The cardiopericardial silhouette is enlarged and globular and the lung fields are clear.

(b) This finding in pericardial effusion can seldom be confidently distinguished from generalized cardiac enlargement with tricuspid incompetence.

(c) Likewise, failure of the heart shadow to decrease during the strain phase of the Valsalva maneuver is not a reliable sign.

(d) Absence of pulsations when the cardiac silhouette is observed by fluoroscopy is highly suggestive of pericardial effusion, but these pulsations may be greatly diminished in a dilated and poorly contracting heart.

(2) Electrocardiography[16]

(a) The voltage is often reduced.

(b) In acute cases, S-T segment elevation may be present.

(c) The T waves may be flat or inverted, reflecting chronic pericarditis.

(d) No pathologic Q waves are observed.

(3) Echocardiography[3]

(a) A properly damped echocardiogram unerringly detects pericardial effusion. A high-quality record on which endocardium, myocardium, epicardium, and pericardium are clearly demarcated is essential.

(b) Fluid appears as an echo-free space between the stationary pericardium and the actively contracting epicardium.

(c) Large effusions are detected over both the anterior and posterior aspects of the heart.

(d) Smaller effusions are confined to the posterior wall.

(e) The technique is exquisitely sensitive and can detect effusion of only 17 ml., far too little to tap.

(f) Meticulous technique is mandatory to avoid diagnosing pericardial effusions that are not there, and to avoid missing considerable pericardial effusion.

(4) Radioisotope angiography

(a) This technique is less often available at the bedside, but in the absence of echocardiography is a simple, dependable means for diagnosing pericardial effusion.

(b) Radionuclide is injected intravenously, and the heart blood pool is scanned.

(c) In the presence of pericardial effusion, cold areas are found between the heart and lung scans and between the liver and heart scans.

(5) Contrast studies

(a) With the patient lying on the left side, 50 to 100 ml. of carbon dioxide are injected into the right atrium via a catheter. Roentgenograms of the heart are made while the patient remains on the x-ray table with the right side up.

(b) The carbon dioxide bubble appears as a radiolucency between the fluid density of the pericardium and that of the right atrium.

(c) Alternatively, 50 ml. of contrast medium may be injected rapidly into the right atrium, whereafter a conventional motion or still film of the angiocardiogram is made. In such studies, it is noted that the catheter tip cannot be made to engage the edge of the cardiopericardial silhouette at the level of the right atrium.

(d) The contrast study shows the contrast-filled cardiac chambers separated from the edge of the cardiopericardial silhouette by the water density of pericardial effusion.

These invasive methods should seldom be necessary at the present time because of the availability of ultrasound and isotope cardiac scanning.

3. *Pathophysiological effects of pericardial fluid* have been discussed under Cardiac Tamponade (see above).

4. *Examination of pericardial fluid*

A. *Indications for pericardiocentesis*

(1) Cardiac tamponade

(2) Suspicion of pus in the pericardium

(3) Culture or tissue diagnosis

Categories (1) and (2) are absolute indications. If pus is found, subsequent management is usually open surgical drainage of the pericardium. Category (3) is a relative indication, e.g., if a patient has a known bronchogenic cardinoma and malignant cells in the pleural fluid, there is no necessity to tap the pericardial effusion to obtain a tissue diagnosis. The yield of tubercle bacillus from pericardial fluid is low.

B. *Assessment of bloody pericardial fluid*

Pericardial effusions of any etiology may be bloody, and even grossly hemorrhagic fluid does not necessarily imply malignancy or tuberculosis. On occasion, when the pericardium is tapped and the yield is at first indistinguishable from blood, the following steps may then be taken.

(1) Empty 5 ml. of the fluid onto a sponge. That the blood is dilute will often be immediately apparent.

(2) Compare the hematocrit with that of a vascular blood sample.

(3) If the patient is in the catheterization laboratory, measure the intrapericardial pressure or inject a few milliliters of contrast medium. The difference between a cardiac chamber and the pericardial space will be immediately obvious. Intrapericardial blood does not usually clot and therefore the Lee White clotting time of pericardial and venous samples can usefully be compared. It must be recalled that acute severe intrapericardial hemorrhage does clot.

5. *Treatment*

A. Tamponade is treated by aspiration.

B. Recurrent tamponade and pus are treated by open surgical drainage.

C. Recurrent pericardial effusion is often benign, but if it is accompanied by systemic signs, fever, or pain, it is best managed by steroid courses.

D. If recurrences persist, the patient benefits from elective pericardiectomy.

CONSTRICTIVE PERICARDITIS

1. *General features and definition*

A. Constrictive pericarditis is a disorder in which the pericardium is scarred and forms a rigid nonyielding encasement around the heart.

B. Classical constrictive pericarditis is a slowly developing chronic disease in which the pericardium may achieve a thickness of over 1 cm., and frequently it eventually calcifies.

C. Constrictive pericarditis may also be subacute. In these cases, constriction may occur in days, weeks, or months.

D. In some cases constriction becomes significant even when pericardial effusion and cardiac tamponade are still present. This is the syndrome of sub-acute effusive constrictive pericarditis.[6]

2. *Etiology*

Virtually any pericarditis, except rheumatic, may evolve into constrictive pericarditis. Two decades ago, the commonest cause of chronic calcific constrictive pericarditis was tuberculosis. Today, the majority of the cases are idiopathic. Some of these may be of unproven tubercular or viral etiology.

Subacute constrictive pericarditis is almost never calcific. This syndrome may occur in rheumatoid arthritis and following H influenzae infection, especially in children.[2]

The most frequently encountered causes of constrictive pericarditis include:

A. Idiopathic pericarditis
B. Tuberculous pericarditis
C. Infectious pericarditis
   (1) Viral
   (2) Bacterial
D. Malignant pericarditis
   (1) Bronchogenic carcinoma
   (2) Carcinoma of the breast
E. Collagen vascular disease
   (1) Rheumatoid arthritis
   (2) Lupus erythematosus
F. Radiation pericarditis
G. Post-traumatic pericarditis.

3. *Pathophysiology*[11]

A. The heart is surrounded by the pericardium, which becomes rigid and unable to stretch.

B. This limits the diastolic volume of the heart.

C. The cardiac volume is not limited at end systole; therefore, cardiac filling occurs rapidly during protodiastole.

D. Toward the end of the period of rapid ventricular filling, the ventricles fill to the limit prescribed by the pericardial encasement.

E. Ventricular diastolic pressure is low during the early part of rapid filling and then rapidly climbs to a plateau that is maintained throughout the remainder of diastole.

F. The venous pressure displays a prominent collapse coincident with rapid ventricular filling but this pressure is greatly elevated during the remainder of the cardiac cycle.

4. *Symptoms*

A. Fluid retention related to elevated systemic venous pressure is an early manifestation of constriction.

B. Ascites may occur early.

C. Ascites is followed by peripheral edema.

D. Patients complain of abdominal swelling, lassitude, and exertional dyspnea.

5. *Signs*

A. Greater or lesser degrees of ascites are present in the chronic cases.

B. Pitting edema may also be found.

C. The jugular venous pressure is greatly increased, and the observer is impressed by the rapid y descent of the jugular venous pulse.

D. The pulse pressure may be decreased.

E. In chronic cases, severe cachexia provides a startling contrast to the swollen abdomen and lower extremities.

F. In chronic cases, jaundice may be present because of liver congestion and/or cardiac cirrhosis.

G. Atrial fibrillation frequently supervenes in chronic cases.

H. Pulsus paradoxus may be present, but it is less common than in cardiac tamponade.

I. Cardiac examination frequently reveals a loud third heart sound, "the pericardial knock."

J. Cardiac murmurs are usually absent.

K. When subacute cases are seen early, the only clues to constriction may be a raised venous pressure in the presence of a small heart. Pulsus paradoxus frequently develops early in the course of rapidly advancing constriction. Ascites and hepatomegaly rapidly make their appearance, but the former is much less pronounced than in chronic constrictive pericarditis and is not accompanied by cachexia.

  6. *Laboratory findings*

    A. *Chest x-ray*

      (1) Chest x-ray may provide the diagnosis when the pericardium is heavily calcified.

      (2) It must by emphasized, however, that not all constrictive pericarditis is calcified and that calcification does not usually occur in the subacute stages.

      (3) Furthermore, calcification of the parietal pericardium may be found without constrictive pericarditis.

      (4) The heart is not necessarily small, particularly in chronic pericarditis in older people who may have underlying heart disease of other etiology.

      (5) The lung fields are usually clear.

    B. *Electrocardiography*[16]

      (1) The P waves may be notched in lead II and display a wide negative component in lead V_1 simulating P-mitrale.

      (2) The QRS voltage is low and the T waves are flattened or inverted: an indication of chronic pericarditis.

      (3) Atrial fibrillation is common in long-standing chronic constrictive pericarditis.

      (4) In some cases, conduction disturbances and Q waves are found due to involvement of the myocardium, conduction system, and coronary vessels in the scarring process.[8]

    C. *Liver function studies*

      (1) Hepatic function is frequently impaired, either by severe congestion or following the development of cardiac cirrhosis.

      (2) Plasma albumin is depressed, and this may be worsened by protein-losing enteropathy.

      (3) Laboratory evidence of hepatic insufficiency varies from mild to extreme.

    D. *Other findings*

    Many laboratory values may be abnormal, depending upon the etiology of chronic pericarditis (e.g., the peripheral blood smear or bone marrow in lymphoma and leukemia and the plasma proteins in rheumatoid arthritis and lupus).

  7. *Diagnosis*

    A. Constrictive pericarditis may be suspected in any patient with a raised venous pressure who does not have cardiac disease.

    B. The absence of cardiac disease is suggested by increased venous pressure without cardiomegaly or cardiac murmur and in the absence of evidence of hypertension, coronary artery disease, or rheumatic heart disease.

    C. In any case in which the jugular venous pressure is increased, edema and ascites should be ascribed, until disproven, to be due either to cardiac or pericardial disease. When the physician has trained himself to a high index of suspicion for the latter, he will not often miss the diagnosis of constrictive pericarditis.

    D. Edema and ascites in the presence of a normal venous pressure are usually of neither cardiac nor pericardial origin.

    E. When in doubt, the central venous pressure should be measured.

    F. Some patients with chronic constrictive pericarditis have been erroneously diagnosed as cirrhosis of the liver. This error is made because the patients present with massive anasarca together with both clinical and laboratory evidence of hepatic insufficiency. Sometimes this diagnosis has been maintained even after liver biopsy when the pathologist fails to distinguish true cirrhosis from cardiac cirrhosis. This diagnostic error can be avoided by the physician who remembers that the central venous pressure is normal in cirrhosis of the liver.

G. The diagnosis of constrictive pericarditis may be rapidly confirmed by cardiac catheterization, which confirms the absence of myocardial and valvular disease and demonstrates restriction of ventricular filling by the constricting pericardium.[11]

8. *Prognosis*

A. Unrelieved constrictive pericarditis leads to progressive congestion of the systemic tissues.

B. The liver bears the brunt of this congestion, and hepatic coma is the terminal event in some patients. The patients eventually succumb to hepatic failure.

C. The lungs, although subject to a high venous pressure, are protected from flooding because of involvement of the right ventricle in the pericardial scar.

9. *Treatment*

A. As soon as the diagnosis of constrictive pericarditis is established, the patient should be subjected to resection of the pericardium.[12] The earlier this operation is performed, the lower the mortality and the greater the benefit.

B. In early cases, the surgeon can easily develop a plane between the myocardium and the constricting pericardium, and the operation is accomplished quickly and easily.

C. In advanced cases, especially those with heavy calcification, the operation proceeds slowly as the surgeons meticulously remove the pericardium bit by bit with the ever present risk of lacerating a cardiac chamber or great vessel.

D. In good hands and with the availability of "pump stand-by," the mortality rate is virtually zero in early cases and less then 10 per cent in well established cases. In severe, long-standing heavily calcified cases, the risk is still high but is much less than the 40 per cent quoted in the literature of 20 years ago.

REFERENCES

1. Bishop, L. H., Estes, E. H., and McIntosh, H. D.: The electrocardiogram as a safeguard in pericardiocentesis. J.A.M.A., *162*:264, 1956.
2. Caird, R., Conway, N., and McMillan, I. K. R.: Purulent pericarditis followed by early constriction in young children. Br. Heart J., *35*:201, 1973.
3. Feigenbaum, H., Waldhausen, J. A., and Slyde, L. P.: Ultrasound diagnosis of pericardial effusion. J.A.M.A., *191*:711, 1965.
4. Fowler, N. O., and Manitsas, G. T.: Infectious pericarditis. Prog. Cardiovasc. Dis., *16*:323, 1973.
5. Franco, E. A., Levine, H. D., and Hall, A. P.: Rheumatoid pericarditis. Ann. Int. Med., *77*:837, 1972.
6. Hancock, E. W.: Subacute effusive constrictive pericarditis. Circulation, *43*:183, 1971.
7. Kriss, J. P.: Diagnosis of pericardial effusion by radioisotope angiography J. Nucl. Med., *10*:233, 1969.
8. Levine, H. D.: Myocardial fibrosis in constrictive pericarditis. Electrocardiographic and pathological observations. Circulation, *48*:1268, 1973.
9. Rebuck, A. S., and Pengelly, D. L.: Development of Pulsus Paradoxus in the presence of airways obstruction. N. Engl. J. Med., *288*:2, 1973.
10. Shabetai, R. et al.: Pulsus paradoxus. J. Clin. Invest., *44*:1882, 1965.
11. Shabetai, R., Fowler, N. O., and Guntheroth, W. G.: The hemodynamics of cardiac tamponade and constrictive pericarditis. Am. J. Cardiol., *26*:480, 1970.
12. Somerville, W.: Constrictive pericarditis with special reference to the change in natural history brought about by surgical intervention. Circulation, *37, 38* [Supp.], 1968.
13. Spodick, D. H.: Pericardial friction. N. Engl. J. Med., *278*:1204, 1968.
14. ———Acoustic phenomena in pericardial disease. Am. Heart J., *81*:114, 1971.
15. ———Differential diagnosis of acute pericarditis. Prog. Cardiovasc. Dis., *14*:193, 1971.
16. Surawicz, B., and Lassiter, K. C.: Electrocardiogram in pericarditis. Am. J. Cardiol., *26*:471, 1970.

9. CARDIOMYOPATHIES

John F. Goodwin, M.D.

DEFINITIONS

1. Cardiomyopathy: heart muscle disease of unknown cause
2. Rare specific heart muscle disease: a disorder of heart muscle arising secondary to disease elsewhere in the body

GENERAL CONSIDERATIONS

The term cardiomyopathy literally means disease of the *heart muscle* as opposed to endocardial, valvular, coronary or hypertensive heart disease. The term *myocardiopathy* has been suggested as being more accurate and preferable, but *cardiomyopathy* now has a firm place in medical nomenclature and will be retained for the purpose of this chapter. It indicates essentially a group of diseases of unknown etiology. Much confusion has been caused by including within the definition of the cardiomyopathies numerous diseases in which the myocardium is involved only as part of disease elsewhere in the heart or in other organs. Examples of confusion are: "rheumatic cardiomyopathy," "thyroid cardiomyopathy," "ischemic cardiomyopathy," and many others. There are of course, important heart muscle diseases arising from disorders which essentially involve other organs. The term *ischemic* or *coronary* cardiomyopathy sometimes is used to describe patients with coronary artery disease in whom heart failure, with diffuse impairment of myocardial function, dominates, replaces, and obscures the usual symptoms of angina and infarction. While useful in emphasizing the myocardial disorder resulting from ischemia, the term is liable to misinterpretation and liable to cause confusion. A striking feature of all true car-diomyopathies is the smooth, regular, unobstructed nature of the coronary arteries, which may actually appear wider than expected. Indeed, hypertrophic cardiomyopathy without obstruction is one of the subgroups of the syndrome, angina with normal coronary arteries.

ETIOLOGY

1. Cardiomyopathy: unknown cause
2. Rare specific heart muscle disease: various systemic diseases (see Table 9-1)

PATHOPHYSIOLOGY

1. *Cardiomyopathy*

A. *Hypertrophic obstructive cardiomyopathy**

(1) Hypertrophic obstructive cardiomyopathy is manifested by massive hypertrophy of the ventricles (mainly the left) with a dominant bulge in the septum; obstruction to outflow from the left ventricle (and not infrequently from the right ventricle) is present in about 80 per cent of patients, though sometimes only on provocation.

(2) The main features are resistance to filling of the hypertrophied, fibrotic, turgid, and stiff left ventricle.

(3) The electron-microscopic lesions of the disease (abnormally oriented and greatly hypertrophied muscle fibers) are found mainly in the septum in patients with marked obstruction but are spread more widely throughout the heart in many patients without obstruction, supporting the suggestion that obstruc-

*It will be noted that hypertrophic obstructive cardiomyopathy, restrictive cardiomyopathy and obliterative cardiomyopathy all have an element of impairment of ventricular filling due in each case to different causes.

***Table 9-1.* Physical Signs in Hypertrophic Obstructive Cardiomyopathy and Their Causes**

	Sign	*Cause*
With outflow tract obstruction	Abrupt, jerky arterial pulse	Powerful contraction of L.V. Sudden onset of outflow gradient after onset of systole causes abrupt collapse of pulse wave.
Major signs	L.V. thrust Palpable atrial beat } cardiac impulse	Powerful contraction of hypertrophied L.V. Powerful contraction of L.A. needed to fill stiff L.V.
	Systolic murmur	L.V. outflow obstruction and mitral regurgitation
	a wave in J.V.P.	Bulging of ventricular septum into R.V.
Minor signs	3rd heart sound	Abnormal papillary muscle tension
	Mid-diastolic murmur	Slow filling of stiff L.V.
Without outflow tract obstruction (No murmur. Other signs less impressive than with obstruction.)	Accentuated pulmonary valve closure	Pulmonary hypertension secondary to high left ventricular end diastolic pressure

tion is associated with a more localized form of the disease. Light microscopy reveals circular collections of whorls of grossly hypertrophied, short, muscle fibers interlaced by fibrous tissue. The abnormal "criss-cross" or lattice arrangement of the myofibrils seen on electron microscopy is thought to account for the irregular contraction and relaxation that occurs and, when found in association with the characteristic light-microscopic features, is probably diagnostic of the disease, although the ultrastructural features have been described in other forms of severe ventricular hypertrophy.

(4) Mitral regurgitation is invariable when obstruction is present but it may be slight. The systolic gradient is produced by apposition of the hypertrophied septum to the anterior mitral valve apparatus. Secondary changes in the mitral valve due to turbulence, infection, or calcification, leading to severe valve damage and further mitral regurgitation, may occur.

(5) Hypertrophic cardiomyopathy is essentially a disorder of diastolic stiffness or compliance and resistance to ventricular filling. Only in the late stages when the disease has become widespread throughout the myocardium does contractile failure develop, and at this stage there is usually no outflow tract obstruction. The left ventricular cavity is unduly small at the end of systole, giving a reduced left ventricular end diastolic volume. This is an important feature of the disease and is emphasized by the massive hypertrophy, giving a "small-cavity/large-muscle" disorder. In the late stages, contractile failure is added to diastolic failure.

B. *Congestive cardiomyopathy*

This condition presents a completely different picture from hypertrophic obstructive cardiomyopathy.

(1) The heart is dilated, the muscle flabby rather than stiff, and while there is no impediment to ventricular filling, there is gross impairment of contractile function.

(2) Hypertrophy, which does occur as a result of dilatation and heart failure, is much less marked than in hypertrophic obstructive cardiomyopathy.

(3) The heart is overweight, pale, and patchy fibrosis and cellular necrosis are present.

(4) The coronary arteries are normal, as are the valves.

(5) There may be antemortem endocardial thrombi, and endocardial fibrosis may result from long-standing heart failure.

(6) The striking excess of dilatation over hypertrophy and the better prognosis of patients with greater hypertrophy has prompted the suggestion that the mechanism (but not necessarily the cause) of pump failure is inhibition of the usual appropriate degree of compensatory hypertrophy.

(7) *Possible causes, associated conditions, or risk factors*

Essentially, congestive cardiomyopathy is a syndrome of heart pump failure of unknown cause and probably represents the end stage of many different diseases. There is no underlying heart disease, toxic factor, or general system disease to be found. Possible causes, associated conditions, or risk factors are: pregnancy and the puerperium, alcohol, systemic hypertension, and virus infections.

(a) *Peripartal cardiomyopathy*

Congestive cardiomyopathy occurring in the third trimester of pregnancy or in the puerperium, especially in underprivileged multiparous women, has been well documented. The cause is unknown, but it has been postulated that multiple causative factors may have summated to produce cardiac damage.

(b) *Alcoholic cardiomyopathy*

This is an extremely difficult entity to define, as there are no diagnostic features other than the intake of alcohol in sufficient quantity, with improvement on withdrawal and recurrence on resumption of alcohol intake. The picture is essentially one typical of congestive cardiomyopathy. It is usually agreed that large quantities of alcohol (beer or spirits or both) are necessary to cause it, but in some cases relatively modest amounts of alcohol may damage further a heart already compromised by some other factor, possibly infective.

(c) *Viruses and the heart*

Acute virus infections of the heart are well documented and may involve pericardium and myocardium. It has even been suggested that they can involve the endocardium and cause valvular disease. The vast majority of viral infections of the heart appear to resolve completely. The commonest viruses to be involved are probably those of the Coxsackie-B group. The crucial question is whether and how often acute virus myocarditis leads to chronic congestive cardiomyopathy. There are a few documented cases, but in general, the evidence is lacking, though the presentation of many patients with congestive cardiomyopathy and an apparent upper respiratory infection encourages the idea that an infective process may have initiated the disease. Intuitively the concept is attractive, and the evidence for and against virus infection as a cause of congestive cardiomyopathy has been summarized recently.

(d) *Systemic hypertension and congestive cardiomyopathy*

It has been argued that congestive cardiomyopathy may represent an unusual response to hypertensive heart failure in which ventricular dilatation and cardiac failure replace the usual progressive hypertrophy. Support for this view has come from West Africa, where Brockington and Edington have noted heart failure with normal blood pressure and dilated left ventricle in patients who were previously hypertensive. An abnormal response to hypertension may well be the cause in some patients with congestive cardiomyopathy but it is unlikely to be so in the majority who do not have hypertension at any time during the course of their disease.

C. *Obliterative cardiomyopathy*[*]

(1) The term is used to describe conditions in which endocardial fibrosis obliterates the ventricles, producing also a restrictive effect.

(2) *The two known causes of obliterative cardiomyopathy are:* endomyocardial fibrosis (EMF) of tropical humid zones and Loeffler's eosinophilic cardiomyopathy, respectively.

(a) In the latter condition, the heart condition may be packed with masses of eosinophils, which appear to damage the endocardium of the left ventricle and impair its function.

(b) Loeffler's disorder may be due in some cases to eosinophilic leukemia or perhaps to the condition known as the *hypereosinophilic syndrome*.

(c) In these conditions there is usually a profuse blood eosinophilia, whereas the eosinophil count is usually only slightly raised in EMF, in which the endocardial obliteration is due not to masses of eosinphils but to fibrous tissue and thrombus.

(d) Emboli are common, and when the right side of the heart is involved by endomyocardial fibrosis, the right ventricle may be completely obliterated and its function replaced by that of the right atrium.

(e) The obliteration essentially involves the apex and inflow tract of the right ventricle and the posterior cusp of the tricuspid valve.

(f) The clinical picture closely resembles constrictive pericarditis, and a pericardial effusion may be present.

(g) When the disease involves the left side of the heart, the body of the left ventricle is involved, as in the posterior cusp of the mitral valve, the anterior being spared.

(h) It has been suggested that

Loeffler's disease is the temperate zone's equivalent of endomyocardial fibrosis, but this view should not be accepted without reservation.

D. *Restrictive cardiomyopathy*[*]

(1) This condition is very rare.

(2) It produces the same hemodynamic effects as constrictive pericarditis with the following differences:

(a) The early diastolic pressure in the ventricles are usually above zero.

(b) The end-diastolic pressures in both ventricles usually differ from each other.

(c) There may be pulmonary hypertension, and the function of the left ventricle is usually impaired.

(3) The condition is produced by infiltration or fibrosis of the myocardium, which restricts the capacity of the ventricle to dilate and thus impairs filling. There is often endocardial thickening also.

(4) The commonest cause is amyloid disease of the heart, with glossy amyloid deposits making the heart rigid and stiff. Chew et al. have defined the characteristics of primary amyloid heart disease and have shown poor contractile function and reduced distensibility of the left ventricle; both early and end diastolic pressures are elevated, the ratio of change in pressure to change in volume is increased. The ventricles fill slowly throughout diastole.

(5) Because of the involvement of small coronary vessels, cardiac pain is common.

(6) Ziady et al. have described a small series of patients with impaired diastolic filling of the left ventricle, abnormal pressure/volume relationships

---

[*]It will be noted that hypertrophic obstructive cardiomyopathy, restrictive cardiomyopathy and obliterative cardiomyopathy all have an element of impairment of ventricular filling due in each case to different causes.

with rapid early filling and slow late filling. Unlike amyloid disease, the pump function of the left ventricle remains good and cardiac enlargement is not a feature.

E. *Cardiomyopathy with less clear-cut forms*

In addition to the four pathophysiological types of cardiomyopathy, there are two less clear-cut forms.

(1) The anginal type

(a) The anginal type (angina with normal coronary arteries) includes some patients with hypertrophic obstructive cardiomyopathy who do not have outflow tract obstruction.

(b) In other cases without hypertrophic obstructive cardiomyopathy, left ventricular dyskinesia may occur and the anginal pain is produced by ischemia of the heart muscle without obvious coronary artery disease.

(c) Evidence of myocardial ischemia (shown by left ventricular dyskinesia in the presence of pain) is required for the diagnosis.

(d) The general definition of ''angina with normal coronary arteries'' probably includes many different conditions, including noncardiac types of pain, neurosis, or hyperventilation syndrome.

(e) In patients where ischemia appears undoubted, a number of causes have been suggested, such as coronary artery spasm, arteriolar disease, a metabolic fault, or abnormal oxygen dissociation.

(2) An ''arrhythmic'' type

(a) An ''arrhythmic'' type of cardiomyopathy, in which multiple arrhythmias cause progressive cardiac enlargement and heart failure, has been suggested.

(b) It is doubtful whether this type can really be defined as an entity.

(c) Specific heart muscle disease such as sarcoidosis should be suspected in any patient with frequent arrhythmias or a conduction defect of unknown cause.

2. *Specific heart muscle disease*

Most specific heart muscle diseases produce a congestive type of cardiomyopathy with a dilated heart and pump failure leading to congestive heart failure.

A. *Glycogen storage disease and Friedreich's ataxia*

(1) Exceptions are the glycogen storage diseases, which may produce a hypertrophic type, simulating hypertrophic obstructive cardiomyopathy, and Friedreich's ataxia, which has features in common with hypertrophic obstructive cardiomyopathy, such as marked ventricular hypertrophy and outflow tract gradients.

(2) There is, however, disease of some of the small coronary arteries in a proportion of patients with Friedreich's disease that has not so far been found in hypertrophic obstructive cardiomyopathy.

B. *Peripheral neuromuscular disorders*

The peripheral neuromuscular disorders commonly cause conduction defects and progressive fibrosis of the ventricles, leading to congestive cardiomyopathy and arrhythmias.

C. *Amyloid heart disease*

Amyloid heart disease produces a restrictive form of cardiomyopathy and when occurring in isolation without associated disease elsewhere (such as lymphoma) should be classified as a ''primary cardiomyopathy.''

D. *Diabetes mellitus*

Cardiomyopathy in diabetes mellitus is difficult to delineate, owing to the common association of diabetes with atherosclerotic disease of the major coronary arteries, but a cardiomyopathy has been said to be due to small coronary vascular occlusion.

E. *Acromegaly*

(1) Similarly, the cardiomyopathy of acromegaly is hard to define in view of the frequency of associated hypertension and coronary atherosclerosis, but personal experience has documented severe congestive cardiomyopathy in acromegalic patients who had no evidence of hypertension or coronary disease.

(2) Improvement does not usually occur even when the acromegaly is successfully treated.

F. *Sarcoid heart disease*

Sarcoid heart disease has recently been reassessed by Ghosh et al., who reemphasized that heart failure, unsuspected arrhythmia, and even cardiac aneurysm can occur.

G. *Hemochromatosis*

(1) Hemochromatosis is an extremely rare cause of cardiomyopathy and usually produces a congestive type of syndrome.

(2) The heart muscle is heavily infiltrated with iron and there is associated fibrosis.

H. *Connective tissue disease*

(1) Specific heart muscle disease with eosinophilia may occur in association with connective tissue diseases such as polyarteritis nodosa.

(2) Cardiac involvement in systemic lupus erythomatosus is well known and usually affects the pericardium, though valvular lesions may occur.

(3) Myocardial sclerosis in diffuse systemic sclerosis produces conduction defects and eventually left heart failure, but right heart failure may result from pulmonary hypertension due to obliterative changes in the pulmonary arterioles and pulmonary fibrosis producing cor pulmonale.

I. *Drugs*

(1) Drugs, such as tricyclic depressants, may cause arrhythmias, as may anesthetics such as chloroform, cyclopropane or halothane.

(2) Daunorubicin can cause fatal cardiac damage (see list below).

Causes of Rare Specific Heart Muscle Disease

INFECTIVE
  Bacterial (diphtheria toxin)
  Protozoal (Schistosoma origin - Chaga's disease)
  Immune response (rheumatic fever)
  Giant cell (Fidler's) myocarditis? (see below)
METABOLIC
  Endocrine
    Thyrotoxic
    Hypothyroidism
    Adrenal cortical deficiency *Addisons*
    Pheochromocytoma *—Tumour*
    Acromegaly *— giant Tumour pituitary?*
    Diabetes mellitus
  Familial Storage Disorders & Infiltrations
    Haemochromatosis *Fett*
    Glycogen storage disease
    Hurler's syndrome (gargoylism)
  Deficiency
    Beri-Beri
  Amyloid
    Myelomatosis
    Paraproteinaemia
    Familial Mediterranean fever
    Chronic sepsis
    Senile
  Carcinoid
  Cancer
HEREDO-FAMILIAL NEUROMUSCULAR DISORDERS
  Muscular Dystrophies
    Pseudohypertrophic
    Limb girdle
    Facio-scapulo-humoral *♂ can't relax Post contract.*
    Dystrophia myotonica —
  Cerebellar Dystrophies
    Friedreich's ataxia
GENERAL SYSTEM DISEASES
  Connective Tissue Disorders
    Systemic lupus
    Polyarteritis nodosa
    Rheumatoid arthritis
    Scleroderma
    Dermatomyositis
  Infiltrations and Granulomata
    Sarcoidosis
    Leukaemia
    Giant cell (Fidler's) myocarditis
    (possibly infective in origin)

SENSITIVITY
  Sulphonamides
  Penicillin - ?
TOXIC
  Antimony
  Cobalt
  Emetine
  Alcohol
  Isoprenalin
  Daunorubicin
  Radiation fibrosis

CLASSIFICATION

1. *Cardiomyopathy*

Cardiomyopathy is classified into four main types based on disordered physiology and pathology.

  A. *Hypertrophic with or without obstruction* (hypertrophic obstructive cardiomyopathy [HOCM]; idiopathic hypertrophic subaortic stenosis [IHSS]; asymmetric hypertrophy of the septum [ASH])

    (1) Hypertrophic cardiomyopathy is characterized by a systolic pressure gradient across the outflow tract of the left ventricle in the majority of patients, who have a pronounced degree of hypertrophy in the region of the septum.

    (2) The stiff, greatly hypertrophied ventricle, is resistant to filling, but there is good contractile function.

  B. *Congestive (COCM)*

This type is characterized by moderate hypertrophy, marked ventricular dilatation, and poor contractile function. There is no diastolic fault.

  C. *Obliterative*

    (1) There is obliteration of the ventricular cavity by fibrous tissue and thrombus, producing both obliterative and restrictive features.

    (2) The commonest form of obliterative cardiomyopathy is endomyocardial fibrosis of humid tropical zones in which there is essentially obliteration of the inflow tracts to both ventricles.

    (3) Another type is Loeffler's eosinophilic cardiomyopathy.

  D. *Restrictive*

    (1) This type is characterized by restriction to filling, which may be accompanied by good contractile function, though sometimes this is impaired.

    (2) Restrictive cardiomyopathy resembles constrictive pericarditis in its hemodynamics.

2. *Rare specific heart muscle disease*

Nearly all specific heart muscle diseases produce a congestive type of cardiomyopathy, with the exception of amyloid disease, which produces a restrictive type with impaired contractile function of the left ventricle.

SYMPTOMS AND SIGNS

1. *Cardiomyopathy*

  A. *Hypertrophic obstructive cardiomyopathy*

    (1) *Symptoms**

      (a) *Dyspnea on exertion*

The commonest symptom is dyspnea on exertion, which is usually mild but occasionally severe.

      (b) Anginal pain

        (i) Anginal pain, usually on effort and relieved by rest, but occasionally occurring in protracted attacks at rest, is well known.

        (ii) Angina is due to disproportion between supply and demand of the hypertrophied ventricle and perhaps to interference with intramural subendocardial blood supply by the abnormal contraction and relaxation.

---

*These symptoms can be related to the abnormal hemodynamics, the most important being the difficulty in filling the stiff left ventricle, which leads to elevated filling pressure and pulmonary venous hypertension. Tachycardia, by decreasing the time available for filling, exacerbates the difficulty and may precipitate syncope or pulmonary edema. Loss of the atrial drive necessary to fill the ventricle may lead to a catastrophic fall in cardiac output or to pulmonary edema.

There is a family history in many cases.

(c) Dizziness, light-headedness and syncope:

(i) Dizziness, light-headedness, and severe syncope, usually but not always on effort, are common.

(ii) Syncope may be due to a sudden fall in cardiac output secondary to rapid reduction in ventricular filling, or less frequently, to outflow tract obstruction.

(iii) Arrhythmia, such as atrial fibrillation or ventricular tachycardia, may be implicated.

(iv) When there is evidence of pre-excitation, atrial fibrillation can lead to instant ventricular fibrillation and this may be the mechanism of sudden death in some patients (see list below).

(2) *Signs*

There are *three major signs,* which permit diagnosis at the bedside. The following signs are due to the rapid powerful contraction of the left ventricle.

Symptoms in Hypertrophic Obstructive Cardiomyopathy and Their Causes

Dyspnea
  High left ventricular end-diastolic pressure; increased on exercise, leading to pulmonary venous hypertension
Angina
  Disproportionate demand for oxygen of hypertrophied muscle
  Possibly, compression of small intramural coronary arteries in the sub-endocardium and reduction of coronary flow by impaired ventricular relaxation
Dizziness and Syncope
  Impaired left ventricular filling, worsened by tachycardia, causing fall in cardiac output
  Arrhythmia
  Outflow tract obstruction (less frequently)
Palpitations
  Arrhythmia: ectopic, paroxysmal atrial fibrillation, ventricular tachycardia, re-entry rhythms (?)
Sudden Death
  Abrupt halt to filling of left ventricle }
  Atrial fibrillation } ventricular fibrillation
  Pulmonary edema

(a) *Abrupt jerky pulse*

(i) the first sign is the abrupt jerky pulse, which is of normal volume but collapsing in quality.

(ii) The rhythm is usually regular and it is uncommon to find ectopic beats on clinical examination.

(iii) The onset of the outflow tract obstruction that occurs after the onset of systole causes the abrupt collapse of the pulse.

(b) *Localized thrust*

(i) The second sign is the powerful localized thrust of the hypertrophied left ventricle, which is preceded by an atrial beat.

(ii) The double impulse is best detected with the patient turned into the left lateral position.

(iii) The palpable atrial beat indicates the forceful contraction of the left atrium required to fill the stiff ventricle.

(c) *Ejection systolic murmur*

(i) The third sign is the characteristic ejection systolic murmur, which is heard at the left sternal edge (over the ventricular septum) and at the apex.

(ii) The murmur starts abruptly after the first sound, there being a short gap in early systole.

(iii) The murmur is due both to outflow tract obstruction and to the mitral regurgitation which is inseparable from it.

(iv) The murmur can be intensified by maneuvers that decrease the volume of the left ventricle, such as inhalation of amyl nitrite, squatting, or the Valsalva maneuver.

(v) Elevation of peripheral vascular resistance, which increases left ventricular afterload and thus left ventricular volume, will cause the murmur to disappear or diminish. Phenylephrine is a useful vasoconstrictor for this purpose.

(d) *Minor signs* that are not always present are:

(i) An early diastolic or third heart sound due to abnormal function of the papillary muscles of the mitral valve

(ii) A prominent "A" wave in the jugular venous pulse when the massive septum bulges into the right ventricle

(iii) A diastolic rumbling murmur of the apex due to abnormal filling of the stiff left ventricle

(iv) A fourth heart sound is usually present but is often too low-pitched for audibility.

When there is no obstruction to outflow, the diagnosis is much more difficult. The arterial pulse, although still jerky, is less impressive; there may be no murmur, and the suspicion of the diagnosis rests on the character of the arterial pulse and the powerful atrial beat. The elevated left atrial pressure may on occasion cause reactive pulmonary arteriolar vasoconstriction and this sign of pulmonary hypertension may dominate the clinical picture. Sometimes, a murmur may be brought out by squatting, the Valsalva maneuver or amyl nitrite inhalation (see Table 9-1).

The general physical condition of patients with hypertrophic obstructive cardiomyopathy is usually excellent, and they are often physically active people who are emotionally as well as physically well developed.

B. *Congestive cardiomyopathy*

(1) *Symptoms* are essentially those of congestive heart failure.

(a) Usually the first manifestation is dyspnea on effort or at night, preceded by orthopnea or an irritating nocturnal dry cough due to left ventricular insufficiency.

(b) Right heart failure may follow shortly. Edema of the ankles, tenderness over the right hypochondrium due to hepatic enlargement and undue fatigue due to low cardiac output are often features.

(c) The history is frequently short and of a few weeks duration though it may not be clear in every patient how long there has been cardiac involvement without obvious symptoms.

(d) Occasionally patients may admit on direct questioning to a longer period of feeling unwell or being excessively tired, presumably as a result of a low cardiac output.

(e) Cardiac pain occurs in a small proportion of patients; perhaps 10 per cent.

(f) Syncope is unusual and may be due to pulmonary embolism.

(2) *Signs*

The clinical signs are, as to be expected, those of heart failure.

(a) Vital signs:

(i) The systemic blood pressure is usually normal but may be elevated in 10 to 15 per cent of patients either as a result of heart failure or as a result of previous hypertension.

(ii) Atrial fibrillation is present in about 20 per cent of patients.

(b) Inspection and palpation

(i) The low cardiac output is manifest by cold extremities with peripheral cyanosis and arterial pulse of small volume with sinus tachycardia at rest.

(ii) The jugular venous pressure is elevated, commonly showing a prominent systolic wave due to tricuspid regurgitation resulting from right ventricular dilatation.

(iii) The cardiac impulse reveals left ventricular enlargement and a poor-quality thrust, suggesting weak muscle.

(iv) There may be a diffuse lifting impulse at the left sternal edge due to right ventricular enlargement.

(v) A palpable gallop rhythm may be found.

(vi) When right ventricular failure is present, there is peripheral edema and hepatomegaly.

(c) Auscultation

(i) On auscultation there is always a gallop rhythm, and usually a third heart sound due to rapid filling of the dilated failing left ventricle and often a fourth heart sound due to the elevated left ventricular end-diastolic pressure. A summation gallop is therefore common, produced by the fusion of third and fourth heart sounds in mid-diastole when there is tachycardia.

(ii) There may be pansystolic murmurs of mitral and tricuspid regurgitation, but these are seldom loud and usually of grade 1 or 2 (of 4) in intensity.

(iii) Pulmonary valve closure is usually slightly accentuated, and

(iv) There may be crepitations at the bases of the lungs due to pulmonary edema, and sometimes pleural effusions.

(v) Less severe degrees of congestive cardiomyopathy may produce only signs of cardiac enlargement and gallop rhythm.

(d) Pericardial involvement

(i) A pericardial effusion may be present as a result of severe congestive heart failure.

(ii) A pericardial friction rub is unusual and its presence points to one of the specific heart muscle diseases, such as systemic lupus erythomatosus.

(e) Thromboembolic phenomenon:

(i) Complications, such as pulmonary embolism or infarction, produce the appropriate signs and may exaggerate the right heart failure.

(ii) Systemic embolism may occur (usually in the presence of atrial fibrillation) and the sudden development of signs of ischemia of any organ are probably due to this cause.

C. *Obliterative cardiomyopathy*

(1) *Endomyocardial fibrosis*

(a) *Symptoms* depend on the site of cardiac involvement.

(i) When the right heart is involved there is fatigue and swelling of the legs and abdomen and often of the face.

(ii) There may be faintness on sitting up or on effort due to a very low fixed cardiac output.

(iii) Atrial fibrillation may cause palpitations.

(iv) When the left heart is involved, there is dyspnea on effort and orthopnea.

(v) Pulmonary edema may occur as a result of mitral regurgitation and damage to the left ventricular muscle.

(vi) Systemic embolism is well known.

(b) *Signs*

(i) *Right-sided endomyocardial fibrosis*

The physical signs of right-sided endomyocardial fibrosis mimic constrictive pericarditis.

(A) There is marked elevation of the jugular venous pulse with a "dip and plateau" pattern due to the sharp x and y descents, although the x descent may be partly obliterated by tricuspid regurgitation.

(B) The cardiac impulse is difficult to feel and the heart sounds may be distant.

(C) A third heart sound is heard.

(D) There may be a soft systolic murmur of tricuspid regurgitation at the lower left sternal edge.

(E) Paradox of the arterial pulse (waning on inspiration) and of the venous pulse (increase in the pressure on expiration) are due to the restrictive effects of the disorder and the pericardial effusion that is often present.

(F) Very occasionally a pericardial friction rub may be heard.

(G) In severely affected patients there is dense ascites and hepatomegaly.

(H) There may be edema of the face, and proptosis is well recognized but edema of the legs may not be marked.

(ii) *Left-sided endomyocardial fibrosis*

In left-sided endomyocardial fibrosis the signs are those of left heart failure and mitral regurgitation.

(A) The apical systolic murmur usually dies away before the second sound as the unaffected anterior cusp of the mitral valve cuts off the reflux at the end of systole.

(B) A third sound and a short mitral diastolic flow murmur are usual.

(2) *Loeffler's cardiomyopathy*

(a) *Symptoms* are usually those of heart failure.

(b) *Signs*

The signs suggest left ventricular disease, and there may be a restrictive picture resembling constrictive pericarditis. Systemic embolism is common.

D. *Restrictive cardiomyopathy*

(1) *Symptoms* are usually those of a low cardiac output:

(a) Fatigue and dizziness on effort, to which dyspnea and swelling of the face may be added

(b) Chest pain is common in amyloid restrictive cardiomyopathy in which there is severe impairment of contractile function.

(c) When restrictive cardiomyopathy is not due to amyloid or other cardiac infiltration, there may be few symptoms because pump function remains good.

(2) *Signs* are those of restriction to ventricular filling:

(a) The jugular venous pressure is raised, the *a* and *v* waves are prominent, and the *x* and *y* descents (particularly the *y* descent) are steep.

(b) The venous pressure may rise on inspiration.

(c) The cardiac impulse may be unimpressive.

(d) There is a third heart sound that may arise from the right or left ventricle.

2. *Specific heart muscle disease*

A. *Symptoms*

Since this group of conditions produces either congestive (in the majority) or restrictive (in a minority) cardiomyopathy, the symptoms are those appropriate to these conditions.

B. *Signs*

In assessing the physical signs, special attention must be paid to evidence of disease outside the heart, such as lymphadenopathy, splenomegaly, scleroderma, Raynaud's phenomenon, joint disease, salivary gland disorder, ocular disturbances, and neurological lesions.

LABORATORY FINDINGS

1. *Hypertrophic obstructive cardiomyopathy*

A. *Blood and urine tests*

(1) No abnormality of the blood count or blood chemistry has been detected.

(2) Enzymes from peripheral or cardiac muscle are not elevated.

(3) Urine excretion of catecholamines has not been shown to be increased unless there is an associated pheochromocytoma.

B. *Electromyography and biopsy*

Electromyography and biopsy of peripheral muscle have not shown any consistent abnormality.

C. *The phonocardiogram and apex cardiogram*

(1) The phonocardiogram confirms the clinical findings.

(2) The phonocardiogram shows the explosive onset of the systolic mur-

mur following the onset of systole as well as its ejection quality.

(3) It may be possible to record a fourth heart sound, which is inaudible to the ear.

(4) The murmur terminates at the aortic valve closure and is heard over the ventricular septum at the left sternal edge and apex.

(5) An apical, diastolic rumbling murmur may be present.

(6) The apexcardiogram shows the large A wave of atrial contraction, which may be as much as 30 per cent of the total displacement of the tracing.

D. *The electrocardiogram*

The electrocardiographic findings vary from normal to grossly abnormal.

(1) The most frequent abnormality is left ventricular hypertrophy, which may be very striking.

(2) In addition there is often left anterior hemiblock.

(3) Q waves may be seen in mid- and even lateral precordial leads, resembling myocardial infarction.

(4) The P waves frequently show a bifid appearance of left atrial hypertrophy and the P-R interval is at the lower range of normal.

(5) Although no delta wave is usually seen, pre-excitation (WPW) syndrome has rarely been shown to be present.

The ECG thus reflects the severe left ventricular hypertrophy, the massive septum, and the left atrial hypertrophy, and hints at the possibility of a disorder of conduction.

E. *The echocardiogram*

Echocardiography has added a new dimension to the diagnostic techniques for hypertrophic obstructive cardiomyopathy. The main findings are:

(1) Greatly increased thickness of the ventricular septum, which may be 1½ times the thickness of the posterior wall of the left ventricle. The maximum thickness of the septum is found midway between the aortic valve and the apex.

(2) Poor septal movement

(3) Displacement of the mitral valve apparatus towards the septum

(4) Decrease in the diastolic closure rate of the anterior cusp of the mitral valve without evidence of mitral obstruction

(5) Systolic anterior movement of the anterior components of the mitral valve, which may approximate the ventricular septum

Many of these features can occur with other forms of ventricular septal hypertrophy, but the association of *all* the features is strongly suggestive of hypertrophic obstructive cardiomyopathy.

F. *The chest radiograph*

(1) The most frequent features are slight left atrial enlargement and signs of raised pulmonary venous pressure (interstitial costophrenic lines; dilatation of upper lobe vessels and narrowing of lower lobe vessels).

(2) The heart may be normal in size or considerably enlarged.

(3) There is not infrequently an appearance like a shelf on the left cardiac border, due to the massive hypertrophy of the free wall of the left ventricle.

(4) The aorta is not dilated and the aortic valve is not calcified.

(5) However, secondary calcification of the mitral valve may occur, due to turbulence or past infection.

G. *Hemodynamics*

(1) The left ventricular end-diastolic pressure is raised, especially on effort.

(2) In 70 to 80 per cent of patients, there is a systolic pressure gradient between the left ventricular outflow tract and the aorta. This is due to apposition of the anterior mitral valve apparatus to the hypertrophied septum.

(3) At the same time mitral regurgitation may be proportional to the degree of obstruction; it occurs due to abnormal forces acting on the mitral valve.

(4) False gradients may be recorded in the cavity of the left ventricle due to squeezing of the catheter by the powerful contraction of the hypertrophied muscle. In this situation the elevated left ventricular systolic pressure is recorded only in the region where the catheter is trapped, whereas with true obstruction all left ventricular systolic pressures, including that in the inflow tract, are elevated.

(5) Only the pressure in the subaortic area distal to the obstruction is normal.

(6) The left ventricle contracts fast and powerfully. Approximately 80 per cent of ejection occurs in the first half of the systole. The ventricle empties completely.

(7) The pressure gradient is exaggerated after an ectopic beat and as a result of an increase in left ventricular systolic pressure without an increase in aortic systolic pressure.

(8) The left ventricular pressure pulse shows a notch in the upstroke at the level of the aortic systolic pressure.

(9) The degree of obstruction is notoriously variable, being increased with inotropic stimulation, exercise, excitement, and fear, and reduced by inotropic suppression.

(10) The gradient is also increased by isoprenalin, digitalis, and tachycardia, and reduced by beta adrenergic blockade with propranolol.

(11) The cardio-selective agent, practolol does not significantly reduce the gradient.

(12) Propranolol has little effect on a persistent gradient but will prevent the development of a gradient under stimulation.

The most important hemodynamic disturbance is the reduction of ventricular elasticity, shown by the high left ventricular end-diastolic pressure and the massive hypertrophy with a normal left ventricular end-diastolic volume. Isoprenalin produces an increase in stiffness, indicated by a rise in left ventricular end-diastolic pressure with reduction in left ventricular end-diastolic volume, but beta adrenergic blockade produces a decrease in stiffness, shown by a fall in left ventricular end-diastolic pressure and a rise in left ventricular end-diastolic volume.

H. *Angiocardiography*

(1) The shape of the left ventricle is severely distorted.

(2) The cavity is elongated, being surrounded by the massive hypertrophied muscle of the septum and free wall.

(3) The papillary muscles are also hypertrophied.

(4) Islands of contrast medium may be isolated in the hypertrophied interstitial muscle bundles or even at the cardiac apex, which may be isolated from the body of the ventricle by the powerful muscle contraction in the middle of the cavity.

(5) The end-systolic left ventricular volume is reduced but the diastolic volume is normal.

(6) Mitral regurgitation is always present when there is outflow tract obstruction but may be relatively trivial. Occasionally it is severe.

I. *Cardiac muscle biopsy*

Biopsy from the septum reveals the characteristic disorientated latticework of myofibrils, simple hypertrophy, or fibrosis, depending on the site of the specimen and the extent of the disease, which is patchy.

2. *Congestive cardiomyopathy*

No consistent abnormalities in blood or urine investigations have been shown unless there is specific heart muscle disease. Attempts to isolate viruses from the blood have been unsuccessful.

A. *The phonocardiogram*

This confirms the auscultatory signs of gallop rhythm and often systolic murmurs of mitral and tricuspid regurgitation. Pulmonary valve closure is commonly accentuated.

B. *The electrocardiogram*

(1) The electrocardiogram usually shows nonspecific abnormalities (flat or gently inverted T waves).

(2) Atrial enlargement

(3) A modest degree of left ventricular hypertrophy

(4) Left bundle branch block is present in about 15 per cent of cases.

(5) The Q waves in precordial leads, with poor R wave progression, may mimic myocardial infarction. The Q waves are due to multiple areas of necrosis or fibrosis scattered through the left ventricle and septum.

(6) Ectopic beats are common and when of multifocal ventricular origin carry a poor prognosis.

(7) Atrial fibrillation occurs in 15 per cent of patients.

C. *The echocardiogram*

(1) The ultrasonic investigation shows dilatation of both ventricles with poor movement of the posterior wall of the left ventricle and paradoxical movement of the septum.

(2) There is a pronounced atrial wave ("kick") of the anterior mitral cusp due to a high left ventricular end-diastolic pressure.

(3) The amplitude of movement of the mitral valve may be increased.

(4) The valve cusp is not thickened and the diastolic closure rate is normal or increased.

(5) The ejection fraction is reduced.

(6) A pericardial effusion may be present.

D. *The chest radiograph*

(1) This shows considerable cardiomegaly involving mainly the ventricles.

(2) The pulmonary vasculature shows evidence of a high left atrial pressure.

(3) The left atrium is slightly enlarged.

(4) Pleural effusions due to right heart failure or pulmonary infarction may be seen.

E. *Hemodynamics*

(1) The changes are those of severe myocardial contractile failure, with high LVEDP, low cardiac index and stroke volume, and commonly elevated pulmonary artery pressure.

(2) The right atrial pressure trace may show evidence of tricuspid regurgitation with a large systolic wave and poor *x* descent.

F. *Angiocardiography*

(1) This shows a dilated, diffusely hypertrophic left ventricle with reduced ejection fraction and increased systolic and diastolic volumes.

(2) Moderate hypertrophy is present, but regional dyskinesia is unusual.

(3) Minor degrees of mitral regurgitation may be found.

(4) The coronary arteries have a wide bore and are smooth and unobstructed.

G. *Cardiac muscle biopsy*

(1) This has so far not revealed any specific changes to indicate etiology.

(2) Fluorescent antigenic material of virus nature has been reported in isolated cases.

(3) Disease of the coronary arterioles has not been a feature.

(4) Current work on enzyme function suggests an increase in LDH and impairment of mitochondrial energy production.

3. *Obliterative cardiomyopathy*

A. *Endomyocardial fibrosis (EMF)*
    (1) *Blood tests*
There is usually a mild eosinophilia.
    (2) *The phonocardiogram*
        (a) The phonocardiogram shows a third heart sound.
        (b) Sometimes wide fixed splitting of the second sound occurs
        (c) If mitral regurgitation is present, an early diminuendo systolic murmur and diastolic rumbling flow murmur at the apex are heard.
    (3) *The electrocardiogram*
        (a) The electrocardiogram usually shows nonspecific appearances with flat T waves.
        (b) Poor R waves progression in the precordial leads is a common finding.
        (c) Low voltage is common due to the presence of a pericardial effusion.
        (d) Right atrial enlargement is notable.
        (e) Atrial fibrillation is common.
    (4) *The chest radiograph*
        (a) In the right-sided type of endomyocardial fibrosis there is a massive cardiac silhouette due to a pericardial effusion and considerable enlargement of the right atrium. The lung fields may appear unduly clear, but pleural effusions may be present.
        (b) In the left-sided type there is usually left atrial enlargement and signs of pulmonary venous hypertension. A linear streak of calcification is often visible in the region of the left ventricle and represents calcium within intracavitary thrombus.
    (5) *Hemodynamics*
        (a) In the right-sided type the pressure tracings show a high end-diastolic pressure in the right ventricle, which approximates that in the pulmonary artery. The early diastolic pressure is also elevated. The systolic pulmonary artery pressure is low or normal. The right atrial trace shows dominant *a* and *v* waves, but the *x* descent may be poor owing to tricuspid regurgitation; the *y* descent remains sharp.
        (b) In the left-sided type, the left atrial pressure is usually considerably elevated. The pulse shows a tall *v* wave with sharp *y* descent when there is mitral regurgitation. The left ventricular end-diastolic pressure is raised. The cardiac index is low in severe patients.
    (6) *The angiocardiogram*
        (a) In the right-sided type this shows obliteration of the inflow tract of the right ventricle, enormous dilatation of the right atrium, and slow transit time through the right heart.
        (b) In the left-sided type, there is usually obliteration of the inflow tract of the left ventricle and often severe mitral regurgitation.
    B. *Loeffler's eosinophilic cardiomyopathy*
    (1) There is usually a profuse blood eosinophilia and evidence is accumulating to suggest that the eosinophils are quantitatively abnormal.
    (2) The electrocardiogram is nonspecific.
    (3) The hemodynamic studies usually show a low cardiac index, high left ventricular end-diastolic pressure, and (often) raised pulmonary artery pressure.
    (4) The angiocardiogram may show a filling defect of the left ventricle due to eosinophilic masses and thrombus.
    (5) Function is usually impaired in systole, although occasionally only diastolic function is abnormal and contraction appears to be good.
    4. *Restrictive cardiomyopathy*
    A. *The phonocardiogram* may show a third heart sound; murmurs are usually absent.
    B. *The electrocardiogram* tends to show low voltage and nonspecific

changes, except in amyloid disease where abnormal Q waves (pseudo myocardial infarction) may be seen.

C. *The chest radiograph* does not usually show cardiac enlargement except in amyloid disease.

D. *Hemodynamics*

(1) Systolic function is normal.

(2) Simultaneous pressure and volume studies of the left ventricle show rapid early ventricular filling, which ceases in late diastole.

(3) Unlike constrictive pericarditis, this disorder is confined to the left ventricle.

(4) In amyloid restrictive cardiomyopathy there is a low cardiac index and ejection fraction, elevated end diastolic pressures in both ventricles (higher in the left than the right) and elevation of early diastolic pressures. Pressure-volume studies show slow ventricular filling.

DIAGNOSIS

Diagnosis of cardiomyopathy depends partly upon the absence or evidence of other heart disease, such as valvular, ischemic, hypertensive, or congenital, but mainly on the many positive features (see list on p. 126 and Tables 9-1 through 9-3) that permit accurate diagnosis, especially in hypertrophic obstructive cardiomyopathy.

DIFFERENTIAL DIAGNOSIS

1. *Differential diagnosis of hypertrophic cardiomyopathy*

A. When obstruction is present the main differential diagnosis lies between aortic, valvular, or discrete subvalvular stenosis, subvalvular mitral regurgitation ("floppy" mitral valve; papillary muscle or chordal dysfunction), rheumatic mitral regurgitation, and ventricular septal defect (Table 9-2).

B. When obstruction is absent, the diagnosis must be made from other forms of myocardial disease (especially ischemic heart disease) and may be very difficult clinically. Signs of pulmonary hypertension with a ventricular filling gallop suggest hypertrophic obstructive cardiomyopathy if the arterial pulse is jerky and there is a palpable left atrial beat.

C. In either form, the presence of a family history is helpful. Angina is unusual in many forms of pulmonary hypertension and points to a left ventricular origin of the symptom. Concealed mitral obstruction due to stenosis, cor triatriatum, or myxoma must be excluded and pulmonary veno-occlusive disease ruled out.

D. The presence of an arcus cornealis, cholesterol deposits on skin or tendons, occult or overt diabetes mellitus, and a high blood cholesterol point to ischemic heart disease rather than hypertrophic obstructive cardiomyopathy, but the differentiation is not absolute. Systemic hypertension occurs occasionally in hypertrophic obstructive cardiomyopathy.

E. When congestive heart failure develops in hypertrophic obstructive cardiomyopathy, the clinical features may be difficult to differentiate from congestive cardiomyopathy, for the impairment of contractile function leads to loss of the abrupt quality of the arterial pulse and also to loss of the outflow tract obstructive murmur. The cardiac impulse, however, still suggests hypertrophic obstructive cardiomyopathy and differs from the feeble left ventricular impulse in congestive cardiomyopathy. The atrial beat is retained in hypertrophic obstructive cardiomyopathy unless atrial fibrillation has occurred. Some of the major differential clues are listed in Table 9-3.

2. *Differential diagnosis of congestive cardiomyopathy*

Table 9-2. Differential Diagnosis of Hypertrophic Cardiomyopathy with Obstruction

Disorder	Family History	History	Atrial Pulse	Systolic Murmur	Diastolic Murmur	Cardiac Impulse	Left Atrial Size	Rhythm
HOCM	+	Angina, often for many years Syncope	Jerky Good volume Ill sustained	L.S.E. & Apex Late onset Ejection A_2 normal	0	Atrial beat. Powerful L.V. thrust.	±	AF 10%
Aortic valve stenosis	0	Angina Syncope	Small volume or anacrotic	Ejection + click. Early onset Base/apex	Often	Well sustained L.V.	0	SR
Aortic subvalvar stenosis (discrete)	0	Rarely angina	Small volume	Ejection, No click. Early onset A_2 inaudible Base & apex	Usual	Well sustained L.V.	0	SR
Rheumatic mitral regurgitation	0	No angina No syncope	Small volume Jerky	Pansystolic Apex to axilla	M.D.M. apex	Ill sustained L.V.	++	AF
Subvalvar mitral regurgitation	+ in "floppy" valve (FV) syndrome	Atypical angina in "floppy" valve syndrome	Small volume Jerky	Apex & base Late onset or ejection. Mid-systolic click & late SM in F.V.	M.D.M. apex	Ill sustained L.V.	+	SR
V.S.D.	0	No angina or syncope	Small volume Jerky	Pansystolic L.S.E.	M.D.M. apex	Ill sustained L.V.	±	SR

A. Since congestive cardiomyopathy is largely a disease of exclusion, it is essential to look for underlying general systemic disease, especially connective tissue disorders, sarcoidosis, hemochromatosis, diabetes mellitus, endocrine disorders (especially thyroid dysfunction and acromegaly), peripheral myopathies, and Friedreich's ataxia. Most of these disorders can be excluded by full clinical examination.

B. Important laboratory investigations are: urine examination, full blood count, serum electrolytes and cholesterol, liver function tests, serum iron, blood sugar or glucose tolerance test, thyroid function tests, and such autoimmune tests as LE phenomena, smooth muscle antibodies, and sheep cell agglutination tests.

C. Where peripheral muscle disease is suspected, an electromyogram or biopsy may be advisable.

D. Differentiation from coronary artery disease:

The most difficult differential diagnosis in congestive cardiomyopathy is from coronary artery disease, and in some cases a final diagnosis can only be made by coronary arteriography. However, the following differential points are of considerable value:

(1) Angina is almost the rule in coronary artery disease, but rare in congestive cardiomyopathy.

(2) Signs of metabolic vascular faults (arcus, cholesterol deposits, abnormal lipids, impaired carbohydrate tolerance, tophi) are common in coronary artery disease but not in congestive cardiomyopathy.

(3) The electrocardiogram shows frank myocardial infarction in many cases of coronary artery disease but only exceptionally in congestive cardiomyopathy.

(4) The left ventricular angiogram shows regional dyskinesia in most patients with coronary artery disease, but diffuse hypokinesia in most with congestive cardiomyopathy, although there is a little overlap.

Some of the differential clinical clues are listed in Table 9-3.

3. *Specific heart muscle disease*

The cardiac features are essentially those of congestive cardiomyopathy, and the diagnosis rests upon the detection of disease elsewhere in the body (see list on p. 124). Examples of important clinical clues are:

A. *Diffuse systemic sclerosis*

Raynaud's phenomenon, teleangiectasis, calcinosis around the terminal phalanges, hypertension.

B. *Systemic lupus erythomatosus*

Hypertension, joint involvement, renal lesions, hemolytic anemia, pericarditis, possibly liver involvement (lupoid hepatitis).

C. *Polyarteritis nodosa*

Neuropathy, hypertension, pericarditis, renal involvement, abdominal pain, pulmonary involvement.

D. *Sarcoidosis*

Arrhythmias, and heart block, lung changes, positive liver biopsy, positive lymph gland biopsy, salivary gland enlargement, occular involvement, negative tuberculin reaction, erythama nodosum.

E. *Hemochromatosis*

Pigmentation, diabetes mellitus, cirrhosis of the liver, high serum iron, family history.

F. *Peripheral myopathy*

Limb girdle weakness.

G. *Friedreich's ataxia*

Cerebellar signs.

4. *Special cardiac features in certain diseases are:*

A. Arrhythmias and heart block point to sarcoidosis or peripheral myopathies.

B. Pericarditis points to polyarteritis nodosa, systemic lupus erythematosus, virus infection, or eosinophilic disorders.

Table 9-3. Some Differential Diagnostic Features of Hypertrophic Cardiomyopathy Without Obstruction, and COCM*

	Family History	History	Arterial Pulse	Cardiac Impulse	3rd Heart Sound	4th Heart Sound	Signs of Disease in Other Systems
Hypertrophic Cardiomyopathy	++	Angina + Dyspnea Syncope	Jerky Good volume Ill sustained A.F. 10%	Atrial beat Powerful L.V.	+	rare	0
Congestive Cardiomyopathy	0	Angina rare Dyspnea ++	Small	L.V. poor quality	++ (L.V.)	+	0
"Primary" Pulmonary Hypertension	±	Dyspnea Syncope Angina rare	Small. S.R.	R.V. ++ L.V. 0	+ (R.V.)	+ (R.V.)	0
Coronary Artery Disease	+	Angina ++	Small or normal. Occ. A.F.	L.V. + Dyskinetic	++ (L.V.)	++	Arcus; May be cholesterol deposits skin and tendons or Diabetes.
Hypertensive Heart Disease	0	Angina +	High tension S.R. or A.F.	L.V. + Atrial beat rare	+ (L.V.)	++	0
Specific Heart Muscle Disease	0	Dyspnea +	Small Occ. A.F.	L.V. poor	+ (L.V.)	+	++
Amyloid Restrictive Cardiomyopathy	0	Dyspnea Angina	Small May be paradoxical	L.V. poor	+ (L.V.) ? (R.V.)	+	(+) i.e. myeloma

*COCM.: Congestive Cardiomyopathy
+: Present
++: Severe

C. Hypertension points to systemic lupus erythematosus or polyarteritis nodosa.

D. Mitral regurgitation points to infiltrative disorders (including sarcoidosis, leukemia, etc.).

Differential diagnosis from other causes of pericarditis, such as tuberculosis, malignancy, rheumatoid arthritis, uremia, etc. is important.

COMPLICATIONS

The complications of the cardiomyopathies are cardiac arrhythmias, sudden death, heart failure, embolism (pulmonary or systemic), and infective endocarditis.

1. *Cardiac arrhythmias*

A. Arrhythmias are not common in hypertrophic cardiomyopathy, although atrial fibrillation occurs in about 10 per cent and ectopic beats and occasionally ventricular tachycardia occur infrequently.

B. Symptoms suggesting arrhythmias are common, however.

C. Multiple ectopic beats are common in congestive cardiomyopathy, while atrial fibrillation occurs more frequently than in hypertrophic cardiomyopathy.

2. *Sudden death*

A. Sudden death is the commonest form of death in hypertrophic cardiomyopathy.

B. Sudden death is due to extreme resistance to left ventricular filling in the presence of tachycardia or atrial fibrillation, to outflow tract obstruction or to malignant arrhythmia, or to a combination of all these factors.

C. Atrial fibrillation is particularly hazardous because it causes both loss of atrial drive and shortening of the time available for ventricular filling.

3. *Congestive heart failure*

Congestive heart failure in hyper-

trophic cardiomyopathy represents a late stage of the disease, often in association with atrial fibrillation, but in congestive cardiomyopathy heart failure is implicit in the diagnosis.

4. *Systemic embolism*

A. Systemic embolism is uncommon in hypertrophic obstructive cardiomyopathy, except when atrial fibrillation has developed, and then it is common.

B. In congestive cardiomyopathy systemic embolism may follow the formation of an atrial or ventricular thrombus, especially if atrial fibrillation is present.

C. Embolism is common in Loeffler's disease and in left-sided endomyocardial fibrosis.

D. Any patient who has a low cardiac output with atrial fibrillation and who is immobilized in bed while on diuretic therapy may produce a systemic or pulmonary embolism.

E. Peripheral edema also predisposes to systemic venous thrombosis and pulmonary embolism.

5. *Infective endocarditis*

Infective endocarditis is well recognized in hypertrophic obstructive cardiomyopathy and usually involves the mitral valve. It can be a cause of calcification of the valve and increase in mitral regurgitation. Similarly patients with subvalvular mitral regurgitation from other causes are prone to infection, which is, however, rare in congestive cardiomyopathy.

MANAGEMENT

A knowledge of prognosis and natural history is essential for rational therapy.

1. *Cardiomyopathy*

A. *Hypertrophic obstructive cardiomyopathy*

The aims of treatment are *the prevention of extension of the disease and of sudden death,* and *the relief of symptoms.* Acute hemodynamic observations indicate that nonselective beta adrenergic blocking agents (notably propranolol) improve ventricular filling characteristics and prevent the development of outflow tract gradients. There is some evidence also that long-term oral treatment may have the same effect.

(1) *Drug therapy*

(a) *Typical phase of the disease*

(i) Propranolol

(A) In the typical phase of the disease, when there is sinus rhythm and good contractile function, beta adrenergic blockade with propranolol is advised.

(B) Propranolol relieves angina and improves dyspnea in the majority, but not in all patients, and may logically be expected to improve the filling characteristics and prevent the development of outflow tract gradients, particularly on effort.

(C) The antidysrhythmic effect is also likely to be important.

(D) Propranolol should be given in the maximum tolerated doses, but it is essential to begin treatment with small doses (10 mg. t.i.d.) in order to detect those few patients who respond with extreme bradycardia or a fall in cardiac output. Most patients, however, tolerate the drug very well, and doses of up to 300 mg. per day should be aimed at. The dose can be increased at intervals of 1 to 2 weeks by increments.

(E) There is no general agreement on whether patients who do not have symptoms should be put on propranolol. There is much appeal in the preventive argument, but it must be noted that propranolol has not so far been shown to prevent sudden death.

(F) Patients with a strong family history should probably start propranolol, irrespective of symptoms if there is other evidence of increasing severity.

(ii) Digitalis and inotropic agents

Digitalis and inotropic agents are not indicated.

(iii) Diuretics

Diuretics are not indicated because they may increase obstruction by reducing blood and left ventricular volumes.

(b) *Heart failure and atrial fibrillation*

When heart failure and atrial fibrillation have developed, the treatment is quite different.

(i) DC conversion under anticoagulant therapy should be attempted as soon as possible.

(ii) Digitalis may be used to control the ventricular rate, since there is now rarely any outflow tract obstruction.

(iii) Diuretics may be used.

(iv) There is no place for large doses of propranolol, but small doses are useful as an adjunct to digitalis to control the ventricular rate if cardioversion fails to achieve sinus rhythm.

(v) In the rare patient who has fascicular block, a pacing wire should be inserted into the right ventricle before conversion is attempted.

(vi) Anticoagulants must be continued indefinitely once atrial fibrillation, whether paroxysmal or established, has occurred (Table 9-4).

(2) *Surgical treatment*

(a) Surgical treatment usually takes the form of resection of the hypertrophied septum.

(b) It is indicated only when there are symptoms unrelieved by propranolol in the presence of severe outflow tract obstruction with a persistent gradient of 50 mm. Hg or more and pronounced septal hypertrophy on echocardiography and angiocardiography.

(c) The operation usually reduces or abolishes the gradient, reduces left ventricular end-diastolic pressure, and improves symptoms.

(d) Its effect on prognosis is unknown but the incidence of sudden death has been reported as half that in patients on propranolol or without treatment.

(e) Heart block, heart failure, and cardiac rupture may follow the operation, whose mortality rate may be as high as 19 per cent.

(f) Mitral valve replacement effectively removes the obstruction and relieves mitral regurgitation. It should be considered when the latter is severe, but should not be used merely to relieve obstruction.

With the possible exception of mitral valve replacement for severe mitral regurgitation, surgical treatment should be regarded as essentially symptomatic and palliative rather than curative.

(3) *Artificial pacemakers*

The use of a permanent pacemaker to create asynchrony of ventricular contraction and thus reduce the gradient in addition to permitting the use of propranolol in patients in whom the drug causes an excessive bradycardia has been suggested, but there is little experience from which to judge the relative success of this measure.

B. *Congestive cardiomyopathy*

(1) The treatment is essentially that for congestive heart failure, with additional use of anticoagulants when embolism is threatened or actual.

(2) Attention should be paid to the control of possible aggravating or causal factors, such as alcohol and cigarette smoking, hypertension, and infections.

(3) Prolonged bed rest for many months may have a beneficial effect, but control studies are not available. It is worth a trial.

(4) Steroids are not indicated unless there is an eosinophilia or evidence of connective tissue disease or sarcoidosis.

(5) Drugs that improve cardiac function:

(a) Drugs that improve cardiac function such as glucagon, phentolamine or salbutamol may be tried.

(b) The most effective of these in the acute stages is salbutamol, which can be given by continuous intravenous infusion at a rate of 2 to 8 μg. per minute.

(c) Improvement in cardiac output and a fall in left ventricular end-diastolic pressure are due probably to a direct inotropic action but possibly to unloading of the left ventricle as a result of peripheral vasodilatation.

Table 9-4. **Medical Treatment of Hypertrophic Obstructive Cardiomyopathy**

Stage or Complication	Treatment
Usual situation with contractile function maintained (gradient in 70-80% patients)	Large doses propranolol. No digitalis or diuretics.
Atrial fibrillation (Usually no gradient)	Anticoagulants. D.C. conversion. *If successful:* Continue large doses propranolol, and anticoagulants. *If unsuccessful:* Small doses digitalis, propranolol, and anticoagulants.
Congestive heart failure ± Atrial fibrillation.	As for unsuccessful conversion of atrial fibrillation. Diuretics in addition.
Infective endocarditis	Full appropriate chemotherapy

(6) Beta adrenergic blocking agents:

(a) A recent suggestion that some of these patients are suffering from endogenous catecholamine cardiac poisoning and should be treated with beta adrenergic blocking agents merits very careful study.

(b) According to Waagstein et al., a group of patients with congestive cardiomyopathy and chronic sinus tachycardia benefitted strikingly from alprenolol or practolol. Clearly this is a most important suggestion, which must be examined intensively.

(c) Selection of patients is obviously most important, because beta adrenergic blockade is usually very dangerous in patients with severely impaired myocardial contractility and heart failure. Great caution should be exercised until the details of selection of patients have been fully evaluated.

C. *Obliterative cardiomyopathy*

(1) *Endomyocardial fibrosis*

(a) There is no specific therapy for endomyocardial fibrosis because its cause is unknown.

(b) The standard treatment for congestive heart failure is employed together with anticoagulants to prevent embolism, especially in left-sided endomyocardial fibrosis with atrial fibrillation.

(c) Operations to bypass the right ventricle, such as those employed for tricuspid atresia, have been suggested in right-sided endomyocardial fibrosis, but there is insufficient experience to permit evaluation.

(2) *Loeffler's disease*

(a) Treatment is essentially for heart failure and embolism, but attempts to reduce the excessive eosinophilic count should be made.

(b) Steroids and immunosuppressive therapy may be tried.

(c) In patients with eosin-ophilic leukemia, appropriate chemotherapy may be helpful also.

(d) Reduction in the eosinophilic count by the cell separator may have a place in therapy.

D. *Restrictive cardiomyopathy*

(1) No specific treatment is available for primary restrictive cardiomyopathy.

(2) In amyloid restrictive cardiomyopathy the treatment is often of little avail.

(3) If myeloma is present, appropriate chemotherapy should be given.

(4) It is not known whether the cell separator would be effective.

2. *Specific heart muscle disease*

A. The underlying disease should be treated with appropriate specific means if available.

B. Steroids are valuable in polyarteritis nodosa and sarcoidosis but not usually in scleroderma.

C. Leukemia and reticuloses may respond to appropriate chemotherapy.

D. Otherwise, the treatment is for congestive cardiomyopathy.

PROGNOSIS AND NATURAL HISTORY

1. *Hypertrophic obstructive cardiomyopathy*

A. Most patients have a long uneventful course with only minor symptoms or sometimes none at all.

B. Angina may be present for many years.

C. A minority of patients develop progressive dyspnea and angina and may lose their signs of outflow tract obstruction, develop atrial fibrillation and congestive heart failure, and die in low output failure with pulmonary edema, or embolism.

D. Loss of outflow tract obstruction indicates that the disease is spreading widely throughout the myocardium and progressively damaging contractile function.

E. Impaired ejection together with impaired filling of the left ventricle result in a drastic fall in cardiac output and rapidly lead to severe and fatal heart failure.

F. The onset of rapid atrial fibrillation constitutes a crisis in which the outflow tract obstruction usually disappears.

G. In some patients the development of outflow tract obstruction can be traced in serial examinations over a period of years.

H. Outflow tract obstruction:
(1) May be present early in life and at first examination
(2) May develop gradually
(3) May disappear gradually
(4) It is present sometime during the course of the disease in 70 to 80 per cent of patients.

I. Sudden death
(1) Sudden death may occur at any stage of the disease, not necessarily in the presence of symptoms, and it is the greatest hazard of the disease.
(2) It is probably a great risk in young children with rapidly increasing symptoms and in the presence of a high left ventricular end-diastolic pressure.
(3) The worst prognosis appears to be in children who have obvious signs of the disease early in life, marked cardiac enlargement, and a strong family history.

J. In very few patients (perhaps 1–2%), severe mitral regurgitation occurs and precipitates heart failure. There is then usually no obstruction of the left ventricular outflow.

K. Systemic embolism is common once atrial fibrillation has occurred.

L. The annual morbidity is around 3.5 per cent, but the disease occurs in a very wide spectrum of age and may be found in newborn infants or in old persons.

2. *Congestive cardiomyopathy*
A. Once the diagnosis has been made, the prognosis is usually poor, and patients are likely to die of heart failure or (less commonly) arrhythmias within 3 years.

B. In a few patients the process appears to be arrested, and survival is possible for very much longer.

C. The presence of hypertension appears to improve prognosis, perhaps because of greater left ventricular hypertrophy.

D. Persistent gallop rhythm, raised jugular venous pressure, and cardiomegaly are usually ominous signs.

E. Some patients make a relatively early recovery from the initial "attack" of left ventricular failure but relapse subsequently and rapidly.

F. Atrial fibrillation marks a further step in a downhill direction.

3. *Obliterative cardiomyopathy*
A. *Endomyocardial fibrosis*
(1) In endomyocardial fibrosis involving the right ventricle, patients often remain remarkably well for many years, but ultimately die in low output heart failure.
(2) When the left ventricle is involved, the prognosis tends to be worse, due to the hazards of embolism and severe mitral regurgitation.
(3) The early stages of the disease are punctuated by episodes of fever, heart failure, or atrial fibrillation, with relatively asymptomatic periods in between.

B. *Loeffler's disease*
(1) The prognosis is not well known, but most patients do badly as the eosinophilia progressively damages the endocardium.
(2) The hazard of embolism is always present.
(3) If the disorder can be arrested

before systolic function has been damaged, the prognosis may be better.

4. *Restrictive cardiomyopathy*

A. *Primary restrictive cardiomyopathy*

This entity probably carries a good prognosis, provided that systolic function remains good, but sufficient information is not available yet on this point.

B. *Amyloid restrictive cardiomyopathy*

(1) There is severe disorder of contractile function of the left ventricle, and the prognosis is especially poor when there are widespread associated disorders, such as myelomatosis.

(2) Patients usually die suddenly or in severe congestive heart failure.

SUGGESTED READINGS

Abelman, W. H.: Virus and the heart. Circulation, *44*:950, 1971.

Braunwald, E. et al.: Idiopathic hypertrophic sub-aortic stenosis. Am. Heart Assoc. Monograph, *10*:64, 1964.

Brockington, I. F. and Edington, G. M.: Adult heart disease in Western Nigeria. A clinical pathological synopsis. Am. Heart J., *83*:27, 1972.

Brockington, I. F. and Olsen, E. G. J.: Loeffler's endocarditis and Davies' endomyocardial fibrosis. Am. Heart J., *85*:308, 1973.

Burch, G. E. et al.: Coxsackie B viral myocarditis and valvulitis identified in routine autopsy specimens by immunofluorescent techniques. Am. Heart J., *74*:13, 1967.

Chew, C. et al.: The functional defect in amyloid heart disease. The "stiff heart syndrome." Am. J. Cardiol., *36*:438, 1975.

Chusid, M. J. et al.: The hypereosinophilic syndrome: analysis of 14 cases with review of the literature. Medicine, *54*:1, 1975.

Davies, M. J., Pomerance, A., and Teare, R. D.: Idiopathic giant cell myocarditis; a distinctive clinico-pathological entity. Br. Heart J., *37*:192, 1975.

Demakis, J. G. and Rahimtoola, S. H.: Peripartum cardiomyopathy. Circulation, *44*:964, 1971.

Epstein, S. et al.: Asymetric septal hypertrophy. Ann. Intern. Med., *81*:680, 1974.

Ferrans, D. J., Morrow, A. G., and Roberts, W. C.: Myocardial ultrastructure in idiopathic sub-aortic stenosis. Circulation, *45*:769, 1972.

Gau, G. et al.: Q waves and coronary arteriography in cardiomyopathy. Br. Heart J., *34*:1034, 1972.

Ghosh, P. et al.: Myocardial sarcoidosis. Br. Heart J., *34*:769, 1972.

Goodwin, J. F.: Prospects and predictions for the cardiomyopathies. Circulation, *50*:210, 1974.

———: The congestive and hypertrophic cardiomyopathies: a decade of study. Lancet, *1*:733, 1970.

Goodwin, J. F. et al.: The clinical pharmacology of hypertrophic obstructive cardiomyopathy. *In* Wolstenholme, G. E. W. and O'Connor, M. (eds.): Cardiomyopathies. Ciba Foundation Symposium. London, Churchill, 1964.

Hamby, R. I., Zonereichs, S., and Sherman, L.: Primary myocardial disease and diabetes mellitus. Circulation, *42*(Supp. III):44, 1970.

Hardarson, T. et al.: Prognosis and mortality in hypertrophic obstructive cardiomyopathy. Lancet, *2*:1462, 1973.

Hernandez, R. R., Greenfield, J. C., Jr., and McCall, B. W.: Pressure-flow studies in hypertrophic sub-aortic stenosis. J. Clin. Invest. *43*:101, 1964.

Hubner, P. J. B. et al.: Double-blind trial of propranolol and practolol in hypertrophic obstructive cardiomyopathy. Br. Heart J., *35*:1116, 1973.

Kawai, C.: Idiopathic cardiomyopathy. A study on the infective immune theory on a cause of the disease. Jap. Circ. J., *35*:765, 1971.

Oakley, C. M.: Debate: That congestive cardiomyopathy is really hypertensive heart disease in disguise. *In* Seminar on Cardiomyopathies. Postgrad. Med., *48*:777, 1972.

Peters, T. J. et al.: Enzyme studies on myocardial biopsies in congestive cardiomyopathy. Br. Heart J., *37*:780, 1975.

Roberts, W. C.: Operative treatment of hypertrophic obstructive cardiomyopathy. The case against mitral valve replacement. Am. J. Cardiol., *32*:377, 1973.

Shah, P. M. et al.: The natural (and un-natural) history of hypertrophic obstructive cardiomyopathy: a multicenter cooperative study. *In* Cardiac Hypertrophy and Cardiomyopathy. Am. Heart Assoc. Monograph, *43*:179, 1974.

Swan, D. A. et al.: Analysis of the symptomatic course and treatment of hypertrophic obstructive cardiomyopathy. Br. Heart J., *33*:761, 1971.

Tobin, J. R. Jr. et al.: Primary myocardial disease in alcoholism: clinical manifestations and causes of the disease in a selected population of patients observed for three or more years. Circulation, *35*:754, 1967.

Waagstein, F. et al.: Effect of chronic beta ad-

renergic receptor blockade in congestive cardiomyopathy. Br. Heart J., *37*:1022, 1975.

Webb-Peploe, M. M. et al.: Cardio-selective beta
adrenergic blockade in hypertrophic obstructive cardiomyopathy. *In* Advances in Adrenergic Beta-Receptor Therapy. Postgrad.
Med., *47*(Suppl.):93, 1971.

Wigle, E. D., Adelman, A. G., and Silver, M. D.:
Pathophysiological considerations in muscular
sub-aortic stenosis. *In* Wolstenholme, G. E.
W. and O'Connor, M. (eds.): Hypertrophic
Obstructive Cardiomyopathy. Ciba Foundation study group, No. 37. London, Churchill,
1971.

Ziady, G. M. et al.: Primary restrictive cardiomyopathy. Br. Heart J., *37*:556 (Proceed-
ings of British Cardiac Society, November,
1974), 1975.

10. CONGENITAL HEART DISEASE

Mary Allen Engle, M.D., Charles S. Kleinman, M.D., and Myles S. Schiller, M.D.

DEFINITION

1. *Congenital heart disease* is that form of cardiovascular disease present at birth and due to a developmental abnormality.

2. The manifestations of some forms of congenital heart disease (CHD) may not appear, however, until later in childhood or even in adult life.

3. Conversely, some severe malformations are incompatible even with fetal life and are responsible for some miscarriages.

INCIDENCE

1. The incidence of CHD reported for most studies is in the range of 8 to 10 per 1,000 live births.

2. Some common kinds of heart disease in the adult are probably congenital, namely the bicuspid aortic valve that may become thick with age so that stenosis or insufficiency occurs, and the apical systolic click syndrome with ballooning mitral valve.

3. If these patients are reckoned in the statistics, the incidence of congenital heart disease probably considerably exceeds 1 per 100 live births, and these two conditions assume the rank of the most common congenital cardiac lesions.

ETIOLOGY

We know from embryology of the heart that the injury or the agent that produces the defect must do its harm in the first 6 to 8 weeks of fetal life, when the cardiovascular structures are forming. A possible exception to this statement is the situation of patent ductus arteriosus, a channel normal for the fetus but one that should close off in the first few hours or days after birth.

1. *Unknown cause*

A. For the largest number (95%) of individuals with CHD, the cause is unknown.

B. Most such parents are healthy adults in the usual childbearing age.

C. The mothers describe their health early in pregnancy and before that as normal.

D. Inquiries about past histories of exposure to radiation or of living at high altitudes have usually been answered negatively.

2. *Medications*

A. Although many women have admitted taking many medications, not always on a physician's advice, it has not been possible to relate the incidence of CHD to a specific medication, except in a very few instances.

B. Some women on long-term anticonvulsant medication, such as trimethadione and paramethadiene[12] have had a higher percentage of babies with heart disease than the average.

C. A few of the infants with malformed limbs due to thalidomide medication in the pregnant mothers also had CHD.

3. *Postnatal environmental factors*

Persistent patency of the ductus may be effected by postnatal environmental factors, such as:

A. The hypoxia of high altitude

B. The respiratory distress syndrome of premature infants

4. *Maternal infection*

In the remaining 5 per cent of infants

145

with congenital heart disease, a portion are due to maternal infection with rubella in the first trimester of pregnancy, and a portion are due to genetic factors and chromosomal abnormalities.

5. *Genetic factors and chromosomal abnormalities*

A. The genetic factors include certain families with clustering of a particular malformation in sibships or members of more than one generation.[2,11]

B. Included also are some heritable forms of cardiovascular disease, as in the Marfan syndrome, Ellis van Creveld syndrome or Noonan syndrome (Turner phenotype with normal karyotype).

C. Chromosomal abnormalities with cardiovascular involvement include the trisomies, such as Down's syndrome (mongolism) and other far less common ones, such as trisomy 18; and monosomy, namely the Turner syndrome, 45 XO.

PREVENTION

Since the key to prevention is the understanding of etiology, it is clear that at the present time we are unable to prevent most forms of this common birth defect.[7]

1. *Maternal rubella*

A. Immunization of children with rubella vaccine, which became available in 1969, helps prevent maternal rubella. This, in turn, reduces the incidence of congenital heart disease due to maternal rubella in the first trimester of pregnancy.

This vaccine is credited with prevention of the nationwide epidemic expected in 1970. It is hoped that the vaccine has broken the 5 to 9 year cycles of mass epidemics of rubella, but there is concern that the public may become complacent or, through apathy or neglect, may fail to have their children immunized.

2. *Genetic factors*

A. For the rare syndromes (combination of defects) that are heritable and are associated with heart disease, better genetic understanding permits counseling of families, and intrauterine detection of some of the conditions can lead to interruption of pregnancy.

B. More knowledgeable counseling is also available for the families with isolated instances of congenital heart disease, heart defect with additional malformation, or familial clustering of heart disease.

3. *Environmental factors and medications*

Until questions about harmful environmental agents are answered, it would seem wise for the future parents to avoid taking drugs unnecessarily.

4. *Birth control*

One way to prevent congenital heart disease is to prevent babies.[20]

PATHOPHYSIOLOGY

Congenital anomalies of the heart and major vessels produce their effects by rerouting or by delaying the course of blood flow. Minor or small lesions produce no symptoms and few signs, whereas severe anomalies produce major derangements that result in symptoms and signs that are usually recognizable, and often treatable, early in life. Moderately severe anomalies are intermediately recognizable, as expected. In the childhood years such anomalies tend to produce more signs than symptoms, but the gradual effects of their continuing presence may become manifest in later life.

1. *Conditions that delay or obstruct the normal course of blood flow*

A. *Ventricular outflow obstruction*

(1) Conditions that delay or obstruct the normal course of blood flow are most often in the form of obstruction to ventricular outflow, such as pulmonic

or aortic stenosis or coarctation of the aorta.

(2) The severity of obstruction, and the precise location (at, above, or below the valve) determine the pathophysiology.

(3) The pressure load on the ventricle leads to concentric hypertrophy of the wall of that chamber.

(4) The hypertrophied ventricle is able to maintain an adequate output on exercise and at rest, unless the obstruction is severe or the myocardial blood flow is impaired.

(5) In severe forms of pulmonic or aortic stenosis, the electrocardiogram (ECG) changes from ventricular hypertrophy (voltage criteria) to hypertrophy with "strain" (depression of S-T segments, flattening or inversion of T waves) when this imbalance of demand and supply occurs.

(6) Dilatation and failure of the ventricle are the next steps in progression of severity.

(7) Until dilatation of the chambers occurs, the work load on the ventricle is better assessed by electrocardiographic evidence of hypertrophy than by radiologic signs of enlargement.

B. *Ventricular inflow obstruction and other A-V valve abnormalities*

(1) Obstruction to ventricular inflow is rare.

(2) Congenital tricuspid or mitral stenosis or cor triatriatum (when severe) is accompanied by elevated pressure in that atrium.

(3) The pressure load is manifest by hypertrophy of atrial wall, assessed electrocardiographically, before dilatation occurs.

(4) Venous drainage into the atrium occurs at an increased pressure.

(5) In the right atrium, jugular venous distention and hepatomegaly are evidence of severe obstruction, and peripheral edema is a late sign thereof.

(6) When obstruction to left atrial outflow is marked, there is elevation of pulmonary venous, capillary, and then arterial pressure.

(7) Pulmonary edema and/or right-sided failure follow if this situation goes unrelieved for a long time.

(8) Less common anomalies that interfere with normal forward flow of blood include lesions such as Ebstein's anomaly of the tricuspid valve, in which there is downward displacement of the leaflets and thinning of the atrialized right ventricle.

(9) Even less common are congenital pulmonic, aortic and mitral insufficiency. These last-named impart a volume overload on the ventricle with the regurgitant flow so that, depending on severity of the regurgitation, chamber dilatation and wall hypertrophy occur, and these may be judged by roentgenogram and electrocardiogram.

2. *Endocardial fibroelastosis*

A. In unusual instances the endocardium is thickened (endocardial fibroelastosis).

B. The chamber wall is hypertrophied, and the chamber itself may either be restricted and small or (more often) dilated.

3. *Congenital complete A-V block*

A. Another type of congenital cardiac anomaly that delays the passage of blood is congenital complete A-V block.

B. The slow ventricular rate is associated with a large diastolic volume and often, therefore, with slight to moderate cardiomegaly.

C. In the ECG of patients with congenital complete A-V block, P waves are often tall and peaked, consistent with right atrial hypertrophy. This change is probably due to the extra work the atria have as they attempt to pump blood through incompletely opened atrioventricular valves.

4. *Abnormal communication between left and right sides of the heart*

In these conditions there is abnormal

communication between the left and right sides of the heart, and the direction of blood flow depends on the relative resistances in the two circuits and/or on the manner in which the major vessels are attached.

   A. *Left to right shunts (Fig. 10-1)*

   (1) The abnormal communication may be at the atrial, ventricular, or aorticopulmonary level.

   (2) The physiologic effect is to in-

DIFFERENTIATION OF LEVEL OF A-V SHUNT.

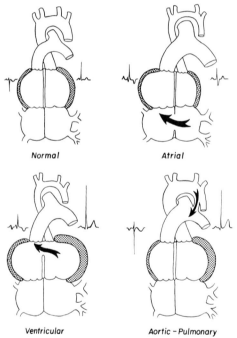

crease the pulmonary blood flow and sometimes to increase the pulmonary arterial pressure, because of the large volume of blood (hyperkinetic hypertension) or because of secondary effects in the pulmonary vascular bed (hyperresistant hypertension; pulmonary vascular obstructive disease).

   (3) When the pulmonary pressure is normal and the shunt is small, there are no pathophysiologic abnormalities.

   (4) Larger shunts produce larger effects so that cardiac chamber enlargement is an accompaniment of the volume overload. If the large volume is pumped at an elevated pressure for the right ventricle, or at the systemic pressure that normally exists in the left ventricle, or at a suprasystemic left ventricular pressure, then the wall of that chamber hypertrophies.

   (5) Shunts at atrial level

      (a) Shunts at atrial level are most often through a secundum-type atrial septal defect in the fossa ovalis region, but may occur through an ostium primum defect related to the atrioventricular valve region, or a sinus venosus defect high in the atrium near the orifice of the superior vena cava. In the last situation, anomalous pulmonary venous return from the right lung is usually present.

      (b) Total or partial anomalous pulmonary venous return may be the primary cause of a left to right shunt at atrial level.

      (c) The abnormal drainage may occur above or below the diaphragm. Such drainage is regularly obstructed when infradiaphragmatic and is occasionally so when supradiaphragmatic.

   (6) Shunts at ventricular level

      (a) At ventricular level, the left to right shunt is due to defective or absent ventricular septum.[4]

      (b) Most often the defect is single and is high in the membranous septum, an infracristal defect.

Fig. 10-1. Schematic diagram of cardiac chambers and great arteries and electrocardiographic right and left ventricular forces in the normal situation and when a large left to right shunt occurs at atrial, ventricular, or aorticopulmonary level. Cardiac chamber enlargement or hypertrophy and relative sizes of the great arteries are indicated as a consequence of whether the shunt is proximal or distal to the atrioventricular valves. The aorta is enlarged if the shunt is distal to the aortic valve.

(c) Sometimes the opening is subpulmonic and supracristal.

(d) The muscular septum may contain one or more defects.

(e) It is the size of the defect more than its location that determines pathophysiology. A small, restrictive ventricular septal defect (VSD) causes no cardiac nor pulmonary burden. A large, nonrestrictive defect permits equalization of systolic pressure in the two ventricles; the effect is tantamount to a single ventricle.

(f) If pulmonary resistance to flow is normally low, a torrential pulmonary flow results.

(g) Increase in obstruction to pulmonary flow, either within the right ventricle or in the pulmonary arterial tree, restricts somewhat this left to right shunt. In this situation, marked obstruction converts the flow through the defect to minimal shunting or to a right to left shunt (Eisenmenger syndrome).

(7) Shunts at aorticopulmonary level

(a) Abnormal communication at aorticopulmonary level is almost always a patent ductus arteriosus between the descending aorta and pulmonary artery (P.A.), but it may be between the ascending arch and P.A. in the form of an aorticopulmonary window (sometimes called an aortic septal defect), or there may be an anomalous origin of the pulmonary artery from the aorta, or a common truncus arteriosus.

(b) Just as with a ventricular septal defect, the volume of shunt depends on the size of the opening and on the resistance to flow into the lungs. A small shunt and normal P.A. pressure cause no cardiopulmonary burden. A large shunt or high resistance to flow causes trouble.

B. *Right to left shunts*

(1) Right to left (R-L) shunts combine an abnormal connection between the two circulations with severe intracardiac or intrapulmonary obstruction to flow or else obligatory venoarterial shunting because of abnormal connection of vessels.

(2) The pathophysiology of R-L shunts involves the presence of cyanosis, with the accompanying clubbing of fingers and toes, polycythemia, and exercise intolerance.

(3) Additional features depend on whether the anomaly results in diminished or in excessive pulmonary blood flow.

(4) Reduction of pulmonary flow

(a) When pulmonary flow is diminished, that is because there is pulmonary stenosis or atresia (as in tetralogy of Fallot) or tricuspid stenosis or atresia together with a rudimentary right ventricle. A portion of blood is shunted so as to bypass the lungs.

(b) The patient may be deeply cyanotic and experience shortness of breath on exertion and sometimes, attacks of paroxysmal dyspnea.

(c) Cardiac enlargement and cardiac failure, however, are not a consequence of this kind of set-up.

(d) In tetralogy, the pressure-loaded right ventricle produces right ventricular hypertrophy on ECG. In roentgenograms the heart has an abnormal contour, but it is not enlarged.

(5) Excessive pulmonary flow

(a) When pulmonary flow is excessive and a R-L shunt is predominant, the patient may be only minimally cyanotic, yet have considerable cardiac enlargement and often cardiac failure.

(b) These conditions are characterized by abnormal mixing at atrial, ventricular, or aorticopulmonary level because of absence of that septum, or by anomalous drainage of veins or origin of arteries.

(c) Examples include total anomalous pulmonary venous return or complete transposition of the great arteries.

5. *Abnormalities of cardiac positions*

A. In any of the above situations, the heart and viscera may be in normal position (situs solitus), or there may be abnormalities of position of one or both of these.

B. These malformations of position may exist alone without any associated cardiac defect.

C. There may, for instance, be dextrocardia due to inversion (mirror-image dextrocardia) or to rotation of the heart (dextroversion or mesoversion).

D. These abnormal positions of the heart may occur in situs solitus, situs inversus, or in that mixed-up situation referred to as visceral heterotaxy (scrambled viscera).

E. Abnormalities of cardiac position per se have no pathophysiologic consequence.

CLASSIFICATION

Although there are many anomalies, singly or in combination, only nine are common. If they are understood, then the various permutations are similar in analysis.

1. It is convenient to classify congenital heart disease into cyanotic and noncyanotic malformations. This is the first step in classification according to presence or absence of cyanosis.

A. In the noncyanotic ones are those with no shunt and also those with a left to right shunt.

B. The cyanotic group includes the malformations with a right to left shunt.

2. The second step relates to the degree of pulmonary blood flow, whether average, increased, or decreased.

3. The third level of a classification notes whether the cardiac burden falls chiefly on the left or on the right ventricle.

Utilizing this schema, the following outline of classification emerges (Table 10-1).

SYMPTOMS AND SIGNS

In infancy and childhood there are very few symptoms of the congenital anomaly unless it is one that causes cyanosis or congestive heart failure. One must look beyond symptoms to the signs that the patient shows. This lack of complaint of symptoms is due not only to the remarkable energy characteristics of the growing child but also to the fact that for the individual born with a defect, it is hard to know what is normal. The way he feels is normal for him. Sometimes it is not until after an operation has improved the situation that a child or his parents realize in retrospect that he had indeed been limited or unusually thin before the operation. A child characterized as "quiet" and one who preferred indoor activities may emerge after operation as a noisy, sports-minded youngster who has to be hauled in from play.

The cyanotic individual is easy to pick out. He may be able to walk on a level at his own pace for quite a distance, but climbing upstairs, walking into the wind, or hurrying cause fatigue and breathlessness. The child with tetralogy of Fallot typically squats or rests at these times.

1. *Blood pressure*

Blood pressure, when measured in the upper and lower extremity with a snug cuff of appropriate size, is an essential component of a physical examination of any individual suspected of having congenital heart disease.

2. *Radial pulses*

Palpation of both radial pulses simultaneously, and of a radial and femoral pulse simultaneously, gives information about aortic obstruction or runoff.

3. *Venous pulsations*

Venous pulsations indicate elevated right atrial filling pressure or obstruction to right atrial outlet.

4. *Cardiac failure*

A. Cardiac failure is most apt to occur in babies in the first weeks or months of life. Symptoms include rapid

Table 10-1. Differential Diagnosis of Most Common Congenital Cardiac Anomalies

COLOR	NONCYANOTIC		CYANOTIC	
PULMONARY BLOOD FLOW	AVERAGE	INCREASED	DECREASED	INCREASED
CATEGORY	NO SHUNT	L → R SHUNT	R → L SHUNT c̄PS	R ⇌ L SHUNT
L.V. ↑	COARCTATION AORTIC STENOSIS	PATENT DUCTUS VENTRICULAR SEPTAL DEFECT	RUDIMENTARY RIGHT VENTRICLE WITH TRICUSPID AND PULMONIC STENOSIS/ATRESIA	
R.V. ↑	PULMONIC STENOSIS	ATRIAL SEPTAL DEFECT	TETRALOGY PULMONIC STENOSIS WITH R → L ATRIAL SHUNT	COMPLETE TRANSPOSITION GREAT ARTERIES OR PULMONARY VEINS HYPOPLASTIC LEFT HEART SYNDROME

and even labored breathing, fatigue on feeding, and slow weight gain.

(1) Labored respirations in the infants are evidenced by retractions of the suprasternal notch and level of the diaphragms.

(2) Wheezing is a symptom of markedly congested lungs, and such a patient is susceptible to lower respiratory infections.

(3) The growing child with a large left to right or with a right to left shunt gains weight slowly and may be retarded in height as well.

B. Mental impairment is not a symptom though for the infant, motor milestones may be delayed.

5. *Cyanosis*

Signs of cyanosis include not only the blue coloration of nails, mucous membranes and skin, but often a ''high color'' to the cheeks, suffusion of conjunctivae, and clubbing of fingers and toes.

6. *Cardiomegaly*

A. A sign of cardiomegaly in the infant and young child is a precordial bulge, just to the left of the sternum if the right ventricle is enlarged, and at the apex, which is often displaced downward and outward, if the left ventricle is too big.

B. On palpation a right ventricular lift accompanies these visible evidences of enlargement.

7. *Heart murmurs*

The timing and location of heart murmurs have especial significance in diagnosis of congenital heart disease.

A. A holosystolic murmur implies an abnormal communication between the ventricle and some other chamber throughout the whole of systole.

B. An ejection-type systolic murmur at the base of the heart is caused by the ejection of a normal amount of blood through a narrowed orifice, or the flow of an abnormally large quantity of blood through a normal semilunar valve.

C. Murmurs of pulmonic origin radiate to the lung fields posteriorly, while those of aortic origin radiate to the suprasternal notch and arteries of the neck.

D. Diastolic murmurs are less common than systolic ones in congenital heart disease.

E. An early and mid-diastolic murmur at the base and along the left sternal border is due to semilunar valve insufficiency.

F. A mid-diastolic murmur lower over the precordium is due to relative tricuspid or mitral stenosis, secondary to excessive flow of blood across that valve.

G. A continuous systolic and diastolic murmur is due to an arteriovenous communication.

H. A thrill often is palpable when the murmur is grade 3 or more (out of 6) in intensity.

8. *Heart sounds* also are important signs in diagnosis.

A. The second sound in the second left interspace (S_2) is especially important. Normally this sound is split, and the aortic component precedes the pulmonic. These two sounds separate in inspiration and come closer together on expiration. The louder the pulmonic component and the narrower the splitting, the greater the pulmonary artery pressure.

(1) Conversely, delay and diminution of the pulmonary component, even to the point of inaudibility, signify increasingly severe pulmonic stenosis.

(2) Wide and fixed splitting of the second heart sound can be heard when there is pulmonary stenosis and also when there is relative pulmonic stenosis with greatly increased pulmonary blood flow and normal pulmonary artery pressure, as in atrial septal defect.

B. A third heart sound at the apex is heard in many normal children.

C. A fourth heart sound is pathologic.

D. In the failing heart, these become S$_3$, S$_4$, or summation gallops.

9. *Ejection sound or click*

A. Early systolic ejection sound, or click, is of valvular or vascular origin.

B. When one finds an ejection-type systolic murmur at the base of the heart, an early systolic ejection sound suggests that the stenosis is valvular rather than sub- or supravalvular.

C. Such clicks can also be heard when the aorta or pulmonary artery is dilated.

D. Mid-systolic click in association with a late systolic murmur at the apex characterizes the mitral click syndrome with prolapsing valve. There is growing reason to think that this may be one of the most common congenital anomalies.

10. *Edema*

A. Edema in an ambulatory subject is dependent, but in a young infant who cannot yet even sit, it is generalized.

B. Its presence may then first be detected as puffiness of the eyelids, if he sleeps prone, or as a "too-good" sudden weight gain on the scales.

LABORATORY FINDINGS

1. *Noninvasive studies*

A. *Electrocardiogram*

(1) Electrocardiogram gives evidence concerning rhythm, rate and conduction, electrical axis, cardiac chamber dilatation, or hypertrophy and strain (Fig. 10-2).

(2) This is the simplest laboratory test, for long-term followup of patients with CHD.

(3) The findings must be interpreted in comparison with the normal standards for infants, children, adolescents, and adults.

B. *Vectorcardiogram* interprets the above information in a three-dimensional display.

C. *Cardiac series of chest roentgenograms*

(1) Cardiac series of chest roentgenograms forms part of the initial evaluation and may be repeated at indicated, infrequent intervals.

(2) This series consists of 6-foot teleoroentgenograms in frontal, right anterior-oblique, left anterior-oblique, and lateral views with barium swallow in all four views.

(3) The series is used to evaluate not only the overall heart size and position but each cardiac chamber, the ascending and descending aorta, the possibility of retroesophageal vessels, and the main pulmonary artery and pulmonary vascularity (Fig. 10-3).

D. *Phonocardiogram* makes a permanent recording of heart sounds and murmurs and helps to clarify confusion in timing of auscultated events.

E. *Echocardiogram*[10,13]

(1) Echocardiogram is the newest informative diagnostic technique to join the four above as valuable in initial diagnosis and in follow-up.

(2) It translates intracardiac anatomy and function into a display of "slices" of the beating heart and into a sweep from one area to adjacent ones.

(3) Presence or absence of ventricular septum, over-riding of the aorta, aortic-mitral continuity, enlargement of either ventricle or the left atrium or aorta are among the many pieces of information that can thereby be analyzed.

(4) In addition ventricular function can be assessed.

F. *Apexcardiogram*[18] records movement of the heart in relation to the simultaneous ECG.

G. *Systolic time interval*[17] provides information about pre-ejection and ejection periods.

H. *Indirect pressure tracings*

Indirect pressure tracings of arterial pulsations record the palpated events in a display that, in high fidelity, mimics intra-arterial recordings for analysis of pulse waveform in systole and diastole.

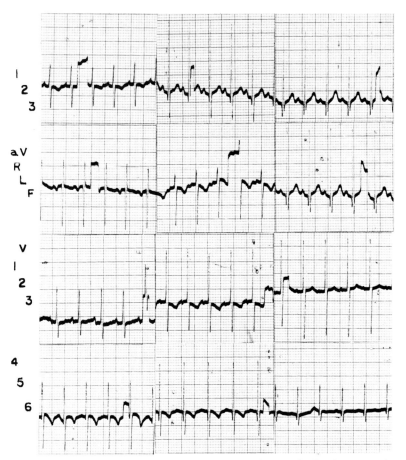

Fig. 10-2. Electrocardiographic evidence of left ventricular hypertrophy (large voltage R wave in V5, AVF, leads 2 and 3) and "strain" (inversion of T waves in V4-6 and in lead I) together with right ventricular hypertrophy (Rs in VI). This ECG was recorded prior to treatment in a 4-month-old infant in severe cardiac failure from a large left to right shunt. The ECG is consistent with a shunt distal to the AV valves. It was through a patent ductus arteriosus in this instance.

2. *Invasive techniques*

A. *Cardiac catheterization with selective contrast visualization*[14]

(1) Cardiac catheterization with selective contrast visualization affords hemodynamic analysis together with biplane display of cardiovascular structures on radiograph or cineradiograph.

(2) Not only can pressures, flows, and resistances be measured but also ventricular function can be assessed.

(3) In the well-equipped and well-staffed laboratory, with personnel experienced in design and interpretation of the study, this investigation affords valuable information to confirm or to clarify

Fig. 10-3. (*A*) Pre-treatment roentgenogram. Frontal view of cardiac series obtained on admission of infant whose ECG is shown in Fig. 10-2. Note cardiomegaly with enlargement of border-forming of right atrium. Rightward deviation of barium filled esophagus indicates left atrial enlargement. Left heart border is full due to enlargement of main pulmonary artery, right ventricular outflow tract, and left ventricle (downward-directed apex). Right and left ventricular enlargement was confirmed on oblique views, not shown here. Pulmonary arterial markings are engorged, and the haziness in right upper lobe is due to pulmonary venous congestion. (*B*) Post-treatment film. After medical management of cardiac failure with digitalization and diuretics, and establishment of diagnosis, early surgical obliteration of the ductus by suture-ligation was carried out a month later; this roentgenogram shows an average-sized heart with normal pulmonary vascularity.

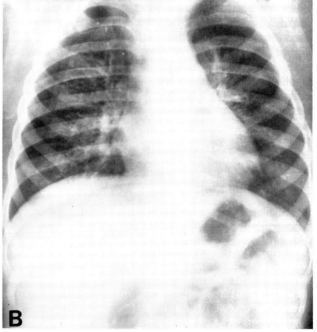

a diagnosis and to evaluate a patient prior to and following reparative surgery.

B. *His bundle electrogram*[1] obtained at right heart catheterization is valuable in delineation of complex arrhythmias and disorders of conduction.

C. *Blood gas studies*

Measurement of pH, pO_2 and PCO_2 on microaliquots of arterial or of venous blood is essential in diagnosis and management of the critically ill patient with congenital heart disease.

D. *Serum electrolyte and glucose* may be altered in metabolic or respiratory acidosis or longterm diuretic therapy for congestive heart failure.

E. *Hemoglobin and hematocrit* determinations are especially helpful in diagnosis and management of cyanotic patient.

F. *Comprehensive coagulation survey* is indicated for patients prior to, and sometimes following, cardiac surgery, particularly when extracorporeal circulation is employed or when there is a history of unusual bleeding.

G. *Blood cultures* (about four in number) should be taken when the patient with congenital heart disease has a fever that is unexplained. The possibility of infective endocarditis is thus evaluated.

H. *Neurologic studies*

(1) Neurologic studies, such as electroencephalogram, EMI brain scanning or carotid arteriography should be considered when the cyanotic patient has a sudden, severe, persistent headache or a stroke.

(2) The presence of a brain abscess or cerebrovascular event may be defined in this way.

DIAGNOSIS

1. The diagnosis of congenital heart disease is entertained for a patient at any age when some of the signs and symptoms described earlier are present.

2. The younger the subject with an organic murmur, the more likely is the condition to be congenital, but the diagnosis of CHD may not be made until late adult life. This is true for such classical forms of CHD as atrial septal defect, for instance, as it is for the two anomalies that are increasingly being identified as congenital but with late onset of signs and symptoms, namely bicuspid aortic valve and the mitral click syndrome.

3. Once the diagnosis is suspected, usually because of a murmur, the precise anomaly and its severity can often be recognized at the bedside and confirmed by the simple and easily available laboratory tests of ECG, and cardiac series of chest roentgenograms. Echocardiography will likely be used more and more at this initial evaluation.

4. We reserve cardiac catheterization with contrast visualization for specific indications:

A. The distressed cyanotic newborn

B. The infant treated for cardiac failure

C. The child or older subject being evaluated before and after cardiac surgery

D. For clarification of an obscure diagnosis.

DIFFERENTIAL DIAGNOSIS

1. *Innocent heart murmurs*

In the pediatric age group, the finding of a heart murmur calls for a differentiation of innocent murmurs from those due to heart disease, either acquired or congenital. An innocent murmur is a normal finding in most healthy children at some time. There are four common kinds of normal or innocent murmurs:

A. *Midsystolic murmur over the midprecordium*

(1) Midsystolic, short, vibratory, buzzing murmur over the midprecordium does not originate at any valve area.

(2) The murmur does not radiate along the course of pulmonary or of aortic blood flow.

(3) It is usually grade 1 to 2 out of 6 in intensity.

B. *Venous hum*

(1) Venous hum is a continuous, humming murmur above and sometimes· below the clavicle on one or both sides.

(2) It is heard in the upright position, it varies with respiration and turning the head, and it disappears in the supine position.

(3) It is the one type of innocent murmur that may have an accompanying thrill.

C. *Pulmonary souffle*

(1) Pulmonary souffle is a short, midsystolic murmur in the second left interspace (pulmonary area).

(2) It is more often heard in adolescents than in young children.

(3) It is heard in the straight back syndrome.

D. *Basal soft systolic murmur* may be heard transiently in some high-output states, such as:

(1) Fever

(2) Anemia

(3) Hyperthyroidism

2. *Rheumatic heart disease*

When an innocent murmur has been excluded, it is then necessary to distinguish the organic murmur of acquired heart disease from that of CHD. The most common form of acquired heart disease is rheumatic.

A. *Mitral insufficiency* produces the apical pansystolic murmur in childhood.

B. *Aortic insufficiency:* the high-pitched, blowing early diastolic murmur at the base can be heard in childhood and beyond.

C. *Mitral and aortic stenosis:* more years are required for mitral and aortic stenosis to appear when acquired from rheumatic fever.

3. *Various congenital anomalies*

When the foregoing causes of a murmur have been eliminated and the diagnosis of congenital heart disease is likely, then the differentiation of the type of lesion is carried out as in Table 10-1, and as illustrated for left to right shunts in Fig. 10-1.

A. *General differential features*

(1) The first question concerns presence or absence of cyanosis.

(2) The second considers whether pulmonary blood flow is average, increased, or decreased.

(3) The third question is which ventricle bears the burden of the lesion.

B. *Specific differential points*

Specific identifying information of the type, location, and radiation of the heart murmur and the quality of the heart sounds usually pinpoints the diagnosis.

(1) *Ventricular septal defect*

(a) The hallmark of a ventricular septal defect (VSD) is a holosystolic murmur at the lower left sternal border, overlying the ventricular septum itself.

(b) One then estimates the size of the shunt by the size of the heart and by the character of the pulmonic closure sound.

(c) A moderately large left to right shunt with moderate pulmonary hypertension is indicated by an enlarged, overly active precordium, slightly wide splitting of S_2 and increased intensity of S_2P.

(d) The auscultatory counterpart of the increased pulmonary blood flow and pulmonary venous return and therefore, the flow across the mitral valve is a mid-diastolic murmur of relative mitral stenosis.

(e) When the heart size and heart sounds are normal and the only abnormal finding is a holosystolic murmur at the lower left sternal border, one can say with accuracy that the diagnosis is a small ventricular septal defect of no hemodynamic significance.

(2) *Patent ductus arteriosus*

(a) The diagnosis of a typical patent ductus arteriosus (PDA) is an auscultatory one: a continuous systolic and diastolic murmur with late systolic crescendo and diastolic decrescendo localized to the second and third left parasternal spaces (the pulmonary area).

(b) The diastolic component is better heard in the supine than in the upright position.

(c) The second sound is often obscured by the crescendo systolic component of the machinery murmur.

(d) Just as for a VSD, one judges whether the ductus and therefore the shunt is small, medium, or large by increasing increments of left ventricular enlargement by roentgenogram and hypertrophy by ECG.

(e) The main pulmonary artery and branches enlarge as the flow through them increases. This is characteristic of any left to right shunt (see Figs. 10-1 and 10-3).

(3) *Left to right shunts proximal to the A-V valves*

(a) In contrast to shunts distal to the atrioventricular valves, like VSD and PDA, which cause a left ventricular burden, L-R shunts proximal to the mitral and tricuspid valves cause right ventricular enlargement, evidenced by roentgenograms and in ECG by right ventricular conduction delay.

(b) The systolic murmur is soft, usually grade 2 (of 6) in the pulmonary area and it radiates along the course of pulmonary blood flow into the lungs.

(c) The second sound shows wide, fixed splitting and the pulmonary component is of average intensity throughout the pediatric age group, since pulmonary hypertension in this lesion is usually limited to some adults.

(4) *Pulmonary hypertension due to pulmonary arterial obstructive disease*

If pulmonary hypertension due to pulmonary arterial obstructive disease occurs, the differential diagnosis of shunt level becomes difficult, for all resemble each other.

(a) The heart is no longer volume-overloaded.

(b) The right ventricle is concentrically hypertrophied so the ECG shows right ventricular hypertrophy (RVH).

(c) The pulmonic component of S_2 is loud and early.

(d) Sometimes, a high-pitched, decrescendo murmur of pulmonic insufficiency is heard.

(e) On roentgenograms, the main pulmonary artery is enlarged, but the branches become pruned.

(f) Cardiac catheterization with selective injection of contrast medium is required for differential diagnosis.

(i) The only one of these that can be recognized with certainty prior to that study is shunt reversal through a patent ductus.

(ii) Then the toes are blue and clubbed, in contrast to a lesser amount or no cyanosis in the lips and right hand.

(5) *Right to left shunt with obstruction to pulmonary blood flow*

(a) Shunt reversal in association with high pulmonary vascular resistance is one of the differential diagnoses in patients with cyanotic heart disease (see (4) above).

(b) More often, the shunt is right to left through a large VSD because there is severe pulmonary stenosis (P.S.) or atresia: tetralogy of Fallot.

(c) The heart is average-sized and boot-shaped, and lungfields are unusually clear or radiolucent from the hilar markings outward.

(d) The ECG shows RVH.

(e) When there is severe P.S.

and R-L shunt at atrial level, the heart is larger, and the ECG shows RVH and often "strain," indicating that right ventricular pressure is suprasystemic.

(f) If the R-L shunt at atrial level is due to tricuspid stenosis or atresia and there is inadequate pulmonary flow, the heart is not enlarged, and the ECG shows left axis deviation and left ventricular dominance.

(g) If that shunt is in association with Ebstein's anomaly of the tricuspid valve, the heart is enlarged (sometimes markedly so), right ventricular forces in the ECG are diminished and delayed, and there are typical angiocardiographic and electrocardiographic features at catheterization.

(6) *Bidirectional shunt*

(a) If the cyanotic individual has an enlarged heart and increased pulmonary vascularity, one considers the possible causes of bidirectional shunting.

(b) Radiologic clues aid in differential diagnosis.

(c) A narrow base of the heart in frontal view that widens to double that width in right anterior-oblique view is found with complete D-transposition of the great arteries.

(d) A base that is wide in all views suggests common truncus arteriosus.

(e) Engorgement of the left and right superior venae cavae to form a vascular collar at the base of the heart is characteristic of total anomalous pulmonary venous return to a left vertical vein.

(f) Echocardiography, cardiac catheterization, and selective angiocardiography are needed to define these lesions and their physiologic consequences.

(7) *Malposition or transposition complexes*

The types of malposition or transposition complexes are fascinating malformations to define and differentiate.

(a) D-transposition is a common form of cyanotic heart disease in which the transposed aorta is dextro (D), to the right, of the pulmonary artery.

(b) L or "corrected" transposition

(i) In L or "corrected" transposition, the aorta is anterolateral and to the left of the posteromedial pulmonary artery.

(ii) The ventricles and atrioventricular valves are inverted so that if there is no other anomaly, the course of circulation is physiologically "corrected."

(iii) Commonly, however, there are associated anomalies: high-grade A-V block, downward displacement of the tricuspid valve (left-sided Ebstein's anomaly), defects or absence of ventricular septum, and pulmonic stenosis.

(8) *Congenital anomalies without shunt*

Differential diagnosis of congenital anomalies without a shunt most commonly requires differentiation of right-sided obstruction from left-sided, and then localization of the level and severity of stenosis.

(a) In pulmonic stenosis, the murmur is maximal in the pulmonary area (second left interspace) and radiates into the lung fields.

(b) In aortic stenosis, the murmur is maximal in the aortic area (second right interspace), and radiates to the suprasternal notch and arteries of the neck.

(c) An early systolic ejection sound, or click, denotes valvular stenosis.

(d) With supravalvular stenosis, there is sometimes a peculiar elfin facies and mental retardation. Since the valve closes proximal to the stenosis, valve closure sound is not diminished and may be accentuated if stenosis is marked.

(e) With subvalvular stenosis, poststenotic dilatation of the great artery is uncommon.

(f) Obstruction in the aorta

(i) If obstruction is in the aorta, the differential in pulses and blood pressure above and below the coarctation permits diagnosis and assessment of severity.

(ii) Often a systolic murmur is heard over the narrowed area posteriorly.

(iii) A pressure-loaded ventricle hypertrophies before it dilates with severe or long-standing load.

(iv) So the ECG evidence of hypertrophy is more sensitive than is radiologic evidence of enlargement to judge all but the most severe.

(v) Catheterization, angiocardiography, and echocardiography confirm the diagnosis and effects of the condition.

COMPLICATIONS

1. Common complications include:
   A. Premature death
   B. Disability in the form of easy fatigue or breathlessness
   C. Cardiac failure
   D. Infective endocarditis
2. The last-named is no respecter of severity, whereas the others are consequences of a severe malformation or a long-standing, moderately severe one.
3. The cyanotic individual may have additional complications:
   A. Cerebrovascular accidents are a hazard for the hypoxic and anemic infant or for the very polycythemic older subject.
   B. Brain abscess is a risk after the age of 5 years.

MANAGEMENT

Optimal management rests on accurate diagnosis and good judgment. The latter is based on experience and on awareness of new developments.[5,8]

The newborn with cyanosis and/or respiratory distress is at greatest risk. As an emergency he should be referred to a pediatric cardiac diagnosis and treatment center.

1. *Surgical approach*

A. If he is found to have complete transposition of the great arteries, he will undergo at cardiac catheterization a Rashkind balloon septostomy[19] and be a candidate for open heart surgery, usually in the form of a Mustard procedure,[16] as soon as he becomes symptomatic.

B. If on the other hand, he is found to have severe pulmonary stenosis with tricuspid atresia and a rudimentary right ventricle and an obstructive patent foramen ovale, he will have a Rashkind septostomy to promote right-to-left exit of blood and then will undergo a shunt procedure to create an artificial patent ductus and thus improve pulmonary blood flow.

C. If the anomaly is totally anomalous pulmonary venous return, emergency open heart surgery is called for.

D. *Indications for reparative cardiac surgery*

Reparative cardiac surgery is indicated electively in childhood for conditions such as:

(1) Tetralogy of Fallot
(2) Moderate or severe "pure" pulmonic stenosis
(3) Large shunts at atrial level (e.g., ASD, TAPVR)
(4) Large or moderate ventricular septal defect
(5) PDA
(6) Severe aortic stenosis or moderately severe discrete subaortic stenosis
(7) Significant coarctation of the aorta

Judgment that combines cardiologic and surgical input is needed for the above decisions and follow-through on management, as well as for plans involving surgery on other anomalies.

2. *Medical approach*

A. Patients with mild lesions, such as small ventricular septal defect or mild valvular pulmonic stenosis, are candidates for medical management,[9] with no restriction of activities and with occasional checkups.

B. If a large VSD is found, intensive medical management with close follow-up is the treatment of choice, since many defects spontaneously decrease in size and the baby's condition improves.

C. *Cardiac failure*

(1) When cardiac failure is recognized in an infant,[3] that baby should also be referred for full diagnosis and treatment, including surgery for some.

(2) Immediate therapy includes digitalization and use of diuretics, and then clarification of the lesion producing failure, and correction if feasible.

D. *Prevention of endocarditis*

(1) Any patient with an organic murmur runs a slight risk of infective endocarditis, but this risk can be minimized by having him understand the purpose for penicillin in therapeutic dosage for three days, beginning immediately before dental extraction or oral surgery.

(2) For genitourinary tract surgery or vaginal delivery, an antibiotic for gram-negative coverage should be added as well.

PROGNOSIS

1. The outlook for good health and normal activity is excellent for those with physiologically inconsequential lesions and for those whose anomalies have been surgically repaired with good success.

2. Palliative operations improve activity and longevity, though usually not to normal.

3. It is comforting to know that for most forms of CHD that produce present disability (or that are likely to produce it later on), based on what is known of the natural history of that condition, help is available through medical and often surgical management.

REFERENCES

1. Damato, A. N., Schnitzler, R. N., and Lau, S. H.: Recent advances in the bundle of His electrogram. *In* Yu, P. N. and Goodwin, J. F. (eds.): Progress in Cardiology, II, pp. 181–206. Philadelphia, Lea & Febiger, 1973.
2. Ehlers, K. H. and Engle, M. A.: Familial congenital heart disease. 1. Genetic and environmental factors. Circulation, *34*:503, 1966.
3. Engle, M. A.: When the child's heart fails: Recognition, treatment, prognosis. Prog. Cardiovasc. Dis., *12*:601, 1970.
4. ———: Ventricular septal defect: Status report for the seventies. Cardiovasc. Clin., *4*:281, 1972.
5. ———: Editorial: Optimal cardiac care: achievable? Circulation, *51*:399, 1975.
6. ———: Review article: Cyanotic congenital heart disease. Am. J. Cardiol., *37*:283, 1976.
7. Engle, M. A. et al.: Primary prevention of congenital heart disease. Report of Inter-Society Commission for Heart Disease Resources. Circulation, *41*:A–25, 1970.
8. ———: Resources for the optimal acute care of patients with congenital heart disease. Report of Inter-Society Commission for Heart Disease Resources. Circulation, *44*:A–123, 1971.
9. ———: Resources for optimal long-term care of congenital heart disease. Report of Inter-Society Commission for Heart Disease Resources. Circulation, *44*:A–205, 1971.
10. Feigenbaum, H.: Echocardiography, pp. 239. Philadelphia, Lea & Febiger, 1972.
11. German, J. L., III, Ehlers, K. H., and Engle, M. A.: Familial congenital heart disease. II. Chromosomal studies. Circulation, *34*:517, 1966.
12. German, J. L., III et al.: Possible teratogenicity of trimethadione and paramethadione. (Letter to the editor) Lancet, August: 261, 1970.
13. Gramiak, R. and Waag, R. C. (eds.): Cardiac Ultrasound. p. 308. St. Louis, C. V. Mosby, 1975.
14. Levin, A. R.: The science of cardiac catheterization in the diagnosis of congenital heart disease. Cardiovasc. Clin., *4*:235, 1972.
15. Michelsson, M. and Engle, M. A.: Congenital complete heart block, An international cooperative study, Pediatric cardiology. Cardiovasc. Clin., *4*:85, 1972.
16. Mustard, W. T.: Successful two-stage correction of transposition of the great vessels. Surgery, *55*:469, 1964.

17. Naughton, J.: Systolic time intervals and the evaluation of cardiac performance. Cardiac Rehab., 6:21, 1975.

18. Prewitt, T. et al.: The "rapid filling wave" of the apex cardiogram. Its relation to echocardiographic and cineangiographic measurements of ventricular filling. Br. Heart J., 37:1256, 1975.

19. Rashkind, W. J.: Atrioseptostomy by balloon catheter in congenital heart disease. Radiol. Clin. North Am., 9:193, 1971.

20. Wegman, M. E.: Annual summary of vital statistics—1974. Pediatr., 56:960, 1975.

11. CARDIAC TUMORS

Frank Gerbode, M.D., *and Nicholas Johnson,* M.D.

DEFINITION

1. Tumors of the heart are a group of heterogeneous space-occupying lesions that are due either to abnormal embryonic development or neoplastic proliferation.

2. They involve either the pericardium, the heart, the great vessels, or all three.

3. Neoplastic disease is primary or secondary.

4. Secondary involvement is twenty times that of the primary tumors.

GENERAL CONSIDERATIONS

Knowledge of the classification, manifestation, and diagnosis of cardiac tumors is as important to the physician as is knowledge of cardiopulmonary resuscitation. This has evolved over the past twenty years with the development of cardiac surgery. Surgery affords complete cure in most cases. Prior to this era, these entities were of curiosity to only the pathologist at postmortem examination.

Primary cardiac tumors occur at any age with no predilection to sex. They are either benign or malignant in histological diagnosis. Benign tumors may be potentially lethal, the result of arrhythmiagenesis or embolization of blood clot or tissue fragments. Therefore, any suspicion of their existence should initiate prompt diagnosis and treatment.

Cardiac tumors produce no characteristic symptoms unless they interfere with cardiac function. However, with even extensive myocardial invasion or destruction, only minimal symptoms or malfunction may exist.

Benign or malignant primary tumors as well as metastatic tumors produce indistinguishable symptoms. Secondary tumors invade the pericardium, most commonly presenting with bloodstained effusions. Infrequently they invade the heart muscle, producing space-occupying lesions.

Primary tumors are classified as to location: pericardial, mural, or endocardial. Although this classification serves to explain symptoms, it by no means accounts for the myriad of clinical manifestations that cardiac tumors may exhibit. Their ability to mimic any hemodynamic syndrome explains why they have been described as the "Great Imitators" in cardiovascular disease. Because they can produce symptoms directing attention away from the heart they are often misdiagnosed or overlooked. These oversights, more so than in other organ systems, can prove to be embarrassingly fatal.

With the availability of such sophisticated noninvasive techniques as echocardiography, and of such invasive techniques as angiocardiography, cardiac tumors can be rapidly confirmed. This is possible only if the physician develops a high degree of suspicion in evaluating the patient with less than classical signs of the more common cardiac ailments.

CLASSIFICATION

There are many ways to classify the cardiac tumors: in terms of location, benign versus malignant, and primary versus secondary. However, the most common approach to classification is the primary versus the secondary cardiac tumors (see list below).

Classification of Cardiac Tumors

Primary
  Tumors arising from embryonic maldevelopment
    Teratomas
    Dermoid cysts
    Sequestered lung
    Thyroid, thymic, parathyroid rest tumors
  Benign pericardial and cardiac tumors
    Pericardial cysts
    Mesotheliomas
    Angiomas
    Fibromas
    Lipomas
    Leiomyomas
    Neuromas
  Benign intramural and intracardiac tumors
    Rhabdomyomas
    Myxomas
    Lymphangioendotheliomas
  Malignant tumors of the heart
    Mesotheliomas
    Sarcomas
  Tumors arising from the major vessels
Secondary
  Carcinoma
  Sarcoma
  Lymphogranuloma
  Leukemia

PATHOPHYSIOLOGY

PRIMARY CARDIAC TUMORS

General Features of Primary Cardiac Tumors

1. Primary tumors of the heart have become surgical diseases. In all cases, excluding those of metastatic disease, surgery is indicated for definitive diagnosis and possible cure. Even the most malignant lesions have been palliated for years after prompt and accurate diagnosis, resection, and radiation therapy.

2. Eighty per cent of primary cardiac tumors are benign; 50 per cent of these are intracavitary myxomas.

3. The spectrum of possibilities includes both such neoplastic entities as fibroma, mesothelioma, lipoma, neurofibroma, angioma, and neuroma, and

such non-neoplastic proliferative lesions as pericardial cysts, bronchial cysts, dermoid cysts, and even sequestered lung. These non-neoplastic lesions must be included, for they often produce symptoms related to the pericardium.

4. Thymic, parathyroid, and thyroid rest tumors are mentioned because they may be confused on initial x-ray evaluation with primary cardiac tumors.

5. Thirty-five per cent of all the non-proliferative masses occur in patients under the age of three. Teratomas, hamartomas, and rhabdomyomas also occur most frequently in this age group.

Specific Features of Primary Cardiac Tumors

1. *Rhabdomyomas*

A. Rhabdomyomas are the most common tumor in childhood.

B. They are usually in the form of isolated or multiple nodes: masses in the atria or the ventricles.

C. Tuberous sclerosis of the brain is the most frequently associated lesion, with rhabdomyomas being noted in almost 50 per cent of reported cases.

D. Tumors and cysts of the kidney are also encountered with rhabdomyomas.

E. Rhabdomyomas are intramural and produce no symptoms until they become large enough to compromise cardiac function or produce either supraventricular tachycardias, extrasystoles, or heart block. Death from arrhythmias is often seen, but surgical removal can very often stop the development of arrhythmias.

2. *Fibromas*

A. Fibromas are characteristically solitary, small, villous, pedunculated masses of acellular, hyaline tissue covered by endothelium.

B. They generally arise from the subendothelium of heart valves.

C. These fibrous tissue nodules with no evidence of mitotic activity are very rarely found in the left ventricle or interventricular septum.

D. They almost always occur in children and are usually congenital.

E. On cut section, the appearance is that of a fibroid with the classic "whorled" pattern.

F. Fibromas are usually compatible with long life, since they grow slowly and insidiously.

G. They produce symptoms if they invade the conduction tissues or obstruct flow.

H. The few antemortem diagnoses have been made by angiocardiography and operative biopsy.

3. *Lipomas*

A. Lipomas, which arise from epicardial or pericardial fat, look and behave like lipomas in any other area of the body.

B. They may include both fibrous and muscular tissue.

C. They undergo the common forms of degeneration, such as fat necrosis and calcification.

D. Rarely are they encountered within the heart.

E. Lipomas may be either sessile or pedunculated, and occasionally they produce valvular insufficiency.

F. One of the first successfully removed cardiac tumors was a 3½ pound lipoma attached to the left ventricle in the pericardial sac.

4. *Teratomas*

A. Teratomas of the heart are similar to those occurring elsewhere in the body.

B. Their elements comprise all three germinal layers of the developing embryo.

C. They are more frequent in the mediastinum and pericardium than within the heart.

D. Usually benign pedunculated masses, they are attached to the base of the great vessels.

E. Most occur in infants in the first year of life; a few occur in the first or second decades.

F. Intracardiac teratomas are probably related to epithelial inclusions in the wall of the ventricle, in the region of the atrioventricular node, or near the tricuspid valve ring.

G. In contrast to the ovarian teratomas, those reported in the heart show no hairs, sebaceous glands, or keratinizing squamous epithelium.

H. Complete excision usually results in cure.

5. *Angiomas*

A. Angiomas are generally clustered, sessile, or polypoid subendocardial lesions.

B. Half of the reported cases have been pure hemangiomas, and the rest are classified as lymphangiomas.

C. They are most often located at the rim of the foramen ovale and are asymptomatic.

D. They may occur on the aortic or mitral valves.

E. With endocardial cushion defects they may be found in the tricuspid valve near the ventricular septum.

F. Microscopically, they are endothelial-lined and filled with blood, lymph, or organizing thrombus.

G. The few symptomatic examples have occurred in the ventricular septum and have produced heart block, syncope, or sudden death.

H. With the advent of cardiac pacemakers, death from heart block has become unusual.

6. *Primary pericardial tumors*

A. Primary pericardial tumors may include most of these cell types already mentioned. However, almost half of these primary pericardial tumors are malignant sarcomas or mesotheliomas.

B. They are encountered mainly in adults.

C. Benign lesions rarely produce symptoms, but the malignant majority produce severe cardiac disability.

D. Hemorrhagic pericardial effusions lead to rapid decompensation and tend to reaccumulate rapidly.

E. Superior vena cava obstruction may be caused by malignant pericardial tumors.

F. The major diagnostic problem is to rule out metastatic disease as the cause of pericardial effusion.

7. *Myxomas*

A. Myxomas are the commonest of all cardiac tumors, comprising half of all reported cases of cardiac tumors.

B. They are always intracardiac.

C. They usually occur in the atria, with the left involved three times more often than the right.

D. They can occur on the mitral valve or in the ventricles, where they are usually multiple.

E. Bilateral atrial myxomas have also been reported.

F. Myxomas are rare in children and almost unknown in infants.

G. The age range has been quoted at from 3 to 95 years. Sixty-eight per cent occur between 30 and 70 years.

H. Females are slightly more affected than males.

I. Pathologic findings of myxomas:

(1) Myxomas are almost always pedunculated, with the remainder being sessile.

(2) They are polypoid gelatinous masses, varying in color from greyish-white to red. The red color is caused by hemorrhage into the tumor.

(3) Their long strands wave like seaweed in the blood stream. Their shape is oval and their length may range from 2 to 10 centimeters. Occasionally they show indentation around them from impingement upon a valve orifice.

(4) Myxomas present highly characteristic appearances, which allow for easy identification. They are semi-transparent, gelatinous, and greenish or colorless in hue. They usually form a round, firm mass that is almost always attached by a pedicle to the interatrial septum near the margin of the fossa ovalis.

(5) Microscopically, the mass is composed of poorly defined cells with a thin endothelial layer. These endothelial cells are of uniform consistency with almost no mitotic activity. They are arranged in syncytial groups closely associated with cleft-like thin-walled capillary blood vessels. Larger thick-walled vessels are in the stalk, which contains fibroelastic tissue.

(6) Ultrastructural features and enzyme studies of the tumor cells appear to favor a mesenchymal cell origin more closely allied to that of endocardial lining cells than to smooth muscle cells or fibrocytes.

(7) Studies of a large series of interatrial septa showed that the region around the fossa ovalis contains a large amount of connective tissue and therefore might be more commonly associated with connective tissue tumors.

(8) It is important to distinguish myxomas from ball thrombi. The gelatinous type of myxoma is easily distinguished by its consistency, color, or by its lobular or villous configuration. It is more difficult to distinguish between myxomas and thrombi when the myxoma is smooth and ovoid. In these instances, the pedicle of the myxoma and the lack of lamination are definite characteristics.

J. Myxoma metastases

(1) Since the first report of the recurrence of a well-excised atrial myxoma (1967), other instances of local invasiveness or metastatic spread have been reported.

(2) In the past, the long duration of symptoms associated with myxomas and the histological picture suggested a slow evolution with little potential for invasiveness.

(3) However, the cases of reported recurrence have shown that the

second lesion appears to grow more rapidly than the first.

(4) A review by Read in 1974, with collected data on 12 patients, showed 15 local or metastatic recurrences of cardiac myxomas. These recurrences were attributed to either inadequate initial resection, new tumor foci derived from pretumor cells concentrated close to the foramen ovale, or implantation far from septal origins. Extraseptal occurrences were more frequently multiple and sessile. The extraseptal recurrences may be more infiltrating than the primary tumors, as is the case with noncardiac myxomas.

(5) The eventuality of recurrence or metastatic spread of these myxomas cannot be predicted from the microscopic appearance of the primary tumor.

8. *Malignant primary tumors*

A. Malignant primary tumors of the heart are all sarcomas.

B. They comprise 20 per cent of all cardiac tumors.

C. All cell types may show malignant change. Myxosarcoma, fibrosarcoma, rhabdomyosarcoma, angiosarcoma, and leiomyosarcoma are the usual entities.

D. They are more common in the right atrium than the benign myxoma, which has a predilection for the left atrium.

E. Because of this common occurrence in the right atrium, they often produce superior caval or tricuspid valve obstruction.

F. Intramural malignant lesions are more common than intracavitary lesions.

G. Primary pericardial tumors are also found to have a higher incidence of malignancy.

H. Pathologic findings of malignant primary tumors:

(1) The pathological diagnosis of malignancy does not preclude chance of cure or a reasonably long palliation.

(2) Distinction between smooth and striated muscle tumors is usually impossible among poorly differentiated neoplasms.

(3) Malignant vascular tumors of the myocardium and endocardium are of diverse histiogenesis: they therefore have been classified under the general term *angiosarcoma*.

(4) Although malignant cardiac tumors have been more common in men between the ages of 30 and 50, the malignant vascular tumors have been more frequent in females of the same age group.

SECONDARY TUMORS OF THE HEART

1. Metastic tumors of the heart are 16 to 40 times more common than the primary heart tumors.

2. With the exception of cerebral neoplasms, all tumors can metastasize to the heart.

3. Reports in the past decades have shown consistently that cardiac metastases occur in 3 to 27 per cent of patients with malignancy.

4. This is greater than 25 years ago and probably reflects a greater longevity in patients with a primary neoplastic process.

5. *Cardiac symptoms*

A. Cardiac symptoms from metastatic tumor are relatively uncommon.

B. They are present in approximately 8 per cent of patients with cardiac metastases proven at autopsy.

C. However, in patients with symptoms, the cardiac metastases are the major factors contributing to death.

6. Metastatic cardiac tumors occur mostly in patients over the age of 50, with no tendency toward either sex.

7. There is no correlation between the duration of malignant disease and the subsequent development of cardiac metastases.

8. *Carcinomas versus sarcomas*

A. Carcinomas are much more apt

to develop metastases to the heart than are sarcomas.

B. Those from carcinoma are usually grossly visible, multiple, and discrete.

C. Sarcomas show diffuse infiltration in most cases. Necrosis is uncommon in either type.

9. *Carcinoma of the lung*

A. Carcinoma of the lung is the primary tumor that most frequently invades the heart.

B. Cardiac metastases are found in almost 10 per cent of all carcinomas of the lung.

10. Carcinoma of the breast, lymphoma, renal carcinoma, and malignant melanoma are the next most frequent metastatic tumors found. Malignant melanomas metastasize to the heart in 50 per cent of cases.

11. Leukemia patients show microscopic infiltration in 50 per cent of cases.

12. Reticulum cell sarcoma shows a 16 per cent incidence of cardiac metastases.

13. *Routes of metastasis*

Metastatic disease reaches the heart by three routes. In descending order of frequency, they are embolic phenomena, lymphatic spread, or direct invasion.

A. Carcinoma of the breast and lung invade by lymphatic spread because the heart is close to the mediastinal lymphatics.

B. Lymphomas usually involve the heart by direct extension.

C. Leukemias and melanomas appear to spread by hematogenous means.

14. Pericardial involvement is the most frequent manifestation of secondary heart tumors.

15. Myocardial involvement shows variable areas of greater involvement with some preponderance for right-sided occurrence in most studies. The cardiac venous return going to the right side may explain this phenomena.

16. Implantation of the endocardium and heart valves is seen, but this usually occurs on already abnormal endocardial surfaces. Those endocardial metastases can be polypoid and simulate a benign myxoma, or they can embolize and mimic bacterial endocarditis.

SYMPTOMS AND SIGNS

The range of symptoms by which cardiac tumors may be manifest often traverses the usual signs of organic heart disease; symptoms may be as mild as malaise, fatigue, and abnormal laboratory studies, or as life-threatening as rapidly progressive congestive heart failure or ventricular fibrillation. Although the clinical symptoms may give good evidence that there is a cardiac neoplasm, more definitive studies must be performed for confirmation. The safety and availability of diagnostic facilities can eliminate the surprise of finding a cardiac tumor when operating for another suspected lesion.

Manifestations of cardiac tumors are divided into four groups (Goodwin): (1) hemodynamic disturbances; (2) mechanical hemolysis; (3) biochemical effects; and (4) constitutional symptoms.

1. *Hemodynamic alterations*

Rapidly progressive congestive heart failure that is sudden in onset and intractable to standard measures is the usual presentation of cardiac neoplasia. Of equal importance may be pericardial effusions that are hemorrhagic and rapidly reaccumulating; unexplained rapidly changing arrhythmias; syncope with Stokes-Adams attacks; unexplained embolic phenomena; and those embolic phenomena associated with a picture of bacterial endocarditis with pulmonary hypertension, or with severe effects of valvular obstruction.

A. *Cardiac obstruction*

(1) General features

(a) Most of the tumors previously described can obstruct the cavities of the heart and great vessels.

(b) These may simulate many

forms of valvular and myocardial disease.

(c) Myxomas, fibromas, and sarcomas (the most common) are usually found in the atria.

(d) Left atrial involvement usually shows obstruction to the mitral valve while right atrial involvement shows inflow occlusion symptoms.

(e) The clues to excluding rheumatic or congenital causes of right-sided obstruction are usually found because isolated valvular lesions with rheumatic disease are rare, and congenital lesions have a longer history.

(f) Symptoms may occur abruptly in tumors of the heart, and constitutional effects such as fever or weight loss may be present.

(2) Atrial tumors

(a) Right as well as left atrial tumors may produce obstruction to the atrioventricular valve flow rather abruptly.

(b) This is because the pedicle that usually attaches the tumor to the septum allows free travel from atrium to ventricle in many instances.

(c) The auscultatory findings in tumors of the atria are often very changeable from one examination to the next. A change in posture may be accompanied by a change in the murmur.

(d) The intensity of the murmur is often out of proportion to the degree of symptoms that the patient may possess.

(e) Left atrial myxomas usually give rise to a soft systolic murmur followed by a mid-diastolic murmur.

(f) The first sound is usually widely split.

(g) Occasionally an "endocardial" friction rub, which is believed to be due to physical contact of the tumor with the atrial or ventricular endocardium, is present.

(h) If the tumor is fixed in position relative to the orifice it obstructs, positional changes in auscultatory findings are unlikely to occur.

(i) Obstruction of the flow to the left side of the heart is almost always due to a left atrial myxoma, the most common primary heart tumor.

(j) The picture is most often confused with mitral stenosis with left atrial hypertension, pulmonary venous obstruction, and pulmonary congestion with dyspnea and hemoptysis.

(k) The shortness of the duration of symptoms as well as the episodic occurrence of the symptoms, which may change with posture, give indication of tumor.

(l) Right atrial myxomas may mimic constrictive pericarditis, tricuspid stenosis and regurgitation, pulmonary embolic disease, or cardiomyopathies.

(m) When a tumor of the right atrium or cavae becomes so large as to interfere with ventricular filling, survival of the patient may depend on the presence of a patent foramen ovale or a small atrial septal defect. The patient usually becomes cyanotic and gives a picture of tricuspid stenosis or atresia.

(n) Ten to fifteen per cent of patients who have been reported as having right atrial myxomas have shown right to left shunts.

(3) Ventricular tumors

(a) Tumors in the right and left ventricles cause obstruction to the semilunar valves.

(b) There are usually signs of aortic or pulmonary obstruction of significant degree to cause symptoms mimicking aortic or pulmonary stenoses.

(c) If symptoms of severe right-sided obstruction, such as fatigue, dyspnea, facial swelling or ascites, appear with a murmur of pulmonic stenosis, a tumor is most often the case; pulmonary stenosis is symptomless except in severe cases.

(d) Left ventricular tumors give a clinical picture of subaortic stenosis.

(e) They usually give less than impressive evidence of obstruction to blood flow as compared to the atrial tumors.

(f) Except for the rare pedunculated myxoma, tumors of the left ventricle cause obstruction from enlargement of the muscular wall.

(g) They may involve the coronary circulation.

(h) Sudden death, convulsions, dyspnea, angina, and syncope were among the symptoms of a series of seventeen cases of intramural left ventricular tumors.

(i) In any patient in whom obstruction to the aortic valve is suspected by symptoms of angina, syncope, or convulsions, and a murmur of aortic stenosis is found and diagnosis of aortic valve disease, subaortic stenosis, or cardiomyopathy is not clear, one must suspect a left ventricular tumor.

B. *Pericardial involvement*

(1) Many of the primary tumors of the heart, as well as most of the secondary ones, invade the pericardium.

(2) They commonly produce an effusion with its concomitant roentgenographic picture of cardiac enlargement.

(3) Often there is tamponade with the characteristic pulsus paradoxus, neck vein distention, and decreased voltage on the electrocardiogram.

(4) Aspiration of bloody pericardial fluid is almost always positive evidence of some type of tumor involvement unless strong clinical evidence points to cardiac rupture.

(5) Whether metastatic or primary tumor is involved can often be determined by cytological examination of the fluid.

(6) Tuberculosis of the pericardium must be ruled out because it can give rise to a bloody pericardial effusion.

C. *Cardiac arrhythmias*

(1) Conduction disturbances are the most frequent clinical manifestations of secondary cardiac tumors and a common occurrence with primary tumors as well.

(2) The most common cardiac arrhythmia is atrial fibrillation.

(3) Metastatic tumors from the lung are the most common cause of such fibrillation.

(4) Atrial fibrillation and flutter are common with right atrial disease.

(5) Invasion of the A-V node or the interventricular septum can produce A-V block with classical Stokes-Adams attacks. This is usually the case in sudden death from cardiac tumors.

(6) Repetitive ventricular tachycardia is usually the main feature of primary tumors involving the right ventricle in infants.

(7) In children, arrhythmias are a common first manifestation of cardiac tumors.

(8) Noncardiac tumors, such as pheochromocytomas, may also produce arrhythmias, such as ventricular tachycardia. Pheochyromocytomas also show a picture of myocardial necrosis resulting from an excess of catecholamines.

D. *Embolism*

(1) Intracardiac tumors are the only ones that can give rise to embolization.

(2) This is either due to blood clot on the tumor or to fragments of the tumor itself.

(3) They may embolize to the lungs or peripheral circulation.

(4) Any patient who has unexplained pulmonary emboli or pulmonary hypertension may have a right-sided tumor showering fragments to the pulmonary circulation.

(5) If there is no obvious source in the lower limbs for the emboli, angiography is required of the pulmonary circulation and right-sided heart chambers.

(6) *Peripheral embolization*

(a) Peripheral embolization is very common in tumors of the heart.

(b) Fifty per cent of left atrial myxomas show signs of peripheral embolization.

(c) Many times, these may be silent and may involve many organ systems.

(d) This may simulate a generalized vascular disease with little sign of cardiac involvement, or constitutional symptoms that are common with left atrial tumors.

(7) Where there is embolization in any patient under forty years of age or where there is no apparent cause for embolization, as from mitral stenosis with fibrillation or recent myocardial infarction, cardiac tumors should be looked for.

(8) It is always wise to have histological sectioning of all emboli retrieved from the vascular system, although failure to find evidence of neoplastic tissue does not rule out the presence of a cardiac tumor.

(9) Left atrial myxomas also can give rise to coronary embolism and infarction.

(10) If clear-cut evidence of infarction occurs in a child or young adult, cardiac tumor should be looked for.

2. *Constitutional symptoms* (see list below)

A. Because the myxoma is the most common cardiac tumor encountered primarily, enough cases have been reported to give some indication of the systemic manifestations of their occurrence.

B. Seventy per cent of patients show anorexia, weight loss, and fatigue, with almost the same percentage showing nausea, vomiting, and diarrhea.

C. Febrile episodes occur in almost 40 per cent, with the same number exhibiting joint or muscle pain.

D. Clubbing of fingers has occurred in 20 per cent.

E. To best explain these symptoms and those of the abnormal laboratory evaluations, it has been felt that the

Symptoms of Cardiac Tumors

Rapid unexplained onset of congestive heart failure
Pericardial effusion, tamponade, or syndrome
    simulating constrictive pericarditis
Obstruction of cardiac flow
  Syncope
  Angina
  Pulmonary edema
  Murmurs of aortic or pulmonary stenosis
  Murmurs of tricuspid and mitral stenosis
Arrhythmias
Unexplained atrial fibrillation
Multiple emboli, pulmonary or systemic
Pulmonary hypertension
  Emboli to lungs from right heart
  Systemic from left heart
Symptoms simulating bacterial endocarditis
  Fever
  Anemia
  Clubbing of fingers
  Changing murmurs
  Embolism
Anemia—hemolytic due to destruction of red cells
Constitutional symptoms
  Fever
  Weight loss
  Abnormal liver function tests
  Abnormal globulins
Chest pain—due to invasion of myocardium by
  tumor or due to coronary insufficiency

fragments of the tumor released into the circulation may produce an autoimmune state similar to that seen after myocardial infarction or cardiotomies.

LABORATORY FINDINGS

1. *Electrocardiography and vectorcardiography*

Changes in the electrocardiogram or the vectorcardiogram produced by neoplasms of the heart generally include chamber hypertrophy in the case of intracavitary tumors or conduction disturbances and nonspecific T wave changes resulting from myocardial replacement by neoplasm.

Replacement of myocardial tissue by neoplasm does not often produce any striking electrocardiographic changes. A consistent finding is nonspecific flattening or inversion of the T waves in some of the standard and left precordial leads.

A. *Chamber enlargement*

(1) With chamber enlargement, as in the case of left atrial and right atrial tumors, there are broad and bifid P waves.

(2) If there is left atrial tumor, the concomitant increase in work for the right ventricle can give rise to right ventricular hypertrophy.

(3) Outlet obstruction of the semilunar valves gives a pattern of either right or left ventricular hypertrophy depending on whether the aortic or pulmonary flow is obstructed.

B. *Pericardial involvement*

(1) Pericardial involvement usually gives the low voltage.

(2) The S-T, T wave changes of pericarditis (usually S-T segment elevation followed by T wave inversion) are common.

C. *Cardiac arrhythmias*

(1) Cardiac arrhythmias are uncommonly observed in intracavitary tumors, but are often encountered in intramural as well as metastatic malignant pericardial tumors.

(2) Atrial premature contractions, tachycardia, flutter or fibrillation, and such ventricular arrhythmias as ventricular premature contractions or ventricular tachycardia can accompany intramural atrial or ventricular neoplasms.

(3) Varying degrees of A-V block or fascicular block occur when the tumor is strategically placed in the region of the A-V node or its continuation into the bundle of His and its subdivisions.

2. *Phonocardiography*

A. Phonocardiography is often very valuable in distinguishing the variability of murmurs that are usually evident with cardiac tumors.

B. Decrease in intensity of heart sounds can be ascertained with both pericardial tumors and intracavitary neoplasms.

C. Accurate timing of the opening and closing sounds of the atrioventricular valves can often help in distinguishing mitral stenosis from atrial tumor.

D. "Endocardial" friction rubs, believed to be due to the physical contact of the tumor against the atrial or ventricular endocardium, may also be defined.

3. *Echocardiography and angiocardiography*

A. Echocardiography, a relatively new technique, has adapted well to the diagnosis of cardiac neoplasms.

B. Not only can intracavitary structures be visualized, but abnormalities in wall thickness can be defined.

C. Pericardial effusions and thickening can likewise be found.

D. Echocardiography has become important, for it can, in some instances, eliminate the need for definitive angiography, which has been the backbone of diagnosis in the past.

E. Echocardiography has primary value in serving as an innocuous step to rule in or out the possibility of an intracavitary cardiac neoplasm before proceeding to the more definitive angiography.

F. It should not be considered as just a screening procedure, because only with a high degree of clinical suspicion will the echocardiographer take the time to perform the various manipulations and gain settings on his equipment to demonstrate a cardiac neoplasm.

4. *Angiocardiography*

A. Angiography is essential and is still the most precise and accurate method for obtaining an anatomic diagnosis of cardiac neoplasms.

B. Cineradiography is more useful than rapid film techniques because of its ease. Some fine delineation of the great vessels, which may be necessary, may be done with cut film rapid changers.

C. Angiography is performed by injecting dye into the cavae if suspicion of right atrial tumors exists, into the pulmonary artery when left-sided or pulmonary artery neoplasm is suspected, or directly into the left atrium when left ventricular lesions are suspected.

D. If the cardiac output is low, a pulmonary artery injection may fail to concentrate enough dye into the left side of the heart for accurate visualization.

E. Directly injecting dye into the left atrium via a trans-septal catheter technique could lead to dislodgement of the tumor into the systemic circulation. The same can happen if one manipulates the catheter in the right side of the heart with right atrial and ventricular tumors, although the consequences of pulmonary embolization are perhaps less.

F. Besides demonstrating the cardiac chambers, angiography gives valuable information regarding the pulmonary circulation. If there is malignant invasion of the mediastinum, contrast studies help to outline the major vessels, particularly the pulmonary artery, aorta, and superior vena cava. Compression or displacement of these vessels by tumor mass may be shown.

G. In the rarer types of tumor, which may be too small to appear as a mass, angiocardiograms will reveal such clues as chamber enlargement, cavity contour irregularities, and gross wall thickening.

H. False positive results may be obtained with angiography also. Streaming of nonopaque venous blood, thrombus, atrial septal hematoma, lipomatous deposits in the atrial septum, congenital septal dysplasias, and hydatid cysts of the interventricular septum have all been erroneously pursued as cardiac tumors.

5. *Cardiac catheterization*

Cardiac catheterization is usually employed for evaluation of mitral or tricuspid disease. This is often undertaken without much suspicion of a cardiac tumor being present. However, when performing a catheterization, the investigator must be alert to any abnormal situations that might indicate a cardiac tumor.

A. Difficulties in passing catheters through the right chambers, variable pressure tracings, and a finding of a marked increase in pulmonary vascular resistance should alert one to the possibility of a tumor.

B. Selzer noted that in 70 per cent of left atrial myxomas, the elevation in pulmonary vascular resistance was severe, in contrast to only 20 per cent or less in other causes of reactive pulmonary hypertensions, such as mitral disease or left ventricular failure.

C. Catheterization is useful because it demonstrates the existence and severity of an obstructing lesion as well as absence of shunting. However, the information obtained is not specific and is often interpreted as the findings due to valvular heart disease.

D. An intracardiac tumor is not usually suspected from the catheterization data but from the clinical findings and history. Because of these factors, angiography is the procedure of choice after an echocardiographic examination has been done.

6. *Chest x-ray*

Radiologic appearance of the heart with intracardiac tumors on plain chest films is by no means specific and usually is quite normal. However, in many situations the plain chest film can be suspicious enough of either a cardiac or pericardial tumor to warrant further investigation.

A. Left atrial tumors can produce left atrial enlargement.

B. Tumors of the myocardium often change the contour of the myocardium.

C. Differentiation between mural and pericardial tumors is very difficult. Effusions may be present in both instances.

D. Fluoroscopy may show diminished pulsation if there is a large effusion or may cause excessive pulsation, as is the case with some malignant tumors.

E. Mediastinal widening and hilar and paramediastinal lymphadenopathy are present in some malignant extensions of cardiac tumors.

F. Evaluation of the lung fields is very important because of the nature of cardiac tumors to cause either pulmonary hypertension, pulmonary oligemia, or signs of congestive heart failure.

G. Left atrial tumors usually produce those pictures of pulmonary venous obstruction similar to mitral valve disease, with septal lines at the bases, perihilar haziness, or venous distention in the upper lobes.

H. Pulmonary arterial hypertension may develop further along in the course of this picture or it may be the result of right-sided tumors producing pulmonary emboli. Pulmonary hypertension is evident if there is pulmonary arterial dilatation of hilar areas with normal picture of the upper lobe vasculature and if there is arterial narrowing and pruning at the periphery of the lungs.

I. Pulmonary infarcts must be screened for, as well as metastatic deposits.

J. Pleural effusions are due either to congestive heart failure, occlusive pulmonary vascular disease when the pulmonary veins are obstructed, or malignant exudates if there is involvement of the malignancy in the pleura itself.

K. Calcification is unusual, being found in rhabdomyomas and in teratomas. Very rarely do atrial myxomas show calcification. It must be ruled out in the heart valves, coronary arteries, and the pericardium in all instances. Fluoroscopy and tomography are aids in this endeavor. Calcification of a thrombus usually is very extensive and hugs the wall of the specific cardiac chamber.

7. *Biochemical and hematological findings*

Biochemical and hematological findings are common in patients with cardiac myxomas. Rarely do the other less common tumors exhibit any significant abnormalities of this nature.

A. Elevated erythrocyte sedimentation rates were present in almost 100 per cent of patients with myxomas.

B. Sixty-five per cent showed a leukocytosis of 8,000 to 15,000 without a shift to the left.

C. A finding of anemia with hemoglobin less than 12 gram per cent was present in 50 per cent of patients.

D. Eighty per cent of patients show a decrease in serum iron levels; thrombocytopenia is present in nearly 30 per cent.

E. *Liver function tests* are also abnormal in most patients with myxomas.

(1) Eighty per cent show elevated bilirubin levels or the upper limits of normal.

(2) In one series of 11 patients with myxoma, 2 had clinical jaundice.

(3) Sixty per cent show an elevation in alkaline phosphatase.

(4) Lactic acid dehydrogenase (LDH) is elevated in close to 50 per cent.

(5) Serum glutamic oxalacetic transaminase (SGOT) levels were for the most part normal.

(6) Total serum protein and albumin determinations are below normal in all patients. Electrophoretic fractioning invariably shows abnormalities in the alpha-1 or alpha-2 fractions, but they may be either greater or lower than normal. In those patients who had C-reactive protein determinations, 50 per cent were positive.

DIAGNOSIS

The diagnosis of cardiac tumors can be made from 4 major alterations, as follows:

1. *Hemodynamic disturbances*
   A. Cardiac arrhythmias

B. Pericarditis with or without effusion

C. Intracavitary obstruction

D. Embolization

2. *Mechanical hemolysis*

A. Anemias

B. Low serum iron

3. *Biochemical effects*

A. Abnormal serum protein

B. Abnormal serum enzymes

C. Elevated serum bilirubin

D. Elevated alkaline phosphatase

4. *Constitutional disturbances*

A. Fever

B. Anorexia, nausea, vomiting, and diarrhea

C. Weight loss

D. Fatigue

E. Dizziness and fainting

F. Joint or muscle pain

G. Clubbing of fingers

H. High sedimentation rate

In addition to the above, various diagnostic tests, particularly echocardiography and angiocardiography, often confirm the presence of cardiac tumors.

DIFFERENTIAL DIAGNOSIS

Despite thoughtful appraisal of all symptoms and tests, the physician can still be mistaken in his diagnosis of a cardiac tumor, because many entities can mimic cardiac tumors. Therefore, cardiac tumors must be differentiated from various other cardiovascular disorders.

1. *Pseudotumors*

A. These so-called pseudotumors that present as pericardial, myocardial, or intracavitary masses are usually pedunculated.

B. Endothelialized thrombi, abscesses, and foreign bodies of the heart appear as endocardial tumors.

C. They may also be congenital diverticuli, ventricular aneurysms, or coronary artery aneurysms that may appear as epicardial tumors.

2. *Valvular heart diseases* (see Chap. 5)

3. *Congenital heart diseases* (see Chap. 10)

4. *Cardiomyopathies* (see Chap. 9)

5. *Pericarditis, myocarditis, and endocarditis* (see Chaps. 7 and 8)

6. *Coronary heart disease* (see Chap. 2)

7. *Congestive heart failure due to other causes* (see Chap. 19)

8. *Mitral valve prolapse syndrome* (Barlow's syndrome, see Chap. 6)

MANAGEMENT

Primary cardiac tumors are a surgical disease. Cardiopulmonary bypass must be available in all surgical approaches to these tumors. There should be no delay in undertaking surgery once the diagnosis has been confirmed.

1. In performing surgery, care is taken to prevent any embolization from the tumor, either to the lungs or the peripheral circulation. Even benign myxomas can set up metastatic foci if allowed to embolize.

2. Superior and inferior vena caval cannulation of the right heart, cross-clamping of the aorta, and electrically induced fibrillation are performed to minimize cardiac manipulation before opening the heart.

3. Median sternotomy is used in all cases.

4. Tumors of the ventricles can usually be removed through either a transaortic or transatrial approach.

5. Removal of the base of pedunculated tumors must be complete. It is recommended that in cases of attachment to the atrial septum, as is the case with most myxomas, a large portion of the septum be removed.

A. This is to prevent any chance of recurrence from the atrial septum, where the abnormal cellular growths arise.

B. The septum is then closed either primarily, with pericardium, or prosthetic material.

6. Because mechanical effects of intracavitary tumors can cause significant damage to valvular function, the surgeon must be prepared to perform plastic repairs or valvular replacement on any damaged valves.

7. Pacemaker provisions likewise must be made when necessary.

PROGNOSIS

1. Depending on the preoperative state of the patient, benign cardiac tumors are almost completely curable.

2. Resolution of symptoms with decrease in heart size, reversal of pulmonary hypertension, and return to normal of the hematological and biochemical abnormalities are expected.

3. When malignant disease is encountered, an aggressive surgical resection and reconstruction coupled with radiation therapy can be of great benefit in eliminating symptoms and prolonging life.

4. Mortality rates for the resection of right- and left sided myxomas approaches that of the surgery for adults undergoing closure of atrial septal defects. If the tumor is found to be benign, long-term results are excellent.

5. Procrastination may result in disabling emboli, advancement of deterioration in valvular function, or sudden death.

SUGGESTED READINGS

Emmanuel, R. W. and Lloyd, W. E.: Right atrial myxoma mistaken for constrictive pericarditis. Br. Heart J., *24*:796, 1962.

Engle, M. A. and Glenn, F.: Primary malignant tumor of the heart in infancy. Case report and review of subject. Pediatrics, *15*:562, 1955.

Gerbode, F.: Tumors of the heart. Cardiac Surgery, II, Cardiovasc. Clin., *3*:59, 1971.

Goodwin, J. F.: Spectrum of cardiac tumors. Am. J. Cardiol., *31*:307, 1968.

Griffiths, G. C.: A review of primary tumors of the heart. Prog. Cardiovasc. Dis., *7*:465, 1965.

Harvey, W. P.: Clinical aspects of cardiac tumors. Am. J. Cardiol., *21*:328, 1968.

Heath, D.: Pathology of cardiac tumors. Am. J. Cardiol., *21*:315, 1968.

Kaufman, G. et al.: Heart sounds in atrial tumors. Am. J. Cardiol., *8*:350, 1961.

Lev, M.: Tumors of the heart. *In* B. M. Gasul et al. (eds.): Heart Disease in Children: Diagnosis and Treatment. Philadelphia, J. B. Lippincott, 1966.

Murphy, W. R. C. et al.: Recurrent myxosarcoma of left atrium. Chest, *67*:733, 1975.

Prichard, R. W.: Tumors of the heart. Review of the subject and report of 150 cases. Arch. Pathol., *51*:98, 1951.

Read, R. C. et al.: The malignant potentiality of left atrial myxoma. J. Thorac. Cardiovasc. Surg., *68*:857, 1974.

Segal, B. L.: Introduction to symposium on echocardiography. Am. J. Cardiol., *19*:1, 1967.

Selzer, A., Sakai, F. J., and Popper, R. W.: Protean clinical manifestations of primary tumors of the heart. Am. J. Med., *52*:9, 1972.

Silverman, J. et al.: Cardiac myxoma with systemic embolization. Review of literature and report of a case. Circulation, *26*:99, 1962.

Steinberg, I. et al.: Angiography in diagnosis of cardiac tumors. Am. J. Roentgenol. Radium Ther. Nucl. Med., *91*:364, 1964.

Sterns, L. P. et al.: Intracavitary cardiac neoplasms. A review of 15 cases. Br. Heart J., *28*:75, 1966.

Thurber, D. L., Edwards, J. E., and Anchor, R. W. P.: Secondary malignant tumors of the pericardium. Circulation, *26*:228, 1962.

Trond, H. K., Shiv, R. U. and Gerbode, F.: Dysfunction of the liver in cardiac myxoma. Surg. Gynecol. Obstet., *134*:288, 1972.

Van Der Hauwaert, L. G.: Cardiac tumors in infants and children. Br. Heart J., *33*:125, 1971.

Willman, V. L. et al.: Unusual aspects of intracavitary tumors of the heart. Dis. Chest, *47*:669, 1965.

12. PULMONARY EMBOLISM

Edward Genton, M.D.

DEFINITION

1. A pulmonary embolism is a mass or plug of material that has moved from a peripheral site through a systemic vein and into the pulmonary arterial circulation, and produced obstruction, either partial or complete, of blood flow through the involved vessel.

2. The majority of pulmonary emboli are composed of fibrin and originate from mobile venous thrombi in a lower extremity or pelvic veins, but occasionally arise from the upper extremities or right atrium. Rarely, emboli consisting of material other than thrombus may occur. These include: tumor material that is usually small but that may be very large when the tumor involves major veins, such as the iliac or inferior vena cava; ova, most often schistosoma parasites; foreign bodies, such as bullets or (more frequently) segments of plastic tubing used as catheter material; fat as part of the syndrome associated with fracture of long bones; amniotic fluid; or air, usually resulting from accidents during surgical procedures or with intravenous feeding.

3. The vast majority of pulmonary thromboemboli originate in the deep venous system of the lower extremities. The pelvic plexus of veins serves as a source of embolic material, especially in association with pelvic disease, such as prostatitis in males and pelvic inflammatory disease in females. The right heart chambers are the source of a small percentage of pulmonary emboli and is seen in patients with dilated or infarcted cardiac chambers and especially in the presence of atrial fibrillation. Veins of the upper extremities, while not a rare source of emboli, seldom give rise to large amounts of embolus.

GENERAL CONSIDERATIONS

1. Pulmonary embolism is a condition of major importance because of the frequency of occurrence and of the morbidity and mortality produced by the process. It is estimated that in the United States, more than 500,000 episodes of pulmonary embolism occur each year, causing the death of more than 50,000 patients and contributing to at least an equal number. It is the most common lethal pulmonary disease and in some centers is the single most frequent cause of death.

2. In the natural history of pulmonary embolism, recurrent episodes are frequent and leads to fatal outcome in more than 25 per cent of untreated patients. Death from pulmonary embolism usually develops rapidly, with more than 60 per cent of fatalities occurring within one hour from onset of symptoms.

3. The diagnosis of pulmonary embolism is often difficult and in fewer than half of major emboli discovered at autopsy, has the diagnosis been clinically suspected.

4. If diagnosed and properly treated, the outlook for survival and in fact for complete recovery is excellent. Thus, it is essential for physicians, regardless of their specialty interests, to maintain a high index of suspicion for pulmonary embolism in their hospitalized patients and to remain familiar with developments in diagnosis and treatment of this important condition.

ETIOLOGY

1. Factors which contribute to the development of thrombosis in veins from which pulmonary emboli derive include: *stasis* of venous blood resulting from

partial obstruction or slowing of venous return due to such conditions as immobilization, varicose veins, obesity, pregnancy, or congestive heart failure; *venous wall damage* by soft tissue trauma, fractures or surgery, or infiltration of the vessel wall by malignant cells or microorganisms; *hypercoagulability* related to thrombocytosis or increased platelet reactivity following trauma, surgery or parturition, polycythemia, hemoconcentration, or tissue breakdown, (e.g., myocardial infarction or cancer). Approximately 10 per cent of pulmonary emboli occur in "normal" people in whom no predisposing factors are identifiable.

2. Patients in various groups are in particular likely to have one or more of the thrombogenic stimuli just listed, and these patients should be considered at high risk of developing venous thromboembolism. These groups include patients (a) who are elderly, especially when they have suffered soft tissue or long bone trauma; (b) who have cardiac disorders with myocardial infarction, myocardiopathy or congestive heart failure; (c) who are immobilized for longer than 3 or 4 days; (d) who are postoperative or postpartum; (e) who have neoplasm or blood dyscrasia or (f) infection and malnutrition (g) who are obese; and (h) especially those with prior history of thromboembolism.

PATHOPHYSIOLOGY

The physiological consequences of pulmonary embolism are greatly variable and depend upon the degree of obstruction produced by the emboli and the pre-existing condition of the pulmonary circulation.

1. The normal pulmonary bed requires compromise of more than 50 per cent of the cross sectional area for significant hemodynamic alteration to be produced. However, when the lung has been previously affected by disease, such as congestive heart failure or chronic obstructive pulmonary disease, embolism of lesser magnitude may produce disability.

2. The consequence of pulmonary arterial obstruction is the development of pulmonary hypertension, which, if abrupt in onset and of sufficient severity, may cause decompensation of the right ventricle. Depending upon the degree of obstruction and its rate of development, the patient may tolerate the insult with only mild or transient alteration, or at the opposite extreme may suffer sudden death.

3. If prior cardiopulmonary abnormalities that reduce collateral circulation to affected lung antedate an embolic episode, sufficient ischemia of pulmonary tissue may occur to produce hemorrhagic necrosis (pulmonary infarction). This occurs in no more than 10 per cent of emboli and is associated with occlusion of medium-sized pulmonary vessels (less than 1 mm.) and insufficient collateral flow from bronchial circulation. Most frequently, "infarction" is incomplete and the products of inflammation resolve completely within a few days.

4. Chronic pulmonary hypertension seldom follows a single embolic episode, but may result from multiple emboli, usually involving medium-sized vessels.

5. Several physiological derangements may occur in association with pulmonary thromboembolism. These include bronchoconstriction, vasoconstriction, and hypoxemia. The genesis of these changes has not been precisely elucidated.

CLASSIFICATION

The most useful means of classifying emboli is based upon their size and the resulting degree of obstruction to the pulmonary circulation. On this basis, emboli may be divided into massive and submassive.

1. Massive embolism refers to the occlusion of the main pulmonary artery, or right or left pulmonary artery, or two or more lobar branches. Submassive pulmonary embolism refers to embolization that produces occlusion of a lesser degree of the pulmonary circulation.

2. As noted earlier, the clinical consequences of embolism is not entirely dependent upon the absolute obstruction present, but depends to a considerable extent upon the pre-existing condition of the pulmonary circulation and upon the suddenness with which obstruction occurs.

SYMPTOMS AND SIGNS

1. *Massive pulmonary embolism*

A. Massive pulmonary embolism is often accompanied by crushing substernal chest pain (often indistinguishable from that of myocardial infarction), dyspnea, diaphoresis, cyanosis, apprehension, stupor, or syncope.

B. Blood pressure may be low, or shock may exist.

C. Respirations are gasping or rapid and shallow.

D. The arterial pulse is rapid and of small volume.

E. The jugular venous pulse reveals elevated venous pressure and frequently prominent A and V waves.

F. Rarely is right ventricular activity palpable, but occasionally a shock of pulmonary closure is felt.

G. A scratchy systolic murmur, which may be mistaken for a pericardial friction rub, is sometimes heard in the pulmonary area, where the second heart sound is widely split and the pulmonic component may be accentuated.

H. Rarely a murmur of pulmonary incompetence is heard or a systolic ejection murmur is present at the left base due to obstruction of the pulmonary outflow tract by the embolus.

I. Occasionally, a pansystolic murmur of functional tricuspid incompetence and right ventricular third and fourth heart sounds may be heard along the lower left sternal border.

It must be appreciated that the clinical picture with massive embolism varies widely, and that it is not unusual that minimal or no signs or symptoms betray the existence of major occlusion to the pulmonary circulation.

2. *Submassive pulmonary embolism*

Submassive pulmonary embolism may be associated with few or no symptoms or signs, or any combination of the changes described above under massive embolism may exist. When changes occur, they may be subtle and transient, lasting for no more than a few minutes. The frequency and accuracy of diagnoses depend on a high index of suspicion and thoroughness in the history and physical examination to identify fleeting and variable clinical findings.

A. When embolization of a medium-sized pulmonary artery has occurred, pulmonary infarction may develop. Usually, several hours following the embolization, fever, pleuritic chest pain, cough, hemoptysis, and a pleural friction rub (often with a pleural effusion that may be serosanguineous) develops over a period of hours or days.

B. Patients with small, recurrent emboli often describe brief episodes of pleurisy or mild hemoptysis, but may have no symptoms until pulmonary hypertension has developed.

LABORATORY FINDINGS

1. Routine laboratory tests. It is important that the clinician recognize that no laboratory test is available that reliably establishes or excludes the diagnosis of pulmonary embolism.

A. The white blood count is often normal and seldom elevated above 15,000.

B. Biochemical tests, including lactic dehydrogenase (LDH), serum glutamic oxalacetic transaminase (SGOT), and serum bilirubin may be elevated. However, the early hope that a characteristic pattern of change in these parameters would allow precise diagnosis of embolization has not materialized. Thus, the triad of elevated LDH and bilirubin with normal SGOT is present in fewer than 20 per cent of patients with embolism and in nearly a quarter of patients there is no alteration in any of these parameters.

2. Chest x-ray. While none is specific for the diagnosis, a number of changes occur in the routine chest x-ray that are helpful to suggest the diagnosis and encourage the clinician to obtain more objective studies.

A. Normal chest x-ray is compatible with embolization of both massive and submassive variety.

B. The changes to be looked for in the chest x-ray include parenchymal infiltration, pleural effusion, an elevated diaphragm, prominent proximal pulmonary arteries, focal oligemia, and atelectasis. With pulmonary infarction, changes are best visualized 12 to 24 hours following embolization and present variably shaped (round, linear, or occasional wedge) areas of consolidation.

3. Electrocardiogram. Alterations may occur in about half the patients with major pulmonary embolism, but these changes may be fleeting and disappear within minutes or hours.

A. When embolism is of sufficient magnitude to cause right ventricular dilation or strain, any one of several electrocardiographic changes may be observed. These include (1) sinus tachycardia or supraventricular tachyarrhythmia (atrial tachycardia, atrial fibrillation, atrial flutter). (2) The initial QRS vector often rotates to the left, causing a Q wave to be recorded in lead III and

possibly in lead II and aVF. A terminal rightward and inferior QRS vector produces right axis deviation with a terminal S wave in lead I and a prominent R wave in lead III. (3) The T wave vector is often to the left, giving an inverted T wave in lead III and possibly lead II and aVF. T waves are often inverted in the right precordial leads. (4) Occasionally, a right bundle branch block may occur. (5) In the presence of right ventricular strain, tall peaked P waves may be seen in leads II, III, and aVF.

B. With submassive pulmonary emboli, the electrocardiogram may remain normal, or any combination of the above-noted changes may occur.

C. With pulmonary hypertension from multiple recurrent small emboli, the electrocardiographic changes of right axis deviation and right ventricular and right atrial enlargement usually occur.

4. Radioisotope lung scan.

A. Pulmonary perfusion scans. When radioisotopically labeled particles ranging in size from 10 to 60μ in diameter are injected intravenously, they are distributed throughout the lung in a manner corresponding to the blood flow through the pulmonary circulation. Thus, areas of under-perfusion will be readily detectable. This fast, simple technique, essentially free of morbidity, is valuable for confirming the diagnosis for initial (or recurrent) pulmonary embolism, or for assessing the natural history of the lesion and for evaluating the effectiveness of medical or surgical therapy. It is therefore indicated in all patients in whom pulmonary embolism is suspected. A properly performed scan requires multiple views, including anterior, posterior, and lateral views, and comparison with a routine chest roentgenogram. Using current techniques, the study can be carried out rapidly enough to allow it to be performed even in the critically ill and uncooperative patient.

(1) For all practical purposes, a

technically adequate scan that reveals no perfusion abnormalities excludes the diagnosis of pulmonary embolism.

(2) However, since the scan measures regional perfusion, false positive scans occur in a variety of conditions, including chronic pulmonary disease, pneumonia, asthma, pulmonary edema, and mitral stenosis.

(3) It is important to obtain follow-up scans at several-week intervals in patients with documented pulmonary embolism to establish the extent of resolution or the degree of residual defect. This allows interpretation of later scans at the time of recurrent symptoms, should they occur.

B. Ventilation scan. The evaluation of ventilation in the lungs by the use of inhaled isotopes, such as xenon 133, is valuable to increase the specificity of perfusion scanning. The finding of ventilation defects in the area of perfusion defects suggests the perfusion abnormality to be due to airway or parenchymal disease rather than obliterative vascular disease. On the other hand, identifying normal ventilation in an area of under-perfusion in a setting compatible with pulmonary embolism provides strong support to the diagnosis.

5. Pulmonary angiography. The pulmonary angiogram is the most sensitive means available for identifying the presence and location of emboli. While it does not quantify the amount of embolic material present, it does disclose the effective magnitude of obstruction. When performed within 48 to 72 hours of the suspected embolic episode, false results are unlikely to be obtained if the embolus involves medium- to large-caliber vessels.

A. Angiography is indicated in patients suspected of having a major pulmonary embolus when the diagnosis cannot be otherwise established or to obtain anatomic information for thrombolytic or surgical management. All pa-tients considered for the latter forms of therapy should have confirmation of diagnosis by angiography.

B. The procedure is usually well tolerated even by severely ill patients when carried out by an experienced team, using established techniques.

C. A complete study often requires selective angiography in areas of lung suspected of having an embolus.

6. Venography. In the evaluation of a patient with suspected pulmonary embolism, venography of the lower extremities is often of considerable value. If thrombotic disease is discovered in the setting suggesting acute pulmonary embolism, it often allows a judgment concerning treatment to be made without further diagnostic studies, such as pulmonary angiography.

7. Blood gas measurement. In the majority of patients with pulmonary embolism, partial pressure of oxygen in blood is abnormally low. This fact has led to the widespread determination of arterial PO_2 as a diagnostic tool in the evaluation of patients with suspected pulmonary embolism.

A. The precise mechanism for the hypoxemia is not established with certainty. However, in more than 85 per cent of patients, the abnormality exists. On the other hand, 10 to 15 per cent of patients with established pulmonary embolism have PO_2 values within the normal range.

B. Thus, while this test represents a parameter useful to measure in suspected pulmonary embolism, it is not specific for the diagnosis and both false positives and false negatives may occur, and the results must be interpreted with caution and should never be taken to include or exclude the diagnosis alone.

DIAGNOSIS

In many patients in whom characteristic clinical picture of pulmonary embolism is present, the diagnosis is not difficult. In all cases an "objective" method, such as perfusion lung scan, should be obtained to establish the diagnosis. In other instances, it may be very difficult and at times impossible to determine with certainty whether pulmonary embolism has occurred when co-existing conditions make clinical evaluation useless and negate the value of the objective studies.

A reasonable and fairly successful approach to the diagnosis of suspected pulmonary embolism includes:

1. Careful history and physical examination

2. Performance of routine chest x-ray and electrocardiogram

3. Determination of arterial oxygen tension

4. The performance of a four-view perfusion lung scan, which, when possible or necessary, is accompanied by a ventilation scan

5. Consideration of pulmonary arteriography if the diagnosis remains in doubt after the above studies, or if the patient is in shock or in an unstable condition and thrombolytic therapy or surgical embolectomy is thought necessary

6. Finally, venography may be useful to assist in the development of plans for treatment.

DIFFERENTIAL DIAGNOSIS

Pulmonary embolism may mimic many other conditions and, similarly, a variety of disorders may produce a clinical picture compatible with pulmonary embolism. The type of lesions to be considered depend on whether they simulate massive or submassive embolization.

1. Massive embolism. The differential diagnosis of this condition includes essentially any disorder associated with cardiopulmonary embarrassment. Correct diagnosis is of great importance to avoid delay in institution of proper treatment that may prove life-saving. Conditions in this category include

myocardial infarction or dissecting aneurysm of the aorta, pneumothorax or cardiovascular collapse for any reason, including hemorrhagic or bacterial shock.

2. Submassive embolization may be simulated by conditions that produce pleural pain, hemoptysis, fever, or an abnormality in the roentgenogram or perfusion lung scan. Included in this group are atelectasis of the lung, pneumonitis, or pleural effusion of any cause.

COMPLICATIONS

The type of complications associated with pulmonary embolism are related to the size of the embolus and resultant hemodynamic consequences.

1. With massive pulmonary embolism, obstruction to pulmonary blood flow and resultant pulmonary hypertension may produce right heart failure with its numerous ramifications. Hypoxemia and reduced systemic blood flow may lead to a variety of complications, such as acute tubular necrosis, cerebral vascular accident, cardiac arrhythmias, or myocardial infarction.

2. Submassive emboli are usually not associated with significant complications, although patients with pulmonary infarction may develop lung abscess or sepsis if the lesion becomes infected. Even without infection, the infarcted lung may cavitate and become the source for hemorrhage into the cavity or become a site for later bacterial complications. When pleural effusion is associated with pulmonary embolus, it too may become infected or organize and form an adherent peel to the lung with the complications thereof.

MANAGEMENT

Broadly stated, the therapeutic objectives in pulmonary thromboembolism are prevention of initial or recurrent embolization, elimination of pulmonary vascular obstruction, and relief of symptoms resulting from the embolic episode. Therapy is to be individualized and is based upon the magnitude of obstruction to the pulmonary circulation.

1. Prophylaxis. Optimally, the primary objective of treatment should be prevention of pulmonary embolization. Since patients at high risk of developing pulmonary embolism can be identified, it is possible and desirable to administer prophylactic therapy. Treatment should be begun prior to the thrombogenic stimulus, (such as elective surgery) when possible, or at the earliest possible time, and continued for as long as the patient remains at risk. Methods of proven effectiveness as prophylactic measures include:

A. Oral anticoagulants in dosage to prolong the prothrombin time to 2 to 2.5 times control values

B. Low-dose heparin, 5000 units subcutaneously every 8 to 12 hours

C. Dextran (low molecular weight) 500 ml. for 2 or 3 days followed by a like amount every other day, when the period of risk is brief, such as following elective surgery

D. Mechanical methods, such as pneumatic compression of the calf during and following elective surgery.

2. Prevention of recurrent embolization. In patients who survive to reach medical attention, the major risk is from recurrent embolization and the major objective of treatment is to prevent this event. This can be accomplished with remarkable effectiveness by the administration of heparin, which acts to arrest the thrombotic process at the distal venous site. With this accomplished, organization of the thrombus and the embolus proceeds, and the risk of recurrence is effectively eliminated and resolution of existing embolus occurs. Heparin should be begun when the diagnosis of embolism is entertained and before diagnostic studies are completed.

A. Heparin should be begun by an I.V. bolus of 5000 to 10,000 units with documentation within 30 minutes that anticoagulation has been achieved by establishing that the Lee-White or an equivalent test has been prolonged to therapeutic levels (Lee-White time, 20 to 25 minutes; partial thromboplastin time, 55 to 85 seconds).

B. Anticoagulation should be maintained with continuous heparin infusion or by intermittent bolus at intervals of 4 to 6 hours. If the patient is at high risk of developing bleeding from the anticoagulant therapy, continuous infusion is to be preferred.

C. Heparin should be continued for a period of 5 to 7 days to allow organization of the distal thrombus. After that, the objective becomes prophylaxis, and oral anticoagulants will be effective in the majority of patients.

D. Oral anticoagulants should be begun 3 to 4 days before the heparin is to be discontinued, to achieve their full antithrombotic effect.

E. Oral anticoagulants should be continued for a period of at least 6 weeks, or until the provocation to thrombosis has been eliminated. In patients who return to full activities and in whom no underlying predisposition remains, treatment can be withdrawn after 6 to 8 weeks, while in others it should continue for 3 to 6 months, and sometimes indefinitely in patients with recurrent embolization. During anticoagulation therapy, measures should be taken to protect the patient from manipulations that may lead to bleeding and during oral anticoagulant therapy, and the possibility of drug interactions must be constantly borne in mind.

F. Interruption of vena cava. Surgical means of preventing recurrent embolization include interruption of the inferior cava.

(1) This is seldom indicated even in patients with submassive or massive emboli or those with recurrent episodes.

It is associated with a significant mortality and morbidity and adds little to the results obtained with the proper use of anticoagulants.

(2) Its use should be reserved for the patient with absolute contraindication to anticoagulation or the patient in whom there has been recurrence of a large embolus during optimal heparin therapy where the recurrence has been demonstrated by an objective method.

3. Removal of pulmonary obstruction. For patients with circulatory failure or those who fail to stabilize or those who deteriorate after a trial of supportive therapy and heparinization, removal of the obstruction may be necessary. Means available for removing emboli are the following.

A. Surgical embolectomy is indicated when massive embolization has been demonstrated by angiography. The procedure is seldom indicated because the majority of patients who would theoretically derive benefit from this approach die before the necessary resources can be mobilized.

B. Thrombolytic therapy. The use of such agents as streptokinase or urokinase have been demonstrated to accelerate the rate of embolus dissolution.

(1) The drugs are administered intravenously by sustained infusion for periods ranging from 6 to as long as 24 hours.

(2) Patients who derive greatest benefit from thrombolytic agents are those with marginal cardiopulmonary compensation following an embolic episode.

(3) At this time, thrombolytic drugs are not generally available and their role in the future remains to be determined.

4. Symptomatic therapy in pulmonary embolism. Alterations induced by the embolic episode other than pulmonary obstruction frequently dominate the clinical picture and require the greatest therapeutic effort. These include: pain (pleuritic or angina-like), to be alleviated with narcotics and oxygen; hypoxemia, corrected with appropriate quantities of oxygen; cardiovascular decompensation, which can be improved with treatment of hypoxemia and acidemia and in addition with drugs with positive inotropic effects (used cautiously), such as digitalis and isoproterenol; and bronchoconstriction, usually benefitted by heparin and intravenous aminophyllin.

PROGNOSIS

1. Mortality figures are difficult to obtain, since many and perhaps most pulmonary emboli remain undiagnosed. If patients with symptomatic emboli go untreated, the recurrence rate approximates 50 per cent and the mortality due to recurrence of 20 to 30 per cent.

2. The outlook in patients who have survived to reach the hospital and who receive optimal treatment have an excellent prognosis. The recurrence rate is less than 5 per cent and fatal recurrence is extremely uncommon.

3. In the majority of patients, rapid resolution of the embolus occurs and in about 75 per cent total dissolution through spontaneous lysis occurs.

4. After completion of the prophylactic treatment, there is recurrent embolism in approximately 5 to 10 per cent of cases. In such patients, a repeat course of heparin followed by more prolonged prophylaxis is indicated.

5. All patients with embolization should receive prophylaxis at any time that they are exposed to a thrombogenic stimulus (e.g., bedrest, surgery, leg fractures).

SUGGESTED READINGS

Fratantoni, J. and Wessler, S. (eds.): Prophylactic Therapy of Deep Vein Thrombosis and Pulmonary Embolism. DHEW publication #(NIH) 76-866, 1975.

Sasahara, A. A., Sonnenblick, E. H., and Lesch, M. (eds.): Pulmonary Emboli. New York, Grune & Stratton, 1975.

13. CHRONIC COR PULMONALE

James J. Wellman, M.D., *and Roland H. Ingram, Jr.,* M.D.

DEFINITION

1. *Chronic cor pulmonale* is defined as heart disease secondary to chronic pulmonary parenchymal and/or vascular disease, abnormal chest wall, or a depressed ventilatory drive.

2. Chronic cor pulmonale comprises some combination of hypertrophy and dilatation of the right ventricle due to hypertension of the pulmonary circulation.

3. The cause is initiated by diseases that affect the function and/or structure of the lung, except when these pulmonary alterations are the result of diseases that primarily affect the left side of the heart or congenital heart disease.[4]

4. Chronic cor pulmonale does not necessarily mean that there is right ventricular failure (i.e., increases in right ventricular end-diastolic pressures) although failure is frequently present.

GENERAL CONSIDERATIONS

The term *chronic cor pulmonale* denotes right ventricular enlargement secondary to intrinsic lung perenchymal and/or vascular disease, an abnormal chest bellows, or a depressed ventilatory drive. *Cor pulmonale* does not connote failure of the right side of the heart; however, the presence of signs and symptoms of right ventricular failure are often the clues that lead the clinician to the diagnosis.

Since the pathophysiologic mechanism responsible for cor pulmonale is pulmonary arterial hypertension, a clear understanding of the natural history of the antecedent pulmonary disease is imperative for the recognition and treatment of this disorder. Chronic bronchitis and emphysema are the most prevalent underlying pulmonary diseases that predispose to the development of chronic cor pulmonale in this country and Western Europe, and although the true incidence is difficult to ascertain, many sources state that chronic cor pulmonale comprises 7 to 10 per cent of all heart disease in the United States.

ETIOLOGY (DISEASES ASSOCIATED WITH CHRONIC COR PULMONALE)

One or several mechanisms for pulmonary hypertension may be operative in the various diseases associated with chronic cor pulmonale. The list on page 186 gives the diagnoses according to the primary anatomic site of disease or to the primary process leading to chronic cor pulmonale.

PATHOPHYSIOLOGY

Since there can be few situations in which an understanding of the functional disturbances is more important in management, this section briefly reviews present knowledge of the mechanisms involved.

Elevation of the pulmonary artery pressure is the primary pathophysiologic process common to the entire group of pulmonary vascular and parenchymal diseases that lead to chronic cor pulmonale. There are several mechanisms that may be present singly or in combination to produce pulmonary hypertension. These are:

1. *Anatomic changes*

Anatomic changes in the pulmonary vessels such as destruction, total occlusion or diffuse luminal narrowing, result

185

in a decrease in the total cross-sectional area of the pulmonary vascular bed.

A. Loss of capillaries in association with extensive destruction of the pulmonary parenchyma is found in pulmonary emphysema.

B. Total occlusion of pulmonary vessels occurs in chronic pulmonary thromboembolic disease.

C. Diffuse luminal narrowing of pulmonary arterioles can result from inflammatory changes secondary to allergic vasculitis or diffuse inflammatory arteritis.

D. Intimal thickening from elastosis or fibrosis as well as smooth muscle hypertrophy and hyperplasia in the media of pulmonary arterioles are frequently observed in patients with long-standing pulmonary hypertension. Whether these changes are a primary event or secondary to hypoxia and elevated pulmonary artery pressures, the onset of these changes certainly intensifies existing pulmonary hypertension.

2. *Alveolar hypoxia*

A. Alveolar hypoxia is probably the most potent stimulus for pulmonary vasoconstriction and is clearly the most reversible of the processes contributing to pulmonary hypertension.

B. The bulk of evidence favors a local regional arteriolar constriction rather than a reflex vasoconstriction.

C. Acidemia has been shown to act synergistically with hypoxia in producing pulmonary hypertension.[5]

3. *Erythrocytosis*

A. In some patients with chronic hypoxemia with secondary erythrocytosis it seems probable that if severe enough, it would increase the blood viscosity and produce important alterations in the pressure-flow relationships of the pulmonary circulation.

B. Although theoretical considerations would suggest that increased blood viscosity leads to elevation in pulmonary arterial pressure, clinical evidence is lacking.[10]

CLASSIFICATION

Chronic cor pulmonale is classified in the list below according to the underlying disease processes.

Classification of the Causes of Chronic Cor Pulmonale

1. Diseases primarily affecting the air passages of the lungs and alveoli
   Chronic bronchitis
   Pulmonary emphysema
   Interstitial lung disease with fibrosis
2. Diseases primarily affecting the neuromuscular apparatus and movements of the chest wall
   Amyotropic lateral sclerosis
   Myasthenia gravis
   Kyphoscoliosis
   Thoracoplasty
3. Diseases resulting in inadequate ventilatory drive
   Obesity-hypoventilation syndrome
   Primary alveolar hypoventilation
4. Diseases primarily affecting the pulmonary vessels
   Chronic recurrent pulmonary emboli
   Primary pulmonary hypertension
   Schistosomiasis

SYMPTOMS AND SIGNS

The hallmark of chronic cor pulmonale is enlargement of the right ventricle. Since this is often difficult to detect clinically, particularly in patients with chronic obstructive pulmonary disease (COPD), cor pulmonale is often not recognized until right ventricular failure has occurred. Therefore, the diagnosis of chronic cor pulmonale is based on an understanding of the natural history of the antecedent pulmonary disorder and the following symptoms, signs, and laboratory data.

1. *Symptoms*

A. *Chronic obstructive pulmonary disease*

Unfortunately the symptoms associated with cor pulmonale from COPD are those of the underlying disease and are not specific for pulmonary hypertension with right ventricular enlargement.

B. *Right ventricular failure*

(1) When right ventricular failure is present, the patient may complain of more shortness of breath and fluid accumulation.

(2) Worsening of shortness of breath is probably the most common presenting complaint in all the diseases associated with cor pulmonale.

C. *Diseases of chest wall or ventilatory drive*

(1) In patients with disease of the chest wall, the neuromuscular apparatus and the hypoventilation syndromes, manifestations of hypoxia, hypercapnia and acidosis are common presenting complaints.

(2) They are cyanosis, confusion, drowsiness, and insomnia, which is a result of sleep deprivation.

(3) Historical evidence such as this is most frequently given by a family member since the patient is seldom cognizant of these changes.

2. *Signs*

The physical examination can reveal signs of chronic cor pulmonale with and without right ventricular failure.

A. *Neck veins*

(1) The neck veins may be distended and with overt right ventricular failure giant V waves and rapid Y descents indicate tricuspid valvular regurgitation.

(2) The lack of an inspiratory collapse may aid in identifying those patients with an elevated right atrial pressure.

B. *Cardiac findings*

(1) Right ventricular hypertrophy is associated with a palpable lower left parasternal or subxiphoid systolic heave.

(2) On auscultation an S_3 or S_4 gallop accentuated by inspiration and a loud pulmonic second heart sound are often heard.

(3) A holosystolic murmur may be present as a result of functional tricuspid insufficiency.

(4) Rapid and/or irregular cardiac rhythm may be present depending upon the underlying rhythm.

(5) Distant heart sounds are common, especially in COPD.

C. *Pulmonary findings*

Depending upon the underlying pulmonary diseases, various physical findings (dry or moist rales, diminished breath sounds, hyperresonance on percussion, and increased A-P diameter etc.) may be appreciated.

D. *Abdomen and extremities*

There may be:

(1) Pedal edema

(2) Ascites

(3) Tender hepatic enlargement when there is significant right ventricular failure.

E. *Hypoxemia and acidosis*

The effects of hypoxemia and hypercapnia with acidosis are cyanosis, tachycardia, muscular twitching and systemic hypertension.

F. *Mental status*

As the level of P_{CO_2} rises, mental confusion, matinal headaches, drowsiness, and even coma develop.

LABORATORY FINDINGS

1. *Determination of arterial blood gases*

A. Arterial blood gases are significant not only as aids in diagnosis but also, when performed at intervals, they serve as a guide to therapy.

B. The P_{O_2} of arterial blood provides a direct index of blood oxygenation and, depending on the amount and saturation of hemoglobin along with the cardiac output, an indirect assessment of the oxygen delivery to the tissues can be made.

C. The P_{CO_2} of arterial blood provides the only true index of effective ventilation.

D. Combined hypoxemia and hypercapnia are usual findings in chronic cor pulmonale with failure.

E. Appreciable arterial hypoxemia

and hypercapnia with respiratory acidemia are unusual in left sided failure unless frank pulmonary edema is present.

2. *Roentgenographic findings*

A. The diverse etiologies for chronic cor pulmonale create many patterns of parenchymal, pleural, and chest wall abnormalities, which often give the diagnostic clue to the type of disease present.

B. The roentgenographic findings of pulmonary hypertension, irrespective of the underlying disease, are dilatation of the main pulmonary artery and its major branches with prompt tapering.

C. The heart may either be enlarged or may appear to be normal on posterior-anterior projections.

D. The enlargement that occurs is confined to the pulmonary arteries, right ventricle, and right atrium and is best seen in the lateral projections where the right ventricle is seen to encroach on the retrosternal space.

E. In the patient with pulmonary emphysema the small vertical heart may be dilated but without apparent increase in size, and only by comparison with previous films can this enlargement be detected.

F. When right ventricular failure occurs, the superior vena caval and azygous venous shadows are prominent.

G. Pleural effusions and Kerley's B lines are rarely found in right ventricular failure alone and suggest a complicating pneumonia in the case of pleural effusion or left ventricular failure when both effusions and Kerley's B lines are present.

H. Occasionally when left ventricular failure is present along with right ventricular failure, the enlarged left ventricle and left atrium can be detected by oblique cardiac views with barium in the esophagus.

3. *Electrocardiographic manifestations*

Electrocardiographic evidence of right ventricular enlargement is most convincing in severe unremitting pulmonary hypertension that follows pulmonary vascular or interstitial disease. Conversely in patients with COPD the ECG is often inconclusive because of the hyperinflated lungs and fluctuations of the pulmonary hypertension and right ventricular overload.

The electrocardiographic findings that may be associated with chronic cor pulmonale are:

A. *P-pulmonale*

(1) A P wave axis that is often greater than $+60°$, with peaked P waves in the inferior leads (II, III and aVF), and V_1, (P-pulmonale)

(2) Often prominent Ta waves produce depression of the P-R segment.

B. *Low QRS voltage*

(1) The QRS voltage is often low. (The sum of QRS voltage in leads I, II, and III is less than 15 mm.)

(2) The low QRS voltage is marked when there are severe COPD, advanced heart failure, and pleural or pericardial effusion.

C. *The QRS axis deviation*

(1) Mean QRS frontal axis is often vertical or directed toward the right (more than $+90°$)

(2) Posterior axis deviation is often indicated by rS or QS patterns in the precordial leads.

(3) In some cases, left axis deviation of the QRS may be found (rS or QS patterns in leads II, III and aVF).

D. *Right ventricular hypertrophy*

Less commonly in chronic obstructive pulmonary disease and more commonly in other etiologies one finds tall R waves in leads V_{1-3}.

E. *Right bundle branch block*

Incomplete or complete right bundle branch block is relatively common.

F. *Cardiac arrhythmias*

(1) Patients with chronic cor pulmonale show a greater tendency than other to develop both atrial and ventricu-

lar arrhythmias, particularly associated with episodes of increasing hypoxemia and hypercapnia with acidosis.

(2) Multifocal atrial tachycardia is relatively common in chronic cor pulmonale.

(3) The incidence of digitalis-induced arrhythmias is high in cor pulmonale.

G. *Pseudo myocardial infarction pattern*

Because of posterior axis deviation and marked right or left axis deviation, the ECG findings may resemble anterior or diaphragmatic myocardial infarction.

H. *Normal electrocardiogram*

Normal electrocardiogram does not exclude the diagnosis of chronic cor pulmonale.

4. *Pulmonary function tests*

The various pulmonary diseases may also be differentiated by tests of pulmonary function. In actual clinical practice, after careful history taking and physical and roentgenologic examinations of the chest, sufficient knowledge of pulmonary function may be obtained by performing simple spirometry including forced expiratory flow rates and lung, volumes.

A. *Airway obstruction*

A reduction in the forced expiratory flow rates along with an increase in the functional residual capacity residual volume and total lung capacity are indicative of airway obstruction.

B. *Restrictive lung disease*

A reduction in the vital capacity and total lung capacity with relatively normal flow rates is indicative of a restrictive lung disease such as may occur with disorders of the chest wall and neuromuscular apparatus as well as interstitial lung diseases.

DIAGNOSIS

1. There is no pathognomonic feature diagnostic of chronic cor pulmonale.

2. The most important sign of chronic cor pulmonale is right ventricular hypertrophy. It should be noted, however, that many other disease processes may produce right ventricular hypertrophy.

3. The diagnosis of chronic cor pulmonale is supported by the findings of the underlying pulmonary diseases in many patients.

4. Symptoms and signs of right ventricular failure are often present.

5. Shortness of breath is the most common presenting symptom.

6. Various laboratory studies, including the determinations of arterial blood gases, chest x-ray findings, electrocardiographic abnormalities, and pulmonary function tests, provide supportive evidence for the diagnosis of chronic cor pulmonale.

DIFFERENTIAL DIAGNOSIS

1. Chronic cor pulmonale should be differentiated from many other disorders that produce *dyspnea*.

2. Chronic cor pulmonale should be distinguished from various disorders that produce *right ventricular hypertrophy*. They include:

A. Various valvular heart diseases, such as pulmonic stenosis and tricuspid insufficiency

B. Various congenital heart diseases, such as tetralogy of Fallot and pulmonic stenosis

C. Cardiomyopathies of various etiologies

D. Myocarditis of various etiologies

3. Chronic cor pulmonale should be distinguished from a *true myocardial infarction*, because the ECG finding of cor pulmonale often resembles myocardial infarction.

4. Chronic cor pulmonale with right ventricular failure should be differentiated from other disorders that produce *hepatomegaly, ankle edema and neck vein distention*, such as constrictive pericarditis.

5. Chronic cor pulmonale with a holosystolic murmur due to functional tricuspid insufficiency as a result of right ventricular failure should be differentiated from other disorders that produce a *holosystolic murmur*. They include:

    A. Organic tricuspid insufficiency
    B. Ventricular septal defect
    C. Mitral insufficiency

COMPLICATIONS

Various complications may be observed in patients with chronic cor pulmonale.

1. *Respiratory infection*

Superimposed respiratory infections produce acute or subacute bronchitis or pneumonia, which result in increasing dyspnea, cough, cyanosis, and respiratory acidosis.

2. *CO_2 narcosis*

Neurologic manifestations of CO_2 narcosis are manifested by mental confusion, coma, convulsions, and frequently a fatal outcome.

3. *Secondary erythrocytosis*

Secondary erythrocytosis is common as a compensatory mechanism for hypoxia.

4. *Cardiac arrhythmias*

Various cardiac arrhythmias occur primarily as a result of hypoxia.

5. *Digitalis intoxication*

The high incidence of digitalis intoxication in patients with chronic cor pulmonale is well documented. Hypoxia is considered to be a main factor for this finding, although total body potassium deficiency may contribute, especially if diuretics have been used.

MANAGEMENT

1. *Management of the clinical forms of chronic cor pulmonale*

Reversibility of pulmonary hypertension depends upon the predominant mechanism. To the extent that vasoconstriction secondary to altered alveolar gas composition is operative, improvement in the gas exchanging function of the lung and/or administration of oxygen should prove helpful.

The basic therapeutic principles for the various forms of chronic cor pulmonale are outlined below.

    A. *Diseases primarily affecting the intrathoracic airways*

The common denominator in this group of disorders is the imbalance between alveolar ventilation and pulmonary blood flow, resulting in hypoxemia with or without hypercapnia. Intrinsic lung disease is the basis for the abnormal blood gas values, since these patients have a normal or increased minute ventilation (net alveolar hypoventilation).

In patients with predominantly chronic bronchitis, the compromised alveolar ventilation in relation to a relatively normal pulmonary blood flow leads to hypoxemia, hypercapnia, and pulmonary hypertension and (frequently) chronic cor pulmonale with right ventricular failure. In contrast, patients with predominant emphysema with minimal symptoms of bronchitis rarely experience episodes of overt right ventricular failure except terminally. Relief of the obstructive process particularly in chronic bronchitis is the keystone to therapy in these patients.

    (1) *Bronchodilators*

        (a) Sympathomimetic amines that stimulate primarily the β-2 receptors have proved effective in the relief of bronchospasm and the clearance of secretions.

        (b) Terbutaline sulfate, marketed for oral and subcutaneous administration, metaproterenol, isoetharine, and salbutamol (available in England and Canada, yet soon to be available in the U.S.) are the sympathomimetic bronchodilators most commonly used.

        (c) The xanthines (aminophylline, theophylline and oxtriphylline), which have a different mechanism of action, have gained widespread support in the treatment of obstructive airways disease.

(d) Aminophylline, which has been used mainly as a bronchodilator, also has beneficial hemodynamic effects of lowering the pulmonary artery pressure and the end-diastolic pressure of both ventricles.[9]

(2) *Antibiotics*

(a) In most patients with COPD the use of such broad spectrum antibiotics as ampicillin and tetracycline appears to be efficacious in the treatment of acute respiratory infection.

(b) When a distinct infiltrate is present, along with a temperature elevation and leukocytosis, a gram stain and culture of the sputum are essential in directing the appropriate antibiotic therapy.

(c) For most patients with excessive purulent sputum a 10–14 day course of antibiotics will reduce the duration and severity of exacerbations of acute respiratory insufficiency.

(3) *Humidification*

(a) Large volume aerosols have been used for their humidifying action.

(b) Ultrasonic nebulizers act by producing fine particles and are successful in thinning secretions and facilitating expectoration.

(c) Heated wall nebulizers are helpful in preventing excessive drying of the nasal mucosa when O_2 must be administered by mask.

(4) *Drainage*

The use of postural drainage, particularly after nebulization, remains an essential and effective method of mobilizing and removing secretions.

(5) *Prevention*

(a) A careful explanation to the patient of his physical problem, stressing the need to stop smoking and to avoid other irritants is mandatory in the pre-vention of recurrent respiratory difficulty.

(b) *Sedatives and narcotics are contraindicated.*

B. *Diseases of the lung parenchyma*

Chronic diffuse interstitial pulmonary diseases, especially when complicated by fibrosis of interstitial tissue and secondary vascular changes, can lead to pulmonary hypertension and chronic cor pulmonale. The pulmonary hypertension is due mainly to anatomic changes, and if severe enough to produce cor pulmonale, therapy is rarely effective.

(1) To the extent that inflammatory changes are operative, glucocorticoids may be expected to abate the abnormal gas exchange and pulmonary hypertension.

(2) By the time chronic cor pulmonale with failure is present, there is little to offer except continuous oxygenation, which in carefully selected patients can prove beneficial.[8]

C. *Diseases affecting the chest wall and neuromuscular apparatus*

The abnormal blood gases that result from diseases in this category are a result of general alveolar hypoventilation, since these patients do not have primary lung disease but have a decrease in minute ventilation.

(1) Therefore, some measure to improve chest bellows performance will improve ventilation and hopefully will reverse the hypoxic and hypercapnic pulmonary arterial constriction.

(2) It is particularly important in this group of patients to avoid bronchopulmonary infections. Their cough mechanism is frequently inadequate to clear tracheobronchial secretions and even minor infections can lead to respiratory insufficiency.

(3) *Sedatives and narcotics are contraindicated,* unless the patient is being mechanically ventilated. Even in this situation, if the patient is intermit-

tently off the ventilator, the sedative action continues to depress respirations.

D. *Diseases resulting in inadequate ventilatory drive*

(1) *Obesity*

(a) In obese patients with the alveolar hypoventilation syndrome, the best therapy is weight loss, which usually leads to recovery.

(b) It is well to remember that a majority of patients in this group are immobile and obese, and, consequently, are prone to have pulmonary embolic episodes which must be constantly suspected.

(2) *General alveolar hypoventilation without obesity*

(a) General alveolar hypoventilation in the absence of extreme obesity, chest wall restriction or muscular abnormalities has been attributed to an abnormality in the central nervous system control of ventilation.

(b) The pathogenesis and treatment are similar to the other forms of general alveolar hypoventilation.

(c) Electrical stimulation of the phrenic nerve as a respiratory pacemaker appears to be a promising and rational therapeutic approach to this disorder.

(d) Patients with cervical spinal cord injury or diseases in which the neural transmission is interrupted above the phrenic nerve may also benefit from phrenic nerve pacing.

E. *Diseases primarily affecting the pulmonary vessels*

(1) In this disorder, widespread occlusion of the small pulmonary vessels takes place over months to years.

(2) The most common cause is recurrent pulmonary emboli.

(3) A less common cause is primary pulmonary hypertension.

(4) Of the patients who develop chronic cor pulmonale, those with multiple pulmonary emboli have the highest pulmonary artery pressure.

(5) The therapeutic principle is to prevent further embolic episodes and to allow regression of vascular changes secondary to previous emboli.

2. *Cardiopulmonary failure*

Congestive heart failure as a result of chronic cor pulmonale is almost invariably accompanied by some degree of respiratory insufficiency (i.e., the inability of the lungs to maintain normal arterial blood gas levels). Consequently, the treatment of right sided heart failure per se is less important than restoring the blood gases to tolerable levels. Since pulmonary hypertension in chronic obstructive lung disease (the most prevalent pulmonary disorders) is rarely anatomically fixed but arises in part from hypoxia and acidosis, relief of hypercapnia and improved oxygenation are usually successful in restoring the circulation to normal. The therapeutic measures outlined above to improve alveolar hypoventilation in patients with COPD are applicable in this situation.

A. *Maintenance of adequate oxygenation*

(1) The principle guiding oxygenation is to use the simplest method and the lowest inspired oxygen concentration that will achieve the desired result.

(2) A reasonable objective of O_2 therapy is to achieve a Po_2 of 50 to 60 mm. Hg.

(3) It is not necessary to attempt to achieve a normal or even supernormal Po_2, because there is little to gain in O_2 content of the blood since increments in PO_2 above these levels lead to only modest increments in hemoglobin saturation.

(4) The hazard of respiratory depression with O_2 is confined to patients with the hypercapnic form of respiratory insufficiency in whom the normal stimuli to ventilation are compromised.

(5) Since these patients need O_2 and while fears of respiratory depression should not prevent adequate relief of hypoxemia, use of O_2 should be judi-

cious, with frequent monitoring of P_{O_2} and P_{CO_2}.

(6) There are many methods for delivering O_2. Soft nasal prongs through which O_2 is delivered at the required flow rate are used most commonly. The net fraction of inspired O_2 (FI_{O_2}) entering the trachea will be determined by the minute ventilation of the patient and the flow rate of O_2. Another method of delivery of O_2 involves the use of masks that have been designed to deliver fixed concentrations by the Venturi principle. These Venturi masks can be obtained in rated concentrations (FI_{O_2}s of .24, .28, .35 and .40). They provide the patient with a microenvironment of constant FI_{O_2} regardless of the total ventilation.

B. *Digitalis (see Chap. 22)*

Opinions have varied concerning the efficacy of digitalis in chronic cor pulmonale. In the catheterization laboratory[6] it has been possible to demonstrate an increase in cardiac output associated with reductions in right atrial pressures during acute digitalization in patients with right ventricular failure; however, the elevations in cardiac output also aggravated pulmonary hypertension. Although the patient may present clinically with systemic venous hypertension and edema, it is difficult to ascertain whether the primary mechanism is congestive heart failure or a syndrome of volume overload related to abnormal renal function.[3] Certainly the clinical effects of digitalis are not so obvious in cor pulmonale with right-sided failure as in other forms of congestive heart failure due to left ventricular dysfunction. Moreover, ectopic rhythms due to digitalis toxicity (see Chap. 23) occur more frequently and at lower plasma levels in cor pulmonale, most likely due to hypoxemia[1] and possibly to the depletion of potassium.[2] *We therefore recommend avoiding digitalis or at least delaying the initiation of therapy until hypoxemia and the electrolyte imbal-*

ances accompanying respiratory failure have been corrected.

C. *Diuretics*

The efficacy of diuretics in chronic cor pulmonale with systemic hypertension and edema seems unquestionable. It has also been suggested that the lungs accumulate excess extravascular fluid.[11] *The administration of diuretics, especially the more potent varieties, such as furosemide and ethacrynic acid, must be monitored with more than usual care in patients with respiratory disease since the metabolic alkalosis that frequently results from their use may aggravate ventilatory insufficiency by depressing the effectiveness of the carbon dioxide stimulus as a respiratory stimulant.* In turn, scrupulous attention must also be paid to the prompt correction of hypokalemia and hypochloremia that can result from diuretic administration, since the renal excretion of bicarbonate is diminished unless there is sufficient potassium and chloride.

D. *Phlebotomy*

(1) In the small number of patients with marked erythrocytosis (i.e., hematocrits greater than 55), venesection has been recommended.

(2) This is, however, of doubtful benefit and has not been shown to produce any improvement in physiologic measurements.[10]

(3) A few patients suffer symptoms, including dizziness, sensations of fullness in the head, and headache, which are relieved by a small volume venesection.

3. *Cardiac arrhythmias*

Although various cardiac arrhythmias may occur in patients with chronic cor pulmonale, the arrhythmia per se is usually not the primary problem. The general therapeutic approaches are as follows:

A. The improvement of pulmonary function is often sufficient to eliminate various arrhythmias.

B. Hypoxia is the most important and direct cause of cardiac arrhythmias in chronic cor pulmonale. Therefore, hypoxia should be corrected for the prevention and treatment of various arrhythmias.

C. Multifocal atrial tachycardia (chaotic atrial rhythm) is considered to be an arrhythmia that is almost pathognomonic for cor pulmonale. Hypoxia is the primary cause of this arrhythmia in most cases. Thus, the treatment for hypoxia is usually more beneficial than any antiarrhythmic agent (see Chap. 24).

D. The prevention of digitalis toxicity is extremely important in chronic cor pulmonale, because it is a common and most difficult problem (see Chap. 23). It is recommended that a smaller than usual dosage of digitalis should be administered (see Chap. 22) in chronic cor pulmonale.

E. When either supraventricular or ventricular tachyarrhythmias persist and the ventricular rate is fast, they should be treated immediately by using antiarrhythmic drugs and/or direct current shock depending upon the clinical circumstances (see Chap. 25).

PROGNOSIS

1. Chronic cor pulmonale without significant right ventricular failure carries the same prognosis as the underlying pulmonary disease.

2. When there is a significant right ventricular failure, the average life expectancy is considered to be 2 to 5 years.

3. Prognosis varies markedly depending upon the underlying pulmonary diseases, the patient's age, the presence or absence and the severity of right ventricular failure, and other complications, such as cardiac arrhythmias and superimposed respiratory infections.

REFERENCES

1. Baum, G. L. et al.: Factors involved in digitalis sensitivity in chronic pulmonary insufficiency. Am. Heart J., *57*:460, 1959.
2. ———: Total body exchangeable potassium and sodium and extracellular fluid in chronic pulmonary insufficiency. Am. Heart J., *58*:53, 1959.
3. Campbell, E. J. M. and Short, D. S.: The cause of oedema in cor pulmonale. Lancet, *2*:1184, 1960.
4. Chronic cor pulmonale: Report of an expert committee of the World Health Organization. Circulation, *27*:594, 1963.
5. Enson, Y. et al.: The influence of hydrogen ion concentration and hypoxia on the pulmonary circulation. J. Clin. Invest. *43*:1146, 1964.
6. Ferrer, I. M. et al.: Some effects of digoxin upon the heart and circulation in man—digoxin in chronic cor pulmonale. Circulation, *1*:161, 1950.
7. Ingram, R. H., Jr. and Grossman, G. D.: Chronic cor pulmonale, *In* Hurst, J. W. (ed.): The Heart, Arteries, and Veins. ed. 3. New York, McGraw-Hill, 1974.
8. Levine, B. W. et al.: The role of long-term continuous oxygen administration in patients with chronic airway obstruction with hypoxemia. Ann. Intern. Med., *66*:639, 1967.
9. Parker, J. O., Kelkar, K., and West, R. O.: Hemodynamic effects of aminophylline in cor pulmonale. Circulation, *33*:17, 1966.
10. Segel, N. and Bishop, J. M.: The circulation in patients with chronic bronchitis and emphysema at rest and during exercise, with special reference to the influence of changes in blood viscosity and blood volume on the pulmonary circulation. J. Clin. Invest., *45*:1555, 1966.
11. Turino, G. M. et al.: Extravascular lung water in cor pulmonale. Bull. Physiopathol. Respir., *4*:47, 1968.

14. DISEASES OF THE AORTA

Myron W. Wheat, Jr., M.D., *and David H. Shapiro*, M.D.

GENERAL CONSIDERATIONS

The effect of disease on the aorta can weaken the wall, causing aneurysm formation with the threat of rupture; narrow the lumen, limiting the flow of blood; or change the smooth intimal lining, promoting thrombosis. The ultimate result is compromise of blood supply to the body distal to the disease process, or sudden rupture of the aorta, and death of the patient. Since the aorta is the main channel of blood flow from the heart to the entire body, the signs and symptoms of these lesions are among the most dramatic in clinical medicine, and the patients among the most critically and suddenly ill.

The aorta differs from smaller arteries, not only in relative diameter but in the amount of elastic tissue in its wall as well. The elastic fibers are concentrated mainly in the tunica media and provide the aorta with its resilience. With degeneration and conversion with aging of elastic fibers to fibrous tissue, the aorta loses resiliency and flexibility with resultant effects on blood pressure, especially in the diastolic phase. Changes in shape and contour of the aorta also can occur with increased tortuosity and diameter.

Atherosclerosis, the most common disease of the aorta, is characterized by the formation of local atheromas or focal lipid disparities. The most common site of involvement is the distal abdominal aorta in the region of the bifurcation.

The early atherosclerotic plaque begins with deposition of fine fat droplets and degeneration of the subendothelial tissue. As the plaque grows, the lipid deposit stimulates increased proliferation of connective tissue, most heavily over the luminal aspect of the atheroma. With increasing size, the atheroma protrudes into and compromises the lumen of the aorta. The plaque may convert to a scar containing amorphous debris and cholesterol clefts, or it may became calcified. The thin overlying endothelium may necrose and ulcerate into the lumen. Hemorrhage into the ulcer then frequently occurs, which can result in elevation of the plaque, with complete occlusion of the vessel lumen, or mural thrombus formation.

The distribution of the atheromas is typically patchy with a predilection for points of maximal stress, such as branches and areas of fixation of the aorta. The posterior wall of the aorta is most commonly affected, as well as the lumina of the branches of the aorta. In the early course of the disease, the arch is more severely involved, but this appears to regress, and later the most common area becomes the abdominal aorta, then the descending portion of the arch, and the transverse arch. Characteristically the roof of the aorta is spared.

The most frequent result of atherosclerotic disease of the aorta is aneurysm formation, a localized dilatation. The aorta, of all the body's blood vessels, is the most common site of aneurysm formation. Approximately 80 per cent of aneurysms of the aorta occur in the infrarenal aorta; 5.5 per cent in the ascending aorta; 12 per cent in the descending aorta; and 2.5 per cent are thoracoabdominal aneurysms, extending from the thoracic into the abdominal aorta.

Aneurysms of the aorta also can be congenital, secondary to an inflammatory or infectious process, or traumatic in origin. Congenital aneurysms, such as aneurysms of the sinus of Valsalva, are rare. Poststenotic dilatation, which occurs in patients with coarctation or congenital segmental hypoplasia, may lead to significant aneurysm formation.

Tertiary syphilis, once the most common cause of aneurysms of the aorta, results in destruction of the media, primarily involving the ascending aorta, and may be complicated by calcification of the wall of the aorta, resulting in further weakening. Left untreated, these aneurysms grow to large size, eroding neighboring structures, and even ulcerating the chest wall. Fortunately, luetic aneurysms are rare today.

Cystic medial necrosis, idiopathic or in association with hypertension or Marfan's syndrome, is the underlying disease process leading to dissecting aneurysms of the aorta. In acute trauma, with the rapid acceleration-deacceleration-type injury, often seen in motorcycle and other vehicular accidents, sheering force is exerted, which can result in partial or complete disruption of the aorta. The most common site is in the descending aorta just distal to the left subclavian artery in the region of the ligamentum arteriosum, which is an area of fixation with the relatively mobile aortic arch just cephalad. If the extravasation of the blood is limited, a false aneurysm results, and may chronically expand and require resection. Massive acute extravasation is usually fatal.

A rare cause of aortic aneurysm is giant cell aortitis, which is accompanied by chronic inflammation and giant cell infiltration, and usually involves the ascending aorta.

Mycotic aneurysms, the result of infectious foci in the aortic wall, are false aneurysms. They are most commonly the result of infection in the suture line of a previous graft insertion. Partial disruption of the anastomosis is axiomatic when infection occurs in a vascular suture line, and varying degrees of extravasation of blood occur.

Though the entire aorta is subject to all the disease processes mentioned above, some areas are more susceptible than others, and special diagnostic and therapeutic considerations arise, depending upon whether it is the thoracic or abdominal aorta (or both) which is involved.

ANEURYSMS OF THE SINUS OF VALSALVA

1. *Definition and classification*

A. The sinuses of Valsalva are three dilatations of the aortic wall located immediately above the aortic valve annulus.

B. The left and right coronary arteries arise from the left and right sinuses of Valsalva, respectively.

C. Absence of the elastic tissue at the base of the aorta and in the walls of the sinuses in this condition suggests a congenital etiology.

D. Abnormalities of the sinus of Valsalva may be of three types, including:

(1) Aneurysm of the sinus of Valsalva alone

(2) Aneurysm with fistula

(3) Fistula alone

E. The aneurysmal dilatation may involve any one of the three sinuses or, more commonly, involve all three of them.

F. Fistulae may develop between the aneurysm and the cardiac chambers.

G. Communications with all four cardiac chambers have been reported, and multiple fistulae may be present in any one patient.

2. *Clinical picture*

A. Aneurysms of the sinus of Valsalva occur in all age groups.

B. The typical patient is a 40-year-old male presenting with fatigue, clinical findings of aortic valve insufficiency and a negative past history.

C. The size of the aneurysm and the size of the location of the fistula are the most important determinants of symptomatology.

D. Large aneurysms produce dilatation of the aortic annulus and aortic valve insufficiency.

E. Mild degrees of aortic valve insufficiency may be detected by the presence of a characteristic diastolic murmur to the left of the sternum, whereas more severe aortic valve insufficiency leads to cardiac decompensation.

F. The onset of symptoms may be acute, due to sudden massive aortic valve insufficiency with intractable pulmonary edema.

G. In most instances, however, the aortic valve leaflets lose their integrity more slowly, and the development of dyspnea and fatigue is more insidious.

H. Fistulae to the left ventricle and the left atrium may also produce symptoms of left ventricular overload.

I. Fistulae to the right side of the heart produce left to right shunts of varying severity.

J. Large left to right shunts of this type produce significant overload lesions and may lead to cardiac arrhythmias and decompensation.

K. Aneurysms of this type and their fistulae provide a site for bacterial endocarditis. Therefore, this lesion must be considered in patients who present with signs of sepsis, endocarditis, and a heart murmur without previously known cardiac disease.

3. *Diagnosis and laboratory findings*

A. Symptomatic patients presenting with signs of congestive heart failure show signs of left ventricular overload with widened pulse pressures, bounding pulses, and an aortic diastolic murmur.

B. Cardiac enlargement is present.

C. The electrocardiogram may show signs of left ventricular hypertrophy and ischemia.

D. Chest roentgenographs reveal a right-sided anterior mediastinal mass.

E. A definitive diagnosis can be made only by angiography, which should include complete right and left cardiac catheterization and coronary angiography.

4. *Treatment*

A. Aneurysms of the sinus of Valsalva, with or without fistulas should be corrected surgically.

B. Initial management must be directed toward treatment of the complicating cardiac decompensation with salt restriction, diuretics, and digitalis.

C. *Bacterial endocarditis*

(1) Special mention must be made of the complication of bacterial endocarditis occurring in the aneurysm and fistula of the sinus of Valsalva.

(2) Bacterial endocarditis constitutes a medical and surgical emergency and dictates intensive treatment to salvage the patient.

(3) Vigorous attempts to control infection prior to operative intervention are indicated.

5. *Prognosis*

Using modern techniques of complete cardiac catheterization preoperatively and open heart surgery, repair of aneurysms and fistulas of the sinus of Valsalva can be carried out with an operative mortality of 5 to 10 per cent.

ANEURYSMS OF THE AORTIC ROOT AND ASCENDING AORTA

1. *Definition and etiology*

A. Aneurysms of the aortic root and ascending aorta constitute 22 per cent of the aneurysms of the aorta.

B. These aneurysms are usually the result of cystic medial necrosis leading to an acute Type I aortic dissection, or the more chronic Type II aneurysm.

C. The aneurysm begins just above the orifice of the left coronary artery ostium and extends distally, proximally, or both.

D. In the *acute situation,* the dissecting process continues for varying distances and may proceed as far as the iliac arteries.

E. In the more *chronic process,* if the extension is primarily distally, an aneurysm of the ascending aorta develops.

F. If the extension is in both directions, an aneurysm of the aortic root develops, rarely extending beyond the innominate artery.

G. Atherosclerosis, syphilis, and giant cell arteritis are more rare causes of aneurysms in this portion of the aorta.

2. *Clinical picture, laboratory findings, and diagnosis*

A. Dilatation of the aortic root produces loss of support of the aortic valve cusps and leads to aortic valve insufficiency.

B. Aortic regurgitation also may develop because of acute aortic dissection that extends down into the area of the annulus and produces a direct loss of support of the aortic valve cusps.

C. The patient with an *acute Type I dissecting aortic aneurysm* (66% of acute dissecting aneurysms) is usually a middle-aged male, frequently black, with known hypertension, who experiences the onset of excruciating pain.

D. The pain, sharp, knifelike, often tearing or ripping in nature, occurs most commonly in the anterior chest or back.

E. The pain does not have the characteristic angina pectoris pattern of radiation into the neck, jaws, or upper extremities.

F. There may be murmurs over the origins of the subclavian and carotid arteries.

G. A significant difference in blood pressure between the two upper extremities is common.

H. The electrocardiogram usually shows only the effects of hypertensive heart disease.

I. An anteroposterior chest roentgenogram may show mediastinal widening and a pleural effusion.

J. The patient suspected of having an acute Type I dissecting aneurysm should be placed in an intensive care unit, carefully monitored, and cardiologists and cardiovascular surgeons called in immediate consultation.

K. In the patient with the more *chronic aneurysm* localized to the aortic root and ascending aorta, the most common symptom is cardiac decompensation secondary to aortic valve insufficiency.

L. The decompensation usually is insidious in onset, although in some cases the patient may present with acute overwhelming aortic valve insufficiency and represent an acute surgical emergency.

M. It is more common, however, for patients to present with shortness of breath, chest pain, and/or angina pectoris as a result of aortic valve insufficiency.

N. Superior vena caval obstruction due to the enlarging aneurysm may be a presenting sign.

O. The most important diagnostic procedure is the *aortogram,* which should be performed as soon as possible in the acute case. Visualization should be from the aortic valve to abdominal aortic bifurcation.

P. In the chronic case, right and left heart catheterization and coronary cineangiography should be included.

3. *Treatment*

A. In general, the definitive treatment for aneurysms of the aortic root and ascending aorta is surgical.

B. If the patient with an acute Type I dissecting aneurysm is a reasonable surgical risk, he should be stabilized and operated upon promptly.

C. Patients who are not good surgical risks can be managed with drugs (see "Drug Therapy in Dissecting Aneurysms of the Aorta" below).

D. Chronic aneurysms of the aortic root and ascending aorta should be treated surgically depending upon their size, shape (fusiform or saccular), and symptomatology.

4. *Prognosis*

Today, aneurysms of the aortic root and ascending aorta can be corrected surgically with an acceptable mortality of 10 to 12 per cent, and good long-term results.

ANEURYSMS OF THE TRANSVERSE THORACIC AORTA

1. *Definition*

A. The transverse thoracic aorta is that segment of aorta extending from the innominate artery to the left subclavian artery.

B. Aneurysms of the aortic arch are rarely isolated, usually being associated with aneurysm formation proximally and distally in the aorta.

2. *Etiology*

A. Cystic medial necrosis, atherosclerosis, and syphilis account for most of the aneurysms of the aortic arch.

B. Type I aortic dissection due to cystic medial necrosis involves the aortic arch.

C. False aneurysms secondary to traumatic rupture of the aorta may cause arch aneurysms, although these lesions are more common distal to the left subclavian artery.

3. *Clinical picture*

A. Aneurysms of the aortic arch become symptomatic by virtue of encroachment on the surrounding structures.

B. The superior vena cava and innominate vein can be compressed by the enlarging aorta.

C. Obstruction of venous drainage produces the "superior vena cava syndrome," characterized by plethora and edema of the face, neck, and upper extremities, and the development of large cutaneous venous channels.

D. The trachea and esophagus lie posterior to the aortic arch and can be compressed by aneurysms of this region, producing respiratory stridor and/or dysphagia.

E. Aneurysmal dilatation of the arch also can produce stretching of the left recurrent laryngeal nerve, with resultant paralysis of the left vocal cord and hoarseness.

4. *Diagnosis*

A. The diagnosis of an aortic arch aneurysm, whether in an asymptomatic patient with a large mass discovered by chest roentgenograph or in a patient with symptoms as noted above, includes consideration of mediastinal tumors or cysts, lung tumors, esophageal tumors, and metastatic cancer.

B. Aortography is the most reliable and direct means of making this diagnosis, and for delineating the full extent of the aneurysm.

5. *Treatment*

A. Indications for operative treatment of aneurysms of the aortic arch generally are related to encroachment on surrounding structures and/or progressive enlargement of the aneurysm.

B. The operative treatment involves a moderate risk (operative mortality 20–30%) and rather extensive surgery.

C. For that reason, aneurysms of the aortic arch should be operated upon only when enlarging or symptomatic.

ANEURYSMS OF THE DESCENDING THORACIC AORTA

1. *Definition*

The descending thoracic aorta extends from the origin of the left subclavian artery to the diaphragm, giving rise to several pairs of intercostal vessels.

2. *Etiology*

A. Cystic medial necrosis with aortic dissection is the most common cause of aneurysms in the descending thoracic aorta.

B. The DeBakey Type III aortic dissection begins distal to the left subclavian artery. The re-entry point of this type of dissection can occur above or below the diaphragm.

C. Although dissecting aneurysms usually are cylindrical in shape, the development of a false saccular aneurysm of the descending thoracic aorta may be an acute or late complication of aortic dissection.

D. Atherosclerotic aneurysms can also involve the descending thoracic aorta. These are usually fusiform aneurysms and may be seen along the entire length of the descending thoracic aorta.

E. Descending thoracic aortic aneurysms may be traumatic in origin and most commonly occur following an acute deceleration-type injury.

F. Traumatic aortic disruption ranges from intimal tears to complete transection of the thoracic aorta.

G. In those patients in whom the adventitia remains intact, false aneurysms develop and progress.

3. *Clinical picture*

A. Males predominate 5:1 and are affected most commonly in the fifth, sixth, and seventh decades of life.

B. An aneurysm of the descending thoracic aorta can be an incidental finding on chest roentgenograph.

C. The development of symptoms is due to growth of the aneurysm, with compression and erosion of surrounding structures.

D. Back pain is a common symptom and is due to erosion of the dorsal vertebral bodies, with pressure being applied to the posterior ribs, intercostal nerves, and nerve roots.

E. Hemorrhage due to rupture of the aneurysm into the pleural cavity or into adjacent structures can occur, such as into the esophagus, pericardium, pulmonary artery, and all other surrounding structures.

F. Erosion into the pulmonary tissue may produce hemoptysis.

G. *The DeBakey Type III aortic dissection*

(1) Acute aortic dissection of the DeBakey Type III variety presents as severe interscapular or left chest pain.

(2) The patient, middle-aged, with known hypertension, presents with the sudden onset of severe tearing pain between the scapulae that radiates down into the lower back and into the left side of the chest.

(3) This pain may be confused with the pain of myocardial infarction.

H. *False aneurysm*

(1) The clinical presentation of false aneurysms following chest trauma can be insidious.

(2) Exsanguination due to rupture of the aorta at the time of injury leads to death in about 80 per cent of patients.

(3) Of the 20 per cent who survive to reach the hospital, widening of the mediastinum or obliteration of the aortic shadow on roentgenograph is the usual first indication of aortic injury and formation of false aneurysm.

(4) These lesions may remain silent and heal, or go on to formation of a chronic false aneurysm with progressive enlargement.

(5) The danger of sudden rupture of the aneurysm, however, dictates an aggressive approach to this problem.

4. *Diagnosis and laboratory findings*

A. Evaluation of patients with roentgenographic findings suggestive of aneurysm of the descending thoracic aorta begins with a careful history and physical examination.

B. Special attention should be paid to the presence or absence of hypertension, atherosclerotic vascular disease, symptoms suggestive of previous aortic dissection, and symptoms referable to those structures that are adjacent to the descending thoracic aorta, such as dysphagia or hemoptysis.

C. Chest fluoroscopy, barium swallow with oblique films of the chest, and tomograms provide relatively simple, noninvasive means of evaluating the mass in question.

D. The definitive diagnosis must be made by aortography.

E. In the emergency post-traumatic situation, an aortic rupture must be considered when mediastinal widening is suggested by the chest roentgenograph.

F. Aortography should be performed as soon as possible because of the potentially lethal nature of this lesion.

G. In situations of multiple injuries, the immediate life-threatening problems must be cared for initially.

H. When the patient's condition is stable, he should undergo aortography.

I. Emergency thoracic exploration in the deteriorating patient may be indicated at times, but, in most instances, aortography to confirm the diagnosis of traumatic disruption of the aorta can be carried out.

J. If an acute Type III dissecting aneurysm is suspected, the patient should be placed in an intensive care unit and monitored carefully, and immediate cardiology and cardiovascular surgical consultations should be obtained. Prompt aortography is indicated.

5. *Treatment*

A. Fusiform aneurysms of the descending thoracic aorta should be replaced when they reach a diameter of 6 or 7 cm., or if they become symptomatic.

B. Patients with saccular aneurysms have poor prognoses because of the danger of aneurysm rupture without warning symptoms. The saccular aneurysm should be resected when diagnosed.

C. Once the diagnosis of traumatic aortic aneurysm is made by aortography, the patient should be taken immediately to the operating room, where the aorta is repaired and continuity restored.

D. The primary treatment for acute dissecting aneurysms (DeBakey Type III) involving the descending thoracic aorta is *pharmacologic*. Control of hypertension and the use of negative inotropic agents have been shown to arrest the dissecting process and, once controlled, the dissection goes on to complete healing.

E. The primary and usually definite therapy for the patient with Type III acute dissecting aneurysms is drug therapy.

F. Drug therapy is the initial therapy for stabilizing purposes in the patient with acute Type I dissecting aneurysm, and definitive therapy in the poor risk patient with acute Type I dissecting aneurysm.

G. Place the patient in an intensive care unit.

(1) Monitor electrocardiogram, blood pressure, cardiovascular pressure, and insert Foley catheter to follow urinary output.

(2) Reduce systolic blood pressure to 100 to 120 mm. Hg (if appropriate). Use trimethaphan camsylate, 1 to 2 mg. per ml. or sodium nitroprusside (Nipride) 1 to 8 mg. per kg. per minute, as intravenous drip acutely, and if necessary 24 to 48 hours or longer, with a flow rate to maintain the desired blood pressure. Keep the head of the bed elevated 30 to 45 degrees to gain orthostatic effect of drugs.

(3) Administer reserpine, 1 to 2 mg., intramuscularly every 4 to 6 hours, or propranolol 1 mg., intramuscularly every 4 to 6 hours (these drugs can be used in combination).

(4) Give guanethidine sulfate, 25 to 50 mg. twice daily by mouth.

(5) Continue to monitor elec-

Table 14-1. Drug Therapy in Dissecting Aneurysms of the Aorta

Drug	Mechanisms of Action	Total Effect
Reserpine	Depletes all catecholamines from all tissue stores; neurotransmitter (norepinephrine) release diminished after nerve stimulation.	Decreases myocardial contractility; sedation, depression, bradycardia (reduces cardiac output); reduces peripheral resistance; stimulates gastric secretion.
Sodium nitroprusside (Nipride)	Selectively relaxes vascular smooth muscle.	Rapid lowering of blood pressure; lowers peripheral resistance; reduces cardiac output and contractility indirectly by decreasing venous return.
Trimethaphan camsylate (Arfonad)	Ganglionic blockade; direct relaxing effect on vascular smooth muscle; histamine release.	Rapid lowering of blood pressure; lowers peripheral resistance; reduces cardiac output and contractility indirectly by decreasing venous return. Produces ileus, bladder distention, pupil dilatation.
Guanethidine sulfate (Ismelin)	Selectively depletes catecholamines from postganglionic nerve terminals, particularly in heart, gut, blood vessels, but not central nervous system.	Postural hypotension, diarrhea, bradycardia (reduces cardiac output); decreases peripheral resistance; no CNS effect.
Propranolol HCl (Inderal)	Specifically blocks beta adrenergic stimulation at end organ receptor (blood vessels, heart).	Bradycardia (reduces cardiac output); increases peripheral resistance; mild sedation; little hypotensive effect).
Methyldopa (Aldomet)	Metabolized to alpha-methyl norepinephrine; a weak neuro-transmitter and pressor agent, which replaces the more potent norepinephrine at nerve terminal; other unknown mechanisms.	Sedation, little depression; reduces peripheral resistance; slight bradycardia.
Thiazides (Diuril, Hydrodiuril)	Decreased tubular reabsorption of Cl^- and Na^+; some K^+ is lost; results in salt and/or extracellular fluid volume depletion, with possibly a direct cardiovascular effect.	Decrease in blood pressure.

trocardiogram, blood pressure, pulses, urine output. Examine stools for blood.

(6) Take daily chest roentgeno-graphs to check for mediastinal widening and pleural fluid.

H. Usually the blood pressure response to trimethaphan camsylate or sodium nitroprusside is rapid and can be profound if not carefully regulated. As a rule, when the blood pressure is lowered, the chest and/or back pain is dramatically relieved. The relief of pain is an important clinical guide to the effectiveness of drug therapy in arresting the so-called dissecting hematoma.

I. As soon as the patient is stable, transfer him to a medical center where aortography can be performed to confirm diagnosis and where a cardiovascular surgical team and facilities for management of major cardiovascular problems are available.

J. Indications for operation in patients with the DeBakey Type III aortic dissections include inability to control the blood pressure and the development of an acute saccular aneurysm. Most patients with dissecting aneurysms of the descending thoracic aorta can be managed well with drugs only and do not develop indications for surgery.

6. *Prognosis*

More than 50 per cent of patients with aneurysms of the descending thoracic aorta treated with surgery or with drugs alone (dissecting aneurysms) will survive at least 3 to 5 years.

THORACOABDOMINAL ANEURYSMS

1. *Definition*

Atherosclerotic aneurysms of both the thoracic and abdominal segments in continuity are not uncommon and make up 2.5 per cent of all aortic aneurysms.

2. *Etiology*

A. The distal thoracic aorta and proximal abdominal aorta usually become aneurysmal on an atherosclerotic basis.

B. DeBakey Types I and III dissecting aneurysms may also lead to enlargement of the aorta in this region.

C. Less commonly, one may see post-traumatic aneurysms secondary to iatrogenic or noniatrogenic penetrating wounds in this area.

D. Mycotic aneurysms are rare in the thoracoabdominal aorta.

3. *Clinical picture*

A. Thoracoabdominal aortic aneurysms are more common in men than in women by an 8:1 ratio.

B. The highest incidence is in the fifth, sixth and seventh decades of life.

C. Symptoms produced by thoracoabdominal aortic aneurysms are due to enlargement of the aneurysm and erosion into the contiguous structures, resulting most commonly in back pain.

D. As in aneurysms localized to the thoracic aorta, this pain is due to erosion of, and pressure on, the vertebral bodies and nerve roots.

E. Aneurysms of the thoracoabdominal aorta can also produce a prominent pulsatile epigastic mass.

4. *Diagnosis*

A. The most important single finding on physical examination is detection of a pulsatile epigastric mass.

B. As with aortic aneurysm in the chest, the aortograph is the definitive procedure in delineating these aneurysms.

C. Biplanar aortography is helpful in evaluation of the relationship of these aneurysms to the major branches of the abdominal aorta.

5. *Treatment*

A. The treatment of thoracoabdominal aneurysms is largely dependent on their symptomatology.

B. Asymptomatic aneurysms in this region generally are not resected because of the risk involved in surgery.

C. However, expanding or otherwise symptomatic aneurysms require replacement.

D. Pharmacological therapy of thoracoabdominal aneurysms in high-risk patients is possible, using drugs to decrease the pulsatile nature of the arterial blood flow as well as the mean aortic pressure, and thereby prevent or slow further expansion of the aneurysm.

ANEURYSMS OF THE ABDOMINAL AORTA

1. *Definition and etiology*

A. The abdominal aorta is the most common site of aortic aneurysm formation, most commonly distal to the renal arteries.

B. The most common cause of abdominal aortic aneurysm is atherosclerosis, resulting in destruction of the elastic fibers within the media with gradual stretching of the remaining fibrous tissue and eventual ballooning of the wall.

C. Tension in the wall gradually increases, according to LaPlace's law, as the diameter of the vessel increases, until finally rupture occurs.

2. *Clinical picture*

A. The abdominal aortic aneurysm is usually asymptomatic, although with increased size, the patient may experience the vague discomfort of a space-occupying lesion of the abdomen and perhaps a fullness.

B. Patients will often complain of a "heart beat" in their abdomen.

C. Pain radiating down the legs, to the back and in the abdomen signifies sudden expansion secondary to dissection or leaking of blood into the retroperitoneum and must be considered a prelude to the catastrophic event of rupture.

D. When tenderness is elicited on palpation of any aneurysm, expansion must be considered, and resection, regardless of size, is in order.

3. *Diagnosis and laboratory findings*

A. *Palpation*

(1) Palpation is the initial step in the diagnosis of an abdominal aortic aneurysm.

(2) Palpation is properly performed by placing the hands on the abdomen, fingers extended, and moving them toward each other from either side towards the midline until they meet the sides of the pulsatile mass.

(3) When the fingers are pushed laterally by the mass, the diameter can be estimated as the distance between the fingertips.

B. *X-ray of the abdomen*

(1) A useful diagnostic aid is the lateral roentgenograph of the abdomen, and this study should be a part of the evaluation of every patient presenting with abdominal pain of uncertain etiology.

(2) In the lateral position, calcifications in the atheromata within the media of the aneurysmal wall can be seen.

C. *Arteriography*

(1) The arteriogram is generally of little benefit in making the diagnosis, since the radiopaque material flows within the effective lumen of the aorta.

(2) The aneurysmal dilatation is usually masked by mural thrombus.

(3) Information can be gained about the status of the renal arteries from an arteriograph.

D. *An intravenous pyelogram* can be helpful in delineating the course of the ureters.

E. Perhaps the most exciting radiographic tool recently developed is the *total body scan,* which, by computer analysis, allows the production of a saggital section detailed study of the body in serial cuts, permitting the very accurate diagnosis of aneurysm with a noninvasive technique.

4. *Treatment and results*
  A. *Asymptomatic abdominal aneurysms*
    (1) The critical size seems to be 6 to 7 cm. because 45 to 50 per cent of aneurysms of this size, left untreated, will rupture within ten years, with a mortality of 50 to 80 per cent.
    (2) One-half of these patients, when untreated, will die within one year from the time of diagnosis.
    (3) Elective resection is indicated and is associated with an operative mortality of 3 to 15 per cent, depending upon associated risk factors.
    (4) When the aneurysm is less than 6 cm. in diameter, the risk of rupture is 15 to 20 per cent.
    (5) The five-year survival rate, when the aneurysm is not treated, is about 50 per cent, and with resection, 70 per cent.
    (6) The usual operative mortality for these smaller aneurysms is only 3 per cent.
    (7) *Risk factors*
      (a) Risk factors include the size of the aneurysm and the absence of femoral and popliteal pulses.
      (b) Cerebrovascular disease, chronic lung disease, and significant cardiac disease are considered relative risk factors as well.
      (c) Age alone is not a contraindication to elective resection. It is clear that the healthy sixty-year-old male with a 6-centimeter aneurysm should undergo resection, but consideration must also be given the good risk patient with a small aneurysm.
      (d) Small aneurysms can rupture because of focal necrosis or ulceration irrespective of the usual higher expectation of rupture, the larger the aneurysm.
  B. *Symptomatic abdominal aortic aneurysms*
    (1) Rupture of the abdominal aortic aneurysm is a catastrophic event as-

sociated with mortality of 32 to 85 per cent for the patients who live to reach the operating room.
    (2) The patient often gives a history of sudden lower abdominal pain radiating to the midback, with a feeling of faintness. This represents an initial leak into the retroperitoneum.
    (3) At a variable interval, more massive leak occurs with severe abdominal pain and shock.
    (4) The patient arrives at the emergency room with a distended acute abdomen, in shock, and often unresponsive.
    (5) Diagnosis must be rapid, resuscitation accomplished, and volume restoration attempted with simultaneous prompt surgery.
    (6) It should be remembered that femoral pulses may be intact even with a rupture of the aneurysm.
5. *Complications*
  A. A late and serious complication is aortoduodenal fistula.
  B. Varying amounts of bleeding into the bowel then occurs, depending upon the size of the leak, requiring reoperation and repair.
  C. Frequently the graft is beyond salvage and must be divided.
  D. An extra anatomic bypass, such as the axillo-femoral graft, must then be relied upon to provide blood supply to the lower extremities.
  E. Infection at the anastomosis also requires ligation and extra-anatomic grafting.

OCCLUSIVE DISEASE OF THE ABDOMINAL AORTA

1. *Etiology and clinical picture*
  A. The abdominal aorta, in particular the region of the bifurcation, is one of the most common sites of atherosclerosis and the ischemic syndrome that results from occlusion.
  B. When the aortic lumen is de-

creased by 90 per cent significant reduction in the blood flow occurs to the pelvic viscera and lower extremities.

C. Impotence in men results and, in combination with claudication in the lower legs and buttocks, comprises the Leriche syndrome.

D. The disease is most common in men in the fifth and sixth decades, and commonly associated with coronary and superficial femoral vessel occlusive disease as well.

E. *Physical findings*

(1) Physical findings include markedly diminished to absent femoral pulses and sometimes femoral bruits.

(2) Distal pulses may be absent.

(3) Signs of severe ischemia with ulceration or gangrene of the toes may be present.

(4) Far more advanced signs occur if aorto-iliac occlusion is combined with femoral popliteal occlusion in the same limb.

(5) Dependent rubor, pallor on elevation, delayed venous filling and capillary refill, atrophic changes of the nails, hair loss, muscle atrophy, decreased temperature and varying degrees of ulceration are all signs of ischemia.

F. Claudication indicates insufficient blood supply to muscle and is a result of anoxia.

G. Rest pain indicates ischemia to the point of impending gangrene, since the muscle, even though inactive, is anoxic because of insufficient flow of blood to supply the muscles' metabolic demand, even at rest.

H. The next step in the progression of the disease is gangrene, and the clinician must take active measures to restore flow to avoid limb loss, when rest pain is present.

2. *Diagnosis*

A. The principal diagnostic method to localize the lesion is arteriography.

B. The site of injection in aorto-iliac occlusion may be percutaneous femoral with retrograde injection or, when femoral pulses are absent, translumbar or transaxillary.

3. *Treatment*

A. Arteriography to provide the blueprint for operation should be obtained in the patient who presents with significant signs of aorto-iliac occlusion, and who does not have a major contraindication for elective surgery.

B. If rest pain is present, gangrene is imminent.

C. A major extremity amputation is associated with a long-term mortality approaching 30 per cent and, under any circumstance, limb loss is to be avoided if possible.

D. A particularly aggressive approach is warranted when rest pain is part of the history.

E. When frank ulceration and gangrene, or rest pain, as indicators of impending limb loss are not present, and a major medical contraindication to elective surgery does not exist, then the decision to operate becomes rather subjective.

F. If claudication significantly interferes with the patient's life style, or ability to earn his livelihood, only then should surgery be considered.

G. A retired octogenarian who develops claudication after walking six blocks, with a history of coronary artery disease and no rest pain, is not a candidate for surgery, and should not have an arteriogram simply to document a lesion for the record.

H. Major amputation because of a complication of angiography can be the outcome in a patient who might otherwise have easily adjusted to his disease.

I. Exercises, and walking longer distances may increase tolerance, perhaps with the development of more collateral vessels.

J. Attention should also be directed to careful foot hygiene and weight reduction.

K. Occasionally vasodilator drugs are of benefit.

L. Cessation of smoking is mandatory.

M. Placement of the bed in a "vascular position" with six-inch blocks beneath the head of the bed may increase flow to the foot and eliminate rest pains.

N. *Lumbar sympathectomy*

(1) Although lumbar sympathectomy does not result in increased flow of blood to the muscle mass, it usually does result in enhanced skin circulation that may allay ulceration and, even when present, may aid healing of superficial ulceration, particularly important in the diabetic with aorto-iliac occlusion.

(2) A check for the presence of sympathetic nerve function in the extremity should be done, since a warm, dry foot may indicate absence of sympathetic tone in the cutaneous vessels, not uncommon in patients with long-standing ischemia.

(3) If the foot is cold and sweaty, and the patient is not a candidate for major revascularization, benefit may follow the lesser procedure of sympathectomy.

O. The treatment of choice is to bypass the region of occlusion, to shunt blood to the ischemic extremity.

P. Various extraperitoneal methods have been suggested in the poor-risk patient to avoid the morbidity and higher mortality of a major abdominal procedure.

Q. Transabdominal procedures usually entail bifurcation grafting from the abdominal aorta proximal to the occlusion, to either the iliac or femoral arteries.

R. Endarterectomy is applicable when occlusion is localized to a single well-defined segment of the artery.

4. *Results*

Long-term patency rates vary in reported series from 65 to 90 per cent.

SUGGESTED READINGS

Benjamin, H. B. and Becker, A. B.: Etiologic incidence of thoracic and abdominal aneurysms. Surg. Gynecol. Obstet., *125*:1307, 1967.

Bennett, D. E. and Cherry, J. K.: The natural history of traumatic aneurysms of the aorta. Surgery, *61*:516, 1967.

Bergan, J. J. and Yao, J. S.T.: Modern management of abdominal aortic aneurysms. Surg. Clin. North Am., *54*(1):175, 1974.

Crawford, E. A. et al.: Aneurysm of the abdominal aorta. Surg. Clin. North Am., *46*(4):463, 1966.

Crawford, E. S. et al.: Surgical considerations of aneurysms, atherosclerotic occlusive lesions of the aorta and major artery. Postgrad. Med., *29*:151, 1961.

Crisler, C. and Bahnson, H. T.: Aneurysms of the aorta. Curr. Prob. Surg., Dec. 1972.

Dagher, F. J. et al.: Hemorrhage in normal man. Effects of Mannitol, plasma volume, and body water dynamics following acute blood loss. Ann. Surg., *163*:505, 1966.

DeBakey, M. E. et al.: Abnormalities of the sinuses of Valsalva. Experience with 35 patients. J. Thorac. Cardiovasc. Surg., *54*:312, 1967.

Downs, A. R.: Aorto-iliac occlusive disease. Surg. Clin. North Am., *54*(1):195, 1974.

Fomon, J. J., Kurzweg, F. T., and Broodaway, R. K.: Aneurysms of the aorta: a review. Ann. Surg., *165*:557, 1967.

Humphries, A. W., and Young, J. R.: The severely ischemic leg. Curr. Prob. Surg., June 1970.

The International Surgery Group of the University of Toronto et al.: Surgical treatment of abdominal aortic aneurysms in Toronto: A study of 1013 patients. Can. Med. Assoc. J., *107*:1091.

Szilagyi, D. E. et al.: Contribution of abdominal aortic aneurysmectomy to prolongation of life. Ann. Surg., *164*:678, 1966.

Temes, G. D. and Wheat, M. W., Jr.,: The management of aneurysms of the aorta. D.M., Sept., 1974.

Weintraub, R. A. and Abrams, H. L.: Mycotic aneurysms. AM. J. Roentgenol. Radium Ther. Nucl. Med., *102*:354, 1968.

Wheat, M. W. Jr., and Palmer, R. F.: Dissecting aneurysms of the aorta. Curr. Prob. Surg., July, 1971.

15. TRAUMATIC HEART DISEASE

Panagiotis N. Symbas, M.D., and Charles R. Hatcher, Jr., M.D.

DEFINITION

Trauma to the heart may be due to penetrating or nonpenetrating injury.

1. *Penetrating cardiac trauma* may cause (1) pericardial wounds; (2) wound of the free cardiac wall with or frequently without a wound of the interventricular septum, aortic valve, atrioventricular valves, chordae tendineae or papillary muscles; and (3) injury to the coronary arteries.[20]

2. *Nonpenetrating trauma* to the heart may cause (1) pericardial rupture; (2) myocardial contusion; (3) rupture of the free cardiac wall, interventricular septum, aortic valve, atrioventricular valves, chordae tendineae, or papillary muscles; and (4) injury to the coronary arteries.[20]

GENERAL CONSIDERATIONS

One of the leading causes of death in our society is trauma. Cardiac injury is a major cause for this high mortality. With the increase in traffic accidents and social violence during recent years, there has been a parallel rise of trauma to the heart.

The most common cause of traumatic heart disease is mechanical injury produced by a penetrating or nonpenetrating physical force. Other causes of cardiac injury, which will not be considered in this chapter, are those secondary to diagnostic and therapeutic techniques utilized in the management of heart and other diseases, (i.e., cardiac catheterization, angiocardiography, pacemaker implantation, vigorous cardiopulmonary resuscitation and invasive hemodynamic monitoring).

Traumatic injury to the heart may be overshadowed by more overt manifestations of other thoracic, cerebral, abdominal, or musculoskeletal injury. Consequently, more subtle aspects of cardiac injuries may remain unnoticed to manifest occasionally in an alarming or catastrophic manner, either in the immediate postinjury period or in hours, days, or even months after the injury. Therefore, an awareness of possible cardiac injury in every traumatized patient is a prerequisite to early diagnosis and treatment.

PENETRATING WOUNDS OF THE HEART

The grave prognosis of penetrating cardiac wounds has been recognized since antiquity when Hippocrates described their fatal nature.

1. *Etiology*

A. Penetrating wounds of the heart, seen in civilian practice, are caused by knives, ice picks, bullets, and other projectiles or even rarely by the inward displacement of ribs or sternal fragments.

B. Although in the past the majority of cardiac wounds in civilians were the results of stabbing[5,7] now gunshot wounds to the heart are seen with increasing frequency.[18,22]

C. Penetrating wounds are most often seen with wounds of the precordium, but may be seen in association with wounds of other areas of the chest and with wounds of the neck and upper abdomen.

D. The relative frequency of penetrating wounds to the various cardiac structures coincides with their relative area of exposure on the anterior chest wall.

E. In order of decreasing frequency, the right ventricle, left ventricle, right atrium, and left atrium are involved in penetrating wounds of the heart.[22]

2. *Pathophysiology*

A. The clinical manifestations of penetrating wounds of the heart are usually dependent upon the site and size of the cardiac wound and the state of the pericardial wound.

B. In the cases in which the pericardial wound remains open and allows free drainage of the intrapericardial blood, the cardiac wound manifests with symptoms and signs of hemorrhage and hemothorax.

C. When the pericardial wound is obliterated with blood clot and adjacent lung or prepericardial fat, the escaping blood from the cardiac chamber cannot drain into the pleural space, and cardiac tamponade ensues.

3. *Symptoms and signs*

A. The patient with a penetrating cardiac wound may have symptoms and signs of the following:

(1) Cardiac tamponade

(2) Various degrees of blood loss and hemothorax or hemopneumothorax

(3) Cardiac tamponade and hemothorax

B. The patient with tamponade of the heart may be restless, may complain of air hunger, or may be in shock.

C. His skin may be cold and moist and his lips and digits mildly cyanotic.

D. Visible superficial neck veins may be distended and have paradoxical filling during inspiration (Kussmaul's sign).

E. The blood pressure may be unobtainable or the systolic pressure below normal level with a decrease during inspiration of 10 mm. Hg or more ("paradoxical pulse").

F. The pulse pressure is narrow.

G. The pulse is rapid and hypodynamic.

H. The heart sounds may or may not be distant and muffled.

I. The central venous pressure is elevated.

4. *Diagnosis*

The diagnosis of penetrating cardiac wound should be suspected in a wounded patient in the neck, upper abdomen, and particularly in the chest when he has symptoms and signs suggestive of cardiac tamponade or has significant intrathoracic bleeding (see Symptoms and Signs).

5. *Treatment*

A. *General approach*

(1) When the clinical manifestation of suspected cardiac wound is that of tamponade, immediate pericardiocentesis with a thin-wall metal needle or preferably a plastic #17 or #18 gauge catheter or needle should be performed through the left substernal paraxyphoid route with the patient in a semierect position 35 to 40 degrees, and the needle pointing toward the left shoulder (Fig. 15-1).

(2) During pericardiocentesis, continuous monitoring with the electrocardiogram is desirable but should not be done at the expense of delaying prompt pericardial decompression.

(3) If nonclotting blood is obtained, the diagnosis of cardiac injury and cardiac tamponade is certain and the pericardial space should be decompressed as much as possible.

(4) If a plastic catheter or needle is used for the pericardiocentesis, it should be left in place for continuous drainage of the intrapericardial blood until the cardiac wound is surgically repaired.

(5) When the clinical manifestations of penetrating wound of the heart are hemothorax and signs and symptoms of blood loss are present, the pleural space should be drained with a closed thoracostomy tube and this procedure should be followed by surgical repair of the wound as soon as possible.

(6) Blood drained from the pleural space may be autotransfused,[19] if needed, with the administration of other blood volume expanders. The expansion

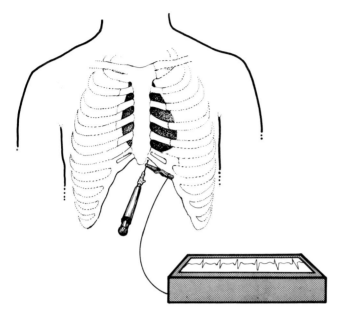

Fig. 15-1. Pericardiocentesis through the paraxyphoid route (Symbas, P. N.: Traumatic Injuries of the Heart and Great Vessels. Springfield, Ill., Charles C Thomas, 1972).

of the circulating blood volume benefits not only the patients with cardiac wound and a clinical picture of blood loss, but also the patients with a clinical picture of cardiac tamponade.[4] However, in patients with cardiac tamponade, the hemodynamic improvement following the administration of blood volume expanders is of short duration. Therefore, definitive treatment of these patients, as well as those with continuous blood loss, should be provided as soon as possible.

(7) The definitive treatment for patients with cardiac wounds and massive unrelenting blood loss is exploratory thoracotomy and cardiorrhaphy. However, the definitive treatment for patients with cardiac wounds and cardiac tamponade has not been uniform.[1,20]

(8) The various treatments for the latter have been:

(a) Pericardiocentesis alone

(b) Surgery after multiple successful pericardiocentesis

(c) Surgery after recurrence of cardiac tamponade following a successful pericardiocentesis

(d) Surgery alone

(9) Presently, pericardiocentesis alone as a definitive mode of therapy is of historical interest only.

(10) Although surgical repair in the face of recurrence of tamponade after one pericardiocentesis has compared quite favorably with immediate surgical repair alone,[22] it should be discouraged, and pericardiocentesis should be used only to provide time for the patient to be operated upon safely.

(11) Since the increasing number of patients with more severe cardiac wounds can only be handled successfully with immediate surgery, and since the unpredictable course of traumatic pericardial tamponade often follows an initial favorable response to pericardiocentesis, immediate surgery for all patients with penetrating wounds of the heart is accepted as the best therapeutic approach. The remarkable advancement in anesthesia and surgery strongly support the policy of immediate surgery.

B. *Surgical treatment*

(1) While light general anesthesia is administered and the entire anterior chest is prepped and draped, the operat-

ing team should be ready for rapid thoracotomy and decompression of the pericardium in case of rapid deterioration of the patient's condition.

(2) An anterolateral submammary incision, performed on the involved side, may be expanded as needed to the opposite side or to the neck.

(3) After the pericardial space is rapidly decompressed, bleeding through the cardiac wound is controlled digitally, and the cardiac wound is usually repaired with ease (Fig. 15-2).

(4) Rarely, projectiles may create a defect in the cardiac wall that is impossible to repair by suture approximation of the wound edges. Under these circumstances, the wound is best managed with or without a prosthesis after establishing cardiopulmonary bypass (Fig 15-3).

(5) Sizable injured branches of the coronary arteries are repaired under cardiopulmonary bypass, either primarily or with the use of a reversed saphenous vein graft, whereas, small severed branches are simply ligated.

(6) After repair of the cardiac wounds, the heart is palpated for the presence of a thrill.

(7) No intracardiac defect thus discovered should be repaired at this time, however, except in the very rare case when the defect is of such magnitude that the patient would not be expected to survive. In such a case, car-

diopulmonary bypass is instituted and the lesion repaired under direct vision.

C. *Postoperative care*

(1) Postoperative management is similar to that of any other critically ill patient, with frequent determinations of hemodynamic parameters and strict attention to intake and output being the hallmarks of good care.

(2) In addition, the patient should be closely observed throughout his hospital stay, and later, for the development of symptoms of residual or delayed sequelae from the penetrating cardiac wound.

(3) Many sequelae may occur following penetrating trauma to the heart, such as:

(a) Post-traumatic or postoperative pericarditis

(b) Ventricular septal defect

(c) Valvular defects

(d) Ventricular aneurysm

(e) Aortocardiac or aortopulmonary communication or communication of coronary artery to coronary vein or to cardiac chamber.[21]

(4) When such sequelae are found, appropriate medical and/or surgical treatment should be instituted.

(5) If a cardiac defect is found that endangers the patient's life, cardiac catheterization should be performed as soon as possible and followed by surgical repair.

(6) If the patient, however, toler-

Fig. 15-2. Closure of penetrating wound (*A*) underneath the wound-occluding finger and (*B*) underneath the wound-occluding finger and underneath the adjacent to the wound coronary artery. (Symbas, P. N.: Traumatic Injuries of the Heart and Great Vessels. Springfield, Ill., Charles C Thomas, 1972).

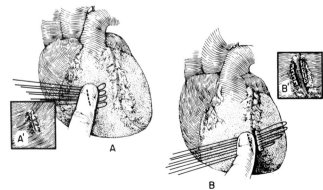

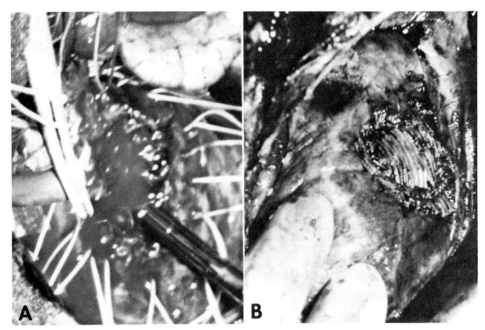

Fig. 15-3. Photograph (*A*) of a large bullet wound of the left ventricle and (*B*) of the left ventricular wound repaired with Dacron graft. (Symbas, P. N.: Traumatic Injuries of the Heart and Great Vessels. Springfield, Ill., Charles C Thomas, 1972).

ates his lesion postoperatively, cardiac catheterization should be performed electively and the hemodynamically significant defects should then be repaired.

CONTUSION OF THE HEART

1. *General features*

A. Initally, the incidence of cardiac contusion was thought to be infrequent, but with the increasing incidence and severity of blunt chest trauma, in addition to the physician's awareness, it appears that such injuries occur in significant numbers.

B. Autopsy studies in unselected auto accident victims have shown myocardial contusion in 15 to 17 percent, while in severe body trauma, an incidence of 76 per cent was found.[9,17]

C. The forces producing the contusion of the heart are of such a nature that

external evidence of injury may be meager or may not even be detectable in about one third of the injured individuals.

D. The lack of external evidence of cardiac trauma, combined with the physician's frequent preoccupation with treating more obvious injuries, is the most common cause of failure to diagnose and evaluate lesions of this type.

2. *Etiology*

A. The etiology of cardiac contusion may vary from a simple blow from a fist to the "steering wheel injury."

B. The steering wheel injury is the most common cause of blunt trauma to the heart.

C. The heart, which hangs freely in the chest cavity between the sternum and thoracic vertebra, is suspended from above by the great vessels. As such, it is subject to trauma by a number of *mechanisms*:[11]

(1) Sudden accelerations or decelerations may cause the heart to be thrust against the sternum or vertebra, injuring the myocardium.

(2) The heart may be compressed between the sternum and vertebra if the sternum is suddenly driven in by a forceful blow (steering wheel injury).

(3) Sudden increase in intrathoracic or intra-abdominal pressure may result in cardiac injury with subendocardial hemorrhage or rupture of the heart.

3. *Pathophysiology*

A. The pathologic lesions in myocardial contusion can be:

(1) Small areas of petechiae or ecchymosis in the subendocardium or subepicardium

(2) Full thickness contusion of the myocardial wall

(3) Rupture of the heart

B. Microscopic examination of an acute myocardial contusion reveals numerous red blood cells in the interspaces between myocardial fibers.

C. The muscle fibers themselves may be edematous, fragmented, or necrotic.

D. Later, polymorphonuclear leukocytes infiltrate the area of hemorrhage and the muscle fibers may appear swollen, may have lumpy cytoplasm, and may show partial loss of transverse striations (Fig. 15-4).

E. In survivors, the areas of damaged myocardium undergoes infiltration of inflammatory cells with or without softening, and eventual healing occurs with or without scar formation.

F. Full-thickness myocardial contusions may be subject to the same complication as myocardial infarction:

(1) Rupture of the softened area

(2) Myocardial failure with or without aneurysm formation.

G. Contusion may cause:

(1) Atrial or ventricular septal defect

(2) Valvular lesions

(3) Coronary artery damage, producing myocardial infarction

4. *Clinical manifestations*

A. Functional disturbances do not always reflect the severity of anatomic damage in the heart, and fatal dysrhythmias can be produced experimentally without demonstrable pathologic changes.[3,12]

B. The clinical picture of myocardial contusion, however, usually does depend, to a degree, upon the extent and type of lesion.

C. Most injuries probably produce no significant dysfunction and go unrecognized, while others are overlooked because of concomitant injuries to other organs.

D. *The most common symptom* of myocardial contusion is pain, which in character, location, and radiation is identical to the pain of myocardial ischemia[3] and is usually unaffected by coronary vasodilators.

E. *Asymptomatic myocardial contusions* may occur[26] or typical descriptions of pain may not be obtained because a detailed history is not available or because of more severe pain from other injuries.

F. With *severe contusions*, cardiac failure, dyspnea, and hypotension may be present.

G. *Auscultation* may disclose:

(1) Pericardial friction rub due to pericarditis

(2) Various heart murmurs, which result from dysfunction of injured myocardium, papillary muscles, chordae tendineae, or valves

H. The majority of the symptomatic patients complain immediately after their injury, although (rarely) their symptoms may be delayed for hours or days.

I. *The most common late symptoms* are congestive heart failure or pain similar to angina pectoris brought on by exertion.

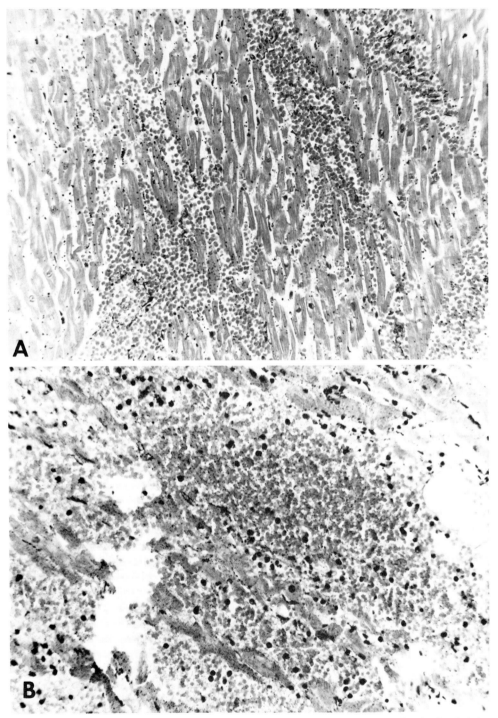

Fig. 15-4. Photomicrographs of a contused heart eight hours before the patient's death (*A*) showing large number of cells crowding the myocardial fibers (H & E; × 176.5) and (*B*) edema fragmentation and loss of transverse striation of myocardial fibers (H & E; × 176.5). (Symbas, P. N.: Traumatic Injuries of the Heart and Great Vessels. Springfield, Ill., Charles C Thomas, 1972).

J. *Cardiac arrhythmias*:

(1) Palpitations and tachycardia are frequent features, with premature atrial or ventricular contractions being the most common rhythm disturbances.

(2) Virtually all types of arrhythmias have been produced experimentally or have been seen in patients with myocardial contusion.

(3) Atrial fibrillation or flutter, sinoatrial block, A-V junctional rhythm, atrioventricular block, and idioventricular rhythm have also been observed.[10,12,17,25]

(4) Paroxysmal atrial tachycardia is uncommon.

(5) Paroxysmal ventricular tachycardia or fibrillation, and idioventricular rhythm are frequent causes of death.

5. *Diagnosis*

A. *Electrocardiography*

(1) Presently, the most readily available diagnostic test for myocardial contusion is the twelve-lead electrocardiogram, which should be obtained in all patients who sustain blunt injury to the chest, particularly involving the precordium.

(2) Electrocardiographic abnormalities that are precipitated by contusion of the heart range from transient to long-lasting disturbances of rhythm, to evidence of pericarditis or focal muscular damage, to changes typical of myocardial infarction.

(3) These ECG abnormalities, which may return to normal in a much shorter time than those produced by frank myocardial infarction, are frequently present shortly after the trauma, but may not appear until 24 to 48 hours later.

(4) Serial electrocardiograms, therefore, should be done in patients who sustain blunt trauma to the thorax to detect the early and late appearing electrocardiographic changes.

(5) Unfortunately, electrocardio-graphic abnormalities other than those indicating muscle damage from cardiac contusion are relatively nonspecific, since they can be precipitated by other conditions not infrequently present in traumatized patients (e.g., hypoxia, hypovolemia, shock).

(6) Despite the error in specificity,[15] repeated twelve-lead electrocardiograms have proven to be the most reliable diagnostic tool in accurately evaluating patients with suspected cardiac contusion.

B. *Other laboratory studies*

Other laboratory studies have not been found to be of great diagnostic value.

(1) Serum enzymes are frequently elevated in liver, lung, and skeletal muscle injuries, or in hemorrhagic shock, and are not very useful in establishing cardiac contusion.

(2) The use of radioisotopes to diagnose myocardial contusion is under investigation.

(3) Coronary injection of technicium albumin microspheres[13] or ^{99m}TC-stannous pyrophosphate[23] clearly outlines the experimentally contused myocardium.

6. *Treatment*

A. The treatment of myocardial contusion, like that of myocardial infarction, is expectant and symptomatic.

B. Early recognition and treatment of cardiac arrhythmias is paramount.

C. A period of bed rest for 2 to 4 weeks is equally important.

D. Anticoagulants are to be avoided, as they may precipitate intramyocardial or intrapericardial hemorrhage.

E. Oxygen should be administered if hypoxemia is present.

F. Digitalis is of value in cardiac failure or atrial fibrillation with rapid ventricular response, although reversion to sinus rhythm with bed rest alone is the rule.

G. Digitalis is ineffective in sinus tachycardia and may accentuate the electrical instability of contused ventricular myocardium.

H. Lidocaine, procainamide, and quinidine may be useful for control of ectopic beats or tachyarrhythmias.

I. Coronary vasodilators have virtually no effect on pain, which is best treated with narcotics.

7. *Prognosis*

A. The prognosis of patients with myocardial contusion for partial or complete recovery is good.

B. The sequelae vary from no cardiac disability to death from complications, particularly ventricular arrhythmias or cardiac rupture.

C. Clinical improvement and reversion of the electrocardiogram to normal usually occur within a month, although this is variable.[17]

RUPTURE OF THE HEART

1. *Etiology*

A. Forceful compression against the vertebral column may cause rupture of the heart at the time of injury.

B. Immediate myocardial discontinuity may also be caused by laceration from a sharp rib or sternal bone fragment.

C. Delayed rupture may occur at the site of a myocardial contusion as late as 2 weeks following the initial blunt trauma.

D. Very rarely, the heart may be ruptured by violent compression applied to the abdomen and legs.

2. *Pathophysiology*

Congestive heart failure is commonly observed. The cardiac rupture may involve the following:

A. The free wall,[2] with clinical manifestations of hemopericardium and cardiac tamponade

B. The interventricular septum[14] with symptoms and signs of interventricular shunt

C. Aortic, mitral,[16] or tricuspid valves,[8] with symptoms and signs of valvular regurgitation.

3. *Symptoms and diagnosis*

A. The diagnosis of rupture of the heart should be suspected when a patient experiences severe blunt injury and has a clinical picture of cardiac tamponade.

B. In the face of symptoms and signs of cardiac tamponade, massive myocardial contusion must be considered as the clinical manifestations, which may be identical to those of cardiac rupture.

C. The diagnosis of rupture of the cardiac valves or interventricular septum should be suspected in patients who sustain severe blunt trauma and develop congestive heart failure.

D. The symptoms of cardiac decompensation in these patients may appear immediately (Fig 15-5) after the injury or following a relatively asymptomatic period of days or even years.

E. The diagnosis of rupture of the cardiac valves or ventricular septum is almost certain in patients who develop a valvular regurgitation murmur, or murmur of ventricular septal defect following severe blunt trauma.

4. *Treatment*

A. In patients with rupture of the free cardiac wall, pericardiocentesis should be performed immediately to relieve the cardiac tamponade and be followed with emergency thoracotomy to close the cardiac defect.

B. In symptomatic patients with rupture of the cardiac valves or interventricular septum, however, the treatment should be supportive, before and after the diagnosis is established.

C. *Common measures* used include:

(1) Assisted ventilation

(2) Good pulmonary toilet

(3) Careful administration of digitalis and diuretics

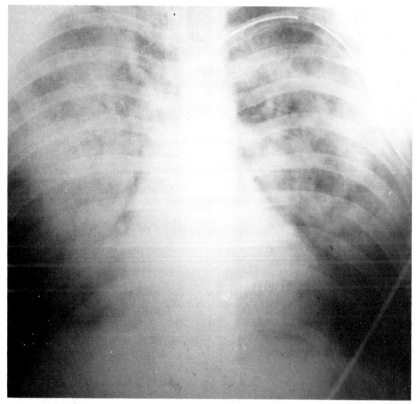

Fig. 15-5. Chest roentgenogram of an eighteen-year old man who was involved in a severe automobile accident two hours earlier. (Symbas, P. N.: Traumatic Injuries of the Heart and Great Vessels. Springfield, Ill., Charles C Thomas, 1972).

D. *Cardiac catheterization and surgical management*

(1) If the patient fails to respond to this treatment, cardiac catheterization should be performed as soon as possible.

(2) The clinical deterioration combined with the specific data of cardiac catheterization will serve as indicators for emergency surgical repair.

(3) In patients with compensated congestive heart failure, cardiac catheterization and angiography should be performed following recovery from the initial trauma.

(4) If the cardiac lesion is found to be hemodynamically significant, elective repair should then be performed.

INJURIES TO THE PERICARDIUM (SEE ALSO CHAP. 8)

1. *Classification*

A. The pericardium may be injured from blunt or penetrating trauma.

B. Its injury may vary from contusion to laceration or rupture.

C. The delayed manifestations of pericardial injury include:

(1) Post-traumatic pericarditis

(2) Suppurative pericarditis

(3) Constrictive pericarditis

2. *Symptoms and signs and diagnosis*

A. Pericardial trauma commonly associated with major cardiac trauma is usually manifested by the signs and symptoms of the coexisting cardiac injury.

  B. Isolated contusions or small lacerations of the pericardium are usually unrecognized.

  C. Pericardial trauma may lead to hemopericardium and cardiac tamponade in rare occasions.

  D. Rupture of the pericardium from lethal or sublethal blunt chest trauma is quite frequent but is usually associated with cardiac injury.

  E. Infrequently, when an isolated lesion occurs, its clinical manifestations are the result of herniation of the heart through the pericardial defect.[6]

  F. *Post-traumatic pericarditis*

    (1) Post-traumatic pericarditis is a frequent complication of blunt or penetrating injury to the heart and pericardium.

    (2) It may appear shortly after the injury or after a few days, weeks, or even months, and it may recur.[24]

    (3) Fever, sweats, and precordial or retrosternal chest pain radiating to the neck, left shoulder or intrascapular area are symptoms of post-traumatic pericarditis, which may be intensified by deep inspiration or recumbency and relieved by sitting upright.

    (4) Friction rub is frequently heard, and muffling of the heart tones and even paradoxical pulse may be present when a significant amount of pericardial fluid has accumulated.

    (5) *Treatment*

      (a) The course of post-traumatic pericarditis is usually self-limited.

      (b) Symptomatic treatment is initially provided with acetylsalicylic acid.

      (c) If this fails, corticosteroids are adminstered.

      (d) Suppurative or constrictive pericarditis and delayed hemopericardium are very rare late complications of trauma to the pericardium.

REFERENCES

1. Blalock, A. and Ravitch, M. M.: A consideration of the nonoperative treatment of cardiac tamponade resulting from wounds of the heart. Surgery, *52*:330, 1962.
2. Borja, A. R. and Lansing, A. M.: Traumatic rupture of the heart: A case successfully treated. Ann. Surg., *171*:438, 1970.
3. Bright, E. F. and Beck, C. S.: Nonpenetrating wounds of the heart. A clinical and experimental study. Am. Heart J., *10*:293, 1934.
4. Cooper, F. W., Jr., Stead, E. A., Jr., and Warren, J. V.: The beneficial effect of intravenous infusions in acute pericardial tamponade. Ann. Surg., *120*:822, 1944.
5. Elkin, D. C.: The diagnosis and treatment of cardiac trauma. Ann. Surg., *114*:169, 1941.
6. Hoffman, K. T.: Traumatic rupture of the pericardium with heart luxation. Thoraxchirurgie, Chir. *14*:62, 1966.
7. Isaacs, J. P.: Sixty penetrating wounds of the heart. Clinical and experimental observations. Surgery, *45*:696, 1959.
8. Jahnke, E. J. et al.: Tricuspid insufficiency. The result of nonpenetrating cardiac trauma. Arch. Surg., *95*:880, 1967.
9. Kissane, R. W.: Traumatic heart disease. Circulation, *6*:421, 1952.
10. Kissane, R. W., Fidler, R. S., and Doons, R. A.: Electrocardiographic changes following external chest injury to dogs. Ann. Intern. Med., *11*:907, 1937.
11. Liedtke, A. J., and DeMuth, W. E., Jr.: Nonpenetrating cardiac injuries: A collective review. Am. Heart J., *86*:687, 1973.
12. Louhimo, I.: Heart injury after blunt trauma. Acta Chir. Scand., [Supp. 380]: 1:1968.
13. Martin, L. G. et al.: Myocardial perfusion imaging with ^{99m}Tc-albumin microspheres. Radiology, *107*:367, 1973.
14. Miller, D. R., Crockett, J. C., and Potter, C. A.: Traumatic interventricular septal defect-review and report of two cases. Ann. Surg., *155*:72, 1962.
15. Reid, J. M., and Baird, W. L. M.: Crushed chest injury: some physiological disturbances and their correction. Br. Med. J., *1*:1105, 1965.
16. Sanders, C. A. et al.: Severe mitral regurgitation secondary to ruptured chordae tendineae. Circulation, *31*:506, 1965.
17. Sigler, L. H.: Trauma to the heart due to nonpentrating chest injuries. Am. Heart J. *30*:459, 1945.
18. Sugg. W. L. et al: Penetrating wounds of the heart. An analysis of 459 cases. J. Thorac. Cardiovasc. Surg., *56*: 531, 1968.
19. Symbas, P. N.: Autotransfusion from hemothorax. J. Trauma, *12*:689, 1972.
20. ———: Traumatic Injuries of the Heart and

Great Vessels. Springfield, Charles C Thomas, 1972.

21. Symbas, P. N. et al.: Penetrating cardiac wounds. Significant residual and delayed sequelae. J. Thorac. Cardiovasc. Surg., 66:526, 1973.
22. Symbas, P. N., Harlaftis, N., and Waldo, W.: Penetrating cardiac wounds: What appears to be the best management. Ann. Surg. *183*:377, 1976.
23. Symbas, P. N., Gonzalez, A., Harlaftis, N., and Waldo, W.: Cardiac scanning and echocardiography for diagnosis of experimental myocardial contusion. (in preparation.)
24. Tabatznik, B., and Isaacs, J. P.: Postpericardiotomy syndrome following traumatic hemopericardium. Amer. J. Cardiol, 7:83,1961.
25. Warburg, E.: Traumatic Heart Lesions. pp. 1676–1868. London, Oxford University Press, 1938.
26. Watson, J. H. and Bartholomae, W. M.: Cardiac injury due to nonpenetrating chest trauma. Ann. Intern. Med., *52*:871, 1960.

16. PERIPHERAL VASCULAR DISEASES

David I. Abramson, M.D.

GENERAL CLASSIFICATION

Depending upon the site of primary involvement, disorders affecting the various types of vessels in the extremities can roughly be placed into 3 categories: (1) arterial diseases; (2) venous diseases; and (3) lymphatic diseases. However, not infrequently an entity falling into one group may at some time in its course also demonstrate associated pathologic alterations in vessels of another group.

1. *Disorders affecting the arterial tree*

Entities affecting the arterial tree can be divided into 2 major groups: functional and organic.

A. *Functional disorders*

The functional disorders are further subdivided into 2 groups: excessive vasoconstriction and excessive vasodilatation.

(1) *Primary vasospastic conditions*

(a) Raynaud's disease

(b) Raynaud's syndrome or phenomenon

(c) Acrocyanosis

(d) Livedo reticularis

(2) *Purely vasodilator reaction*

(a) Primary erythromelalgia

(b) Secondary erythromelalgia

Some conditions, like trench foot, frostbite, and post-traumatic vasomotor disorders, may demonstrate both vasospasm and excessive vasodilatation, but at different periods of their clinical course.

B. *Organic disorders*

The organic disorders can also be divided into 2 groups: occlusive type (which includes chronic occlusive disorders and acute occlusive disorders) and nonocclusive type.

(1) *Occlusive disorders*

(a) Chronic occlusive:

(i) Arteriosclerosis obliterans (with or without diabetes mellitus)

(ii) Thromboangiitis obliterans

(iii) Connective tissue diseases (polyarteritis nodosa, progressive systemic sclerosis, systemic lupus erythematosus and dermatomyositis)

(b) Acute occlusive

(i) Arterial embolism

(ii) Sudden thrombosis of a critical artery

A superimposed state of vasospasm may coexist in these two conditions, as well as in thromboangiitis obliterans.

(2) *Nonocclusive disorders*

(a) Arterial aneurysm

(b) Dissecting arterial aneurysm

(c) Congenital and acquired arteriovenous fistula

2. *Disorders affecting the veins*

Diseases affecting the veins in the extremities can also be divided into 2 major groups: functional and organic.

A. *Functional disorders*

The functional disorders are of minor importance, and hence they will be only briefly mentioned here and not described below. They consist of 2 categories: venospasm and venoparalysis.

(1) *Venospasm*

(a) Venospasm is the transient excessive constriction of the circular muscle fibers of the venous wall, producing a reduction in lumen size.

(b) Such a state may result from direct mechanical trauma to a vein or from the effect of a disease process involving neighboring arteries or nerves.

(c) It may also occur in certain systemic disorders, as in shock, where it is a compensatory response to a marked reduction in circulating blood volume.

(2) *Venoparalysis*

(a) Venoparalysis represents an absence of venous tone.

(b) It is typically noted in true postural hypotension, a condition in which a prompt and precipitous fall in blood pressure occurs when the patient changes from the horizontal to the upright position.

(c) Nitrites can also produce venoparalysis because of their direct relaxing action on the circular muscle fibers in the venous wall.

(d) In the severe, uncontrolled shock states, venoparalysis may replace venospasm.

B. *Organic disorders*

The organic disorders can be subdivided into 2 groups: obliterative and nonobliterative.

(1) *Obliterative*

(a) Superficial thrombophlebitis

(b) Deep thrombophlebitis

(c) Venous obstruction due to neoplastic invasion and external compression

(2) *Nonobliterative*

(a) Primary and secondary varicosities

(b) Venous anomalies

(c) Phlebosclerosis

(d) Rupture of veins

3. *Disorders of the lymphatic system*

Diseases of the lymphatic system can likewise be divided into 2 major groups: functional and organic.

A. *Functional disorders* are generally due to:

(1) Malfunction of the lymphatic vessels

(2) Alterations in the distribution or composition of body fluids due to local factors

For example, the rate of lymph formation, which is dependent upon the hydrostatic pressure in capillaries and veins and upon the environmental temperature, increases if there is an elevation in either of these factors, thus producing a concomitant rise in the amount of lymph fluid produced. The rate of lymph flow is also altered by such mechanisms as the concentration of local metabolites, variations in osmotic pressure, and the pumping action on the thin-walled lymphatic channels supplied by contraction of voluntary muscles in the limb. For these reasons, prolonged dependency and immobility predispose to lymphedema. Since no abnormal clinical entities fall into the category of functional lymphatic disorders, this subject will not be discussed below.

B. *Organic disorders*

The organic lymphatic conditions are subdivided into 2 groups: obstructive and nonobstructive.

(1) *Obstructive*

(a) Primary and secondary lymphedema

(b) Occlusion of lymphatics by fibrosis and scarring from radiation therapy or prolonged venous stasis

(c) Surgical removal of lymph channels and lymph nodes

(d) Fibroedema

(2) *Nonobstructive*

(a) Lymphatic fistulas causing lymphedema

(b) Lymphangiectasis

(c) Benign lymphatic tumors

(d) Lymphangiosarcoma

ARTERIAL DISORDERS OF THE LIMBS

FUNCTIONAL ARTERIAL DISORDERS

The functional arterial disorders are entities characterized by temporary and generally reversible alterations in blood flow into the limbs due primarily to changes in vasomotor control over the peripheral blood vessels. Typical of functional vasospastic arterial disorders is Raynaud's disease, which is a relatively common condition.

Raynaud's Disease

Definition

Raynaud's disease is characterized by intermittent episodes of color changes limited to the fingers and, less often, to the toes, elicited by exposure to cold and/or emotional excitation. Essential to a proper diagnosis is the absence of any possible underlying etiologic factor.

Pathophysiology and Clinical Characteristics

1. *Color sequence*

The usual color sequence is first pallor, followed by cyanosis, and then rubor on termination of the attack. However, variations in this order are not uncommon.

A. *Pallor*

(1) Pallor is the typical initial color change and is due to spasm of the digital arteries supplying the involved fingers or toes.

(2) As a consequence, the cutaneous capillaries and venules are soon emptied of blood, and blanching ensues.

(3) Pulsations in the arteries at the wrist or ankle are not affected during the attack.

(4) Basis for transient functional obliteration of the digital arteries has not been elucidated.

(5) It may be that an inherent increased sensitivity to cold of the involved vessels is responsible for the change, possibly associated with an abnormality of the local sympathetic innervation.

(6) The best assumption is that the digital arteries in Raynaud's disease tend to react excessively to normal vasoconstrictor impulses and to circulating catecholamines

B. *Cyanosis*

(1) The exact mechnism responsible for cyanosis of the involved digits is likewise unknown.

(2) One theory is based on the belief that the spasm of the digital arteries is intermittently released during the attack, allowing blood to enter the capillaries at a slow rate and hence permitting a greater than normal quantity of oxygen to be removed from each unit of blood.

(3) As a consequence of the higher concentration of reduced hemoglobin in the venous blood, the skin is colored blue.

(4) The possibility of blood being trapped in the superficial vessels or of an associated venospasm has also been raised.

C. *Rubor*

(1) The rubor of the skin is a manifestation of reactive hyperemia, a state of dilatation of arterioles, capillaries, and venules, occurring immediately upon release of the digital spasm.

(2) The rubor represents an attempt to repay rapidly the oxygen debt incurred during the period when no blood was entering the digit.

Certain symptoms are associated with the color changes. When pallor exists, there is a sense of numbness in the fingers, this continuing into the period of cyanosis. However, on termination of the attack and re-establishment of the local circulation, the patient generally immediately experiences paresthesias, especially in the fingertips. In between episodes of color changes, in most instances, there are no symptoms in the digits, other than a feeling of coldness. This type of response may occur even when the environmental temperature is only slightly below a physiologic level, thus reflecting the increased responsiveness of the vessels to cold in Raynaud's disease.

Differential Diagnosis

1. *Raynaud's syndrome*

The most important differential diagnosis is the distinction between Raynaud's disease and Raynaud's syndrome or phenomenon, since in both categories the color changes in the digits are similar.

A. The main difference consists of the existence of some type of etiology in Raynaud's syndrome and its absence in Raynaud's disease.

B. In Raynaud's syndrome, there may be any one of a large number of unrelated causative factors:

(1) Occupational trauma (e.g., prolonged use of vibrating tools—"pneumatic hammer disease"—or a chain saw, typing, or playing the violin or piano)

(2) Certain neurologic disorders (e.g., multiple sclerosis, tabes dorsalis, and syringomyelia)

(3) Neurovascular syndromes of the shoulder girdle (e.g., costoclavicular, cervical rib, hyperabduction, and scalenus anticus syndromes)

(4) Connective tissue disorders (e.g., progressive systemic sclerosis or scleroderma, polyarteritis nodosa, systemic lupus erythematosus, dermatomyositis, rheumatoid arthritis)

(5) Chronic occlusive arterial disorders (e.g., arteriosclerosis obliterans and thromboangiitis obliterans)

(6) A sequel of cold injury produced either by trench foot, immersion foot, or frostbite

2. Vasospastic states

A. Raynaud's disease must also be differentiated from such primary vasospastic conditions as livedo reticularis and acrocyanosis and from nonspecific vasospasm.

B. In livedo reticularis, there is the characteristic reticular or blotchy appearance of the skin.

C. In acrocyanosis there is the persistent uniform cyanosis affecting the distal and (at times) the proximal portions of a limb.

D. Color sequence of pallor, cyanosis, and rubor, typically limited to the digits in Raynaud's disease, is never noted in acrocyanosis or livedo reticularis.

Complications

1. *Mild complications*

Mild trophic or nutritional changes in the involved digits are fairly common in Raynaud's disease.

A. Abnormal growth of nails with widening of the cuticle

B. Thickening of the skin at the tips of the fingers

C. Loss of subcutaneous tissue followed by dimpling of the skin on pressure

D. Deposits of calcium (calcinosis) in the skin and subcutaneous tissue

2. *Severe complications*

A. Atrophic arthritis

B. Sclerodermatous alterations in the skin of the involved digits (sclerodactylia)

C. Ulceration and superficial gangrene of the fingers

Treatment

1. The most important step in the treatment of Raynaud's disease is minimizing or eliminating those factors which precipitate the attacks of color change.

2. Exposure of the body to cold should be reduced as much as possible.

A. Various types of hand warmers are generally fairly effective in preventing the episodes of digital pallor if the patient must go outdoors in the winter months.

B. Electrically-heated mittens and socks that receive their energy from 6-volt batteries are also useful in this regard, as are fur-lined "stadium boots" or overshoes.

C. If possible, residence in a warm climate in which there are only minor variations in temperature, associated with low humidity, is the most ideal approach to the control of the condition.

3. Fingers should be protected from trauma, even of slight degree, since this may precipitate the one serious complication of Raynaud's disease, ulceration or gangrene of the digits.

4. Duties that expose the hands to injury should also be eliminated.

5. Complete abstinence from tobacco smoking should be emphasized, since this habit ordinarily produces vasoconstriction of cutaneous small arteries, arterioles, and capillaries. The fact that the blood vessels in Raynaud's disease are hyperresponsive to all types of vasoconstricting stimuli, including smoking, makes it even more imperative to eliminate this habit.

6. Drug therapy

Certain medications are helpful in controlling or reducing the severity of the attacks of digital pallor.

A. Among these are phenoxybenzamine hydrochloride (Dibenzyline), an alpha receptor blocking agent, and cylandelate (Cyclospasmol), a myovascular relaxant, both given orally, and Nitrol ointment (2% nitroglycerine ointment in a lanolin base), applied to the skin at the base of the involved fingers.

B. The Nitrol ointment is useful primarily when trophic changes, like ulceration or gangrene of the fingertip, are present.

C. Reserpine (Serpasil) has also been proposed as therapy on the basis that it impairs catecholamine retention, with subsequent loss of physiologic effectiveness by degradation. Reserpine, besides being given orally, has also been injected into the brachial artery, with reported clinical improvement lasting for as long as 7 months.[3]

7. Whiskey and other alcoholic beverages may have a beneficial action because of their vasodilating effect on cutaneous blood vessels.

8. Thoracic sympathectomy

A. Thoracic sympathectomy has only a limited application as a therapeutic agent in patients with mild or even moderate Raynaud's disease in whom there are no trophic changes.

B. It has some basis when it is used in the control of severe and disabling attacks of color changes and in the treatment of ulcers and gangrene of the fingers which are nonresponsive to conservative therapy. Under the latter circumstances, the operation may produce prompt demarcation of the necrotic tissue and healing of the lesions.

It is important to point out, however, that sympathectomy will not necessarily prevent recurrence of ulcers or gangrene.

Prognosis

1. As compared with chronic organic arterial disorders, Raynaud's disease is a relatively benign condition.

2. It may cause great inconvenience to some patients during the winter months and may interfere with their general activity.

3. Number and severity of the attacks can be controlled to some extent by eliminating the agents initiating them, and hence the prognosis is relatively good as far as progression of the condition is concerned.

4. Even in the presence of the relatively rare complication of ulceration or superficial gangrene of fingertips, medical or surgical therapy can generally limit the involvement to the distal portion of the digits, with no need for further loss of limb.

5. At no time is the patient's life in jeopardy.

ORGANIC ARTERIAL DISORDERS

The organic arterial disorders are entities in which a permanent and irreversible pathologic change has occurred in the arterial or arteriolar wall, leading either to a narrowing or complete obstruction of the lumen (occlusive type) or to a weakness, dilatation, and thinning of the vessel wall (nonocclusive type).

Arteriosclerosis Obliterans

Definition

1. Arteriosclerosis obliterans is the typical and the most common chronic organic occlusive disorder affecting the arterial tree in the extremities.
2. Since the pathologic process is generally progressive, eventually tissue needs are satisfied primarily by blood flow through collateral vessels.
3. This type of circulation develops in response to a moderate state of chronic ischemia of distal structures, resulting from slow obliteration of the main arterial channels and their branches.
4. Arteriosclerosis obliterans occurs primarily in patients between the ages of 45 and 70 years. However, when associated with diabetes mellitus, this disorder may be noted as early as the first decade of life.

Etiology

No view as to its cause has received general acceptance, although a large number of theories have been proposed. These include:
1. Error in the metabolism of fat and other lipids
2. A coagulation defect in the blood, which is responsible for thrombosis
3. Alterations in blood supply to the arterial wall
4. Normal and abnormal stresses on the arterial wall
5. Inherited characteristics

Pathology

1. Typical of the histologic changes in arteriosclerosis obliterans is the atheromatous plaque in the subintima, which extends into the lumen of the involved artery.
2. The lesion consists of proliferating endothelial cells, fibroblasts, foam cells, and large quantities of cholesterol and sudanophilic materials.
3. Due to the resulting distortion of the intima, thrombus formation is favored.
4. A sudden hemorrhage into the plaque, a predisposition that exists in atherosclerosis, may produce rapid arterial thrombosis.
5. Plaque formation may be associated with thickening of the intima, due to deposition of excess fibrous material in this structure.
6. There may also be degenerative changes in the media, consisting of atrophy and necrosis of muscle and replacement by collagenous fibers and later by calcium deposits.

Clinical Characteristics and Diagnosis

1. Diagnosis is based, in part, on the history of intermittent claudication, either in the small muscles of the feet, the calf muscles of the legs, or the large muscles of the thighs or buttocks.
2. Following rapid progression of the disorder, leading to thrombosis of critical arteries without the formation of adequate collateral circulation, rest pain may be experienced.
3. When unassociated with trophic changes, the symptom (ischemic neuritis) represents a state of severe ischemia of the peripheral nerves.
4. Complaints may include:
   A. Paresthesias or a sense of numbness, coldness, or burning that is experienced in the toes soon after the patient assumes a horizontal position in bed.

B. Complaints disappear on sitting up or on standing and walking, only to recur when lying down again. They are due to further worsening of the local ischemia by the loss of the hydrostatic mechanism, which tends to increase blood flow in the lower extremities on standing or with the legs in dependency.

C. Another rest pain occurs when either ulcers or gangrene exists in the limb.

(1) This pain is located in the area of the lesion and is due to marked ischemia of nerve endings in the junctional zone between viable and necrotic tissue.

(2) Severity depends upon the patient's threshold for pain; it becomes less with dependency of the involved limb but may be exaggerated by movement, as in walking, because of stretching of inflamed structures.

5. Associated with the above symptoms are definite findings indicating the presence of an impaired local blood flow. There are usually reduced or absent pulsations in the main arteries of the lower extremities:

A. The femoral in the groin

B. The popliteal in the popliteal fossa

C. The dorsal pedal and posterior tibial in the foot

6. The oscillometric readings at the different levels of the lower extremity (thigh above the knee, calf, and leg above the ankle) are likewise reduced or absent.

7. There may also be signs of impaired nutritional blood flow to the skin, particularly of the toes, manifested by:

A. Decreased or absent hair or nail growth

B. Distortion, pigmentation, and friability of toenails

C. Lowered skin temperature

D. Decreased or absent sweating of the feet

E. Changes in skin color (cyanosis, cyanotic rubor, or pallor)

8. With further reduction in cutaneous circulation or following even minor trauma to the skin, trophic changes may appear, such as ulceration, with or without superimposed infection, and gangrene.

Differential Diagnosis

1. *Thromboangiitis obliterans*

Arteriosclerosis obliterans (AO) must first be differentiated from thromboangiitis obliterans (TAO), which is a definite and distinct clinical entity.

A. Of importance in this regard is the average age of the patient at the time of onset of the disorder, this being 58.9 years for AO and 29.3 years for TAO.[1]

B. In AO there is frequently the presence of generalized arteriosclerosis, a finding not observed in TAO.

C. A history of total abstinence from tobacco smoking tends to negate a diagnosis of TAO, while this is not so for AO.

D. The history or presence of superficial migratory thrombophlebitis is firm support for the diagnosis of TAO, this state never being observed in AO.

E. The appearance of ulcers or gangrene in the fingers is also in favor of this diagnosis, for such a response is infrequently noted in AO.

F. In the case of TAO, arteriography usually visualizes a patchy segmental distribution of the disease process in the brachial artery and its branches in the upper extremity and in the popliteal artery and its branches in the lower extremity. Rarely is involvement seen in more proximal vessels, like the common femoral, superficial femoral, and deep femoral arteries, or above.

G. In AO, in contrast, partial or complete occlusions may be found in the entire vascular tree supplying the lower extremities, including the abdominal aorta and its main subdivisions.

H. Finally, the histologic findings

are entirely different in the two conditions. In TAO, during the acute stage the
microscopic lesions in the peripheral arteries are of an inflammatory nature,
while in AO the predominant change is
that of a degenerative process, primarily
in the form of intimal formation (see
above).

2. *Mönckeberg's* sclerosis is a benign
arteriosclerotic process.

A. Calcium is deposited in the
media of large muscular arteries, which
is readily visualized by soft-tissue x-ray
technique.

B. Such a change causes some decrease in the distensibility of the involved vessels, resulting in a slight reduction in pulsations and oscillometric
readings, but no material decrease in
blood flow through the arteries.

C. There are no signs of ischemia of
distal tissues of the type noted in TAO
and AO.

3. *Miscellaneous states*

Other conditions that must be considered in the differential diagnosis include:

A. Cystic adventitial disease of the
popliteal artery

B. Raynaud's disease

C. Peripheral embolism

D. Infectious processes

Treatment

1. Medical therapy

Since effective means to prevent the
formation and growth of atherosclerotic
plaques in the main arteries of the lower
extremities are not available at present,
the medical therapeutic approach to arteriosclerosis obliterans, in general, consist of: (1) the maintenance of the continuity and viability of the skin of the
lower limbs; and (2) treatment of the
complications of the condition, such as
ulceration and gangrene.

A. *The maintenance of the continuity and viability of the skin of the
lower limbs*

(1) Abstinence from smoking

and local care of the feet are the most
essential.

(2) The use of various types of
cutaneous vasodilating drugs is of questionable value. This also applies to
pharmacologic agents advocated for the
purpose of increasing claudication distances.

(3) In reference to claudication:

(a) It is very important to emphasize to the patient that he must walk
frequently and to continue to do so for a
short distance after the pain in the exer-
cising muscles has been experienced.

(b) Such a step, by placing
stress on the local vascular tree in the
muscles, may accelerate the rate of
growth of a collateral arterial system,
due to the resulting production of a state
of ischemia in these structures.

B. *Treatment of the complications
of the condition, such as ulceration and
gangrene*

(1) When either ulcers or gangrene exists, medical therapy involves
steps to delimit and localize the lesion.

(2) Bed rest is advisable in order
to prevent the spread of infection.

(3) Soaks with mild antiseptics
help to free the area of noxious secretions.

(4) Cultures and sensitivity
studies are necessary if the proper antibiotics are to be administered by
mouth, parenterally, or locally.

(5) The goal of developing an
adequate concentration of the medication in the area of the lesion is very
difficult to achieve with the parenteral or
oral route because of the reduced local
blood flow.

(6) The use of sympathetic blocking agents may play a minor role in increasing cutaneous circulation to the
foot. Such a response can be expected
only when the skin vessels are still capable of dilating on elimination of vasomotor control.

(7) It is necessary to remove ne-

crotic tissue repeatedly by debridement, for as long as such material remains in the wound, healing is prevented. A preliminary period in the whirlpool helps to carry out this step more effectively.

2. *Surgical therapy*

The surgical approach to arteriosclerosis obliterans is still a controversial subject. For the patient who complains only of intermittent claudication and has no signs of impending or existing ulceration or gangrene, the question of whether a venous graft procedure or thromboendarterectomy is warranted depends upon a number of factors.

    A. Factors influencing surgery

        (1) The age of the patient

        (2) Patient's general physical state

        (3) The degree of disability resulting from the symptom

        (4) Rate of its progression

        (5) Psychological effect on the patient of being limited in his physical efforts

        (6) Need to be gainfully employed in a job requiring extensive walking

When there are impending or existing trophic changes that have not responded to medical means or that appear to be extending, then one or all three of the following procedures are indicated in order to prevent a major amputation.

    B. Lumbar sympathectomy

        (1) In the case of a lumbar sympathectomy, it must first be demonstrated that temporary removal of vasomotor tone, by a paravertebral sympathetic block, will be followed by definite signs of a temporary increase in cutaneous circulation in the feet.

        (2) Lumbar sympathectomy has no role as therapy in the patient with intermittent claudication alone.

    C. Venous graft or thromboendarterectomy

The decision whether to insert a venous graft or to perform a thromboendarterectomy depends in great part upon the information derived from an arteriogram, such as:

        (1) The location of the occlusion or occlusions

        (2) Their number and length

        (3) The state of the remaining vascular tree

        (4) The extent and profusion of the "runoff" below the distal block

Prognosis

1. In order to discuss prognosis in arteriosclerosis obliterans, it is necessary first to point out that this condition is progressive and frequently has its counterpart in a similar involvement of such vital organs as the heart, brain, and kidneys.

2. Therefore, longevity is markedly influenced by the severity of the coexisting atherosclerotic changes in sites other than the limbs.

3. The fact that the complication of gangrene of a limb may require a major amputation also affects prognosis, because such an approach is associated with an element of danger to the patient. This is particularly so since most individuals in whom it is necessary to perform this operation are in the 5th and 6th decades of life and hence are relatively poor surgical risks.

4. In recent years, the popularization of surgical vascular procedures for the preservation of a limb has also contributed to some increase in mortality in arteriosclerosis obliterans.

5. In view of the fact that the pathologic process in arteriosclerosis obliterans is progressive, eventually the maintenance of viability of local tissues may depend upon the rate of growth of the collateral circulation. If this does not parallel the rate of obliteration of the main arteries by atherosclerotic plaque formation, nutritional disturbances will

develop, leading to the need for amputation.

6. Trauma to the skin of the feet, even of a minor degree, may rapidly accelerate the production of gangrene.

7. On the other hand, if sufficient time is available for the formation of an adequate blood flow to the various structures via the collateral circulation, the patient will be able to lead a fairly normal life, except for some difficulty in walking.

8. Such a prognosis is applicable to the great majority of persons suffering from arteriosclerosis obliterans, provided that they abstain from smoking and pay strict attention to the local care of their feet.

Arterial Embolism

Definition

1. Sudden occlusion of a main artery to a limb by an organized clot or a mass of tissue formed elsewhere (embolus) is a typical and dramatic example of an acute organic occlusive arterial disorder.

2. More than any other entity in the field of vascular disorders, it is a real emergency, requiring immediate clinical recognition and institution of proper treatment, generally embolectomy. Otherwise, if the obstructed vessel is a critical artery, loss of viability of distal structures can usually be expected.

Clinical Characteristics and Diagnosis

1. *The origin of emboli*
Arterial emboli may arise from a number of different sites:
   A. The cavity of the left atrium
   B. The endocardial surface of the left ventricle following a myocardial infarction
   C. The cavity of an aneurysm of the abdominal aorta or of a main artery to a limb
   D. The ulcerated endothelial surface of a large vessel (generally being the source of microemboli)
   E. Very rarely, emboli may originate in the deep veins of the legs, enter the right side of the heart, and pass through a patent foramen ovale to reach the systemic circulation (paradoxical embolus).
   F. Fat emboli may be liberated into the bloodstream from areas of fractured bone.

2. *Symptoms*
The early symptoms of an arterial embolic occlusion are related to the sudden onset of a severe degree of acute ischemia of tissues.
   A. There is generally an abrupt onset of pain in the distal structures, particularly the digits.
   B. This is followed by a sense of numbness and paresthesias.
   C. In some patients, there is no sudden appearance of symptoms, the severity of the complaints gradually building up in intensity.
   D. The associated findings consist of the following:
      (1) Markedly reduced arterial inflow occurs. Because of emptying of the subpapillary venous plexuses of blood, the skin assumes a cadaveric pallor, with islands of cyanosis.
      (2) The superficial veins are collapsed.
      (3) No pulsations are noted in the peripheral arteries, together with absent oscillometric readings at the lower levels of the involved limb.
      (4) Skin temperature is reduced.
      (5) There are neurologic signs of acute ischemia of the peripheral nerves, such as anesthesia and hypesthesia; the location and extent of the changes cannot be related to any anatomic nerve distribution (stocking-glove type).
      (6) There may be a reduction in motor function, consisting of difficulty or inability to move the toes and varying degrees of foot-drop.

Differential Diagnosis

1. Arterial thrombosis

There must be no delay in making a differentiation between arterial embolism and arterial thrombosis, since the two conditions require different therapeutic approaches.

A. One important point is that in arterial thrombosis there is frequently a long history of intermittent claudication due to the underlying arteriosclerosis obliterans.

B. Also, there may be signs of chronic arterial occlusive disease in the other apparently uninvolved limb.

C. In the case of an embolic occlusion of a normal artery, such findings are absent. At the same time, a potential site for the origin of emboli must exist.

D. The clinical signs in arterial embolism are generally more abrupt in onset and more marked in degree, the state of acute ischemia of distal tissues being of a severe degree.

E. In most cases of arterial thrombosis, the changes are not as dramatic, since more collateral vessels are available for transporting blood to the various local structures when complete occlusion of the main artery now occurs. This is due to the fact that the chronic ischemia resulting from the previously slowly-progressive arteriosclerosis obliterans acted as a stimulus for the growth of this secondary circulation.

F. Such a situation is not present in the case of arterial embolism, because in most instances no collateral network is available at the time of the sudden block of the main arterial channel by the embolus.

2. *Vasospasm*

A. Vasospasm produces a marked reduction in arterial circulation to a limb, such as occurs when a large artery is traumatized or the tissues in the vicinity of the vessel are injured.

B. In the vasospastic state, there is frequently a proximal border of pallid or mottled cyanotic skin, which is irregular and not as sharply delineated as in organic arterial occlusion.

C. If the vasospasm is neurogenic in origin and dependent upon the integrity of the sympathetic nervous system, then the changes that follow a paravertebral sympathetic block are diagnostic, since such a procedure produces an almost immediate improvement in the clinical picture.

D. In the case of an arterial embolism, only slight alterations occur with removal of vasomotor tone.

3. *Occlusion of a main vein*

A. The most important differential point between this condition and acute arterial embolism is the rapid onset of edema involving the entire limb.

B. In contrast, in arterial embolism, if anything, the limb appears thinner than normal because of the reduced arterial inflow.

C. Moreover, the superficial veins are collapsed, while in the case of occlusion of a main collecting vein, the vessels distally are distended.

D. The only finding that may mimic an arterial embolism is the superimposed vasospasm that occurs with iliofemoral thrombophlebitis.

Treatment

1. *Embolectomy*

If at all possible, the ideal treatment for sudden occlusion of a critical artery by an embolus is embolectomy with a Fogarty intravascular balloon catheter.[2]

2. *Heparin administration*

A. The first step after the diagnosis is made is the immediate intravenous administration of heparin in order to prevent propagation of the clot into distal branches of the involved vessel or into arteries arising proximal to the site of occlusion.

B. Such a step will in no way interfere with the subsequent surgical approach, for the therapeutic effect of the medication is generally dissipated by the time preparations for embolectomy are completed.

3. *Preoperative care*

A. Preoperatively, the limb is wrapped in several layers of cotton padding to form a protective boot.

B. The limb is placed slightly below heart level by raising the head of the bed about 8 inches.

C. At no time should the limb be maintained in the elevated position.

4. *Contraindication to local heat or cold application*

A. Neither local heat nor local cold is indicated, since the application of either agent to the skin may precipitate gangrene.

B. Cold has this effect because of its vasoconstricting action on the collateral circulation, now the only available means for transporting blood to the distal structures.

C. Heat produces a significant increase in metabolic needs of the tissues, in the face of an already existing dangerously low blood supply.

Prognosis

Whether the distal tissues will remain viable after an arterial embolism depends upon a number of factors:

1. The size and role of the occluded vessel in supplying blood to the limb
2. The interval between the onset of the process and removal of the embolus
3. The general physical state of the patient
4. The degree and duration of the superimposed local vasospasm
5. The capability of the surgeon to perform the operation with facility and dispatch
6. The severity of the underlying cardiovascular disease responsible for the embolism
7. The ultimate state of the circulation in the involved limb

Arterial Aneurysm

Definition and Classification

1. An aneurysm located in a critical artery in a limb is representative of the category of spontaneous, chronic, non-occlusive organic arterial disorders.

2. A similar clinical picture may result from trauma to an artery, producing weakening, stretching, or actual perforation of the wall of the vessel.

3. There are two types of arterial aneurysm: the true and the false.

A. In true aneurysm, continuity of the vessel wall is still intact, but there is dilatation due to thinning of the muscle layer.

B. In false aneurysm, complete rupture of the artery has taken place, followed by bleeding into the neighboring tissues and eventual production of a wall over the clotted material. A communication exists between the interior of the sac thus formed and the vessel through the original site of rupture.

4. The spontaneous arterial aneurysm, generally a complication of arteriosclerosis obliterans, is frequently a true type, at least one of the coats of the affected artery being intact. In the limbs the lesion is most commonly found in the popliteal artery and (less often) in the superficial femoral artery in its course through Hunter's canal.

**Clinical Characteristics
and Diagnosis**

1. Most often the physical signs of an arterial aneurysm are responsible for making the diagnosis of the clinical entity, while the symptoms are of minor importance in this regard.

2. The most significant finding is the presence of an expansile and pulsatile mass in the location of a large artery in a limb.

3. A thrill and a bruit are inconstant abnormalities, due to the fact that the frequent deposition of layers of clot in

the sac damps the transmission of vibrations resulting from the eddy currents set up in the bloodstream by the lesion.

4. There may be pain locally as a consequence of compression of neighboring structures, particularly peripheral nerves, by the enlarging mass.

5. Unless the artery at the site of the lesion becomes obliterated, there is no reduction in blood flow to distal structures, and hence there are no symptoms or signs related to ischemia of tissues.

6. If the associated vein becomes occluded because of injury to the intima by pressure from the aneurysmal sac, then signs of interference with venous outflow appear, such as edema, distention of cutaneous veins, and pain locally over the site of involvement.

Differential Diagnosis

1. *Pulsating and nonpulsating masses*

A. Any mass in the vicinity of a large artery must be differentiated from an arterial aneurysm.

B. In most instances, this can be done readily, since lesions of other origins do not expand and pulsate with each heart beat.

C. At times, however, a mass may overlie a large artery and hence pulsations may be transmitted to the examiner's fingers.

D. The absence of pulsations may be misleading as a distinguishing point, since such a situation may exist in the case of a thrombosed arterial aneurysm.

E. When there is doubt as to the etiology of a mass, then arteriography should be performed.

2. *Arteriovenous fistula*

Differential diagnosis between arterial aneurysm and arteriovenous fistula is not difficult if one considers the cardinal signs of the two conditions.

A. In arteriovenous fistula, there is almost invariably a continuous bruit over the lesion, with systolic accentuation.

B. The same type of bruit is also heard proximal and distal to the fistula.

C. There are numerous dilated and varicose veins above the lesion, demonstrating a very high venous pressure.

D. In the distal portion of the limb, arterial pulsations and oscillometric readings are diminished or absent, and the tissues appear to be suffering from chronic ischemia.

E. In contrast, in uncomplicated arterial aneurysm, there are no signs of impaired arterial circulation in distant structures, and dilated veins are not noted proximal to the lesion. If a bruit exists, it is only systolic in timing, and it is not transmitted along the course of the vessels.

F. In both conditions a pulsatile, expanding mass is present in the vicinity of an artery.

Treatment

Therapy for arterial aneurysm is surgical. This applies to traumatic as well as spontaneous lesions. The various techniques consist of:

1. Aneurysmectomy
2. Endoaneurysmorrhaphy
3. Reestablishment of the continuity of the lumen using a venous graft or a plastic prosthesis

The graft procedure is indicated whenever an aneurysm involves an essential artery to a limb, in the absence of an adequate collateral circulation. Such an approach is more readily utilized in the treatment of a traumatic aneurysm than in the case of a spontaneous lesion, for in the latter, there is the technical disadvantage of dealing with a vessel in which generally extensive atherosclerotic changes exist.

Prognosis

The outlook with regard to an arterial aneurysm in the limbs depends upon a number of factors.

1. If a successful arterial graft has been performed, then the prognosis is good and the patient will have no

symptoms or signs of local impairment of arterial circulation so long as the transplant remains patent.

2. If a surgical approach cannot be utilized, the prognosis regarding the maintenance of viability of the involved limb depends upon:

A. The complications that may arise, such as thrombosis of the artery at the site of the aneurysm

B. Liberation of emboli from the aneurysmal sac, causing occlusion of critical arteries distally

C. Rupture of the aneurysmal sac internally or externally

D. Compression of neighboring veins with the production of thrombophlebitis

E. Pressure on peripheral nerves

A number of these conditions can seriously jeopardize the preservation of the limb.

ORGANIC VENOUS DISORDERS OF THE LIMBS

Deep Venous Thrombosis and Thrombophlebitis

Definition

A typical obliterative venous disorder is thrombosis or thrombophlebitis affecting the deep venous system of a limb. In the lower extremities, the condition has been arbitrarily divided into two clinical entities: phlebothrombosis and popliteal and iliofemoral thrombophlebitis depending upon the original site of occlusion. Such a category has been criticized because, not infrequently, one state is followed by the other. Moreover, there appears to be little or no difference in the pathologic changes observed in the two disorders. However, because the clinical picture, the treatment, and the prognosis are generally dissimilar, it appears of value to continue utilizing the two designations.

Classification

1. Phlebothrombosis

A. The term is applied to a state in which there is a partial or complete occlusion by a bland thrombus of the small deep venous plexuses in the muscles of the calf or sole of the foot.

B. When a propagation occurs, the clot usually enlarges without apparently becoming firmly adherent to the wall of the involved vessel.

C. Because of this tendency, it develops a jellylike consistency and is a frequent source of pulmonary emboli (see Chap. 12).

D. The veins involved are of a small caliber, at least initially, and hence there are very few signs of venous stasis. At the same time, systemic responses are minimal.

2. Iliofemoral or popliteal thrombophlebitis is a state in which the thrombus is located in the iliofemoral or the popliteal vein. It is strongly attached to the vessel wall as a result of an inflammatory (phlebitic) response in the intima.

A. Associated with this reaction is a local periphlebitis affecting such tissues as the neighboring lymphatic channels.

B. Because of the changes in the interior of the vessel, the tendency for the liberation of emboli is not very great unless propagation of the clot is extensive.

C. In contrast with phlebothrombosis, the local changes in the limb and the systemic responses are both marked.

Etiology

The causes for intravenous clotting are many, and only a listing of them will be attempted in this section.

1. Local changes, such as adhesion of thrombocytes to the intima of a blood vessel at a site of injury, resulting in platelet damage, occur first, followed by release of procoagulant and thrombin.

2. Venous stasis, particularly in valve pockets, contributes to the growth of the thrombus.

3. Trauma

A. How trauma of any type to a vein predisposes to thrombus formation is not clear, although there is little doubt that it does. It is possible that after injury to the vessel wall, the "stickiness" of the cement substance in the intima increases, and hence there is a tendency for the blood platelets to adhere to the area of involvement, producing platelet thrombi.

B. Trauma to the intima can result from:

(1) Crush injuries

(2) Fractures

(3) Deep wounds

(4) The intravenous administration of irritants like sclerosing and hypertonic solutions

(5) Indwelling venous catheters

(6) Neoplastic infiltrations

(7) Prolonged pressure on calf veins during immobility

(8) Severe physical exertion or strain involving the muscles of the lower extremity

4. Hypercoagulability of the blood due to:

A. Trauma to distant tissues

B. Visceral carcinoma

C. Hematologic abnormalities, which may also play a significant role in the formation of clots in veins

5. Contraceptive agents likewise have been implicated (see Chap. 18).

Clinical Characteristics and Diagnosis

1. *Phlebothrombosis*

As has already been implied, the diagnosis of a thrombotic process in the venous plexuses of the calf is very difficult to make, and frequently the condition becomes apparent in retrospect, only after a pulmonary embolism has occurred.

A. The symptoms and signs are meager because the veins occluded play a minor role in removing blood from the lower limb.

B. There is no gross swelling of the foot, ankle, and lower part of the leg.

C. The venous pressure in the superficial vessels is not raised.

D. Some local discomfort may be experienced in the calf, consisting of an aching or cramp-like complaint at rest.

E. The calf muscles are tense or spastic, and the circumference of the upper part of the leg is generally larger than that of the opposite normal limb.

F. Pain is frequently elicited on dorsiflexion of the foot (positive Homans' sign).

G. Deep palpation of the calf muscles may reveal an indefinite, tender, indurated mass between the bellies of the gastrocnemius muscle.

H. Associated with such findings are slight systemic reactions, such as a mild increase in body temperature and in pulse and respiratory rates.

2. *Iliofemoral or popliteal thrombophlebitis*

In contrast to phlebothrombosis, the diagnosis of iliofemoral or popliteal thrombophlebitis is generally readily made.

A. First, there is a severe aching, a cramp, or a throbbing pain in a portion or the whole involved limb, associated with tenderness in Scarpa's triangle and in the groin.

B. Usually swelling appears soon after the onset of the pain, due to the marked interference with venous outflow from the limb, because of complete occlusion of the main collecting vein.

C. In the case of popliteal thrombophlebitis:

(1) The swelling extends from the foot to the knee

(2) The change is first noted on the dorsum of the foot and ankle.

D. In iliofemoral thrombophlebitis:

(1) The edema also involves the thigh up to the groin.

(2) It generally develops to its maximum in 6 to 12 hours.

(3) Although the superficial veins

are distended as a result of the increased venous pressure, usually this is not apparent early in the disorder because of the masking effect of the edema fluid.

E. Associated with local symptoms and signs are systemic changes, such as:

(1) A fever of up to 102° F. (38.9° C)

(2) Tachycardia

(3) Malaise

(4) Chilly sensation

Laboratory Findings

1. *Phlebothrombosis*

A. *Venography*

In the presence of a normal venous pattern, one can eliminate the possibility of clots in the venous plexuses. Unfortunately, early in the disease the test frequently produces false positive results.

B. *Radioactive fibrinogen test*

This is based on the premise that since fibrinogen is incorporated into a forming clot, the radioactivity in the affected area of the leg will thus increase if thrombosis exists.

C. *Other approaches incude*

(1) Impedance phlebography

(2) The determination of skin temperature in the region of the calf

2. *Iliofemoral thrombophlebitis*

The value of the laboratory procedures for making the diagnosis is not as essential as in phlebothrombosis because the clinical signs are much more apparent. Nevertheless, the following diagnostic methods are used:

A. *Doppler ultrasound technique* has been used and considered to be a valuable tool for the diagnosis of popliteal thrombophlebitis.

B. *Venography* may be helpful in identifying the location of the occluded segment of vein.

Differential Diagnosis

1. *Phlebothrombosis*

This condition must be distinguished from symptoms caused by a number of different states and clinical entities.

A. *Pain caused by continuous pressure to the calf area* occurs when a patient's leg rests in a stirrup during the course of a long surgical procedure. As a consequence, there may be pain locally, which persists for days afterward.

B. A similar type of symptom may follow a protracted period of bed rest while the patient is recovering from an operative procedure. During that time, the full weight of the limb is transmitted to the calf resting on the mattress.

C. *Popliteal (Baker's) cyst*

(1) This is due to osteoarthritis or rheumatoid arthritis of the knee.

(2) This entity may elicit findings that mimic those associated with phlebothrombosis, including a positive Homans' sign, an increase in circumference of the calf, a rise in local cutaneous temperature, and tenderness and pain in the muscles of the calf.

(3) Arthrography of the knee is helpful in determining whether a dissecting popliteal cyst exists.

D. *Sudden occlusion of the popliteal artery at its bifurcation by an embolus*

(1) This generally results in a periarterial inflammatory reaction and the production of pain and swelling in the calf muscles.

(2) Of importance as differential points are the associated findings of a marked reduction in arterial circulation in the foot, such as absent pulsations and oscillometric readings in the distal portions of the limb and reduced cutaneous temperature and sensation in the toes.

(3) Such signs are not noted in phlebothrombosis, since the local arterial blood supply is intact in this disorder.

E. *Other conditions that may resemble phlebothrombosis*

(1) Superficial thrombophlebitis located subcutaneously in the vicinity of the calf muscle

(2) Rupture of the plantaris tendon

(3) Chronic and acute cellulitis involving the posterior portion of the leg

(4) Dermatitis in the same site

(5) A shortened Achilles tendon

(6) Myofibrositis

(7) Local trauma—producing rupture of a vein, hematoma formation, or contusion—and laceration and rupture of the gastrocnemius muscle may result in findings that also mimic phlebothrombosis.

(8) Herniation of intact muscle through a defect in the sheath can likewise be mistaken for this clinical entity, a distinguishing point being the disappearance of the mass when the muscle contracts. The bulge of a ruptured muscle, on the other hand, becomes more noticeable under such conditions.

(9) Finally, an acute alcoholic myopathic syndrome must be considered in the differential diagnosis, since in this state there may be muscle pain, tenderness, and swelling in the area of involvement—findings also present in phlebothrombosis. However, the presence of an elevated serum transaminase level gives support to the former diagnosis. This change is related to the extensive muscle fiber degeneration and necrosis resulting from imbibing large quantities of alcoholic liquors.

2. *Iliofemoral or popliteal thrombophlebitis*

Although there is generally no difficulty determining that either one of these conditions exists, still on occasion several clinical entities may mimic them.

A. *Posttraumatic vasomotor disorders (Sudeck's atrophy)*

(1) There may be vasospasm and edema of a limb, and therefore this condition may mimic iliofemoral or popliteal thrombophlebitis.

(2) Generally no history is elicited of an acute onset of marked swelling affecting most of an extremity.

(3) There are no signs indicating the presence of a block in a main collecting vein.

(4) Invariably, a close relationship is noted between an injury to the limb and the appearance of the clinical findings associated with posttraumatic vasomotor disorders.

B. *Acute cellulitis of the leg*

(1) Local swelling is a common finding in this state; however, it is usually nonpitting. Furthermore, it is limited to the area of involvement and does not encompass the entire circumference of the limb.

(2) Other local findings of inflammation are noted, including redness of the skin, an increase in cutaneous temperature, bounding pulses in the foot, and possibly lymphangitis and lymphadenitis.

(3) In iliofemoral thrombophlebitis, none of these changes is present.

C. *Superficial thrombophlebitis*

(1) Signs of inflammation are limited to the area in which the superficial thrombosed vein is located.

(2) The rest of the limb appears normal.

(3) No systemic responses are observed, in contrast to the rise in temperature, the sensation of malaise, and the increase in white blood count and sedimentation rate almost always present in iliofemoral thrombophlebitis.

D. *Acute arterial occlusion*

(1) Iliofemoral thrombophlebitis may superficially resemble acute arterial occlusion because in the former there may be a superimposed arterial vasospasm, producing a reduction or even an absence of pulses in the foot and other signs of reduced arterial circulation, such as cyanosis, pallor, and a low cutaneous temperature.

(2) At times, in the severe degree of iliofemoral thrombophlebitis (phlegmasia cerulea dolens), there may actually be necrosis of the tissues of the foot and leg.

(3) The main differential point, however, is that in acute arterial occlu-

sion, the limb, if anything, is thinner than normal because of the reduced arterial inflow, while in iliofemoral thrombophlebitis, it is significantly enlarged because of the presence of edema.

Treatment

1. For deep venous thrombosis of the lower extremities:
   A. All patients should be immediately hospitalized
   B. Placed at complete bed rest (no bathroom privileges)
   C. Given anticoagulants
2. For phlebothrombosis:
   A. Intermittent intravenous administration of heparin using an indwelling catheter, or continuous intravenous drip is indicated. This regimen should be maintained all during the hospital stay.
   B. Bed rest is maintained in the case of phlebothrombosis until all local symptoms and signs have disappeared. Then the patient is started on an ambulation program using an Ace bandage.
3. In the case of iliofemoral thrombophlebitis:
   A. Both heparin and oral Coumadin or dicumarol should be given simultaneously for at least 6 or 7 days and then the heparin is discontinued.
   B. The oral anticoagulant should be continued until the patient is discharged from the hospital.
4. For iliofemoral or popliteal thrombophlebitis:
   A. The patient remains at complete bed rest until all signs of local inflammation have disappeared and edema is completely controlled.
   B. At this point, he is measured for an elastic stocking that will possess a gradient of pressure, the greatest force being exerted at the ankle.
   C. In the period of time required for the manufacture of the support, the patient begins to walk for 15-minute periods, using an Ace bandage.
   D. The leg is measured at several levels before and after each session.

(1) If no enlargement of the limb occurs with the physical exertion, the number of periods of ambulation is increased.
(2) Should the edema return, the patient is again placed at complete bed rest.
   E. After a week of repeated short periods of walking without any untoward effects, the patient is discharged from the hospital with his elastic stocking. He is instructed on how and when to apply the elastic support and on what other steps to carry out to prevent the reappearance of edema.

Prognosis

1. *Phlebothrombosis*
   A. If there are no complications of this condition, such as pulmonary embolism, then there will be no subsequent disability or sequelae once the acute phase has been controlled.
   B. If pulmonary embolism has developed, the prognosis depends upon the degree of involvement in the pulmonary bed and whether recurrences have taken place or can be expected.
2. *Iliofemoral thrombophlebitis*
   A. In this disorder, the incidence of pulmonary complications is much less than in the case of phlebothrombosis.
   B. If pulmonary embolism occurs, then again the prognosis depends upon the severity of the pathologic process in the lungs.
   C. In the absence of such a complication, the outlook for the properly treated limb suffering from acute iliofemoral thrombophlebitis is good.
   D. In the presence of an adequate local venous collateral circulation and the use of a well-fitting elastic stocking and with observance of simple rules to control the swelling, the patient will subsequently be very little inconvenienced by his affliction. However, he may have to continue on his therapeutic regimen for years, learning when he can discard his elastic stocking with impunity only

by utilizing trial periods of ambulation without it and determining whether edema recurs.

Complications

In those instances in which proper treatment was not instituted early in the inception of the condition or in those patients in whom originally extensive intravascular clotting took place despite adequate therapy, the post-phlebitic syndrome may develop.

This is a disabling condition, since it results in the need for frequent periods of hospitalization for the treatment of the various changes associated with the entity, such as:

1. Secondary varicosities
2. Stasis dermatitis
3. Pigmentation of the skin
4. Chronic indurated cellulitis
5. Severe ulceration in the lower portion of the leg

Primary Varicosities

Definition and Pathophysiology

1. Primary varicosities are typical of the nonocclusive chronic organic disorders affecting the venous tree of the lower extremities, as well as being one of the most common peripheral vascular afflictions.

2. The condition develops when the valves in the superficial veins of the lower extremity become incompetent, thus allowing regurgitant flow in the great and small saphenous venous systems.

3. The reflux occurs either through the saphenofemoral junction, through the junction of the small saphenous and popliteal veins, or through communicating or perforator vessels which join the superficial veins with the deep circulation at various levels in the leg and thigh.

4. As a consequence, there is distention of the superficial vessels, which then enlarge and become tortuous.

5. Such changes, in turn, produce incompetency of the valves in the veins.

6. The fact that the superficial vessels possess poor support, being surrounded mainly by fat, contributes significantly to the formation of varicosities.

Etiology

Several factors have been implicated in the production of varicosities.

1. *Inherent factor*
   A. An inherent structural weakness of the veins themselves, a type of congenital defect, is an important etiologic factor.
   B. Of interest in this regard is the anatomic finding that in some patients with varicosities, smooth muscle and an internal elastic membrane may be absent in the valve area of the great saphenous vein at the sapheno-femoral junction.[4]

2. *Mechanical or hemodynamic factors*
   A. There is little question that mechanical or hemodynamic factors associated with the erect position also play a role in the production of varicosities.
   B. In accord with this view is the anatomic finding that on standing, the column of blood in the abdomen is supported solely by valves located in the external iliac and femoral veins, for normally such structures are not present in the inferior vena cava and common iliac veins.
   C. In individuals in whom valves are also absent in the external iliac and femoral veins, prolonged standing places a very great load upon the valve at the saphenofemoral junction, a structure that is almost invariably incompetent when varicosities exist.
   D. Heavy muscular work, straining at stool, and constriction of the lower limb by poorly fitting elastic stockings, girdles, or garters may all raise venous pressure in the lower extremities and thus contribute to the appearance of varicosities.
   E. Obesity has a similar effect,

since excess subcutaneous fat supplies little support to superficial veins and hence predisposes to venous pooling.

Clinical Characteristics and Diagnosis

1. In general, the patient with an uncomplicated moderate or even severe degree of primary varicosities has very few complaints referable to this condition.
2. There may be a sense of aching, heaviness, fullness, and easy fatigue in the affected limb, particularly at the end of a day of physical activity involving prolonged standing.
3. The patient may also experience night cramps.
4. Because of their unsightly appearance and their prominence, varicosities are frequently considered by patients to be the cause of various unrelated symptoms in the legs.
5. At times, the pain due to marked pooling of blood in the distended vessels, which at first is dull in character, can become acutely sharp and stabbing, and require the patient to lie down and elevate his legs in order to obtain relief.
6. Generally, there is no correlation between the severity of the various symptoms and the size and extent of the varicosities.
7. Physical findings:
 A. The signs associated with the condition are mainly the appearance of prominent, tortuous, and dilated superficial veins on the leg and thigh with assumption of the upright position.
 B. In the long-standing case the vessels remain enlarged even when the patient is lying down.
 C. The important point in diagnosis is the demonstration of a regurgitant flow of blood in the involved veins on assumption of the upright position.
 (1) For this purpose, it is necessary to perform the single or multiple tourniquet test (Trendelenburg test). This procedure not only is essential in

making the diagnosis of primary varicosities, but it also gives information as to the location of the incompetent valve or valves (i.e., whether the abnormality is in the fossa ovalis alone, in the various levels of communicating vessels, or in both sites).
 (2) There may be pitting edema of the ankles and lower portion of the legs, the severity of which is related to the length of the period of standing. In most instances, the swelling disappears after a night's rest.
 D. Other changes are brown pigmentation of the skin of the medial aspect of the distal part of the leg and increased vasomotor tone.

Differential Diagnosis

Primary varicosities must be differentiated from a number of conditions.
1. *Secondary Varicosities*
The first is secondary varicosities following acute thrombophlebitis in a main collecting vein of the lower extremity (popliteal or iliofemoral thrombophlebitis).
 A. In both conditions a regurgitant flow can be demonstrated in the superficial veins, the appearance of the vessels also being similar.
 B. The main differential points are:
 (1) In secondary varicosities, there is the history of sudden swelling of the limb during the acute stage of iliofemoral or popliteal thrombophlebitis, with the onset of varicosities months or years later.
 (2) In primary varicosities, such a clinical picture is absent.
 C. Secondary varicosities may also be present in an arteriovenous fistula due to the large quantity of blood entering the superficial venous system proximal to the lesion through the fistulous tract. Distal to the arteriovenous opening, the superficial veins are less prominent than normally.
 D. In contrast, primary varicosities are almost always present in the legs as

well as elsewhere. Moreover, there are no signs of an arteriovenous communication in primary varicosities, such as a pulsating mass, a bruit and a thrill over it, an increase in skin temperature proximal to the lesion and a decrease distal to it, and absent or reduced arterial pulsations in the foot.

2. *Klippel-Trenaunay syndrome*

A rare condition that must be differentiated from primary varicosities is Klippel-Trenaunay syndrome.

A. In this entity unilateral varicosities have been present since birth, associated with cutaneous hemangioma and lengthening of the limb.

B. It may be necessary to resort to venography and arteriography in order to distinguish this disorder from primary varicosities.

C. Such a diagnostic approach generally reveals agenesis of portions of the deep venous system and the existence of small congenital arteriovenous fistulas that open into typical vascular pools.

D. Similar tests when carried out in the presence of primary varicosities visualize a normal architecture of the deep venous circulation.

Treatment

1. *Medical therapy*

A. *General approach*

(1) Conservative management of primary varicosities has limited value, since this type of therapy in no way cures the disorder. All that can be hoped for by such an approach is the prevention of further progression of the condition.

(2) It can be used, however, as a temporary measure in the case of non-symptomatic minor varicosities and in the presence of marked obesity until weight loss can be achieved.

(3) It should be used as a permanent procedure for an individual in whom recurrences have taken place after several corrective operations or in whom

there is an associated arteriosclerosis obliterans in the involved limb.

(4) Elderly patients frequently should also be treated conservatively because of the possible risk associated with the administration of an anesthetic of several hours' duration required for the surgical approach.

B. *Specific approach*

General conservative management of primary varicosities consists of:

(1) Elastic stocking

(a) An elastic stocking, which possesses a gradient of pressure built into it, is made to the order of the patient.

(b) The greatest force (about 40 mm. Hg) is applied at the level of the ankle, with the exerted pressure becoming gradually less in the proximal portion of the stocking.

(c) It should always be placed around the limb before the patient arises in the morning, so that its elasticity will maintain the superficial veins in a collapsed state on standing.

(d) On walking, the gradient of pressure incorporated in the stocking tends to pump the blood out of the local venous system with each contraction of the voluntary muscles of the limb.

(e) A compression support that may be used on a temporary basis is an Ace bandage.

(f) If there is edema of the leg and foot at the end of the day, it is advisable to raise the foot of the bed about 6 inches by placing books, blocks, or bricks under its two legs.

(2) Sclerotherapy

(a) The injection of a sclerosing solution into the involved veins is another medical therapy for primary varicosities, but this approach has only limited application.

(b) Either empty-or-full vein technique may be used.

(c) It is necessary to be aware of the fact that the intravenous injection of a sclerosing solution may produce an allergic response, in the form of either minor urticaria, a severe degree of angioneurotic edema, asthmatic dyspnea, or even severe anaphylactic shock.

(d) The advantage of sclerotherapy is that it permits the patient to be ambulatory. As a primary treatment, it should be used only in the case of mild involvement of the venous system, provided the valves are competent. It also has a role as a supplement to surgical therapy for the obliteration of residual varices.

2. *Surgical therapy*

A. In most cases of uncomplicated primary varicosities, a surgical approach is indicated.

B. Vein stripping is by far the preferred technique since the rate of recurrence is the least with this procedure.

C. The surgical therapy may involve:

(1) High ligation of the great saphenous vein at its junction with the femoral vein

(2) High ligation of the great saphenous vein with retrograde injection of a sclerosing solution into the distal portion of the vessel

(3) High ligation of the great saphenous vein with multiple interruptions by ligation and division of the vessel among its course

(4) High ligation of the great saphenous vein and extirpation of part or all of this channel using a stripper.

Complications

1. Prolonged venous stasis due to primary varicosities may result in the appearance of several abnormalities, which may have serious consequences.

2. Various complications may include:

A. Repeated attacks of superficial thrombophlebitis

B. Hemorrhage from eroded superficial veins

C. Ulceration

D. Dermatitis

E. Pigmentation of the skin

F. Chronic indurated cellulitis

3. The presence of any of these complications of varicosities is an indication for surgical treatment, provided that there are no systemic or local contraindications to such an approach.

Prognosis

1. The outlook for primary varicosities depends in great part upon whether the complications (discussed above) can be prevented, or if present, whether they can be controlled and eliminated.

2. Ordinarily, the existence of primary varicosities does not affect the general physical activity of the patient. However, if some of the more serious complications, like venous stasis ulcers, exist, then repeated periods of hospitalization may be required in order to heal the lesions.

3. The patient who has undergone a successful vein stripping is generally asymptomatic subsequently.

ORGANIC LYMPHATIC DISORDERS OF THE LIMBS

Primary and Secondary Lymphedemas

Definition and Etiology

Since, aside from their respective etiologies, the clinical picture of the two groups is, for the most part, similar, both will be discussed in the same section.

Primary and secondary lymphedemas are examples of the obstructive type of lymphatic disorders.

1. *The primary type* is due to some congenital anomaly of the lymphatic system, such as:

A. An absence of formed lymph trunks (aplasia)

B. Unconnected lymph spaces

C. A reduced number or size of lymph channels (hypoplasia)

D. Widening and tortuosity of lymph channels (hyperplasia) producing incompetency of the vessels.

2. *A secondary type of* lymphedema may follow from a number of different states or diseases resulting in obstruction or destruction of critical lymph vessels and lymph nodes. Among the causative factors are:

A. Trauma to or excision of critical lymph nodes and lymph channels

B. Fibrotic changes in the vessels following irradiation or chronic venous insufficiency

C. Metastatic infiltration of lymph nodes

D. Various inflammatory processes, such as streptococcal infections and filariasis.

Clinical Characteristics

1. *Primary (idiopathic) lymphedema*

A. In primary (idiopathic) lymphedema, whether it is the simple congenital type, in which there is diffuse swelling of a leg or legs present at birth, or whether it is Milroy's disease, in which more than one member of a family is found to be suffering from the condition, the gradual enlargement of the limb is not associated with any pain.

B. At times, the swelling pits on pressure, but usually it is firmer than ordinary edema.

C. The general health of the patient remains unaffected by the local difficulty.

D. The involved limb may demonstrate a susceptibility to streptococcal infections; this may manifest itself in the form of recurrent attacks of lymphangitis, lymphadenitis, and systemic responses, such as fever, chills and malaise.

E. Lymphedema praecox

Lymphedema praecox is a disorder of lymphatic drainage, observed in girls around the time of puberty. Whether it is due to an endocrine factor, to congenitally undeveloped lymphatic vessels, or to a slowly developing lymphatic system, incapable of functioning adequately in the face of rapidly growing tissue needs, can not be determined on the basis of available evidence.

(1) The condition is characterized by progressive intractable, painless swelling of one or both lower limbs.

(2) At first, the degree of edema appears to be increased by prolonged physical exertion in the upright position, the menstrual period, and hot weather, the swelling being reduced by bed rest with the foot of the bed elevated.

(3) However, late in the disease, the effect of recumbency is much less marked.

(4) The edema is associated with a sense of heaviness in the involved limb and an unpleasant sensation due to stretching of the skin by edema fluid.

(5) Also, the embarrassing disfigurement of the limb in a young girl or woman leads to emotional trauma.

2. *Secondary lymphedema*

In secondary lymphedema, the clinical picture will vary somewhat depending upon the etiologic factor.

A. In the case of a streptococcal infection, generally there is an underlying dermatophytosis in the feet, which acts as the portal of entry for the bacteria. This is followed by lymphangitis, lymphadenitis, and a systemic response, all the abnormal changes generally being readily controlled by a course of an appropriate antibiotic. However, the condition frequently recurs, eventually causing permanent fibrosis of the affected lymphatics and the appearance of slow-forming permanent edema.

B. Other fibrosing agents, like irradiation therapy and protracted chronic venous stasis, produce a progressive nonpainful type of nonpitting edema.

C. Destruction of lymph channels or nodes by trauma or surgical excision also causes slow-forming swelling of the involved limb.

D. Metastasis of malignant cells to regional lymph nodes elicits a similar clinical picture, the nonpitting, firm edema first being noted below the level of the affected nodes and then, with time, progressing in a distal direction.

Diagnosis

1. *Primary lymphedema*

A. Primary lymphedema is diagnosed on the basis of the appearance of nonpitting, nonpainful edema either at the time of birth or shortly thereafter or at puberty or several years beyond that period.

B. The patient is usually a female, in whom no etiologic factor capable of producing edema can be identified.

2. *Secondary lymphedema*

A. Secondary lymphedema occurs in a limb in which there exists a mechanism responsible for interference with or elimination of proximal lymph flow.

B. The clinical appearance of the involved extremity is somewhat similar to that observed in the one suffering from primary lymphedema.

C. The edema is slow-forming, painless, and nonpitting in nature, at least, later in the disease.

D. Elevation of the limb, even for prolonged periods, has very little effect on the degree of swelling.

3. *Lymphangiography*

A. Lymphangiography is the only procedure that can clearly distinguish between lymphedema due to an intrinsic abnormality of lymphatic channels (primary lymphedema) and that which is secondary to obstruction, obliteration, or absence of lymphatic channels and lymph nodes due to an extralymphatic process.

B. The procedure is also helpful in differentiating the secondary lymphedema that follows the postphlebitic syndrome from the swelling due to primary lymphatic involvement.

Differential Diagnosis

1. *Lipedema*

A. Since in this condition there is painless, insidious, symmetrical swelling of the lower extremities, it must be distinguished from primary and secondary lymphedema.

B. The disorder is invariably noted in obese individuals.

C. The swelling is not particularly affected by elevation of the lower limbs.

D. Of help is the occasional finding of fibrous trabeculations in the soft tissues of the lymphedematous limb and the absence of such changes in lipedema.

E. In lipedema, the skin is not thickened or altered in any manner, as contrasted with lymphedema.

2. *Miscellaneous states*

A. Unilateral lymphedema may be mimicked by a number of unrelated conditions, such as:

(1) Congential arteriovenous fistula

(2) Acute iliofemoral thrombophlebitis

(3) Postphlebitic syndrome

The history of the type of onset, venography, and lymphangiography may all be important in making the differential diagnosis.

B. In the presence of bilateral edema of the lower extremities, it is necessary to exclude such systemic conditions as:

(1) Congestive heart failure
(2) Nephrosis
(3) Myxedema
(4) Cirrhosis of the liver
(5) Nutritional disorders

Treatment

1. *Medical therapy*

A. The conservative management of primary and secondary lymphedema consists, in great part, of care of the involved limb.

B. The patient is warned against sustaining any type of local injury in order to prevent subsequent streptococcal infections.

C. In the case of postmastectomy lymphedema, the patient should be careful not to burn her fingers with a lighted cigarette and should not carry heavy packages using the affected upper extremity. In fact, she should take precautions at all times not to traumatize her hand.

D. Meticulous foot hygiene is indicated if a lower limb is involved, in order to minimize dermatophytosis followed by bacterial infections.

E. Control of the swelling is attempted by means of elevation of the limb and the use of various means to prevent reaccumulation of fluid, such as a pure gum rubber bandage applied and removed several times a day.

F. As an adjunct, the patient should be placed on a low-salt diet and on parenteral and oral diuretics.

G. Mechanical methods can also be used, including treatment with a vasopneumatic apparatus or a compression cuff and later the application of an elasticized Dacron sleeve or stocking fabricated according to the size of the limb.

H. In some patients in whom repeated attacks of cellulitis, lymphangitis, and lymphadenitis occur, it is essential to control the dermatophytosis of the feet by obtaining a culture of the fungi or molds in the lesion and then institution of the proper therapy.

I. Also of value is the prophylatic administration on a long-term basis of the antibacterial agent found useful in the treatment of acute episodes of streptococcal infection. Such an approach may help prevent subsequent attacks of lymphangitis and lymphadenitis and further enlargement of the limb by pooled lymph fluid.

2. *Surgical therapy*

The operative approach to the control of primary or secondary lymphedema has a limited use and should be attempted only when all other measures have failed and the involved limb is so large as to be disabling. The surgical therapy consist of the following:

A. Lymphangioplasty is generally unsuccessful in achieving growth of new lymphatic channels.

B. The Kondoleon operation frequently results in an unsatisfactory cosmetic appearance of the leg.

C. Superficial lymphangiectomy (Charles' operation) is a major surgical undertaking.

D. Recently the process of omental transposition has been attempted, but there are too few cases in the literature to allow for proper evaluation of the procedure.

Prognosis

The outlook for the patient suffering from either primary or secondary lymphedema is not good as far as eliminating the condition is concerned. However, in many instances the rate of enlargement can be slowed or even stopped with proper therapeutic procedures, such as the prevention of recurrence of streptococcal infections.

Aside from the incapacity, inconvenience, and local and systemic symptoms associated with the acute attacks of cellulitis, the patient has no handicaps other than the effect the heavy limb has on his ability to ambulate. As already mentioned, in the case of the female patient, there is the added psychological trauma consequent to the marked changes in the appearance of the limb, a response that may completely alter her outlook on life.

The effect of primary or secondary lymphedema on longevity is minimal unless the episodes of streptococcal infections cannot be controlled by medications, with the result that serious systemic reactions ensue.

Lymphatic Tumors

Typical of nonobstructive lymphatic disorders is the group of lymphatic tumors, nonmalignant and malignant.

Definition and Etiology

1. *Benign tumors*

The benign tumors probably represent an anomalous formation of lymphatic vessels rather than being true neoplasms. They can be divided into the simple, the cavernous, and the cystic types.

A. *The simple lymphatic tumor* is usually congenital, consisting of small lesions made up of large networks of lymphatic spaces connected to lymphatic channels.

B. *The cavernous lymphatic tumor*, also of congenital origin, appears at birth or shortly thereafter and grows slowly. It consists of numerous large dilated sinuses containing lymph.

C. *The cystic type (hygroma)* is considered to arise from embryonal rests and is generally composed of several cysts.

2. *Malignant tumors*

A. The lymphangiosarcoma is a rare primary malignant lymphatic tumor that may be a complication of longstanding lymphedema of a limb.

B. It is most often seen in women suffering from postmastectomy lymphedema, generally 5 to 15 years after the operation.

Clinical Characteristics and Diagnosis

1. *Benign tumors*

A. *The simple type* of benign lymphangioma is generally located in the skin and mucous membrane and is slow growing.

B. *Cavernous lymphangioma* is noted in the skin and subcutaneous tissue and less frequently in the tongue, lips, and cheeks.

C. *The cystic type*

(1) The cystic type is most often found in the neck and rarely in the axilla, groin, and pelvis.

(2) Histologically, the thin-walled cystic masses have walls of endothelium, connective tissue, fat, smooth muscle, nerves, and lymphoid tissue.

(3) The lesion is filled with a clear or straw-colored fluid containing white blood cells, phagocytes, and cellular debris.

2. *Malignant tumors (lymphangiosarcoma)*

A. Lymphangiosarcoma may be first observed as spontaneous, purplish bruise marks or tender nodules on the anterior surface of the lymphedematous arm.

B. The lesion then may break down to form ulcerations or areas of necrosis, involving the skin and subcutaneous tissue.

C. Histologic examination of a biopsy specimen reveals the tissues to be comprised of neoplastic endothelial cells, forming solid layers of tissue or poorly defined lymph spaces.

D. Spread may take place to neighboring structures, including venous channels.

E. Some spaces may contain blood.

Prognosis

1. The outlook for benign lymphangiomas is excellent.

2. On the other hand, that for lymphangiosarcoma is very poor, rapid progression of the malignant lesion generally occurring.

REFERENCES

1. Abramson, D. I. et al.: Thromboangiitis obliterans: a true clinical entity. Am. J. Cardiol., *12*:107, 1963.
2. Fogarty, T. J. et al.: A method for extraction of arterial emboli and thrombi. Surg. Gynecol. Obstet., *116*:241, 1963.
3. Romeo, S. G., Whalen, R. E., and Tindall, J. P.: Intra-arterial administration of reserpine: its use in patients with Raynaud's disease or Raynaud's phenomenon. Arch. Intern. Med., *125*:825, 1970.
4. Wagner, F. B., Jr., and Herbut, P. A.: Etiology of primary varicose veins: histologic study of 100 saphenofemoral junctions. Am. J. Surg., *78*:876, 1949.

17. CARDIOVASCULAR DISORDERS IN SYSTEMIC DISEASES

Nanette K. Wenger, M.D.

GENERAL CONSIDERATIONS

Cardiovascular involvement in systemic diseases may present to the clinician as cardiac enlargement; varying degrees of severity of congestive heart failure; cardiac arrhythmias, including those leading to sudden cardiac death; embolic phenomena, both pulmonary and systemic; chest pain syndromes (due to myocardial ischemia or to pericarditis); valvular disease with varying obstruction to blood flow or valvular incompetence; pericardial disease, inflammatory and noninflammatory, with and without effusion; or detection may be based on abnormalities on the electrocardiogram.

The specific etiologic diagnosis is often dependent on the extracardiac manifestations of the disease, in that the cardiovascular clinical syndromes and pathologic alterations are often strikingly similar for many different etiologic systemic diseases. Cardiovascular manifestations constitute a variable proportion

Classification of Systemic Diseases

Infectious*	Hematologic
Endocrine	Sarcoidosis
Neuromuscular	Pregnancy and heart disease††
Collagen vascular	Chemical, toxic, hypersensitivity§
Metabolic	Physical agents
Nutritional	Complications of oral contraceptive use‡
	Complications of drug abuse
Neoplastic†	Miscellaneous systemic syndromes

*See Chapter 7.
†See Leukemia in Hematologic section, and also Chapter 11.
††See Chapter 31.
§See also Chapter 18.
‡See also Chapter 18.

of the presenting signs and symptoms of the illness; although they are usually over-shadowed by the other components of the systemic illness, they may, on occasion, be the major evidence of disease. At times, cardiovascular involvement is documented only as an incidental finding at postmortem examination. This chapter will emphasize those systemic diseases which commonly present with clinical cardiovascular manifestations, rather than with only pathologic evidence of cardiovascular involvement.

ENDOCRINE DISORDERS

1. *Thyroid*
    A. *Thyrotoxicosis*
        (1) *General features*
It is controversial whether an excess of thyroid hormone per se produces heart disease; or whether antecedent or concomitant heart disease is requisite for the patient with thyrotoxicosis to develop cardiovascular manifestations. The young patient generally has more florid manifestations of thyrotoxicosis; in the older patient, evidence of thyrotoxicosis is often less prominent than the cardiovascular manifestations; indeed, clinical evidence of heart disease is unusual before age 40 in the thyrotoxic patient.

        (2) *Pathology and pathophysiology*

            (a) Thyrotoxicosis does not alter myocardial anatomy, although cardiac dilatation and hypertrophy may occur.

            (b) The thyrotoxic heart is physiologically hyperactive, with an increased heart rate and oxygen consumption; most myocardial structural alterations are attributed to complicating heart disease or hypertension.

(c) Thyrotoxic cardiovascular disturbances appear due to the combined effects of thyroid hormone and of sympathetic stimulation; tachycardia and an increased stroke volume result in augmentation of the cardiac output, left ventricular work, coronary blood flow, and myocardial oxygen consumption.

(d) Augmentation of myocardial contractility is not sympathetic in origin, as it does not abate with beta blockade, which decreases the tachycardia and narrows the pulse pressure.

(e) In addition to the myocardial hypermetabolism per se, an increased peripheral blood flow (due both to the decreased peripheral resistance and the arteriovenous shunting) imposes added work on the heart.

(f) The tachycardia is not sufficient to cause congestive heart failure in a normal heart, but the combination of tachycardia and the increased cardiac output (due to increased blood volume, increased circulatory velocity, increased venous return and arteriovenous shunting) can produce congestive heart failure in a patient with underlying cardiovascular disease.

(g) Neither the atrial fibrillation nor the congestive heart failure can be attributed to a direct effect of thyroid hormone.

(h) Dyspnea, in the absence of heart failure, probably is due both to the decreased lung compliance and to the respiratory muscle myopathy.

(3) *Signs and symptoms*

(a) The cardiovascular manifestations of a hyperdynamic circulation —(a) resting tachycardia, (b) a widened pulse pressure, (c) brisk arterial cardiac apical pulsations, (d) a loud S-1, and (e) flow murmurs—must be differentiated from the cardiovascular complications of thyrotoxicosis.

(b) Unexplained atrial fibrilla-tion, often unresponsive to digitalis; unexplained tachycardia or congestive heart failure (the latter often with a normal circulation time); and congestive heart failure that responds poorly to therapy are clues to thyrotoxic heart disease.

(c) Tachycardia during sleep particularly suggests thyrotoxicosis.

(d) Angina pectoris is common, probably due to increased myocardial work in a patient with underlying coronary atherosclerotic heart disease.

(e) Congestive heart failure occurs more frequently in the female, with increased age, with atrial fibrillation, and with a longer duration of the thyrotoxicosis; a major clue to thyrotoxic congestive heart failure is the rapid or normal circulation time.

(f) Digitalis toxicity is not uncommon prior to cardiac compensation or slowing of the heart rate.

(4) *Laboratory findings*

(a) *Chest x-ray and fluoroscopy*

(i) The chest roentgenogram is usually normal in the absence of atrial fibrillation or congestive heart failure, although pulmonary artery dilatation with prominent pulsations and evidence of increased cardiac contractility may be observed fluoroscopically.

(ii) When congestive heart failure occurs, the cardiac silhouette becomes globular, but the lung fields often show no congestion, probably due to the increased pulmonary blood flow and rapid circulation time.

(b) *Electrocardiography*

(i) There are no distinctive electrocardiographic features, except the sinus tachycardia or atrial fibrillation.

(ii) The P-R interval prolongation and Q-T interval shortening may occur.

(iii) The increased QRS voltage appears due to cardiac hypermetabolism rather than to hypertrophy.

(iv) All electrocardiographic abnormalities characteristically resolve with control of thyrotoxicosis.

(v) The majority of electrocardiographic abnormalities in the thyrotoxic patient are related to the underlying cardiovascular disease.

(5) *Management*

(a) Propranolol or reserpine aid in controlling either the sinus tachycardia or the rapid ventricular response to atrial fibrillation until the hypermetabolism can be reversed.

(b) Larger than usual doses of digitalis are often required to slow the ventricular response to atrial fibrillation.

(c) Stable iodine, administered as a saturated solution of potassium iodide, is initially recommended when severe thyrotoxic heart disease is present.

(d) The alternatives for long-term therapy include:

(i) Antithyroid drugs

(ii) Radioactive iodine

(iii) Subtotal thyroidectomy

(6) *Prognosis*

(a) The prognosis for the remission of the atrial fibrillation, cardiac enlargement, and congestive heart failure is excellent with control of the hypermetabolic state.

(b) The functional and laboratory abnormalities, related to associated cardiovascular disease, cannot be expected to regress.

B. *Myxedema*

(1) *General features*

(a) The cardiac enlargement in myxedema is commonly due to pericardial effusion.

(b) Clinical evidence of cardiac failure is unusual except in long-standing myxedema.

(c) Myxedema tends to predispose to coronary atherosclerotic heart disease, but symptomatic evidence of this problem usually appears only after thyroid hormone replacement therapy has been instituted.

(d) Most patients with myxedema are extremely sensitive to digitalis, leading to digitalis toxicity (see Chap. 23).

(2) *Pathology and pathophysiology*

(a) The myxedematous heart is dilated, pale, and flabby with swollen myofibers, increased interstitial fluid, and a mucoprotein myocardial infiltrate.

(b) The latter regress, in the early stages, with thyroid hormone replacement; the later cardiac fibrosis is usually not reversible.

(c) There is frequent associated coronary atherosclerosis.

(d) A major cardiovascular alteration in myxedema is a decreased cardiac output, due both to the bradycardia and the diminished stroke volume.

(e) The bradycardia and diminished peripheral blood flow parallel the reduction of oxygen consumption; however, the ability to increase the heart rate appears unimpaired, as is the ability to increased cardiac output with exercise.

(f) With normal intracardiac pressures, it is evident that cardiac failure is not present, despite the cardiac enlargement.

(g) The arterial blood pressure is usually normal, although the pulse pressure may be narrowed.

(h) The arteriovenous oxygen difference is augmented, reflecting increased tissue oxygen uptake; the diminution in cardiac work is greater than the diminution in oxygen consumption, providing an adequate cardiac reserve.

(3) *Signs and symptoms*

(a) Myxedema without cardiovascular involvement may simulate congestive heart failure because of (a) dyspnea, (b) fatigue, (c) edema, (d) serous effusions, and (e) cardiac enlargement.

(b) Cardiovascular symptoms are unusual in the absence of underlying cardiovascular disease.

(c) A normal response to a Valsalva maneuver differentiates the uncomplicated myxedematous patients from those with cardiac failure.

(d) This is important as the latter usually have underlying cardiovascular disease, and the heart failure may increase with restoration of the normal metabolic state after thyroid hormone replacement.

(4) *Laboratory findings*

(a) *Chest x-ray*

(i) The globular enlarged cardiac silhouette on chest x-ray is more suggestive of pericardial effusion than of true cardiac enlargement.

(ii) Absence of pulmonary congestion is noteworthy.

(iii) However, serous effusions can occur both in the pleural and peritoneal cavities, due to increased capillary permeability, even in the absence of heart failure.

(b) *Echocardiogram*: Pericardial effusion can be confirmed by echocardiography.

(c) *Serum cholesterol*: The serum cholesterol is generally elevated.

(d) *Electrocardiogram*

(i) Characteristic electrocardiographic abnormalities include sinus bradycardia and low voltage of all electrocardiographic complexes.

(ii) T wave abnormalities are common.

(iii) The electrocardiographic abnormalities may relate to the pericardial effusion, to the edema, or to the myxedematous myocardial infiltrate.

(iv) Regression of the ECG abnormalities with thyroid hormone replacement suggests a direct relationship to myxedema effect on the myocardium.

(5) *Management*

(a) Thyroid hormone should be administered cautiously, particularly to the patient with associated heart disease.

(b) An average daily dose of 0.05 mg. of thyroxine is increased by 0.05 mg. every 2 to 3 weeks until a daily maintenance dose of 0.2 to 0.3 mg. is reached.

(c) If angina pectoris occurs:

(i) The thyroid dosage may be decreased.

(ii) Alternatively, propranolol can be added to the therapeutic regimen.

(d) It should be remembered that the myxedematous patient has increased sensitivity to morphine, to digitalis, and to numerous other drugs.

(6) *Prognosis*

(a) Thyroid hormone therapy restores myocardial contractility, cardiac output, and reverses the bradycardia.

(b) Resorption of serous effusions occurs, the heart size returns to normal, the electrocardiographic pattern returns to the premyxedematous state, and the serum cholesterol level decreases.

(c) The cardiovascular status should return to normal in the absence of underlying heart disease.

2. *Pituitary*

A. *Acromegaly*

(1) *General features*

Excessive growth hormone in the prepubertal individual causes giantism without disproportionate cardiac enlargement; in the adult, disproportionate cardiac enlargement occurs.

(2) *Pathology and pathophysiology*

(a) Marked cardiac hypertrophy, particularly left ventricular, and disproportionate to the hypertrophy of other viscera, is characteristic of acromegaly.

250   *Cardiovascular Disorders in Systemic Diseases*

(b) Severe coronary arterial and other vessel atherosclerosis, with associated myocardial infarction, occur commonly.

(c) The cardiac enlargement probably reflects both a direct pituitary hormone effect on the heart and the increased cardiac work required to supply blood to an enlarged body; the associated thyrotoxicosis, diabetes mellitus, and/or hypertension also play a role.

(d) Hypertension does not occur with increased frequency in the acromegalic patient, but, when present, hypertension is poorly tolerated.

(e) Chronic congestive heart failure probably relates both to the myocardial hypertrophy and dysfunction and to the associated coronary atherosclerosis.

(3) *Signs and symptoms*

(a) Symptomatic cardiac failure occurs in about one-fourth of patients, with dyspnea as the most common presenting symptom.

(b) Dyspnea may be secondary both to the congestive heart failure and to the associated kyphoscoliosis.

(c) Weakness, palpitations, and syncope have been reported.

(d) Cardiac enlargement is almost universal.

(4) *Laboratory findings*

(a) *Electrocardiography*

There are no diagnostic electrocardiographic abnormalities, but left ventricular hypertrophy and left axis deviation are common.

(b) *Chest x-ray*

On chest x-ray, there is generalized disproportionate cardiac enlargement, even in the enlarged thoracic cavity.

(5) *Management and prognosis*

(a) Therapy involves control of excessive growth hormone secretion by pituitary irradiation or, occasionally, by neurosurgical removal of the tumor.

(b) The hypertension and congestive heart failure respond to standard management.

(c) The prognosis is related to the degree of control of the acromegaly.

B. *Hypopituitarism*

(1) *General features*

Anterior pituitary failure usually occurs gradually, except with the precipitous panhypopituitarism complicating pregnancy in Sheehan's syndrome.

(2) *Pathology and pathophysiology*

(a) Adrenocortical, gonadal, and thyroid function failure occur because of the absence of stimulatory trophic hormones.

(b) The most common cardiac changes are those of myxedema and/or Addison's disease.

(c) The patient with panhypopituitarism has cardiac atrophy, with loss of ability to respond to cardiac pressure or volume loads.

(3) *Signs and symptoms*

(a) Clinical manifestations are predominantly those of myxedema, except that pericardial effusion is unusual.

(b) The blood pressure is often low and the heart size small.

(c) Atherosclerosis is rare.

(4) *Laboratory findings*

(a) *Chest x-ray*: There are no specific radiographic features.

(b) *Electrocardiography*

The electrocardiographic abnormalites are primarily those of myxedema:

(i) Low voltage

(ii) Q-T interval prolongation

(iii) Nonspecific S-T, T wave changes.

(5) *Management and prognosis*

(a) With replacement of the target gland hormones—cortisone, thyroid hormone, and gonadal hormones—the clinical and electrocardiographic abnormalities revert.

(b) Thyroid hormone restores normal electrocardiographic voltage.

(c) Cortisone, however, is

necessary to reverse the S-T, T waves, and Q-T abnormalities.

  3. *Adrenal*
    A. *Cushing's syndrome*
      (1) *General features*
  Cushing's syndrome is a rare problem, occurring predominantly in women, with a peak incidence in the 30s and 40s, particularly following a pregnancy.
      (2) *Pathology and pathophysiology*
        (a) The syndrome may be due to adrenal hyperplasia or to carcinoma.
        (b) The major morphologic changes reflect the end organ damage of systemic hypertension:
          (i) Cardiac hypertrophy
          (ii) Advanced coronary atherosclerosis
          (iii) Cerebral hemorrhage
          (iv) Renal insufficiency
          (v) The changes secondary to congestive heart failure
        (c) The mechanism of the hypertension remains obscure.
        (d) The accelerated atherosclerosis is attributed to:
          (i) Hypertension
          (ii) Hypercholesterolemia
          (iii) Associated diabetes mellitus
      (3) *Signs and symptoms*
        (a) The major cardiovascular complications of Cushing's syndrome are:
          (i) Hypertension
          (ii) Cerebrovascular accident
          (iii) Chronic renal failure
          (iv) Cardiac hypertrophy
          (v) Congestive heart failure
        (b) The hypertension is severe, and occurs in 75 to 90 per cent of patients.
        (c) Atherosclerosis appears related both to the duration of the Cushing's syndrome and the severity and duration of the hypertension.
        (d) If untreated, a cerebrovascular accident or severe congestive heart failure usually occurs in the patient with Cushing's syndrome within 3 to 5 years.
      (4) *Laboratory findings*
        (a) *Chest x-ray*
  Characteristic radiologic abnormalities include:
          (i) Cardiac enlargement with left ventricular hypertrophy
          (ii) The pulmonary changes of congestive heart failure.
        (b) *Electrocardiography*
  The electrocardiographic findings are of (a) left ventricular hypertrophy and/or (b) hypokalemia.
      (5) *Management and prognosis*
        (a) Management may involve (1) pituitary irradiation (2) total bilateral adrenalectomy, (3) long-term adrenocortical-suppressant drugs, or (4) tumor removal, depending on the etiology of the Cushing's syndrome.
        (b) The hypertension, however, may not regress completely, even after treatment of the Cushing's syndrome.
    B. *Primary aldosteronism*
      (1) *General features*
        (a) This problem is due to either an adrenocortical adenoma or to bilateral adrenal hyperplasia.
        (b) Hypertension and electrolyte abnormalities are the characteristic cardiovascular disturbances.
      (2) *Pathology and pathophysiology*
        (a) Myocardial hypertrophy occurs secondary to the hypertension.
        (b) The extent of coronary atherosclerosis varies.
        (c) Most clinical and chemical abnormalities are secondary to the chronic potassium depletion.
        (d) Overt edema is rare, since the retained sodium enters the potassium-depleted cell.
      (3) *Signs and symptoms*
        (a) The major changes, muscular weakness, polyuria, and polydypsia, relate to chronic potassium depletion.

(b) Hypertension is almost universal.

(c) Clinical evidence of atherosclerosis and congestive heart failure is rare.

(4) *Laboratory findings*

(a) *Chemical data:* The serum potassium level is characteristically low with high blood and urine aldosterone and low plasma renin levels.

(b) *Chest x-ray and electrocardiography*

(i) There are no characteristic radiologic or electrocardiographic alterations.

(ii) Electrocardiographic abnormalities, when present, are those of hypokalemia: S-T segment depression, flattened or inverted T waves, and prominent U waves.

(iii) Cardiac arrhythmias may occur secondary to the hypokalemia.

(5) *Management and prognosis*

(a) Surgical removal of the tumor and correction of the hypokalemia usually relieve the mild hypertension and revert the hypokalemic syndromes and most electrocardiographic abnormalities.

(b) Minor residual electrocardiographic abnormalities may be due to a hypokalemic cardiomyopathy.

(c) The subsidence of arrhythmias is dramatic.

C. *Addison's disease*

(1) *General features*

In past years, tuberculosis was the major etiologic factor in Addison's disease. Today, primary idiopathic adrenal cortical atrophy is etiologic.

(2) *Pathology and pathophysiology*

(a) The myocardium shows brown atrophy, due to an increase in hemofuscin pigment.

(b) There is decreased myofiber size and impaired myocardial contractility.

(c) Hypovolemia appears to be the primary determinant of the decreased heart size and the hypotension.

(d) Mineralocorticoid deficiency explains both the hypovolemia and the hyposensitivity to pressor amines, with failure of vasoconstriction.

(3) *Signs and symptoms*

(a) Cardiac manifestations usually appear insidiously. They include:

(i) Dyspnea

(ii) Palpitations

(iii) Arterial hypotension with considerable orthostasis

(iv) A small cardiac size with feeble pulsations

(b) Hypotension, consistently below 100 mm. Hg systolic pressure, demands evaluation for Addison's disease.

(4) *Laboratory findings*

(a) *Chest x-ray and fluoroscopy*

(i) The heart size on chest x-ray is small and parallels the severity of the disease.

(ii) Cardiac pulsations at fluoroscopy are hypodynamic.

(b) *Electrocardiography*

(i) Electrocardiographic abnormalities are nonspecific. They include: generalized low voltage, bradycardia, and S-T segment and T wave alterations.

(ii) At times, electrocardiographic evidence of hyperkalemia may occur during Addisonian crises.

(5) *Management and prognosis*

(a) Specific cardiovascular therapy is rarely warranted.

(b) The management involves steroid hormone replacement, which causes the clinical, radiologic, and electrocardiographic abnormalities to regress.

D. *Pheochromocytoma*

(1) *Pathology and pathophysiology*

(a) These adrenal medullary

tumors may result in fixed or paroxysmal hypertension, due to excessive plasma catecholamine secretion.

(b) Additionally, the catecholamines may produce myocardial damage: (a) interstitial inflammation, (b) myofiber necrosis and degeneration, and (c) subsequent fibrosis, due to failure of the coronary circulation to meet the increased myocardial metabolic demand.

(2) *Signs and symptoms*

(a) In addition to the hypertension, the picture of cardiomyopathy (cardiac enlargement with heart failure) may ensue.

(b) Cardiac arrhythmias are common.

(3) *Laboratory findings*

(a) *Electrocardiogram*: The electrocardiographic S-T, T wave changes are nonspecific.

(b) *Chest x-ray*: Cardiomegaly is noted on the chest film.

(4) *Management and prognosis*

(a) Adrenergic blocking agents and subsequent tumor removal result in clinical and electrocardiographic improvement.

(b) The hypertension characteristically resolves.

4. *Parathyroid*

A. *Pathology and pathophysiology*

(1) The major cardiovascular manifestations of parathyroid disorders relate to the effect of hypocalcemia or hypercalcemia on the electrocardiogram.

(2) Cardiac failure occasionally occurs in the patient with hypoparathyroidism, possibly related to the adverse effect of hypocalcemia on myocardial excitation-contraction coupling.

(3) Hypocalcemia may also sensitize the heart to cardiac arrhythmias.

B. *Laboratory findings*

(1) *ECG findings in hyperparathyroidism*

The characteristic electrocardiographic abnormality of hypercalcemia—a short Q-T interval, with the S-T segment appearing to fuse with the upstroke of the T wave—is encountered in the patient with hyperparathyroidism.

(2) *ECG findings in hypoparathyroidism*

The Q-T interval prolongation, primarily because of S-T segment prolongation, and nonspecific T wave abnormalities, are encountered with hypoparathyroidism.

(3) Electrocardiographic abnormalities subside following correction of the serum calcium level.

NEUROMUSCULAR DISORDERS

1. *Progressive (Duchenne's) muscular dystrophy*

A. *General features*

(1) Cardiomyopathy is a major feature of Duchenne's muscular dystrophy, occuring in more than half of these patients.

(2) Indeed, the cardiovascular manifestations may antedate the diagnosis of the neuromuscular disease.

(3) However, there is no correlation between the severity of the muscular disease, the cardiomyopathy, and the extent of electrocardiographic abnormalities.

B. *Pathology and pathophysiology*

(1) Fibrous and fatty replacement of the myocardium occurs selectively in the posterobasal left ventricle and the posteromedial papillary muscle, consistent with the electrocardiographic abnormalities.

(2) Additionally, degenerative changes occur in the small myocardial arteries, including those supplying the A-V and sinus nodes; James suggests this as the basis for the frequently encountered arrhythmias.

C. *Signs and symptoms*

(1) Various cardiac arrhythmias, and cardiomegaly with congestive heart

failure are the most common clinical findings.

(2) The tachycardia may persist during sleep, but there is usually little difficulty differentiating this from the comparable finding in thyrotoxicosis.

(3) Symptomatic evidence of heart failure is rarely present because of the patient's prolonged immobilization by the neuromuscular problems.

(4) Sudden death, presumably secondary to arrhythmias, occurs frequently.

D. *Laboratory findings*

(1) *Electrocardiography*

(a) Distinctive electrocardiographic changes occur in 40 to 90 per cent of patients:

(i) Tall R waves are present in the right precordial leads, with deep Q waves in the limb leads and left precordial leads.

(ii) Identical electrocardiographic abnormalities occur in affected family members.

(b) P wave abnormalites, conduction defects, and nonspecific T wave changes are also encountered.

(2) *Chest x-ray*

Evaluation of the cardiomegaly and the pulmonary congestive changes is complicated by the elevated diaphragms and frequent thoracic deformities.

E. *Management and prognosis*

(1) Both the neuromuscular and cardiovascular diseases tend to be progressive.

(2) There is no known therapy.

2. *Friedreich's ataxia*

A. *General features*

(1) Cardiovascular problems occur in ⅓ to ½ of patients with Friedreich's ataxia and, as with Duchenne's muscular dystrophy, may be the initial manifestation of illness.

(2) Congestive heart failure is a major cause of death.

B. *Pathology and pathophysiology*

(1) The myocardium is hyper-trophic, with diffuse fatty degeneration and interstitial fibrosis.

(2) Fibrous disruption of the conduction system may explain the frequent arrhythmias, as may involvement of the smaller intramural coronary arteries, particularly those supplying the sinus and A-V nodes.

(3) Chest deformity may accentuate the cardiovascular problems.

C. *Signs and symptoms*

Common findings include:

(1) Inappropriate sinus tachycardia

(2) Other arrhythmias

(3) Cardiac enlargement

(4) Congestive heart failure

(5) Nonspecific cardiac murmurs

D. *Laboratory findings*

(1) *Electrocardiography*

(a) Nonspecific S-T, T wave changes occur frequently; indeed, electrocardiographic abnormalities occur in the majority of patients with Friedreich's ataxia and cardiac disease.

(b) As in Duchenne's muscular dystrophy, affected family members tend to show comparable electrocardiographic alterations.

(c) Atrioventricular block, bundle branch block, and other arrhythmias are frequent.

(2) *Chest x-ray:* There are no distinctive radiologic features.

E. *Management and prognosis*

(1) The disease tends to be progressive.

(2) Routine management for the arrhythmias and the congestive heart failure is recommended.

3. *Myotonia atrophica (Steinert's disease)*

A. *General features*

(1) Cardiovascular involvement is a late occurrence in myotonia atrophica, but is usually responsible for the sudden death.

(2) There is no correlation between the severity of the cardiovascular

disease, the electrocardiographic abnormalities, and the muscular disorder.

B. *Pathology*: There is diffuse myocardial fibrosis.

C. *Signs and symptoms*

(1) Dyspnea and palpitations are common.

(2) Cardiac arrhythmias, particularly supraventricular, occur frequently; and Stokes-Adams syncope has been described.

(3) Cardiac enlargement and congestive heart failure are late findings.

D. *Laboratory findings*

(1) *Electrocardiography*

(a) Electrocardiographic abnormalities occur in 70 to 85 per cent of patients, and serve as the most sensitive index of cardiac involvement.

(b) Atrioventricular and intraventricular conduction defects are the characteristic abnormalities, and may progress with time.

(c) The electrocardiogram may mimic that of myocardial infarction.

(2) *Chest x-ray*: There are no specific radiographic abnormalities.

E. *Management and prognosis*

(1) The disease tends to be progressive.

(2) In addition to the usual arrhythmia treatment, Stokes-Adams syncope has been successfully managed with artificial pacemaker implantation.

4. *Myasthenia gravis*

A. *General features*

Many patients with myasthenia gravis have no clinical or electrocardiographic cardiovascular abnormalities.

B. *Pathology*

Myofiber necrosis is seen, with a secondary inflammatory infiltrate.

C. *Signs and symptoms*

Various arrhythmias, dyspnea, and precordial discomfort are reported.

D. *Laboratory findings*

Nonspecific electrocardiographic S-T, T wave abnormalities and terminal QRS notching are described.

COLLAGEN VASCULAR DISEASES

1. *Scleroderma (progressive systemic sclerosis)*

A. *General factors*

It is difficult to differentiate the manifestations of primary cardiac scleroderma from those secondary to the pulmonary and systemic hypertension, the latter due to underlying renal disease.

B. *Pathology*

(1) Fibrous replacement of the myocardium occurs, associated with pericarditis, with and without effusion.

(2) Aortic and mitral valve deformity and nodularity have been described.

C. *Signs and symptoms*

(1) Cardiovascular symptomatology is a late occurrence in scleroderma.

(2) Exertional dyspnea is the most frequent complaint.

(3) Cardiac murmurs may relate to either anemia or to valve deformity.

(4) Nonspecific chest pain, apparently unassociated with coronary artery obstruction, occurs, as does the classical pain of pericarditis.

(5) Cardiac failure may be due to the myocardial disease; but as previously mentioned, may also be explained by right ventricular failure due to pulmonary hypertension or myocardial dysfunction secondary to systemic hypertension.

D. *Laboratory findings*

(1) *Electrocardiography*

(a) Electrocardiographic findings are extremely variable.

(b) They include bundle branch blocks, supraventricular and ventricular arrhythmias, and variable atrioventricular block.

(c) The electrocardiographic abnormalities do not correlate with the severity of the myocardial disease.

(d) Low voltage may suggest pericardial effusion.

(2) *Chest x-ray*

The cardiac silhouette on chest x-ray varies in size with cardiac enlargement due either to myocardial disease or to pericardial effusion.

E. *Management and prognosis*

(1) There is no specific therapy for scleroderma.

(2) Symptomatic myocardial involvement indicates a poor prognosis.

(3) Routine management of the congestive heart failure and rhythm abnormalities is warranted.

(4) Corticosteroid hormones may be of value in pericarditis, with or without effusion.

2. *Periarteritis nodosa*

A. *Pathology*

(1) This necrotizing vasculitis of unknown etiology commonly involves the major coronary arteries, with resultant myocardial fibrosis and infarction.

(2) Pericarditis may be secondary to myocardial infarction or to the concomitant uremia.

B. *Signs and symptoms*

(1) Tachycardia is a common feature of this multisystem febrile illness.

(2) Anginal pain is rare, despite the occurrence of myocardial infarction.

(3) Hypertension is common, and is a major contributory factor to the heart failure.

(4) Nonspecific cardiac murmurs probably relate mainly to the anemia.

(5) The incidence of pericarditis is variable.

C. *Laboratory findings*

(1) *Chest x-ray*

The routine chest film usually shows only generalized cardiac enlargement or left ventricular enlargement.

(2) *Electrocardiography*

(a) Electrocardiographic changes of left ventricular hypertrophy are common.

(b) Bundle branch blocks, atrioventricular block, and supraventricular arrhythmias have been described.

(c) Classical changes of myocardial infarction may be seen.

D. *Management and prognosis*

Massive corticosteroid hormone therapy in the acute phase, with subsequent maintenance suppressive therapy, may dramatically improve the heart failure and the pericarditis.

3. *Lupus erythematosus*

A. *General features*

Endocardial, myocardial, and pericardial involvement may be present.

B. *Pathology*

(1) The endocardial abnormality, Libman-Sachs endocarditis, occurs in about 50 per cent of cases.

(2) Verrucous lesions are present, particularly on the mitral and aortic valves.

(3) Fibrinoid material is deposited in the myocardium, and there is arteritis of the intramyocardial coronary arteries.

(4) The left ventricular hypertrophy probably reflects both this arteritis and the systemic hypertension.

(5) Pericarditis is common, with or without effusion, and constriction has been reported.

C. *Signs and symptoms*

(1) Cardiovascular signs and symptoms may be the presenting manifestations of lupus erythematosus.

(2) About 33 per cent of patients have clinical evidence of pericarditis: pain, rub, and/or electrocardiographic changes; tamponade may occur.

(3) Cardiac murmurs may be due to the Libman-Sachs endocarditis or may relate to the anemia, fever, and tachycardia.

(4) Bacterial endocarditis may occur and should be considered in the setting of unexplained fever and changing cardiac murmurs.

(5) Significant arrhythmias are unusual.

(6) The congestive heart failure

usually is related to severe, sustained hypertension.

D. *Laboratory findings*

(1) *Chest x-ray*

There may be generalized cardiac enlargement on x-ray, due to varying combinations of left ventricular hypertrophy and pericardial effusion.

(2) *Electrocardiography*

(a) Electrocardiographic abnormalities, particularly S-T, T wave changes of pericarditis are common.

(b) Low voltage has been reported, often associated with pericardial effusion.

(c) Changes of left ventricular hypertrophy are common.

E. *Management and prognosis*

(1) Corticosteroid hormones have been valuable in controlling the pericarditis and in managing some cases of refractory cardiac failure.

(2) Hypertension and congestive heart failure respond moderately well to the usual therapy.

4. *Dermatomyositis*

A. *Pathology*

(1) Cardiac involvement is uncommon in dermatomyositis.

(2) Myocardial abnormalities include:

(a) Degeneration

(b) Fibrosis

(c) Lymphocytic infiltration

B. *Signs and symptoms*

(1) There is usually little clinical evidence of cardiac involvement.

(2) However, cardiac failure has been reported as a cause of death.

C. *Laboratory findings*

(1) Electrocardiographic changes may be due to pericarditis or myocarditis.

(2) Atrioventricular block and atrial arrhythmias have been described.

D. *Management*: Corticosteroid hormones may be of value.

METABOLIC DISORDERS

1. *Amyloidosis*

A. *General features*

(1) Cardiac amyloidosis is a common cause of cardiomyopathy, particularly in the older patient.

(2) Cardiac amyloidosis should be considered in any patient with unexplained heart failure; about 50 per cent of patients have associated significant systemic amyloidosis.

(3) The senile form is unusual before age 80, and occurs primarily in the male.

B. *Pathology and pathophysiology*

(1) Amyloid is an amorphous glycoprotein that may diffusely or in a nodular distribution infiltrate the myocardium, often extending onto the heart valves and the chordae tendineae; the rigid heart valves may be stenotic, insufficient, or both.

(2) Loss of myocardial distensibility causes a restrictive cardiomyopathy, characterized by intractable heart failure, and often mimicking constrictive pericarditis.

(3) Amyloid infiltration of the atria, particularly the left atrium, is characteristic, often with selective involvement of the sinus node; this explains the arrhythmias and atrioventricular conduction abnormalities.

(4) Additionally, amyloid may narrow the coronary arteries, producing chest pain syndromes and, on occasion, true myocardial infarction.

C. *Signs and symptoms*

(1) The classical presentation is of intractable congestive heart failure, often with digitalis intolerance, in an elderly patient.

(2) Atrial arrhythmias and atrioventricular conduction disturbances, at times with syncope, are common.

(3) Cardiac murmurs are frequent.

(4) The hypotension primarily reflects the decreased cardiac output, but an orthostatic component may relate to amyloid infiltration of the autonomic nervous system.

D. *Laboratory findings*

(1) *Chest x-ray*

(a) There is characteristic diminution of cardiac pulsations at fluoroscopy.

(b) Heart size varies considerably.

(2) *Electrocardiography*

(a) Low voltage is present on the electrocardiogram in the majority of cases.

(b) Cardiac arrhythmias are common.

(c) QRS abnormalities may mimic myocardial infarction, or true myocardial infarction may occur and be evident on the electrocardiogram.

E. *Management and prognosis*

(1) There is no specific therapy for amyloidosis.

(2) Arrhythmias and congestive heart failure require the usual therapy, but sensitivity of the patient to digitalis should be noted.

(3) The prognosis is poor after the onset of congestive heart failure.

2. *Hemochromatosis*

A. *General features*

(1) Cardiac involvement in hemochromatosis is usually encountered in patients presenting with the disease early in life.

(2) Cardiac failure is the leading cause of death in patients with hemochromatosis.

B. *Pathology and pathophysiology*

(1) The disease is characterized by myocardial infiltration with iron pigment granules, and resultant myocardial damage and fibrosis.

(2) Arrhythmias, including atrioventricular conduction disturbances, may be explained by iron pigment deposition, with secondary tissue damage in the A-V node.

(3) However, there is little correlation between the extent of myocardial iron pigment deposition, the extent of myocardial fibrosis, and the impairment of cardiac function.

C. *Signs and symptoms*

(1) Arrhythmias including atrioventricular block are frequent.

(2) The most common finding is a progressive congestive heart failure that responds poorly to the usual management.

(3) Pericarditis with and without effusion may be seen.

D. *Laboratory findings*

(1) *Chest x-ray*: At radiologic examination the heart is large and cardiac pulsations are feeble.

(2) *Electrocardiography*

Electrocardiographic abnormalities are nonspecific:

(a) Diminished QRS voltage

(b) T wave changes

(c) Conduction disturbances

(d) The arrhythmias previously mentioned

E. *Management and prognosis*

(1) Therapy involves repeated venesection, designed to remove tissue iron stores.

(2) Chelating agents may also be of value.

(3) Nevertheless, despite this approach and the usual therapy for congestive heart failure, the patient usually succumbs within months to a few years after the onset of cardiovascular symptoms.

3. *Cardiac glycogenosis (glycogen storage disease of the heart)*

A. *General features*

(1) Five categories of glycogenosis have been delineated, but cardiac involvement occurs predominantly in Type II.

(2) This autosomal recessive dis-

order of carbohydrate metabolism is characterized by excessive glycogen accumulation, due to the absence of the enzyme alpha glucosidase, in cardiac and skeletal muscle.

B. *Pathology and pathophysiology*

(1) There is massive left ventricular hypertrophy, with the interventricular septum often encroaching on the right and left ventricular outflow tracts.

(2) The myofibers are enlarged, with a characteristic lacework appearance due to extensive vacuoles filled with normal glycogen.

(3) The atria are normal.

C. *Signs and symptoms*

(1) Heart failure occurs in early infancy, with extreme dyspnea, cyanosis, and tachycardia.

(2) There is associated generalized muscle weakness.

(3) The picture of outflow tract obstruction may be evident clinically, and is, at times, accentuated by digitalis therapy.

D. *Laboratory findings*

(1) *Chest x-ray and angiography*

There is massive cardiac enlargement with a rigid, thick, left ventricular wall demonstrable at angiography.

(2) *Electrocardiography*

The electrocardiographic pattern is almost pathognomonic, with excessive increase of the QRS voltage and a short P-R interval.

E. *Management and prognosis*

(1) The congestive heart failure tends to be difficult to manage.

(2) Surgical approach to the outflow tract obstruction is generally unsuccessful.

(3) The prognosis is uniformly poor, with death usually occurring by the end of the first year of life.

4. *Mucopolysaccharidosis*

A. *General features*

Hurler's syndrome (gargoylism), the most common of the mucopolysac-

charidoses, is an inherited disorder characterized by multisystemic abnormal glycoprotein deposition.

B. *Pathology*

(1) The heart is enlarged.

(2) The heart valves, particularly the mitral valve, are thickened and nodular.

(3) There is endocardial sclerosis, and coronary and pulmonary artery intimal disease occur.

C. *Signs and symptoms*

(1) The early abnormalities are the murmurs of valve dysfunction.

(2) These lead to cardiac enlargement and subsequent congestive heart failure.

(3) Hypertension and pulmonary disease secondary to thoracic deformities occur.

(4) Evidence of myocardial ischemia is uncommon.

D. *Laboratory findings*

(1) *Chest x-ray*

The heart is enlarged, with frequent mitral annular calcification; this and the Marfan syndrome are the commonest causes of mitral annular calcification at a young age.

(2) *Electrocardiography*

The electrocardiogram is abnormal, but not diagnostic.

E. *Management and prognosis*

(1) There is no specific therapy.

(2) Death characteristically occurs during childhood, usually related to heart failure.

5. *Fabry's disease (angiokeratoma corporis diffusum universal)*

A. *General features*

This sex-linked inherited disorder is due to a deficiency of ceramide trihexosidase, which results in abnormal glycolipid deposition in the myocardium and the blood vessels.

B. *Pathology*: Glycolipid deposition causes:

(1) Myofiber fragmentation

(2) Coronary artery narrowing

(3) Heart valve abnormalities

C. *Signs and symptoms*

(1) Angina pectoris and myocardial infarction are due to the coronary artery narrowing.

(2) Cardiac failure probably results both from the myocardial damage and the associated hypertension, secondary to renal failure.

D. *Laboratory findings*

(1) *Chest x-ray*

There is generalized cardiac enlargement, particularly of the left ventricle, at x-ray examination.

(2) *Electrocardiography*

The electrocardiographic abnormalities are nonspecific.

E. *Management:* There is no specific therapy.

6. *Gout*

A. *Pathology and pathophysiology*

(1) Urate deposition may occur in:

(a) The heart valves

(b) The myocardium

(c) The pericardium

(d) The coronary arteries

(2) Rarely, a classic tophus is seen in the heart.

B. *Signs and symptoms*

Arrhythmias have been described, possibly related to urate deposition.

C. *Management and prognosis*

Arrhythmias have been reported to subside in association with uricosuric therapy.

7. *Oxalosis*

A. *Pathology*

This hereditary disease is characterized by calcium oxalate deposition in the myofibers, coronary arteries, and cardiac conduction system.

B. *Signs and symptoms*

Arrhythmias and conduction abnormalities, including complete A-V block, have been described.

C. *Management:* There is no specific therapy for the underlying disease.

8. *Hypokalemia* (see also Chap. 31)

A. *Pathology and pathophysiology*

(1) The myocardial lesions of hypokalemia are myofiber vacuolation and fragmentation, with necrosis and fibrosis most evident in the subendocardial layer.

(2) Abnormalities are unusual unless the serum potassium level falls below 3 mEq per liter.

(3) The actual serum potassium level correlates poorly with the electrocardiographic changes, which probably reflect the intracellular potassium concentration.

B. *Signs and symptoms*

Clinical manifestations, other than occasional hypertension and heart failure, are unusual.

C. *Laboratory findings*

(1) The characteristic electrocardiographic abnormalities include prominent U waves, T wave flattening, and S-T segment depression.

(2) Pseudo P-pulmonale pattern is usually a late manifestation of hypokalemia.

(3) The P-R interval is often prolonged and the QRS voltage may be low.

D. *Management and prognosis*

Potassium repletion reverses the electrocardiographic abnormalities, but the myocardial lesions, if of long duration, appear irremediable.

9. *Uremia*

A. *General features*

With the advent of renal hemodialysis, cardiovascular complications of uremia have markedly increased, as patients with this problem survive for a longer period of time.

B. *Pathology and pathophysiology*

(1) A combination of hypertensive cardiovascular disease, electrolyte imbalance, fluid overload, anemia, and pericarditis explain the frequently encountered heart failure, arrhythmias, and left ventricular hypertrophy.

(2) The high fat, low protein renal failure diet also increases the incidence

of coronary atherosclerotic heart disease.

C. *Signs and symptoms*

(1) Manifestations of congestive heart failure and the pain of pericarditis occur commonly.

(2) The massive cardiomegaly may be related either to the uremic cardiomyopathy or to the pericardial effusion, which occasionally may produce tamponade.

D. *Laboratory findings*

(1) *Chest x-ray*: The cardiac silhouette is increased in size.

(2) *Electrocardiogram*: The electrocardiographic abnormalities are nonspecific.

E. *Management and prognosis*

(1) Hemodialysis markedly improves the uremic cardiomyopathy and the pericardial effusion.

(2) Indomethacin is also of value in pericarditis with effusion.

(3) Pericardiocentesis and/or pericardiectomy may occasionally be required.

NUTRITIONAL DISORDERS

1. *Beriberi*

A. *General features*

Beriberi heart disease is most commonly encountered in the patient with generalized malnutrition or in the alcoholic patient.

B. *Pathology and pathophysiology*

(1) The myocardial alterations include:

(a) Myofiber and conduction system degeneration

(b) Myocardial edema

(c) Biventricular dilatation and hypertrophy

(2) However, the cardiovascular manifestations probably relate not to these anatomic alterations, but to the derangement of carbohydrate metabolism, with lack of cocarboxylase producing the picture of hypoxia.

(3) High cardiac output failure in-

creases the oxygen demand on a myocardium with impaired oxygen utilization.

(4) Oriental beriberi, characterized by a marked diminution of the peripheral resistance, is a fulminant disease with high cardiac output failure.

(5) The occidental form has little or none of the hyperdynamic component and is characterized by biventricular failure with a low cardiac output.

C. *Signs and symptoms*

(1) Cardiovascular involvement is more evident in patients with minimal neurologic derangement, who are able to continue at physical activity.

(2) Sinus tachycardia is almost universal; but other arrhythmias are unusual.

(3) Common manifestations include:

(a) Cardiac enlargement

(b) Pulmonary congestion

(c) Evidence of high output cardiac failure

(4) Physical findings of high output failure may include:

(a) Peripheral vasodilatation

(b) Full bounding pulses

(c) Hemic murmurs

(d) Gallop rhythm

(5) Patients with occidental beriberi are usually alcoholics; they do not have evidence of a hyperdynamic circulation, but manifest cardiac enlargement, pulmonary congestion, serous effusion, and edema.

D. *Laboratory findings*

(1) There is generalized cardiomegaly on chest x-ray.

(2) The circulation time is usually rapid or normal.

(3) Electrocardiographic abnormalities are nonspecific, but sinus tachycardia is characteristic. The Q-T interval may be prolonged.

E. *Management and prognosis*

(1) Thiamine, bedrest, adequate diet, supplementary vitamins, and sodium restriction classically reverse all

symptoms and abnormal laboratory findings, particularly the electrocardiographic derangements, after a variable duration of therapy.

(2) Digitalis and diuretic agents, in the absence of thiamine replacement, have little effect.

2. *Pellagra*

A. *General features*

Most cardiovascular abnormalities in pellagra are probably due either to underlying heart disease or to the frequently associated beriberi.

B. *Pathology*: No specific cardiovascular lesions have been demonstrated.

C. *Signs and symptoms*: Typical abnormalities include tachycardia, palpitations, dyspnea, and edema.

D. *Laboratory findings and prognosis*

Electrocardiographic abnormalities are nonspecific, but often resolve with niacin therapy and after control of the beriberi with thiamine.

3. *Scurvy*

A. *Pathophysiology*

Vitamin C deficiency is considered responsible, via an unknown mechanism, for the cardiovascular symptoms.

B. *Signs and symptoms:* Chest pain, dyspnea, and sudden cardiac death are encountered.

C. *Laboratory findings and prognosis*

Nonspecific electrocardiographic abnormalities revert with the administration of ascorbic acid.

4. *Kwashiorkor*

A. *General features*

The disease is encountered in the South African Bantu child and is assumed to be due to the low-protein-high-carbohydrate diet.

B. *Pathology*

(1) There is biventricular dilatation and hypertrophy, with myofiber atrophy and extensive endocardial mural thrombosis.

(2) Marked degeneration of the conduction system occurs.

C. *Signs and symptoms*

(1) The patients have progressive evidence of cardiac failure, edema, and peripheral and pulmonary embolization.

(2) Atrioventricular conduction disturbances are frequent, and probably explain the high incidence of sudden cardiac death.

D. *Laboratory findings*

(1) There is gross biventricular cardiac enlargement on chest x-ray.

(2) Nonspecific electrocardiographic changes are encountered, most generally S-T, T wave abnormalities.

E. *Management and prognosis*

Both the clinical and the electrocardiographic abnormalities resolve, except in the latest stages of the disease, with bed rest, an adequate diet, digitalis, diuretic therapy, and sodium restriction.

HEMATOLOGIC DISORDERS

1. *Leukemia*

A. *General features*

(1) The cardiovascular manifestations of leukemia may be due to (a) anemia, (b) pericarditis, or (c) the myocardial infiltration and hemorrhage secondary to the leukemic process.

(2) Myocardial infiltration is more common with an increased duration of survival.

B. *Pathology and pathophysiology*

(1) Leukemic cellular infiltrates occur in the atria, the ventricles, and in the pericardium.

(2) Muscle compression by leukemic infiltration may result in myofiber necrosis.

(3) However, cardiac hypertrophy is usually secondary to the anemia and the high cardiac output state.

C. *Signs and symptoms*

(1) Common manifestations include:

(a) Cardiac enlargement
(b) Congestive heart failure
(c) Pericarditis
(d) Tachycardia and other arrhythmias
(2) It is difficult to differentiate between the effect of the anemia and of the myocardial infiltration in the production of the symptoms.
  D. *Laboratory findings*
(1) There is cardiac enlargement on chest x-ray.
(2) The electrocardiogram shows nonspecific S-T, T wave abnormalities, and various arrhythmias, including conduction abnormalities.
  E. *Management and prognosis*
(1) Both parameters depend primarily on the type of leukemia and the response to chemotherapy.
(2) However, electrocardiographic abnormalities and cardiovascular symptoms tend to subside during clinical remissions of the disease.
  2. *Sickle cell anemia*
  A. *General features*
Cardiovascular problems in sickle cell anemia may result from:
(1) The anemia
(2) The cor pulmonale secondary to pulmonary vascular thrombosis
(3) The cardiomyopathy
  B. *Pathology*
There is biventricular hypertrophy with thrombosis of the small intracardiac blood vessels, and secondary myocardial degeneration.
  C. *Signs and symptoms*
(1) Dyspnea is common early in the clinical course, with congestive heart failure a late manifestation.
(2) Cardiac murmurs are frequent, in part related to the anemia.
  D. *Laboratory findings*
(1) The heart is often diffusely enlarged.
(2) The electrocardiogram is abnormal, but the changes are nonspecific.
  E. *Management and prognosis*

(1) Standard therapy is recommended for the congestive heart failure.
(2) The cardiovascular disease tends to be slowly progressive, but is accentuated during sickle-cell crises.
  3. *Polycythemia vera*
  A. *Pathology*
Myocardial infarction occurs frequently, probably related to coronary artery intravascular thrombosis.
  B. *Signs and symptoms*: Myocardial infarction and systemic hypertension are encountered.
  4. *Anaphylactoid purpura*
  A. *Pathology*: Myocardial arteriolar and capillary arteritis and periangitis are encountered.
  B. *Signs and symptoms*: Cardiac arrhythmias, retrosternal pain, and heart failure have been described.
  C. *Laboratory findings*
(1) The electrocardiogram may show atrial fibrillation, A-V block, A-V junctional arrhythmias, and nonspecific S-T, T wave changes.
(2) The ECG finding often resemble those of myocardial infarction.
  D. *Management*: The therapy of choice is corticosteriod hormone administration.

SARCOIDOSIS

  1. *General features*
  A. Cardiovascular involvement is frequent in sarcoidosis, particularly in younger patients.
  B. Cor pulmonale is the most common cardiovascular manifestation of systemic sarcoidosis.
  C. Myocardial involvement with sarcoid occurs equally in whites and in blacks, despite the predilection of the blacks to sarcoidosis.
  2. *Pathology and pathophysiology*
  A. Sarcoid granulomas of varying size occur in the myocardium, often impinging on the conduction system and heart valves.

B. Pericardial granulomas are less frequent.

3. *Signs and symptoms*

Common clinical presentations are:

A. Various cardiac arrhythmias including complete A-V block and other conduction abnormalities

    B. Cardiac enlargement

    C. Congestive heart failure

    D. Cardiac murmurs

4. *Laboratory findings*

    A. *Chest x-ray*

The cardiac enlargement varies with the degree of myocardial involvement, resultant congestive heart failure and valvular dysfunction.

    B. *Electrocardiography*

Electrocardiographic abnormalities are characteristically nonspecific, but may mimic myocardial infarction.

5. *Management and prognosis*

A. Corticosteriod hormone therapy is recommended for myocardial sarcoidosis.

B. Because of the high incidence of sudden cardiac death in myocardial sarcoid, permanent artificial pacemaker implantation should be considered for patients with high degree atrioventricular block.

C. Beta-adrenergic blocking agents may control apparent life-threatening tachyarrhythmias.

D. The congestive heart failure responds poorly to conventional therapy.

CHEMICAL AND TOXIC HYPERSENSITIVITY

1. *Ethyl alcohol*

    A. *General features*

(1) In addition to the high output cardiac failure of beriberi seen in the chronic alcoholic patient with severe nutritional deficiency, a toxic alcoholic cardiomyopathy may have two different presentations.

(2) The earlier phase characteristically occurs in obese, well-nourished, middle-aged men who habitually drink to excess, but who are not generally recognized as alcoholics.

(3) The late picture is that of a low cardiac output, chronic alcoholic cardiomyopathy.

    B. *Pathology and pathophysiology*

(1) In the early stages of alcoholic cardiomyopathy, left ventricular dysfunction, particularly depression of left ventricular contractility, is evident at cardiac catheterization.

(2) As the disease progresses, cardiac output decreases, intracardiac pressures and volumes become abnormally increased, and the ejection fraction is progressively depressed.

(3) The heart is dilated, with patchy necrosis and fibrosis, and there is left ventricular endocardial fibroelastosis with frequent mural thrombosis.

(4) At electron microscopy, extensive degeneration of the contractile elements and of the mitochondria is seen.

    C. *Signs and symptoms*

(1) The earliest symptoms of alcoholic cardiomyopathy are palpitations and breathlessness.

(2) Tachycardia occurs, with frequent ventricular ectopy and/or atrial fibrillation; sudden death has been reported.

(3) A corneal arcus, in the presence of a normal serum cholesterol level, suggests alcoholic cardiomyopathy in the young patient.

(4) In the late stage of the illness, the findings of severe left ventricular and then biventricular failure appear:

    (a) Cardiac enlargement

    (b) A narrow pulse pressure

    (c) Tachycardia

    (d) Atrial and ventricular gallop sounds

    (e) An abnormal left ventricular impulse

    (f) Murmurs of mitral and tricuspid regurgitation

(g) Edema and pericardial effusion may occur.

D. *Laboratory findings*

(1) *Chest x-ray*

(a) The heart size is normal early in the illness.

(b) As the disease progresses, there is increasing cardiomegaly, particularly left ventricular, with pulmonary congestion and pleural and pericardial effusions.

(2) *Electrocardiography*

(a) The characteristic early electrocardiographic abnormality, in addition to the sinus tachycardia, ectopic ventricular beats, and/or atrial fibrillation, is a cloven, spinous, dimpled, or narrowly inverted T wave.

(b) This T wave abnormality reflects disparity in the rate of repolarization, the same problem that predisposes to arrhythmias.

(c) Late in the disease, the electrocardiogram is abnormal, but nonspecific, with changes of left ventricular hypertrophy commonly encountered.

E. *Management and prognosis*

(1) Early in the illness, the management includes:

(a) Abstinence from alcohol

(b) A sodium-restricted and B-vitamin-supplemented diet

(c) Bedrest

These measures effect a dramatic regression of the clinical symptoms and the electrocardiographic abnormalities, but the illness recurs if alcohol intake is resumed.

(2) Even at this early stage, anticoagulant therapy is recommended because of the high incidence of pulmonary and peripheral thromboembolism and sudden cardiac death.

(3) In the late stage illness, the standard therapy for congestive heart failure and thromboembolic complications is only minimally effective.

(4) Even with bedrest and abstinence from alcohol, the clinical, electrocardiographic, and radiologic abnormalities fail to regress in the late stage.

(5) However, prolonged bedrest has been reported to effect a major improvement in some patients adhering to this regimen.

2. *Beer-drinker's cardiomyopathy*

A. *General features*

This fulminating toxic cardiomyopathy, due to a cobalt additive in beer, occurred primarily in individuals drinking excessive quantities of beer. Since cobalt is no longer added to beer, the syndrome may be only of historical interest. However, it illustrates the problem of cobalt cardiomyopathy.

B. *Pathology and pathophysiology*

(1) Cobalt interferes with the myocardial respiratory enzymes and results in myocardial dysfunction, which may proceed to heart failure, often with pericardial effusion.

(2) Myofiber vacuolation and degeneration occur, with damage to the contractile elements and mitochondria seen at electron microscopy.

C. *Signs and symptoms*

(1) Patients who drank excessive quantities of cobalt containing beer presented with:

(a) Anorexia

(b) Nausea

(c) Vomiting

(d) Subsequent sudden severe cardiac failure

(2) Early mortality was extremely high.

(3) The characteristic physical findings include:

(a) Facial and truncal cyanosis

(b) Hypotension

(c) Tachycardia

(d) Elevation of the jugular venous pressure

(e) Gallop sounds

(f) Edema

(g) Evidence of pericardial effusion

D. *Laboratory findings*

(1) *Chest x-ray and fluoroscopy*

(a) Cardiac enlargement is due both to the cardiomyopathy and the pericardial effusion.

(b) Cardiac pulsations are poor.

(2) *Electrocardiography*

The electrocardiogram is characteristic. In addition to the sinus tachycardia, the QRS voltage in the limb leads is low, nonspecific S-T segment and T wave changes and bizarre P waves are present.

E. *Management and prognosis*

(1) With abstinence from the cobalt-containing beer, the standard therapy for congestive heart failure, and administration of an adequate diet with thiamine and vitamin supplementation, there occurred a gradual regression of the heart failure, the cardiac enlargement, and the pericardial effusion.

(2) Electrocardiographic abnormalities resolved more slowly.

(3) The disease did not recur, in the patients who recovered, with subsequent beer drinking, once the cobalt additives had been removed.

(4) A number of patients had residual heart failure, and all of these had persistent electrocardiographic abnormalities.

3. *Arsenic*

A. *General features*

Arsenic trioxide poisoning is the most common cause of acute heavy metal poisoning.

B. *Pathology and pathophysiology*

Myocardial hypoxia results from interference with the respiratory enzymes; and subepicardial myocardial hemorrhages may occur.

C. *Signs and symptoms*: There are no clinical manifestations.

D. *Laboratory findings*: The electrocardiogram shows changes compatible with myocardial ischemia.

E. *Management and prognosis*

(1) Therapy with British anti-

lewisite (BAL) reverses the electrocardiographic abnormalities.

(2) There are no residual cardiovascular manifestations.

4. *Carbon monoxide*

A. *General features*

Damage from acute carbon monoxide poisoning is attributed to both of the following:

(1) The decreased oxygen-carrying capacity of the blood, with resultant hypoxemia

(2) A direct toxic effect of carbon monoxide on the myocardial mitochondria

B. *Pathology*

The subendocardium of the left ventricle, especially the area of the papillary muscles, shows hypoxemic lesions.

C. *Signs and symptoms*

Presenting complaints include:

(1) Dyspnea

(2) Palpitations

(3) The pain of angina pectoris and/or myocardial infarction

D. *Laboratory findings*

Ischemic S-T, T wave changes, various arrhythmias including conduction abnormalities are seen on the electrocardiogram.

E. *Management and prognosis*

(1) One hundred per cent oxygen should be administered.

(2) Hyperbaric oxygen and bedrest should be considered when there is electrocardiographic evidence of myocardial damage.

(3) Electrocardiographic changes only of ischemia usually resolve within a day or so.

5. *Lead*

A. *General features*

(1) Lead poisoning may be an occupational problem, or it may be encountered in moonshine-whiskey drinkers whose source of alcohol is a lead-contaminated still.

(2) Electrocardiographic evaluation should be part of the assessment of

all patients with chronic lead poisoning.

B. *Pathology and pathophysiology*

The anatomic changes are those of myocarditis, and the cardiac dysfunction may reflect both this direct toxic effect on the myocardium and/or the hypertension associated with lead nephropathy.

C. *Signs and symptoms*

(1) Chest pain and the symptoms of heart failure are described.

(2) Pulmonary edema is occasionally encountered.

D. *Laboratory findings*

Electrocardiographic alterations include:

(1) Nonspecific S-T, T wave abnormalities

(2) Sinus bradycardia

(3) A shortened P-R interval

(4) Occasionally, other arrhythmias

E. *Management and prognosis*

Therapy with ethylene diamine tetraacetic acid (EDTA) is usually associated with resolution of the cardiomyopathy and the electrocardiographic abnormalities.

PHYSICAL AGENTS AFFECTING THE CARDIOVASCULAR SYSTEM

1. *Radiation*

A. *General features*

Since the advent of high dosage radiation therapy for intrathoracic neoplasms, cardiovascular manifestations are encountered with increasing frequency as the therapy becomes more widespread and patient survival increases.

B. *Pathology and pathophysiology*

(1) The myocardium tends to be radiation-resistant.

(2) However, coronary artery narrowing secondary to radiation has resulted in myocardial infarction.

(3) Pericardial fibrosis is the most common problem, although endocardial fibrosis and valve damage may produce cardiac murmurs.

(4) Conduction system fibrosis has resulted in complete A-V block.

C. *Signs and symptoms*

The usual symptoms are those of pericarditis, often with pain and occasionally with the picture of acute tamponade or constrictive pericarditis.

D. *Laboratory findings*

(1) Cardiac catheterization and pericardiocentesis are often necessary to differentiate between radiation effusion and malignant effusion, and to determine whether constrictive pericarditis is present.

(2) The electrocardiographic abnormalities of pericarditis are usually transient.

E. *Management*

(1) Pericardiocentesis is often indicated, and on rare occasions, surgery for constrictive pericarditis.

(2) The role of corticosteroid hormones remains controversial.

(3) Acute pericarditis may progress to pericardial constriction.

2. *Trauma*

For discussion of trauma as it affects the cardiovascular system, see Chapter 15.

COMPLICATIONS OF ORAL CONTRACEPTIVE USE

1. *Pathophysiology*

A. The major problem with oral contraceptive use appears to be related to estrogen effect.

B. Estrogen increases platelet stickiness and inhibits fibrinolysis, increasing the tendency to intravascular thrombosis, particularly in a setting of venous stasis.

C. Estrogen also decreases vascular smooth muscle tone, increasing the predisposition to venous stasis, particularly in the lower extremities.

D. Additionally, estrogen and progesterone effects on the renin-angiotensin-aldosterone system may predispose to hypertension.

E. The possibility of myocardial infarction seems to be increased and this may relate to the acceleration of normal atherogenesis; to the associated hypertension, hyperglycemia, and hyperlipidema; or to local intimal changes that, associated with an increase in platelet function, result in thrombus formation.

2. *Specific complications*

A. *Hypertension*

(1) Hypertension occurs in a small percentage of patients taking oral contraceptive drugs, is characteristically mild, and usually disappears when oral contraceptive use is stopped.

(2) It occurs more commonly with the estrogen compounds of higher dosage.

(3) The exact mechanism remains speculative.

B. *Cerebral vascular occlusion*

(1) There is an increased incidence of cerebral arterial occlusion and cerebral venous thrombosis with the use of oral contraceptive agents.

(2) They are not recommended for patients with a history of migraine headaches or other neurologic events, particularly transient ischemic episodes.

C. *Acute myocardial infarction*

(1) There is an increased occurrence of acute myocardial infarction, particularly in women over age 40.

(2) Current recommendations are that an alternate form of contraception be considered for patients in this age group.

D. *Venous thrombosis and pulmonary embolism*

(1) The question still remains whether pulmonary thromboembolism is increased with oral contraceptive use, although there is a definite increase in the incidence of leg deep-vein thrombosis.

(2) Patients with a history of thrombophlebitis and/or pulmonary embolism should not receive oral contraceptive agents.

(3) Pulmonary embolism appears more common with estrogen compounds of higher dosage.

CARDIOVASCULAR COMPLICATIONS OF DRUG ABUSE

1. *Cardiac complications of heroin (opiate) overdose*

A. *Pathophysiology*

(1) Heroin pulmonary edema may reflect the hypoxia of respiratory depression, a direct opiate effect, or an allergic response to impurities in the opiate preparation.

(2) The combination of hypoxia and intravenous impurities may also produce cardiac arrhythmias.

B. *Signs and symptoms*

(1) There is loss of consciousness, with respiratory depression which progresses to apnea.

(2) Cyanosis, pinpoint pupils, loss of reflexes, and pulmonary edema without congestive heart failure are seen.

C. *Management and prognosis*

(1) Nalorphine therapy, intubation, and oxygen administration are indicated.

(2) Arrhythmias respond to standard management.

(3) A favorable outcome is usual.

2. *Thrombophlebitis with and without pulmonary embolization*

This common complication of intravenous drug abuse may also result in mycotic aneurysms, secondary to infected emboli.

3. *Bacterial endocarditis* (see also Chap. 7)

A. *Pathophysiology:* Right-sided endocarditis is frequent.

B. *Signs and symptoms*

The clinical findings are of septic pulmonary emboli and tricuspid and occasionally pulmonic valvular insufficiency.

4. *Cardiac arrhythmias*

A. These occur with glue and

solvent sniffing; sudden death is not infrequent.

B. Phenothiazine and other psychotropic agents are also associated with both a high incidence of arrhythmias and frequent electrocardiographic abnormalities.

C. Amphetamine compounds may produce both arrhythmias and hypertension.

5. *Pulmonary hypertension secondary to intravascular thrombosis*

A. *Pathophysiology*

Arterial and capillary thrombosis, usually secondary to intravenous talc or starch particles, produce this problem.

B. *Laboratory findings*

The chest x-ray shows a characteristic interstitial reticulondoular infiltrate.

MISCELLANEOUS SYSTEMIC SYNDROMES

1. *Progeria*

A. *Hutchinson-Gilford syndrome*

(1) In previously healthy infants who develop premature aging, the cardiovascular complications are primarily those of accelerated atherosclerosis.

(2) Hypertension, myocardial infarction, heart failure, cerebrovascular accident and premature death, usually cardiovascular in origin, occur.

B. *Werner's syndrome*

Adult progeria is similarly characterized by severe atherosclerosis with resultant myocardial infarction and cerebrovascular accident.

2. *Rejection cardiomyopathy*

A. *General features*

This new clinical syndrome is seen in the cardiac transplantation patient. The exact mechanism is not understood.

B. *Pathology*

Myocardial abnormalities include:

(1) A fibrinoid and necrotizing arteritis

(2) Myofiber damage

(3) Edema

(4) A mononuclear cellular infiltrate

C. *Signs and symptoms*

(1) Cardiac enlargement is due both to dilatation and to pericardial effusion.

(2) There is decreased exercise tolerance and early heart failure.

(3) Some patients, however, may be asymptomatic.

D. *Laboratory findings*

(1) The sedimentation rate is elevated.

(2) Decreased electrocardiographic voltage is a characteristic finding.

(3) Early abnormalities may be detected on endomyocardial (transcatheter) biopsy.

E. *Management and prognosis*

Response to immunosuppressive and corticosteroid hormone therapy is associated with an improvement in cardiac function.

3. *Rheumatoid disease*

A. *General features*

Rheumatoid heart disease is more frequent in the patient with long-standing rheumatoid arthritis.

B. *Pathology and pathophysiology*

(1) Rheumatoid granulomas occur in the myocardium, the epicardium, and at the bases of the cardiac valves.

(2) Pericarditis is encountered in almost 50 per cent of the cases at postmortem examination.

(3) Clinical manifestations of pericardial effusion, tamponade, or constrictive disease are less frequent.

(4) Small artery coronary arteritis is not uncommon.

C. *Signs and symptoms*

(1) The pericardial disease is usually asymptomatic.

(2) Heart failure and valvular insufficiency, particularly aortic insufficiency, may be encountered.

(3) Cardiac arrhythmias, particu-

larly complete A-V block, have been attributed to rheumatoid nodules infiltrating the interventricular septum.

D. *Management and prognosis*

(1) Artificial pacemaker therapy has been of value in patients with complete A-V block.

(2) Pericardiocentesis may be indicated for the pericardial effusion, as may pericardiectomy for constrictive pericarditis.

(3) The heart failure and other arrhythmias respond to standard management.

4. *Ankylosing spondylitis*

A. *General features*

Cardiovascular complications occur late in the course of this illness, more commonly in the older patient with extensive peripheral joint involvement.

B. *Pathology and pathophysiology*

The aortic valve and the aortic root are involved by focal medial inflammation, arteritis, and subsequent fibrosis, which often extends into the interventricular septum to involve the conduction system.

C. *Signs and symptoms*

(1) Aortic regurgitation is characteristic.

(2) Both atrioventricular and intraventricular conduction defects are frequent, at times occurring before the evidence of valvular dysfunction.

(3) Cardiomyopathy and congestive heart failure have also been described.

D. *Laboratory findings*

Considerable prolongation of the P-R interval and intraventricular conduction disturbances are common.

E. *Management and prognosis*

(1) Artificial pacemaker implantation has, at times, controlled the complete A-V block.

(2) Other arrhythmias are treated in the usual fashion.

5. *Reiter's disease*

A. *General features*

Cardiac involvement is seen in the pa-

tient with recurrent episodes of the illness.

B. *Pathology*

(1) The aortic valve is most commonly involved, with thickening and rolling of the valve cusps and valve ring dilatation.

(2) Myocarditis and pericarditis may also occur.

C. *Signs and symptoms*

(1) The murmur of aortic regurgitation is frequent.

(2) The pain and rub of pericarditis may be encountered.

(3) Evidence of congestive heart failure may be present.

D. *Laboratory findings*

(1) The electrocardiographic abnormalities are nonspecific.

(2) The ECG findings may include first degree A-V block progressing to complete heart block and intraventricular conduction disturbances.

E. *Management*

(1) Heart failure and rhythm disturbances require the standard therapeutic approach.

(2) Corticosteroid hormones may control the pericarditis.

6. *Marfan's syndrome*

A. *General features*

This heritable disorder of connective tissue is inherited as an autosomal dominant, but variable degrees of severity are evident.

B. *Pathology and pathophysiology*

(1) Aortic medial cystic necrosis, often with aneurysm or dissection; valve cusp deformity with redundant chordae tendineae and resultant valvular abnormalities; and pulmonary artery dilatation and/or dissection are encountered.

(2) Myocardial and coronary artery cystic and noncystic medial degeneration are probably the basis for the conduction abnormalities and the sudden cardiac deaths.

(3) Thoracic skeletal deformities may contribute to the cardiovascular symptomatology.

C. *Signs and symptoms*

(1) The clinical presentation may be of:

(a) Aortic dissection

(b) Pulmonary artery dissection

(c) More rarely, coronary artery dissection

(2) Aortic regurgitation is frequent.

(3) Mitral regurgitation is also encountered.

(4) The hemodynamic severity is variable.

(5) Cardiac arrhythmias, secondary to sinus and A-V node artery abnormalities, probably explain the sudden cardiac deaths.

D. *Laboratory findings*

(1) The cardiac silhouette on chest x-ray varies considerably with the degree of aortic, aortic and mitral valve, and myocardial involvement.

(2) The electrocardiogram frequently shows arrhythmias, including conduction abnormalities.

E. *Management and prognosis*

(1) The management for aortic dissection, congestive heart failure, and arrhythmias follows standard guidelines.

(2) Valve replacement may be required.

(3) Endocarditis prophylaxis is important.

(4) Many patients with Marfan's syndrome with cardiovascular involvement have minimal and often asymptomatic disease at times detected only at a routine clinical examination.

7. *Pseudoxanthoma elasticum* (Gronblad-Strandberg syndrome)

A. *General features*

Cardiac abnormalities are unusual in this heritable connective tissue disorder.

B. *Pathology*

(1) Endocardial fibroelastosis may extend onto the heart valves and entrap the cardiac conduction system.

(2) The myocardial arteries have a fragmented and calcified elastica.

C. *Signs and symptoms*

The clinical presentations may be of:

(1) Cardiac enlargement with heart failure

(2) The murmurs of valve deformity

(3) Arrhythmias including those resulting in Stokes-Adams syncope.

D. *Management*: There is no specific therapy.

8. *Ehler-Danlos syndrome*

A. *General features*

This collagen-vascular disorder is inherited as an autosomal dominant.

B. *Pathology*

(1) Redundant chordae tendineae and valvular abnormalities may result in aortic and mitral valve disease.

(2) Aortic dissection and spontaneous arterial rupture are described.

C. *Signs and symptoms*

Aortic and mitral valve murmurs, heart failure, and the picture of aortic dissection occur.

D. *Management*: There is no specific therapy.

9. *Wegener's granulomatosis*

A. *Pathology*

The myocardial lesions include necrotizing vasculitis, fibrinoid degeneration, and granulomatous lesions.

B. *Signs and symptoms*

Cardiac enlargement, heart failure, and pericarditis with effusion have been described.

C. *Management*: Standard therapy for these entities is recommended.

10. *Lentiginosis*

A. *Pathology and pathophysiology*

(1) Progressive, massive atrioventricular septal hypertrophy results in bilateral outflow tract obstruction.

(2) The cardiomyopathy is often mild at onset, but increases in severity.

(3) Because skin melanin and myocardial norepinephrine are chemically related, an enzymatic or precursor substance defect has been suggested as etiologic.

B. *Signs and symptoms*

(1) The patient may present increasing severity of cardiomyopathy, with bilateral outflow tract obstruction.

(2) At times, increase in the disease severity is associated with an increase in the number of lentiform moles.

(3) Cardiac murmurs may be heard.

C. *Laboratory findings*: Electrocardiographic abnormalities are nonspecific.

D. *Management and prognosis*

(1) Surgical septectomy is often recommended.

(2) Propranolol therapy is effective to manage the outflow tract obstruction.

11. *Q-T Interval syndrome*

For discussion of cardiovascular complications of Q-T Interval syndrome, see Chapter 31.

SUGGESTED READINGS

Bailey, G. L., Hampers, C. L., and Merrill, J. P.: Reversible cardiomyopathy in uremia. Trans. Am. Soc. Artif. Intern. Organs, *13*:263, 1967.

Baker, G. et al.: Pheochromocytoma without hypertension presenting as cardiomyopathy. Am. Heart J., *83*:688, 1972.

Barth, W. F.: Amyloidosis: review of cardiac and renal manifestations. Med. Ann. D.C., *36*:228, 266, 1967.

Biran, S., Hochmann, A., and Stern, S.: Therapeutic irradiation of the chest and electrocardiographic changes. Clin. Radiol., *20*:433, 1969.

Bottiger, L. E., and Edhag, O.: Heart block in ankylosing spondylitis and uropolyarthritis. Br. Heart J., *34*:487, 1972.

Collaborative Group for the Study of Stroke in Young Women: Oral contraceptives and stroke in young women: associated risk factors. J.A.M.A., *231*:718, 1975.

Ehlers, K. H. et al.: Glycogen-storage disease of the myocardium with obstruction to left ventricular outflow. Circulation, *25*:96, 1962.

Ghosh, P. et al.: Myocardial sarcoidosis. Br. Heart J., *34*:769, 1972.

Hamolsky, M. W., Kurland, G. S., and Freedberg, A. S.: The heart in hypothyroidism. J. Chronic Dis., *14*:558, 1961.

Hejtmancik, M. et al.: The cardiovascular manifestations of systemic lupus erythematosus. Am. Heart J., *68*:119, 1964.

Jaffe, R. B. and Koschmann, E. B.: Intravenous drug abuse, pulmonary, cardiac, and vascular complications. Am. J. Roentgenol., *109*:107, 1970.

James, T. N. and Fisch, C.: Observations on the cardiovascular involvement in Friedreich's ataxia. Am. Heart J., *66*:164, 1963.

Krovetz, L. J., Lorinez, A. E., and Schiebler, G. I.: Cardiovascular manifestations of the Hurler syndrome: hemodynamic and angiocardiographic observation in 15 patients. Circulation, *31*:132, 1965.

Leonard, J. J. and DeGroot, W. J.: The thyroid state and the cardiovascular system. Mod. Concepts Cardiovasc. Dis., *38*:23, 1969.

McKusick, V. A.: A genetical view of cardiovascular disease. Circulation, *30*:326, 1964.

Morin, Y., Tetu, A., and Mercier, G.: Cobalt cardiomyopathy: clinical aspects. Br. Heart J., *33*:175, 1971.

Perloff, J. K., DeLeon, A. C., Jr. and O'Doherty, D.: The cardiomyopathy of progressive muscular dystrophy. Circulation, *33*:625, 1966.

Perloff, J. K., Lindgren, K. M. and Groves, B. M.: Uncommon or commonly unrecognized causes of heart failure. Prog. Cardiovasc. Dis., *12*:409, 1970.

Riley, T. R. et al.: Werner's syndrome. Ann. Intern. Med., *63*:285, 1965.

Roberts, W. C., Bodey, G. P., and Wertlake, P. T.: The heart in acute leukemia: a study of 420 autopsy cases. Am. J. Cardiol., *21*:388, 1968.

Sachner, M., Heinz, E., and Steinberg, A.: The heart in scleroderma. Am. J. Cardiol., *17*:542, 1966.

Shanoff, H. M.: Alcoholic cardiomyopathy: an introductory review. Can. Med. Assoc. J., *106*:55, 1972.

Shapiro, S.: Oral contraception and myocardial infarction. N. Engl. J. Med., *293*:195, 1975.

Somerville, J. and Bonham-Carter, R. E.: The heart in lentiginosis. Br. Heart J., *34*:58, 1972.

Uzsoy, N. K.: Cardiovascular findings in patients with sickle cell anemia. Am. J. Cardiol., *13*:320, 1964.

Vessey, M. P. et al.: Investigation of relation between use of oral contraceptives and thromboembolic disease. A further report. Br. Med. J., *2*:651, 1969.

Wasserman, A. J. et al.: Cardiac hemochromatosis simulating constrictive pericarditis. Am. J. Med., *32*:316, 1962.

18. DRUG-INDUCED CARDIOVASCULAR DISORDERS

James P. O'Neil, M.D., and Edward K. Chung, M.D.

GENERAL CONSIDERATIONS

As improved and more effective drugs are produced, the price has to be paid in drug-induced adverse effects. It is unfortunate that there are no harmless drugs, and all physicians are becoming more and more aware of this fact. Consumer groups, the Federal government, and the courts have also become concerned about iatrogenic diseases because of increasing incidence of such events.

It is not the purpose of this chapter to discuss the side effects and toxicity of all drugs, but rather to describe adverse effects on the cardiovascular system due to commonly used drugs. These drugs will be discussed according to the following classification: cardioactives, antihypertensives, diuretics, anesthetics, hormones, antineoplastic agents, autonomics, and central nervous system (CNS) stimulants and depressants.

1. *Cardioactive drugs*
   A. *Digitalis*
   (1) Of the cardioactive drugs, digitalis is the most widely used and best known to produce adverse cardiovascular effects.
   (2) The toxicity is identical or very similar for the various digitalis preparations.
   (3) It can be said that digitalis intoxication is probably the most common drug-induced disorder encountered in our practice.
   (4) It is also true that digitalis toxicity is one of the most common causes to produce almost every known type of cardiac arrhythmias. (Detailed description of digitalis toxicity is found in Chap. 23.)

B. *Quinidine*
   (1) Quinidine is well known to depress myocardial contractility. This is a dose-related phenomenon, but in an occasional patient, may be present in low dosage and necessitate withdrawal of the drug.
   (2) Hypotension during quinidine therapy is due principally to a direct vasodilating effect although a decreased cardiac output due to a depression of myocardial contractility is a contributory factor. This again is most often dose-related and especially hazardous when given parenterally.
   (3) Sinus arrest, sinoatrial block, ventricular tachycardia, ventricular fibrillation, complete A-V block and atrial or ventricular standstill are also dose-related adverse side effects. The above toxic manifestations of quinidine often follow such signs of mild toxicity as prolongation of the P-R interval and widening of the QRS complex.
   (4) Syncope or sudden death during quinidine therapy is most likely due to the initiation of ventricular tachycardia or fibrillation from the R-on-T phenomenon (Fig. 18-1). The R-on-T phenomenon is commonly observed during quinidine therapy because the drug produces wide T wave with prolonged Q-T interval. Unusual hypersensitive reaction to quinidine has also been considered in some cases with quinidine syncope.
   (5) Atrial flutter with 2:1 A-V response may become 1:1 A-V conduction by quinidine when digitalis is not given simultaneously. This is observed because A-V conduction is accelerated and the atrial rate slows by quinidine.

273

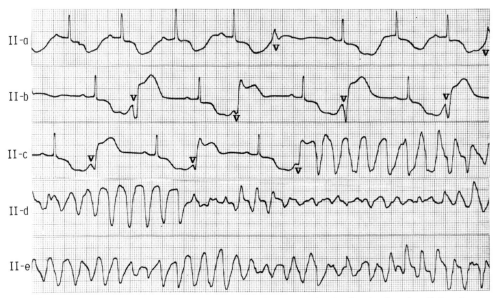

Fig. 18-1. Leads II-a, b, c, d and e are continuous. The basic rhythm is slight sinus bradycardia (rate: 58 beats per minute) with first degree A-V block (The P-R interval: 0.24 second). Ventricular fibrillation is provoked by the R-on-T phenomenon when the ventricular premature beat (marked V) is superimposed during the vulnerable period. The R-on-T phenomenon is observed because of markedly prolonged Q-T interval with very large T wave due to quinidine.

C. *Procainamide (Pronestyl)*

(1) Procainamide closely resembles quinidine in such toxic effects as depression of myocardial contractility and hypotension and is dose-related.

(2) Arrhythmias induced by procainamide resemble those due to quinidine and again are preceded by similar electrocardiographic evidence of toxicity.

(3) Syncope or sudden death due to procainamide is unusual.

(4) Widening of the QRS complex is much more common in procainamide toxicity.

(5) The widening of the QRS complex in procainamide toxicity is usually due to diffuse and nonspecific intraventricular block rather than left or right bundle branch block.

(6) Precipitation of a lupus-like syndrome may cause pericarditis and even pericardial tamponade in patients with even relatively small doses.

D. *Lidocaine (Xylocaine)*

(1) Toxicity of lidocaine is relatively uncommon, but caution should be employed in the repeated use of the drug in patients with severe liver or renal disease because accumulation may lead to toxicity. This is because the drug is metabolized primarily in the liver and excreted by the kidney.

(2) Lidocaine should also be administered with caution in patients with hypovolemia and shock because the drug may aggravate the existing problems.

(3) Lidocaine often produces cardiorespiratory depression.

(4) Lidocaine may aggravate the pre-existing cardiac arrhythmias such as sinoatrial block, sinus arrest, sinus bradycardia, A-V block and/or intraventricular block.

(5) Marked sinus bradycardia (rate: 14–20 beats per minute) following a small (50 mg.) intravenous injection of lidocaine has been reported.

E. *Diphenylhydantoin (Dilantin)*

(1) Diphenylhydantoin toxicity is relatively uncommon unless very large dosages are used.

(2) Diphenylhydantoin, like lidocaine, procainamide, and quinidine, may produce cardiac and respiratory depression.

(3) Untoward cardiovascular effects of diphenylhydantoin may include hypotension, marked sinus bradycardia, S-A or A-V block of varying degrees.

F. *Propranolol (Inderal)*

(1) The cardiac effects of propranolol are a combination of depression in the myocardial excitability and contractility and blockade of cardiac beta receptors.

(2) The most frequent untoward effect of propranolol is slowing of heart rate, particularly marked sinus bradycardia. It can be said that sinus bradycardia is most commonly due to propranolol at present.

(3) Propranolol may also produce sinus arrest, S-A block, and varying degree A-V block, and in certain cases, propranolol-induced arrhythmias may be fatal.

(4) Hypotension is commonly produced by propranolol, especially when large doses are used because of negative inotropic action of the drug. For the treatment of hypotension large amounts of isoproterenol (Isuprel) or glucagon may be required to reverse it.

(5) The development of pulmonary edema, congestive heart failure, or shock during propranolol therapy is not uncommon in patients with advanced heart disease.

(6) Recent clinical experiences indicate that it is difficult to resuscitate during cardiac surgery when the patient is taking relatively large amounts of propranolol. Therefore, it is recommended to discontinue propranolol 2 to 3 days prior to the surgery.

(7) The development of acute myocardial infarction following abrupt discontinuation of propranolol has been reported recently. Thus, a gradual reduction of propranolol is recommended when the drug has to be discontinued.

G. *Glucagon*

(1) The cardiotonic properties of glucagon have been useful in the treatment of acute myocardial infarction and cardiogenic shock.

(2) Large doses of glucagon by intravenous injection may produce small pulmonary emboli.

(3) Glucagon-induced ventricular tachycardia and fibrillation have been reported.

(4) The property of glucagon to promote catecholamine synthesis and storage may lead to the development of cardiac arrhythmias.

(5) In addition, small pulmonary emboli produced by glucagon may also provoke cardiac arrhythmias.

H. *Bretylium tosylate*

(1) Bretylium tosylate has been found to be effective in the prevention and treatment of supraventricular as well as ventricular tachyarrhythmias.

(2) Some investigators have proposed that the drug is found to be the agent of choice for ventricular tachyarrhythmias, particularly in acute myocardial infarction.

(3) However, marked supine hypotension frequently develops in patients treated with bretylium tosylate.

(4) The occurrence of supine hypotension was found to be well correlated with a poor initial hemodynamic state.

(5) Occasionally, hypotensive episodes may be associated with ventricular premature beats.

(6) Bretylium tosylate is not recommended for routine use in the preven-

tion of ventricular arrhythmias associated with acute myocardial infarction because of the substantial and unpredictable circulatory effects of the drug.

I. *Verapamil*

(1) Verapamil (intravenous route) has been found to be effective in the treatment of supraventricular tachycardia.

(2) Prolongation of the A-V nodal conduction appears to play an important role as an antiarrhythmic agent.

(3) It has been suggested that the antiarrhythmic effect of verapamil may be related to its action in blocking the movement of ionized calcium across the myocardial cell membrane and this property may constitute a new, fourth class antiarrhythmic action.

(4) In spite of the antiarrhythmic property of verapamil, the drug may provoke ventricular tachyarrhythmias including frequent ventricular premature contractions and ventricular tachycardia.

2. *Drugs affecting the autonomic nervous system*

A. *Sympathetic catecholamines*

(1) *General features*

(a) In discussing catecholamines it is useful to divide them into those that have primarily alpha stimulation, beta stimulation, or a mixture of both.

(b) From the cardiovascular standpoint, alpha stimulation causes vasoconstriction of small arterioles, arteries, and veins with a resultant elevation of intravascular pressure, especially in the vascular beds of the skin, kidney, and splanchnic region.

(c) Beta stimulation causes vasodilatation in the same areas, although to a variable degree. Its direct cardiac effect is to increase contractility (inotropism), increase pacemaker automaticity (chronotropism) and increase conduction in the A-V node. Induction of ectopic arrhythmias by catechola-

mines is due primarily to the amount of beta stimulation which that particular drug possesses.

(d) Of the naturally occurring amines, epinephrine and norepinephrine have combined alpha and beta stimulation with epinephrine's beta effect predominating and norepinephrine's alpha effect predominating.

(e) The synthetic vasopressors, phenylephrine and methoxamine, have no direct cardiac effect since they stimulate only alpha receptors, although cardiac slowing can occur through reflex vagal stimulation.

(f) The synthetic beta stimulators are isoproterenol, mephenteramine, and metaraminol.

(g) A less commonly known effect on the heart is the anatomic damage to heart muscle and to blood vessels.

(2) *Untoward effects*

(a) Catecholamines may induce various tachyarrhythmias, particularly ventricular ones.

(b) Necrosis and fibrosis of the myocardium due to epinephrine infusion have been shown in the laboratory and in man. The exact cause is unclear.

(c) An indirect cause of atherosclerosis due to catecholamines is felt to be due to ultrafiltration of plasma into vessel walls and by the increase in turbulence around areas of vessel branching.

(d) Another possible deleterious action of catecholamines is the relation of catecholamines to intravascular clotting, which is felt to be the earliest stage of arteriosclerotic plaques.

B. *Parasympathomimetic drugs*

(1) Edrophonium chloride (Tensilon), which is a rapid acting anticholinesterase drug of short duration, has been used in the treatment of paroxysmal supraventricular tachyarrhythmias.

(2) Edrophonium chloride, however, may produce bradyarrhythmias including marked sinus bradycardia and A-V block.

(3) On rare occasions, ventricular

standstill (arrest) may be produced by edrophonium chloride.

    C. *Autonomic blocking drugs*

        (1) Atropine sulfate (intravenous injection) and related drugs have been commonly used in the treatment of bradyarrhythmias, especially marked sinus bradycardia, during acute myocardial infarction.

        (2) Atropine sulfate may, however, induce ventricular tachyarrhythmias, and even fatal ventricular fibrillation.

        (3) Small doses of atropine (≤ 0.4 mg.) may produce parodoxical sinus slowing.

        (4) In addition, atropine sulfate has been reported to increase the area of ischemia in acute myocardial infarction immediately following intravenous injection.

        (5) On rare occasions, atropine may precipitate re-entrant (reciprocating) atrial tachycardia through facilitation of A-V nodal conduction.

        (6) Therefore, atropine should be used with caution during acute myocardial infarction only when the hemodynamic situation clearly warrants its use and/or when a serious bradyarrhythmia exists.

    3. *Antihypertensive drugs*

    A. Drugs that reduce arterial blood pressure may produce symptoms due to hypotension, especially on sudden standing (postural hypotension).

    B. The most common untoward effect of various antihypertensive drugs such as reserpine (Serpasil), methyldopa (Aldomet) and guanethidine (Ismelin) is marked sinus bradycardia. Reserpine may also produce increased sensitivity to vagal stimuli, A-V block, and various other arrhythmias.

    C. Antihypertensive drugs may inactivate the baroreceptors, the carotid sinuses and aortic arch, and produce sinus tachycardia, which may aggravate symptoms of coronary insufficiency.

    D. Fluid retention can be trouble-some with the majority of antihypertensives if not administered with a diuretic.

Hydralazine, ganglionic blocking agents such as trimethaphan (Arfonad), alpha-methyldopa, guanethidine, and diazoxide (Hyperstat) exhibit these cardiovascular side effects to various degrees.

    4. *Diuretic drugs*

    A. Thiazides and the more potent "loop" diuretics such as furosemide (Lasix) and ethacrynic acid (Edecrin) may cause severe fluid shifts and produce hypotension, hyponatremia, hypokalemia, hypochloremia, and alkalosis.

    B. The adverse side effects of diuretics are related entirely to the hypovolemia and electrolyte disturbances that result from administration.

    C. The most important and the most frequent side effect of diuretics is hypokalemia, which commonly predisposes to digitalis-induced arrhythmias (see Chap. 23).

    D. Hypokalemia induced by diuretics may also produce various cardiac arrhythmias.

    5. *Hormones*

There is significant controversy regarding cardiovascular disorders produced by hormones, but there appears to be a definite relationship between some hormonal preparations and cardiovascular disease.

    A. *Oral contraceptives*

There is a well known relationship between oral contraceptives and thromboembolism. However, the less well known fact is the increasing incidence of coronary heart disease and strokes in women on oral contraceptives.

A recent report (see Suggested Readings, Lehrman 1976) described the occurrence of pulmonary embolism in a healthy man taking estrogen to alter his secondary sex characteristics. The exact relationship between the thromboembolic phenomenon and contraceptives is not clearly understood. Mild elevations of blood pressure may be caused by oral contraceptives.

High incidence of liver-cell adenomas associated with the use of oral contraceptives has been reported recently.

   B. *Thyroid preparations*

Thyroid preparations are known to precipitate myocardial infarction, especially when given parenterally to the myxedematous patient with coronary artery disease.

   C. *Hypoglycemic agents*

Controversy still exists concerning the increased risk of cardiovascular disease associated with the use of sulfonylureas such as tolbutamide.

   6. *Antineoplastic agents*

   A. *Doxorubicin hydrochloride (Adriamycin)*

Doxorubicin hydrochloride has received wide publicity concerning its cardiotoxicity. Tachycardia, hypotension, and congestive heart failure have all been reported in patients treated with adriamycin. This toxic effect appears to be dose-related.

   B. *Other antineoplastic agents*

There has been experimental work suggesting that other antineoplastic agents such as amphotericin B and 5-fluorocytosine can be toxic to the heart, but this has not been proven in man.

   7. *General anesthetics*

Nearly all the commonly used anesthetics can cause cardiac arrhythmias.

   A. *Halothane*

   (1) Arrhythmias due to halothane have been reported to range from 32 to 66 per cent. The incidence tended to increase if the patient was taking digitalis.

   (2) It is known that halothane has a direct stimulant action on the beta receptors in the heart, which probably accounts for the wide variety of arrhythmias produced by this anesthetic.

   B. *Barbiturates*

Intravenous barbiturates can produce various tachyarrhythmias by releasing epinephrine.

   C. *Ketamine*

Ketamine, which is a widely used anesthetic, causes a release of catecholamines, specifically norepinephrine, which can cause blood pressure elevation.

   D. *Curareform drugs*

   (1) Curareform drugs such as succinylcholine and d-tubocurarine can produce brady- or tachyarrhythmias.

   (2) All the curareform drugs can have complex interactions with other drugs that might be used during anesthesia.

   8. *Central nervous system (CNS) stimulants and depressants*

   A. *Amphetamine*

   (1) Amphetamine has powerful CNS stimulant actions in addition to the peripheral alpha and beta actions common to sympathomimetic drugs.

   (2) Amphetamine raises both systolic and diastolic blood pressure with increased pulse pressure.

   (3) Heart rate is often reflexly slowed.

   (4) Cardiac arrhythmias may develop when large doses are given.

   B. *Tricyclic antidepressants*

   (1) Tricyclic antidepressants frequently cause various tachyarrhythmias.

   (2) The incidence of other arrhythmias is increased when imipramine and amitriptyline are used, even in therapeutic doses when the patient is taking digitalis.

   (3) The development of 2:1 A-V block in a patient with right bundle branch block during imipramine therapy has been reported.

   C. *Levodopa*

   (1) Levodopa can cause various cardiac arrhythmias in approximately 10 per cent of patients (most commonly with parkinsonism) who are taking this drug.

   (2) Atrial arrhythmias are most common during levodopa therapy.

   (3) This can be decreased substantially if a decarboxylase inhibitor is used concomitantly.

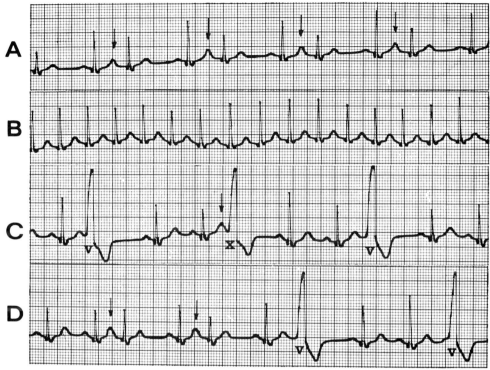

Fig. 18-2. Holter monitor rhythm strips during Atromid-S therapy show sinus rhythm with atrial as well as ventricular premature contractions (strips A, C, D) and paroxysmal atrial tachycardia (strip B). Rhythm strips A, B, C and D are *not* continuous. Note that all atrial premature contractions show aberrant ventricular conduction.

9. *Miscellaneous drugs*

   A. *Clofibrate (Atromid S)*

   (1) Clofibrate (Atromid S), which is used to lower serum lipid levels, has been reported to have caused various supraventricular as well as ventricular arrhythmias (Fig. 18-2).

   (2) Clofibrate-induced arrhythmias have been reported to be difficult to control with the usual antiarrhythmic agents.

   (3) It therefore should be considered a potential arrhythmia-inducing agent and should be withdrawn if this occurs after beginning the drug.

   (4) The fundamental mechanism responsible for the genesis of cardiac arrhythmias during clofibrate therapy is not well understood.

   (5) It has been reported that an-gina may be increased or decreased during clofibrate therapy.

   (6) Clofibrate has been found to act synergistically with anticoagulants of the coumarin series.

   B. *Aminophylline and related compounds*

   (1) Aminophylline and related compounds used in various bronchodilators can lower the threshold for ventricular fibrillation as well as induce other tachyarrhythmias.

   (2) In large intravenous boluses, they can have a hypotensive effect.

   C. *Anticoagulants*

   Anticoagulants have no true cardiovascular toxicity other than their inducement of a hemmorrhagic diathesis. They have been reported to have caused cardiac tamponade when associated with some underlying conditions such as myocardial infarction, pericarditis, or cardiac trauma.

D. *Iodide*

Recently, there has been a report indicating cardiac irritability during acute iodide intoxication. Namely, a 54-year-old male developed frequent ventricular premature contractions producing ventricular bigeminy and ventricular group beats following accidental ingestion of large amounts of iodide. Ventricular arrhythmias, in iodide intoxication, did subside after saline diuresis with consequent reduction of the serum iodide level.

E. *Fluorescein*

Recently, it has been observed that a patient (64-year-old woman) developed acute diaphragmatic (inferior) myocardial infarction soon after the intravenous injection of fluorescein. The exact mechanism for the development of acute myocardial infarction following fluorescein angiography is not clearly understood. Two cases of cardiac arrest following fluorescein injection had been reported previously.

F. *Diazepam*

Diazepam, which is an antianxiety agent, has been used (intravenous injection) frequently for direct current shock or bronchoscopy. The development of ventricular arrhythmias following intravenous injection of diazepam has been reported during or after cardioversion. Diazepam may produce hypotension.

G. *Heroin*

(1) Heroin overdosage is a relatively common problem in our practice. Very serious consequences of heroin overdosage include acute pulmonary edema and acute respiratory failure. Fortunately, most patients respond satisfactorily to narcotic antagonists, intubation, mechanical ventilation, oxygen therapy, digitalis, and diuretic therapy.

(2) In addition, heroin overdosage may also produce various cardiac ar-

rhythmias, gallop rhythm, cardiac enlargement, elevated central venous pressure and reduction of cardiac output.

SUGGESTED READINGS

Aviado, D.: Drug action, reaction, and interaction. II. Iatrogenic cardiopathies. J. Clin. Pharmacol., *15*:641, 1975.

Aviado, D. and Salem, H.: Drug action, reaction and interaction. I. Quinidine for cardiac arrhythmias. J. Clin. Pharmacol., *15*:477, 1975.

Bissett, J. K. et al.: Electrophysiology of atropine. Cardiovasc. Res., *9*:73, 1975.

Chung, E. K. and Dean, H. M.: Diseases of the heart and vascular system due to drugs (Chapter 15) *In* Meyler, L. and Peck, H. M. (eds.): Drug-Induced Diseases, vol. 4. Amsterdam, Excerpta Medica, 1972.

Das, G., Talmers, F. N. and Weissler, A. M.: New observations on the effects of atropine on the sinoatrial and atrioventricular nodes in man. Am. J. Cardiol., *36*:281, 1975.

Deglin, S. M., Deglin, E. A. and Chung, E. K.: Acute myocardial infarction following fluorescein angiography. (In press), 1976.

Edmondson, H. A., Henderson, B. and Benton, B.: Liver-cell adenomas associated with use of oral contraceptives. N. Engl. J. Med., *294*:470, 1976.

Ghose, M. K.: Pericardial tamponade. A presenting manifestation of procainamide-induced lupus erythematosus. Am. J. Med., *58*:581, 1975.

Goodman, L. S. and Gilman, A.: The Pharmacological Basis of Therapeutics, ed. 5. Chapts. 6, 7, 8, 9, 12, 14, 23, 24, 26, 31, 32, 33, 35, 39, 61, 67, 68. New York, Macmillan, 1975.

Haft, J.: Cardiovascular injury induced by sympathetic catecholamines. Prog. Cardiovasc. Dis., *17*:73, 1974.

Hurst, J. W., and Logue, R. B.: The Heart, ed. 3. Chapter 101. New York, McGraw-Hill, 1974.

Kantor, S. J. et al.: Imipramine-induced heart block. A longitudinal case study. J.A.M.A., *231*:1364, 1975.

Karlsson, E.: Procainamide and phenytoin. Br. Heart J., *37*:731, 1975.

Klein, H. O., Jutrin, I., and Kaplinsky, E.: Cerebral and cardiac toxicity of a small dose of lignocaine. Br. Heart J., *37*:775, 1975.

Lehrman, K.: Pulmonary embolism in transsexual man taking Diethylstilbestrol. J.A.M.A., *235*:532, 1976.

Luomanmäki, K., Keikkila, J., and Härtel, G.: Bretylium tosylate. Adverse effects in acute myocardial infarction. Arch. Int. Med., *135*:515, 1975.

Medical Letter on Drugs and Therapeutics. Drug and Therapeutic Information, Published by the

Medical Letter, Inc., New Rochelle, N.Y., 1969–1975.

Miller, R. R. et al.: Propranolol-withdrawal rebound phenomenon. Exacerbation of coronary events after abrupt cessation of antianginal therapy. N. Engl. J. Med., *293*:416, 1975.

Moser, R. H.: Diseases of Medical Progress. Chap. 2. Springfield, Charles C Thomas, 1969.

Paranthaman, S. K. and Khan, F.: Acute cardiomyopathy with recurrent pulmonary edema and hypotension following heroin overdosage. Chest, *69*:117, 1976.

Richman, S.: Adverse effect of atropine during myocardial infarction. Enhancement of ischemia following intravenously administered atropine. J.A.M.A, *228*:1414, 1974.

Rossen, R. M., Krikorian, J., and Hancock, E. W.: Ventricular asystole after edrophonium chloride administration. J.A.M.A., *235*:1041, 1976.

Tresch, D. D. et al.: Acute iodide intoxication with cardiac irritability. Arch. Int. Med., *134*:760, 1974.

Vohra, J. et al.: Verapamil induced premature ventricular beats before reversion of supraventricular tachycardia. Br. Heart J., *36*:1186, 1974.

19. CONGESTIVE HEART FAILURE AND ACUTE PULMONARY EDEMA*

Richard R. Miller, M.D., and Dean T. Mason, M.D.

DEFINITION

1. Congestive heart failure (CHF) is defined as the pathological state in which a severe abnormality of cardiac function results in the inability of the heart to pump blood at a rate commensurate with the systemic requirements at rest or during normal activity.

2. Compensated congestive heart failure may be defined as the condition in which cardiac pump function is depressed but heart and peripheral circulatory compensatory mechanisms are utilized to prevent a fall in cardiac output to less than systemic requirements in the resting state.

3. The clinical expressions of congestive heart failure that afford bedside definition of the abnormality are related to evidence of impaired organ perfusion, most notable of which are sodium retention, with consequent increase in extracellular fluid, and elevation of pulmonary venous pressure, and increase in sympathetic stimulation.

GENERAL CONSIDERATIONS

Congestive heart failure represents the final clinical expression of deteriorating cardiac function and results from a primary impairment of myocardial contractile units or a primary mechanical abnormality, or a combination of the two. The clinical manifestations of congestive heart failure are principally related to resultant dysfunction of vital organs other than the heart, such as the lungs, kidneys, and liver. The intelligent therapy of congestive heart failure is based on a firm knowledge of the pathophysiology of advance heart failure, the specific types of cardiac disease responsible, and contributory extracardiac factors. Because of frequent extracardiac organ involvement, often associated with serious metabolic and electrolyte disturbances that may be compounded by overzealous or inappropriate use of therapeutic agents, thorough understanding of multiple system dysfunction and knowledge of the actions and potential adverse effects of drug therapy are also essential. Finally, by careful history and physical examination and appropriate use of diagnostic procedures, cardiac lesions that are potentially surgically correctable may be identified.

ETIOLOGY

1. The causes of congestive heart failure are varied and may be primarily cardiac or extracardiac; this discussion will concern the more common forms of the cardiac etiologies.

2. Congestive heart failure may result from:

A. Mechanical abnormalities (valvular stenosis or incompetence, ventricular aneurysm, intracardiac shunt, pericardial restriction or tamponade)

B. Depression of the contractile performance of cardiac muscle, resulting in myocardial dysfunction (cardiomyopathy of idiopathic, infectious, metabolic, familial or ischemic origin)

3. Commonly, mechanical and myocardial functional disorders coexist, as, for example, in longstanding aortic valvular stenosis in which case, despite se-

*Supported in part by Research Program Project Grant HL 14780 from the National Heart and Lung Institute, NIH, Bethesda, Maryland

vere stenosis, the left ventricular myocardium may maintain an adequate cardiac output for many years.

4. Eventually, however, myocardial contractile performance deteriorates and cardiac output can be maintained only at the expense of elevation of left ventricular filling pressures via utilization of the Frank-Starling compensatory mechanism with resultant symptoms of pulmonary congestion. Thus, both a mechanical abnormality and impairment of myocardial contractile units are present.

5. Persistent tachyarrhythmias may precipitate or greatly aggravate CHF by reducing ventricular filling time, loss of atrial contribution to ventricular filling when atrioventricular dissociation occurs, and disordered synchrony of ventricular contraction.

6. Marked bradyarrhythmias may result in an inadequate cardiac output when the ventricles are unable to greatly augment stroke volume.

PATHOPHYSIOLOGY

1. The performance of the intact heart normally is regulated by the integration of four principal determinants that govern stroke volume and cardiac output:
    A. Preload (ventricular end-diastolic volume or pressure)
    B. Afterload (intraventricular systolic tension, which is principally determined by preload and peripheral vascular resistance)
    C. Contractility (force of contraction independent of loading)
    D. Heart rate
2. A disturbed sequence of ventricular contraction, dyssynergy, may also be a factor in certain types of heart disease.
3. While the fundamental abnormality in CHF resides in depression of myocardial contractility, circulatory decompensation can result from three general types of cardiac abnormalities:
    A. A primary defect in contractil-

ity, as in primary or ischemic myocardial disease
    B. Diastolic mechanical inhibition of cardiac performance in which left ventricular hypertrophy does not occur, as in restricted ventricular filling in mitral stenosis
    C. Systolic mechanical overloading characterized by excessive pressure loading, as in systemic hypertension or aortic stenosis, or in systolic volume overloading, as in mitral regurgitation.
4. When pressure or volume overloading or a primary defect in contractility is imposed on the heart, there are three principal compensatory mechanisms for the direct support of cardiac function and its fundamental goal of maintaining normal cardiac output:
    A. The Frank-Starling principle, which relates ventricular performance to preload
    B. Ventricular hypertrophy
    C. The sympathetic nervous system
5. Reduced cardiac output (CO) causes a decline in renal blood flow and glomerular filtration rate, which promotes sodium retention. Further, through the renal release of renin the angiotensin-aldosterone system is activated, resulting in increased sodium reabsorption in the distal tubules. In addition, a humoral but as yet undefined third factor appears to play an important role in sodium-water retention in congestive heart failure. Thus, a major consequence of lowered cardiac output is sodium and water retention, which may result in edema and ascites.
6. An important correlate of a lowered cardiac output is the decline in the fraction of left ventricular end-diastolic volume ejected (ejection fraction), which results in an increase in end-diastolic volume, causing the ventricle to initiate systole at a higher point on the Frank-Starling curve and affording utilization of this important intrinsic mechanism of maintaining cardiac output. Although

CO may be augmented by this pathway, it is done so at the cost of increased pulmonary venous pressure and the likelihood of congestive symptoms.

7. Concomitant with a lowered cardiac output, the sympathetic nervous system is activated, leading to elevation of circulating levels of norepinephrine at rest and particularly with exercise. Although cardiac muscle remains responsive to circulating norepinephrine, in advanced CHF, myocardial stores of the catecholamines are depleted, impairing the function of the cardiac sympathetic nerves, and thus augmenting the contractile state. Heightened activity of the sympathetic nervous system in CHF leads to increased heart rate, redistribution of regional blood flow with a decline in renal, splanchnic, and skin blood flow, and diaphoresis.

CLASSIFICATION

Although inadequate cardiac output is the final abnormality common to all forms of CHF, a wide variety of classes of heart failure exist.

The New York Heart Association Functional Classification provides an extremely useful framework for categorizing patients with CHF:

Class I:	Patients with heart disease who are asymptomatic.
Class II:	Slight limitation of physical activity. Symptoms only with more than ordinary physical activity.
Class III:	Marked limitation. Symptoms with ordinary physical activity.
Class IV:	Symptoms at rest.

1. *Cardiac heart failure*
  A. *Myocardial failure*
    (1) Myocardial dysfunction occurs when the number and/or quality of ventricular contractile units is inadequate to produce muscle shortening sufficient to provide a stroke volume capable of meeting the body's demands.
    (2) Examples of myocardial failure include:
      (a) Extensive myocardial infarction in which a major portion of the left ventricle becomes necrotic and is replaced by noncontracting fibrous tissue
      (b) Hypertensive cardiomyopathy
      (c) Primary myocardial disease
  B. *Mechanical disorder*
    (1) Cardiac output may be drastically impaired despite relatively normal left ventricular contractile function.
    (2) Serious forms of congestive heart failure may be produced by:
      (a) Mitral valve stenosis
      (b) Pulmonary embolism
      (c) Cardiac tamponade with normally preserved myocardial contractility
  C. *Mixed myocardial failure and mechanical disorder:*
  The majority of patients with CHF resulting from (a) acquired valvular disorders and (b) adult congenital heart disease develop important abnormalities of myocardial contractile function consequent to the mechanical abnormality.
2. *Extracardiac heart failure*
  A. *Systemic disease*
    (1) High output heart failure may be due to:
      (a) Hyperthyroidism
      (b) Arteriovenous fistula
      (c) Anemia
      (d) Paget's disease
    (2) In these settings a cardiac abnormality may not be apparent; however, the heart is unable to meet the excessively increased systemic demands.
  B. *Mechanical disorders*
  Inadequate venous return to the heart with subsequent extracardiac heart failure may result from obstruction by tumor of the inferior or superior vena cava.

SYMPTOMS AND SIGNS

1. Although the rate of progression of symptoms varies, depending on the etiology of CHF, the majority of patients develop remarkably similar complaints during the course of heart failure.

2. Symptoms of dyspnea occur initially in left-sided failure and indicate elevated pulmonary venous pressures, which may reflect compensatory measures.

3. Fatigue is a late symptom, indicating inadequately compensated reductions of cardiac output.

4. *Symptoms*: dyspnea (effort, rest, nocturnal, orthopnea), edema (lower extremities, ascites), nocturia, hepatic pain and tenderness, fatigue, hemoptysis, diaphoresis, and cachexia.

5. *Signs*

   A. General: tachycardia, pulsus alternans, tachypnea, diaphoresis, cool skin, cyanosis, jaundice, edema, Cheyne-Stokes respiration, confusion, cachexia.

   B. Chest: fine moist inspiratory rales (alveolar fluid), coarse inspiratory rales (bronchiolar fluid), wheezes (peribronchiolar edema), pleural effusion (right-sided or bilateral).

   C. Abdomen: hepatomegaly, hepatic pulsation, splenomegaly, ascites.

   D. Jugular venous pulse: reflects elevated right atrial pressure; increased A and V waves; with tricuspid insufficiency there are large CV waves.

   E. Precordial palpation: Position and quality of apical impulse is dependent on etiology of CHF, usually large and displaced to left. Occasionally there is a palpable ventricular filling impulse in early diastole.

   F. Auscultation: third heart sound in early diastole; summation gallop when third heart sound and fourth heart sound coexist with tachycardia; holosystolic murmur of mitral or tricuspid insufficiency (functional murmur).

LABORATORY FINDINGS

1. *Routine laboratory studies*

   A. Electrolytes are dependent upon duration and severity of CHF and previous diuretic therapy.

   B. Hyponatremia and reduced urinary sodium concentrations are expected.

   C. Peripheral blood studies may be normal.

   D. Serum enzymes may be normal or reflect hepatic congestion and dysfunction.

   E. Blood urea nitrogen may be elevated indicating reduced renal blood flow.

2. *Chest x-ray*

   A. Cardiac dimensions are dependent on the etiology of CHF.

   B. In chronic left ventricular failure, enlargement of this chamber is to be expected.

   C. Common findings include:

   (1) Increased pulmonary vascular markings consist of bilateral prominence of the superior pulmonary veins (antler effect)

   (2) Dilatation of the central right and left pulmonary arteries

   (3) Interstitial density of the central lung markings

   (4) Interlobar fluid

   (5) Kerley B lines

3. *Electrocardiography*

   A. There are no electrocardiographic findings specific for CHF.

   B. Rather, the ECG alterations are those of the underlying disease process (e.g., myocardial infarction, left ventricular hypertrophy).

4. *Cardiac catheterization*

   A. Cardiac output is usually depressed with CHF; however, occasionally cardiac output is found to be within the lower limits of normal.

   B. Invariably normal cardiac output is only achieved at the expense of elevated left ventricular filling pressures.

C. The pulmonary artery wedge and pulmonary artery diastolic pressures are usually greater than 15 mm. Hg as determined by right heart catheterization and reflect the elevated ventricular end-diastolic pressure.

D. Cardiac catheterization should afford definition of the underlying cardiac abnormality.

DIAGNOSIS

1. The diagnosis of CHF is established by careful interpretation and integration of the history, physical examination, and laboratory findings.

2. Understanding the underlying cardiac lesion is of paramount importance.

3. Of particular value are a history of progressive dyspnea initially limited to exertion but gradually occurring at rest, paroxysmal nocturnal dyspnea, weakness, and diaphoresis.

4. The constellation of physical findings consisting of tachycardia, cool moist skin, jugular venous distention, peripheral edema, cardiac enlargement, a third heart sound, and bilateral moist basilar pulmonary rales is essentially diagnostic of CHF.

5. X-ray evidence of cardiac enlargement, pulmonary venous distention, and laboratory evidence of reduced organ perfusion or congestion are extremely helpful.

6. Prolongation of the arm to tongue circulation time is highly suggestive of a depressed cardiac output.

DIFFERENTIAL DIAGNOSIS

The diagnosis of congestive heart failure may be straightforward when the underlying cardiac lesion is obvious and occurs in concert with the findings described above. However, occasionally primary pulmonary, renal, or hepatic disease may closely mimic certain of the peripheral manifestations of CHF and must be considered in the differential diagnosis.

1. *Pulmonary disease* (see also Chap. 13)

A. In chronic primary pulmonary disease, dyspnea may be aggravated by the supine position like CHF; however, patients with pulmonary disease rarely have paroxysmal nocturnal dyspnea.

B. Evidence of reduced organ perfusion is lacking in primary pulmonary disease until serious cor pulmonale occurs.

C. Pulmonary function tests and cardiac examinations, including x-ray and cardiac catheterization, will determine the underlying disease in difficult cases.

D. Occasionally pulmonary infection may be confused with the radiologic findings of CHF. Clinical and laboratory confirmation of infection and response to antibiotic therapy will distinguish from CHF.

2. *Renal disease*

A. Primary renal disease may cause generalized edema but rarely is associated with elevated venous pressure.

B. Urine analysis and renal function tests are usually diagnostic.

3. *Liver disease*

A. Primary liver disease may result in hepatic enlargement, ascites, and elevations of enzymes similar to passive liver congestion.

B. However, elevation of pulmonary venous and right atrial pressures rarely occurs.

COMPLICATIONS

The severity and nature of complications of CHF are related to the type of underlying cardiac lesion and may be categorized as occurring consequent to: (1) reduced cardiac output and inadequate organ perfusion, (2) passive venous congestion and (3) complications of treatment.

1. *Reduced cardiac output and inadequate organ perfusion* may result in:

A. Renal failure with attendant metabolic and electrolyte disturbances

B. Massive fluid retention

C. Serious confusion and disorientation

D. Marked weakness, eventuating in cachexia

2. *Passive venous congestion*

A. Pulmonary venous congestion leads to:

(1) Increased work of respiration

(2) Hypoxia

(3) Carbon dioxide retention

(4) Pulmonary infection

B. Systemic venous congestion results in:

(1) Hepatic engorgement

(2) Portal hypertension

(3) Small bowel malabsorption

(4) Renal vein thrombosis

(5) Pelvic and lower extremity venous stasis with pulmonary emboli

3. *Complications of treatment*

Frequent complications include (a) digitalis toxicity with resultant cardiac arrhythmias (see Chap. 23) and (b) potassium depletion subsequent to diuretic therapy.

MANAGEMENT OF CONGESTIVE HEART FAILURE

1. *General measures*

A. The underlying cardiac lesion responsible for CHF should be defined at the initial examination. This knowledge allows intelligent definitive treatment and aid in recognition and alleviation of factors precipitating or aggravating the CHF.

B. Bed rest alone reduces cardiac work and promotes diuresis.

C. Sodium restriction is mandatory in preventing new edema formation. A 2.5 g. salt diet is equivalent to 1000 mg. Na and is palatable and generally adequate. When hyponatremia is present in the presence of edema, rigid water restriction is also required.

D. Prophylactic anticoagulation is indicated to reduce the high risk of pulmonary emboli when there is long-standing lower extremity edema, elevation of systemic venous pressure, or when prolonged bed rest is anticipated.

2. *Specific measures*

A. Diuretics

The class, dose, and route of administration of diuretics depends on the severity and duration of CHF, previous diuretic therapy, and knowledge of the serum electrolytes.

(1) Furosemide and ethacrynic acid

(a) Furosemide and ethacrynic acid, which block sodium reabsorption in the ascending loop of Henle, are the most potent diuretics in current usage.

(b) Their rapid onset of action and potency make them the preferred diuretics in the initial management of severe CHF.

(c) Furosemide is the more suitable intravenous agent because of fewer adverse effects.

(d) Potassium replacement is required during administration of these agents.

(2) Thiazide diuretics

(a) The thiazide diuretics are excellent oral agents useful in the chronic management of CHF.

(b) Potassium supplementation is generally required.

(3) Potassium-sparing diuretics

Potassium-sparing diuretics, such as the spironolactones, which are direct aldosterone antagonists, and triamterene, which is a noncompetitive inhibitor of aldosterone, are somewhat less potent agents that are most useful in the chronic management of CHF when used in combination with a thiazide or furosemide.

B. Digitalis (see also Chap. 22)

(1) Digitalis exerts two major pharmacologic actions on the heart: (i) a

direct positive inotropic effect, and (ii) an increase in the functional refractory period with slowed rate of impulse transmission in conduction tissue.

(2) Thus, myocardial contractility is increased and conduction through the A-V node is slowed.

(3) The agent is indicated in the majority of patients with low-output failure consequent to myocardial dysfunction.

(4) By reducing the frequency of ventricular response in supraventricular tachyarrhythmias, particularly atrial fibrillation, digitalis may relieve congestive symptoms.

(5) Contrary to earlier beliefs, complete digitalization is not necessary to achieve pharmacologic effect, so the risks of toxicity associated with rapid full digitalization may be avoided.

C. Afterload reduction

(1) Nitroprusside, phentolamine, and nitroglycerin effectively lower left ventricular filling pressure and may afford prompt relief in pulmonary congestive symptoms.

(2) Cardiac output is augmented in certain patients with CHF by nitroprusside and phentolamine through reduction in impedance to left ventricular ejection.

(2) These agents are ideally suited for management of CHF in hypertension and may be used in normotensive patients with low-output CHF when monitoring of intra-arterial and pulmonary artery wedge pressures may be performed.

(4) Chronic administration of long-acting nitrates, used in conjuction with digitalis and diuretics, frequently affords additional improvement in congestive symptoms.

3. *Management of pulmonary edema*

A. Morphine sulfate induces a central sympatholysis with beneficial relief in anxiety, decrease in tachypnea, and decline in peripheral vascular resistance,

resulting in less venous return to the heart.

B. Oxygen is indicated when the arterial Po_2 is depressed.

C. Aminophylline relieves bronchospasm and, through its inotropic effect on the heart, increases cardiac output. This agent should be used with caution, as many cases of serious ventricular tachyarrhythmias have been documented to result from the too-rapid administration of aminophylline.

D. A rapid-acting potent diuretic should be administered parenterally. Intravenous furosemide is probably the most useful drug in this setting.

E. Rotating tourniquets and phlebotomy may be helpful but are less often required when furosemide is used because of the rapidly effective action of the agent.

F. Digitalization should be carried out with a rapidly acting agent, such as ouabain or digoxin.

G. Afterload reducing agents administered intravenously may afford prompt improvement that precedes the beneficial effects of diuretics and digitalis. In addition, careful titration of these drugs allows more rigid control of dose-response than is possible with digitalis or diuretics.

4. *Management of arrhythmias* (see also Chap. 24)

A. When the precipitating course of CHF is an arrhythmia, primary attention should be directed toward correction of the rhythm disturbance.

B. The sudden appearance of atrial fibrillation with rapid ventricular response in mitral stenosis may cause immediate decompensation despite relatively normal left ventricular function.

C. In this setting, restoration of sinus rhythm or slowing of the ventricular response may be lifesaving.

D. Thus, direct current cardioversion or rapid digitalization may be required.

PROGNOSIS

1. Prognosis in CHF relates to the nature and severity of the underlying cardiac lesion.

2. The majority of patients with CHF will improve with modern medical management.

3. Failure to do so reflects either end-stage myocardial failure with an extremely poor early prognosis or a mechanical lesion requiring immediate surgical correction.

4. In patients refractory to medical therapy, vigorous effort should be made to define a surgically correctable lesion.

SUGGESTED READINGS

Brest, A. N.: Management of refractory heart failure. Prog. Cardiovasc. Dis., *12*:558, 1970.

Guiha, N. H. et al.: Treatment of refractory heart failure with infusion of nitroprusside.N. Eng. J. Med., *291*:587, 1974.

Kim, K. E. et al.: Ethacrynic acid and furosemide. Am. J. Cardiol., *27*:407, 1971.

King, J. F. et at.: Recent advances in therapy for refractory congestive heart failure. Geriatrics, *28*:94, 1973.

Laragh, J. H.: The proper use of newer diuretics. Ann. Intern. Med., *67*:606, 1967.

Mason, D. T., Spann, J. F. and Zelis, R.: New developments in the understanding of the action of digitalis. Prog. Cardiovasc. Dis., *11*:443, 1969.

Mason, D. T. et al.: Alterations of hemodynamics and myocardial mechanics in patients with congestive heart failure: Pathophysiologic mechanisms and assessment of cardiac function and ventricular contractility. Prog. Cardiovasc. Dis., *12:*507, 1970.

Mason, D. T. et al.: Current concepts and treatment of digitalis toxicity. Am. J. Cardiol., *27*:546, 1971.

Miller, R. R. et al.: Clinical use of sodium nitroprusside in chronic ischemic heart disease. Circulation, *51*:238, 1975.

Ramirez, A. and Abelmann, W. H.: Cardiac decompensation. N. Eng. J. Med., *290*:499, 1974.

Spann, J. F., Mason, D. T., and Zelis, R. F.: Recent advances in the understanding of congestive heart failure I and II. Mod. Concepts Cardiovasc. Dis. *39*:73 and 79, 1970.

Vismara, L. A., Mason, D. T., and Amsterdam, E. A.: Cardiocirculatory effects of morphine sulfate: Mechanisms of action and therapeutic application. Heart and Lung, *5*:495, 1974.

20. CARDIOGENIC SHOCK*

Charles E. Rackley, M.D.

DEFINITION

1. Cardiogenic shock is the clinical syndrome accompanying acute myocardial infarction of arterial hypotension with evidence of impaired circulation to the skin, kidneys, and central nervous system.

2. The definition of cardiogenic shock employed by the Myocardial Infarction Research Unit Program has been an arterial blood pressure less than 90 mm. of mercury or a systolic fall of greater than 80 mm. mercury in a patient previously known to have hypertension.

3. In addition to hypotension, evidence of cold, clammy, cyanotic skin, reduced urine production, and altered sensorium must also be evident.

4. Other precipitating causes of shock, such as primary cardiac arrhythmias or hypotension due to administration of pharmacologic agents to a patient with acute myocardial infarction, must be excluded.

GENERAL CONSIDERATIONS

Cardiogenic shock is the most serious complication of patients sustaining acute myocardial infarction, and is attended by a mortality rate exceeding 80 per cent. Despite impaired cardiac performance and reduced circulation, certain patients with this complication of acute infarction

*This research was supported in part by the Specialized Center of Research for Ischemic Heart Disease, Contract #1P17HL17667-02, the Cardiovascular Research and Training Center, Program Project Grant #HL 11, 310 (Division of Heart and Vascular Diseases, National Heart and Lung Institute), NIH Grant #T01LM00154, and the Clinical Research Unit Grant #M01-RR00032-13 (General Clinical Research Centers Program, Division of Research Resources), National Institutes of Health.

do survive. The pathophysiology, differential diagnosis, monitoring facilities, therapeutic interventions, assisted circulation and emergency surgery must be considered in the approach to this clinical problem. While clinically evaluating the patient, the physician must simultaneously consider the pathophysiology, differential diagnosis, appropriate laboratory studies and optimal treatment. Initial therapy must be instituted while laboratory procedures are being performed and data collected. Therefore, knowledge of the alterations in cardiac and circulatory function, clinical pathophysiological features of shock, monitoring systems, medical treatment, and indications for surgery are valuable to the physician.

ETIOLOGY

1. Cardiogenic shock generally results from significant destruction of left ventricular myocardium.

2. This destruction produces impairment of the mechanical performance of the left ventricle to the extent that cardiac output and arterial blood pressure are severely reduced.

3. In addition to major disturbances in left ventricular mechanical performance, imbalances between blood volume and diastolic filling of the left ventricle may develop.

4. Peripheral vascular tone is sometimes inappropriately affected by hormonal and neurogenic mechanisms.

PATHOPHYSIOLOGY

1. Pathological studies in patients who have expired from cardiogenic shock have demonstrated destruction of 40 to 50 per cent of the total mass of the

myocardium of the left ventricle. This is usually composed of a recent or a recent as well as a previous myocardial infarction.

2. In addition to massive destruction of the myocardium, these patients often exhibit severe three vessel coronary artery disease.

3. Generally, the infarction produces transmural necrosis, which involves the full thickness of the ventricular wall.

4. Cardiogenic shock can result from extensive subendocardial infarction limited to the endocardial layers of the left ventricle.

5. Reductions of the cardiac output and arterial blood pressure in the shock state produce further decreases in coronary blood flow that contribute to left ventricular dysfunction and extension of the infarcted area.

CLASSIFICATION

Although cardiogenic shock is considered to result from extreme mechanical dysfunction of the left ventricle, several hemodynamic subgroups have been identified. These subgroups can be considered as mechanical dysfunction, relative hypovolemia, and impaired peripheral vasomotor control mechanisms.

1. *Mechanical dysfunction*

In cardiogenic shock due to mechanical dysfunction, extensive destruction of ventricular myocardium severely impairs cardiac output and systolic emptying of the left ventricle.

2. *Relative hypovolemia*

In patients with relative hypovolemia, the shock state can develop while the filling pressure of the left ventricle is normal or slightly elevated. The condition of these patients resembles the shock condition produced by blood loss or inadequate venous return to the heart.

3. *Impaired peripheral vasomotor control mechanisms*

The third category of shock may result from hormonal and neurogenic mecha-

nisms that disproportionally alter peripheral vasomotor tone. In these patients mechanical impairment of the left ventricle is less and the subsequent course is attended by a higher survival rate.

SYMPTOMS AND SIGNS

The clinical features of patients presenting in cardiogenic shock are a history of recent chest pain, manifestations of reduced organ perfusion, and electrocardiographic changes of acute myocardial infarction. Cardiogenic shock can develop in the absence of chronic heart failure, and the physical findings of chronic volume overload may be present.

1. *Vital signs*

A. Vital signs generally reveal a normal temperature, tachycardia with a thready peripheral pulse, normal or increased respiratory rate, and significantly reduced blood pressure.

B. In some patients there may be difficulty in obtaining blood pressure by the cuff technique.

C. Bradycardia may be present in patients with inferior (diaphragmatic) myocardial infarction and excessive vagal tone or due to complete A-V block.

2. *Inspection and palpation*

A. The patient is restless with altered sensorium, and the skin is pale, cyanotic, cool, and moist.

B. Neck veins are flat but can be distended if right heart failure has been chronic.

C. If the patient has a history of chronic heart failure, neck vein distention, hepatic enlargement, and peripheral edema can be detected.

3. *Auscultation*

A. If the patient has left ventricular failure and pulmonary edema, pulmonary rales are audible but the lungs may be clear to auscultation.

B. Heart sounds are often distant.

C. Atrial and ventricular gallops or a summation gallop may be audible.

D. Detection of a harsh systolic murmur at the apex or along the left sternal border suggests rupture of a papillary muscle or the ventricular septum.

E. If an aortic diastolic murmur is present, this finding should be considered in the differential diagnosis.

4. *Cardiac size*

Heart size may be normal or may be enlarged depending on the presence or absence of chronic left ventricular overload.

5. *Peripheral pulses*

A. Peripheral pulses are generally diminished, thready, or not palpable.

B. Disparity between the right and the left radial, brachial, or femoral pulses should suggest a dissecting aneurysm.

LABORATORY FINDINGS

1. *Routine laboratory studies*

Since cardiogenic shock is usually a sudden complication of acute myocardial infarction, routine laboratory studies of the peripheral blood and urinalysis may be normal.

2. *Serum electrolytes determinations*

If the patient has a previous cardiac condition with a history of diuretic use, serum electrolytes should be determined.

3. *Renal function tests*

Evaluation of renal function will be useful not only for detection of pre-existing renal disease but also to establish a baseline for comparison during management of the shock state.

4. *Arterial blood gas determinations*

Arterial blood gas determinations often reveal hypoxemia, normal CO_2, and varying degrees of acidosis.

5. *Serum enzyme studies*

Cardiac enzymes may not be initially elevated if the patient develops shock shortly after the acute myocardial infarc-

tion. Six or more hours can elapse from the onset of chest pain before the cardiac enzymes are abnormally elevated.

6. *Chest roentgenogram*

A. Chest roentgenogram may reveal a normal cardiac silhouette if there is no prior history of heart failure or hypertension.

B. Cardiomegaly would suggest hypertension or heart failure secondary to coronary disease.

C. Acute myocardial infarction can produce pulmonary vascular congestion and edema in the absence of cardiac enlargement.

7. *The electrocardiogram* is essential in documentation of a recent myocardial infarction.

A. Abnormal Q waves, S-T segments, and T-wave changes of myocardial necrosis confirm myocardial infarction.

B. Although it is generally contended that Q-waves are necessary and transmural infarction required to destroy sufficient myocardium to produce cardiogenic shock, cardiogenic shock can result from subendocardial infarction showing only S-T and T-wave abnormalities in the electrocardiograms.

C. The presence of conduction disturbances, such as left bundle branch block or complete A-V block, may obscure the characteristic electrocardiographic findings of acute myocardial infarction. However, in the absence of left bundle branch block or complete A-V block, characteristic changes of myocardial infarction usually accompany cardiogenic shock.

DIAGNOSIS

1. The diagnosis of acute myocardial infarction is established by history of ischemic chest pain, enzymatic, and electrocardiographic abnormalities.

2. Additional findings of hypotension and impaired skin perfusion, renal blood

flow, and central nervous system function confirm the clinical diagnosis of cardiogenic shock.

3. Primary cardiac arrhythmias may be excluded as the precipitating cause of the shock, and this can be difficult since rhythm disturbances frequently develop as a result of cardiogenic shock and impaired coronary blood flow.

4. Administration of analgesics for the relief of myocardial infarction pain can significantly reduce the blood pressure.

5. Therefore, cardiac arrhythmias and analgesics can result in hypotension in a patient with acute myocardial infarction, and such mechanisms must be excluded in order to confirm the diagnosis of cardiogenic shock.

DIFFERENTIAL DIAGNOSIS

Unless the history, clinical and electrocardiographic findings are unequivocal for recent myocardial infarction and cardiogenic shock, other possible mechanisms must be considered. Shock due to any cause reduces coronary blood flow, and in a patient with preexisting coronary artery disease, hypotension can produce myocardial damage.

1. *Hypovolemic shock*

A. Hypovolemic shock can develop due to blood loss, and a common site of such loss is in the gastrointestinal tract of patients with peptic ulcer disease.

B. Internal bleeding can develop from trauma; occult sites for internal blood loss include the mediastinum and retroperitoneal space.

C. Dissection of the aorta produces intense pain similar to myocardial infarction. Blood loss from a dissecting aorta can accumulate in the mediastinum, plueral space, or retroperitoneal space, with production of the shock syndrome. Rarely the dissection may extend retrograde into the pericardium with cardiac tamponade. In addition to intense pain, blood loss, and cardiac tamponade, aortic dissection can occlude a coronary artery and produce myocardial infarction.

2. *Pulmonary embolism* can produce shock with obstruction of pulmonary blood flow, impaired filling of the left ventricle, and reduction in coronary blood flow.

3. *Bacteremia*

Gram-negative bacteremia is a mechanism for the shock syndrome, but this condition is usually attended by chills and fever. Often bacteremia is secondary to urinary tract manipulation or surgical procedure.

4. *Neurogenic shock*

Shock can develop on a neurogenic basis from intense pain or trauma. However, significant blood loss must be considered under traumatic circumstances.

5. *Anaphylactic shock* can develop in patients who have received medications or intravascular injections for various diagnostic procedures.

Finally, cardiogenic shock can result from any mechanism that reduces arterial pressure with reduction of coronary blood flow in a patient with coronary artery disease.

COMPLICATIONS

The mortality rate is extremely high in patients who develop cardiogenic shock as a complication of acute myocardial infarction. The highest mortality is encountered in those patients who have excessive destruction of left ventricular myocardium. The mortality is slightly lower in patients who exhibit relative hypovolemia as an additional pathophysiological mechanism in cardiogenic shock. Inappropriate peripheral vasomotor disturbances with minimal mechanical impairment of left ventricular function in cardiogenic shock has the most favorable prognosis. The development of a prominent precordial systolic murmur and thrill with the acute infarction and cardiogenic shock suggests either a ruptured papillary muscle or ventricular septum. These mechanical complications can be managed with circulatory support systems and cardiac surgery.

1. *Renal failure* secondary to acute tubular necrosis may occur in patients who remain in cardiogenic shock for prolonged periods.

2. *Cerebral vascular accidents* may be caused by reduced cerebral blood flow in a patient with cerebral vascular disease.

3. Gastrointestinal disorders such as ischemia of the bowel with necrosis and bleeding can be a result of prolonged shock.

4. *Cardiovascular disorders* such as cardiac arrhythmias as well as pulmonary edema and heart failure often accompany cardiogenic shock, and all of these cardiac disturbances can be attributed to a reduction in coronary blood flow.

MANAGEMENT (TABLE 20-1)

1. *General therapeutic approach*
A. The initial management of the patient with cardiogenic shock requires the rapid establishment of an intravenous route for the administration of vasopressor agents.

B. Several vasoactive medications are available but levarterenol (Levophed), dopamine and metaraminol (Aramine) have proved most reliable in the elevation of arterial blood pressure and restoration of vital organ perfusion.

C. The filling pressure of the left ventricle should be elevated and an effective blood volume established for maximum action of the vasopressor agents. The Swan-Ganz catheter can provide this information in the shock patient.

D. Arterial systolic pressure should be maintained above 90 mm. Hg with infusion of a vasopressor.

E. Although isoproterenol has been utilized in the past both to improve the mechanical performance of the ventricle and to increase renal blood flow, this beta-stimulating agent inordinately increases myocardial oxygen demands and damages the viable myocardium.

F. In addition to the prompt administration of vasopressors, a Foley catheter should be inserted to quantitate urine flow.

G. Patients generally maintain respiratory control in cardiogenic shock even though the arterial blood gases are

Table 20-1. **Drugs Commonly Used in Cardiogenic Shock**

Agent	Concentration (mg./250 ml. 5% D/W*)	Infusion Rate (Standard) µg./kg./min.	Adverse Reaction
Dopamine	200	10	Nausea, vomiting, arrhythmia, angina, azotemia.
Norepinephrine	4	0.1	Bradycardia, headache, hypertension, extravasation can cause tissue necrosis.
Epinephrine	4	0.1	Arrhythmia, headache, angina, anxiety.
Isoproterenol	1	0.05	Nausea, vomiting, arrhythmia, tachycardia, angina.
Metaraminol	50	as necessary to maintain BP	Sinus or ventricular tachycardia, arrhythmia.

*D/W = dextrose and water

significantly altered. If the patient does not exhibit spontaneous respiration, intubation and ventilatory support must be supplied.

H. Acute pulmonary edema can occur in the cardiogenic shock syndrome and phlebotomy is the most expedient method for reduction of the blood volume.

I. Cardiac irritability requires intravenous lidocaine to control rhythm disturbances.

J. Metabolic acidosis quickly develops in cardiogenic shock, and infusion of sodium bicarbonate is required to restore acid-base balance.

These initial interventions can stabilize and sometimes restore arterial blood pressure and coronary blood flow.

2. *Specific therapeutic measures*

A. If facilities are available in the coronary care unit, a Swan-Ganz catheter should be introduced through an anticubital cutdown and advanced to the pulmonary artery for measurements of pulmonary end-diastolic or capillary wedge pressure and cardiac output.

B. These measurements can supply valuable information on the prognosis of the patient as well as establish a monitoring system for the selection and regulation of pharmacologic interventions.

C. The Swan-Ganz catheter can provide the necessary data to confirm a ruptured ventricular septum or mitral regurgitation.

D. Patients who develop a loud systolic murmur should be considered potential surgical candidates if the shock state cannot be reversed with pharmacological agents.

E. If facilities are available for insertion of the intra-aortic balloon, diastolic augmentation of cardiac output and coronary blood flow can restore arterial blood pressure.

F. It should be recognized, however, that counter pulsation with intra-aortic balloon pumping is merely pallia-

tive and will not cure the shock condition. Therefore, this clinical intervention requires additional considerations for emergency coronary arteriography and cardiac surgery if indicated.

G. The insertion of a Swan-Ganz catheter, intra-aortic balloon pumping, emergency coronary arteriography, and cardiac surgery require the attendance and availability of a highly trained team of cardiologists, cardiac surgeons, technicians, and nurses.

PROGNOSIS

1. Prognosis in patients who develop cardiogenic shock with acute myocardial infarction is determined by the extent of muscle damage from the acute as well as the previous myocardial infarctions.

2. Patients who exhibit hemodynamic evidence of severe elevation in left ventricular filling pressure and reductions in cardiac index are in a high mortality category despite the use of available pharmacologic agents. Furthermore, these patients have a low probability of survival if emergency surgery and bypass grafting are performed.

3. Patients who present in shock with a normal or modestly elevated left ventricular filling pressure are relatively hypovolemic and approximately one-third of these patients respond to expansion of the blood volume with low molecular dextran or albumin.

4. Patients who reveal minimal alterations in left ventricular filling pressure and cardiac index with cardiogenic shock often respond promptly to vasopressor agents.

5. The overall prognosis for patients with cardiogenic shock remains grave.

SUGGESTED READINGS

Cohn, J. N., and Franciosa, J. A.: Pathophysiology of shock in acute myocardial infarction. *In* Yu, P. N. and Goodwin, J. F. (eds.): Progress in

Cardiology, Chapt. 7, Philadelphia, Lea and Febiger, 1973.

Perloth, G. G., and Harrison, D. C.: Medical therapy for shock in acute myocardial infarction. *In* Yu, P. N. and Goodwin, J. F. (eds.): Progress in Cardiology. Chapt. 8. Philadelphia, Lea and Febiger, 1973.

Rackley, C. E. et al.: Cardiogenic shock in patients with myocardial infarction. Chapt. 10. *In* Rackley, C. E. and Russell, R. O., Jr. (eds.): Hemodynamic Monitoring in a Coronary Intensive Care Unit. New York, Futura Publishing Co., Mt. Kisco, 1974.

Rackley, C. E. et al.: Cardiogenic shock: recognition and management. *In* Brest, A. N. (ed.): Cardiovascular Clinics: Innovations in the Diagnosis and Management of Acute Myocardial Infarction. Philadelphia, F. A. Davis, 1975.

Ratshin, R. A., Rackley, C. E. and Russell, R. O., Jr.: Hemodynamic evaluation of left ventricular function in shock complicating myocardial infarction. Circulation, *45*:127, 1972.

Swan, H. J. C. et al.: Hemodynamic spectrum of myocardial infarction and cardiogenic shock: a conceptual model. Circulation, *45*:197, 1972.

Weber, K. T. et al.: Left ventricular dysfunction following acute myocardial infarction. A clinico-pathologic and hemodynamic profile of shock and failure. Am. J. Med., *54*:697, 1973.

21. CARDIAC ARRHYTHMIAS

Edward K. Chung, M.D.

DEFINITION

Cardiac arrhythmia is defined as disturbances of impulse formation and/or conduction anywhere in the heart. In other words, cardiac arrhythmias include any type of cardiac beats or rhythm other than normal sinus rhythm. Various terms such as *dysrhythmia, ectopic rhythm,* and *disorder of heart beat* have been used to designate cardiac arrhythmias.

ETIOLOGY

Cardiac arrhythmias may be observed in many clinical circumstances including cardiac as well as noncardiac disorders. In addition, various arrhythmias may also occur in apparently healthy individuals.

1. The most common cause of cardiac arrhythmias is coronary heart disease, especially acute myocardial infarction (see Chap. 2).

2. The next most common cause of arrhythmias is digitalis intoxication (see Chap. 23).

3. Hypokalemia alone is capable of producing various arrhythmias and it often predisposes to digitalis-induced arrhythmias.

4. Atrial fibrillation is the most common arrhythmia in rheumatic heart disease (see Chap. 5).

5. First degree A-V block (prolonged P-R interval) is the most common ECG finding in acute rheumatic fever (see Chap. 4).

6. Hyperthyroidism (thyrotoxicosis) is the most common noncardiac disorder that produces atrial fibrillation (see Chap. 17).

7. Sudden appearance of atrial tachyarrhythmias and/or right bundle branch block often indicate pulmonary embolism (see Chap. 12).

8. Multifocal atrial tachycardia (chaotic atrial rhythm) is most commonly found in chronic cor pulmonale (see Chap. 13).

9. The most common cause of non-paroxysmal A-V junctional tachycardia and atrial tachycardia with A-V block is digitalis intoxication (see Chap. 23).

10. Wolff-Parkinson-White syndrome should be suspected when an apparently healthy individual develops paroxysmal supraventricular tachyarrhythmias (most commonly reciprocating tachycardia, so-called paroxysmal atrial tachycardia).

11. Unexplainable arrhythmias, particularly premature beats and paroxysmal atrial tachycardia, are often due to an excessive consumption of coffee, tea, and cola, which contain a high content of caffeine.

12. Sinus tachycardia is frequently present in various high output states such as anemia, beriberi, fever, A-V fistula and hyperthyroidism (see Chap. 17).

13. Acute congestive heart failure (see Chap. 19) is frequently associated with various cardiac arrhythmias, particularly ventricular premature beats and atrial flutter or fibrillation.

14. Cardiomyopathies are frequently associated with various intraventricular conduction disturbances.

15. Hemiblocks, bifascicular block, and trifascicular block of acute onset are most commonly due to acute anterior myocardial infarction.

16. The most common congenital heart disease associated with right bundle branch block pattern is atrial septal defect (see Chap. 10).

17. Left ventricular hypertrophy (most commonly due to systemic hypertension) is almost always found in patients with left bundle branch block.

18. The most common cause of complete A-V block is a degenerative-sclerotic change in the Purkinje network.

19. Hypoxia and various anesthesic agents frequently produce various arrhythmias.

20. Ventricular premature beats are the most common arrhythmia found in mitral valve prolapse syndrome (Barlow's syndrome, see Chap. 6).

21. Sinus bradycardia is commonly due to various drugs, particularly digitalis, propranolol (Inderal), methyldopa (Aldomet), reserpine (Serpasil) and guanethidine (Ismelin).

22. Sick sinus syndrome and chronic bifascicular or trifascicular block are common in elderly individuals.

CLASSIFICATION

Cardiac arrhythmias have been classified in various ways, but in general they are divided into two major categories:

1. Abnormal impulse formation
2. Abnormal conduction

A detailed classification of cardiac arrhythmias is shown on page 299.

DIAGNOSTIC APPROACH

Although there may be many different diagnostic approaches when one is dealing with unknown cardiac arrhythmias, the logical and electrophysiologic approach is discussed below.

1. Obtainment of all available clinical information
2. General inspection of the electrocardiogram
3. Determination of the dominant rhythm

4. Determination of the presence or absence of a P wave
5. Determination of the origin of the QRS complex when atrial and ventricular activities are independent
6. Determination of the nature and origin of beats occurring prematurely or later than usual
7. Determination of ventricular aberrancy vs. ventricular ectopy
8. Classification of arrhythmias
9. Reaching a final conclusion

OBTAINING CLINICAL INFORMATION

It is of great help in interpreting cardiac arrhythmias if clinical information is available. This information should include the patient's age, presence of a previous similar arrhythmia, and its onset and frequency, presence of known heart disease, a previous history of congestive heart failure and such noncardiac diseases as hyperthyroidism, drug administration (particularly digitalis), and electrolyte imbalance. A detailed history of an artificial pacemaker implantation including the approximate date of implantation and type of pacemaker, etc. is important because malfunction of an artificial pacemaker may produce various serious arrhythmias. In addition, one must review all available previous tracings in order to determine whether the patient has had any cardiac disorder such as arrhythmia, left bundle branch block, right bundle branch block or bilateral bundle branch block, Wolff-Parkinson-White syndrome, or myocardial infarction. This information is frequently invaluable in distinguishing between supraventricular and ventricular tachycardia, and enhances the accuracy of the diagnosis.

GENERAL INSPECTION OF THE ELECTROCARDIOGRAM

By a general inspection of a given tracing, it is possible to determine whether the basic rhythm is either normal sinus rhythm or any type of cardiac arrhythmia. If any arrhythmia is present, one should determine whether the arrhythmia occurs occasionally, frequently, continuously, regularly or irregularly, repetitively, or with various combinations. Various artifacts, which may simulate cardiac arrhythmias, must also be detected. It is also possible to determine

Classification of Cardiac Arrhythmias

I. Disturbances of impulse formation
  A. Disturbance of sinus impulse formation
    1. Sinus premature beats (extrasystoles)
    2. Sinus tachycardia
    3. Sinus bradycardia
    4. Sinus arrhythmia
      a. Respiratory
      b. Nonrespiratory
      c. Ventriculophasic
    5. Wandering pacemaker in the sinus node
    6. Sinus arrest (pause or standstill)
  B. Disturbance of ectopic impulse formation
    1. Passive impulse formation
      a. A-V junctional escape beats and rhythm
      b. Ventricular escape beats and rhythm (idioventricular beats and rhythm)
      c. Wandering pacemaker between S-A and A-V nodes
    2. Active impulse formation
      a. Atrial in origin
        (1) Atrial premature beats (extrasystoles)
        (2) Atrial tachycardia
        (3) Atrial flutter
        (4) Atrial fibrillation
        (5) Atrial flutter-fibrillation (impure flutter)
        (6) Wandering pacemaker in the atria
      b. A-V junctional in origin
        (1) A-V junctional premature beats (extrasystoles)
        (2) A-V junctional tachycardia
          (a) Paroxysmal
          (b) Nonparoxysmal
        (3) Wandering pacemaker in the A-V junction
      c. Ventricular in origin
        (1) Ventricular premature beats (extrasystoles)
        (2) Ventricular tachycardia
          (a) Paroxysmal
          (b) Nonparoxysmal
        (3) Ventricular flutter
        (4) Ventricular fibrillation
        (5) Chaotic rhythm

II. Conduction disturbances
  A. Sinoatrial block
  B. Intra-atrial block
  C. Atrioventricular (A-V) block
    1. First degree A-V block
    2. Second degree A-V block
      a. Mobitz Type I (Wenckebach phenomenon, common type)
      b. Mobitz Type II (uncommon type)
    3. High degree (advanced) A-V block
    4. Complete A-V block
    5. Dual A-V conduction
    6. Supernormal A-V conduction
  D. Intraventricular block
    1. Right bundle branch block
      a. Complete
      b. Incomplete
    2. Left bundle branch block
      a. Complete
      b. Incomplete
      c. Hemiblocks
    3. Bilateral bundle branch block (bifascicular block, trifascicular block)
    4. Nonspecific intraventricular block
  E. Exit block
III. Mixed disturbances of impulse formation and conduction, and ill-defined arrhythmias
  A. Atrioventricular (A-V) dissociation
    1. Complete
    2. Incomplete
  B. Wolff-Parkinson-White syndrome (ventricular preexcitation syndrome)
  C. Reciprocal beats, rhythm and tachycardia
  D. Parasystole
    1. Atrial
    2. A-V junctional
    3. Ventricular
    4. Combined
  E. Atrial dissociation
  F. Electrical alternans
  G. Slow atrial rhythm
  H. Coronary sinus rhythm
  I. Coronary nodal rhythm
  J. Lown-Ganong-Levine syndrome
  K. Concealed conduction.
IV. Artificial pacemaker-induced rhythm

whether the arrhythmia is simple or complex, clinically benign or serious.

DETERMINATION OF DOMINANT RHYTHM

After a general inspection of a given electrocardiogram, a determination of the dominant rhythm is the next step. The dominant rhythm may be sinus rhythm, but it could be any type of ectopic rhythm. If an ectopic rhythm is dominant, one should determine whether the ectopic rhythm is due to either active or passive impulse formation. However, in most common and simple arrhythmias, the dominant rhythm is of sinus origin. The second most common dominant rhythm is atrial fibrillation, and, less commonly, atrial flutter. Occasionally, the dominant rhythm may change from one mechanism to another (from sinus to ectopic or vice versa or even from ectopic to ectopic) on the same electrocardiogram. At times, it is difficult to determine the dominant rhythm, particularly when dealing with complex arrhythmias. Even if the dominant rhythm is ectopic in origin, one begins, as a rule, with sinus beats if present even occasionally. It is immensely helpful to determine whether sinus beats are present.

DETERMINATION OF PRESENCE OR ABSENCE OF P WAVES

By knowing whether a P wave is present or absent, one can narrow the differential diagnosis significantly. When a P wave seems to be present, one should be certain that the P wave is a true P wave and not various other waves, such as atrial fibrillation or flutter, T wave, U wave, or even artifacts that look like P waves. If a true P wave is definitely present, one should determine whether the P wave and QRS complex are related or independent.

1. *Presence of P wave*

When a P wave is present, one should determine whether the P wave is of sinus or ectopic origin. In order to reach a conclusion, the following steps should be carried out:

A. Determination of origin of P wave (mean axis of P wave)

B. Inspection of P wave configuration

C. Inspection of regularity of P-P cycle

D. Measurement of P wave rate

E. Determination of the relationship between P wave and QRS complex

By the above process, if the P wave is found to be of sinus origin, one has reached a conclusion as to whether normal sinus rhythm, sinus tachycardia, sinus bradycardia, etc. is present. If the P wave is not of sinus origin, it must be originating from an ectopic focus in the atria or A-V junction or rarely in the ventricles. When the P wave originates in the atria, the P wave may resemble or at times be almost identical to the sinus P wave, but the rate is usually faster when impulses originate in the atria. The P wave may be conducted in a retrograde fashion if it originates from either the A-V junction or ventricle. If this occurs, the P wave will be inverted in lead II but upright in lead aVR and thus have a direction almost opposite to that of a sinus P wave. When the atria are activated in a retrograde fashion from the A-V junction, the P wave may appear before or after the QRS complex, depending upon whether the atria or ventricles are activated first. If the atria and ventricles are activated simultaneously, the P wave will be superimposed on the QRS complex, leading to an absent P wave. When the P wave configuration changes from beat to beat in the presence of a constant P-R interval, a wandering pacemaker is present in the sinus node. The pacemaker may wander in the atria. This may be diagnosed when one observes a changing P-R interval with fluctuations in the P wave configuration. A wandering pacemaker is present between the sinus node and A-V junction when the P wave configuration changes from upright to inverted in the same lead with or without a changing P-R interval. It should be noted that respiration may slightly change the P wave configuration is some leads, and this should be distinguished from a wandering atrial pacemaker. In addition to its influence on the P wave, respiration may also affect the QRS complex and T wave in a similar fashion. Taking of an electrocardiogram during sustained inspiration or expiration eliminates this problem. On rare occasions, the P wave configuration may only change after ectopic beats. This is due to aberrant atrial conduction (Chung's phenomenon). A varying P wave configuration is also observed when atrial fusion beats of varying degree appear on the electrocardiogram.

An irregular P-P cycle is usually due to sinus arrhythmia, but may also occur with sino-atrial block, sinus arrest, or even sinus premature beats. Ectopic atrial beats that appear during sinus rhythm also result in an irregular P-P cycle, but the configuration of the ectopic P wave is usually different from the sinus P wave. The rate of the P wave helps us determine with relative accuracy the cardiac rhythm. A P wave rate between 60 and 100 per minute with the P wave conducted in a forward direction is usually indicative of normal sinus rhythm. Nonparoxysmal A-V junctional tachycardia often produces the same rate as normal sinus rhythm, but the P wave during the former is conducted in a retrograde fashion. In general, nonparoxysmal A-V junctional tachycardia produces retrograde P wave with a rate between 70 and 130 per minute. When the rate of the P wave is between 180 and 250 per minute, the ectopic rhythm present is usually either paroxysmal A-V junctional or atrial tachycardia. The P wave is conducted in a forward fashion in the latter, but in a retrograde fashion

in the former. A-V junctional escape rhythm may produce retrograde P waves, but at a much slower rate (40–60 beats per minute) than A-V junctional tachycardia. Rarely, idioventricular rhythm (ventricular escape rhythm) may show retrograde P waves. These P waves usually occur after the QRS complex. It is not uncommon to find a retrograde P wave following artificial pacemaker-induced ventricular rhythm. A retrograde P wave also can be produced in reciprocal rhythm or reciprocating tachycardia.

The final step in this subgroup is to appreciate the relationship between atria and ventricles. If the P-R or R-P intervals are constant, all the above-mentioned diagnostic possibilities (normal sinus rhythm, sinus bradycardia, sinus tachycardia, atrial tachycardia, A-V junctional escape rhythm and idioventricular rhythm) should be considered. This list should be narrowed after careful observation of the direction and rate of P waves. If the P-R interval varies, one must be certain whether or not the atria and ventricles are related in the cardiac cycle. The degree and frequency of such a relationship must be determined. When no relationship exists between the atria and ventricles, complete A-V dissociation is said to be present. The underlying disorders responsible for A-V dissociation may be (1) a marked slowing of sinus impulse formation; (2) acceleration of ectopic impulse formation in the A-V node or ventricles; and (3) complete A-V block (see list below). Complete A-V dissociation need not always be present, for the atria and ventricles may at times become related (atrial or ventricular captured beats) and this rhythm is known as incomplete A-V dissociation.

When the atrial rate is found to be a multiple of the ventricular rate, a second degree or advanced (high degree) A-V block, such as 2:1, 3:1, is usually

Causes of A-V Dissociation

1. Disturbances of Sinus Impulse Formation & Conduction
   A. Sinus Bradycardia
      (1) With A-V Junctional Escape Rhythm
      (2) With Ventricular Escape Rhythm
   B. Sinus Arrest
      (1) With A-V Junctional Escape Rhythm
      (2) With Ventricular Escape Rhythm
   C. S-A Block
      (1) With A-V Junctional Escape Rhythm
      (2) With Ventricular Escape Rhythm
2. Acceleration of Impulse Formation in the A-V Junction or Ventricles
   A. A-V Junctional Tachycardia
      (1) With Sinus Rhythm
      (2) With Atrial Fibrillation
      (3) With Atrial Flutter
      (4) With Atrial Tachycardia
      (5) Multiple A-V Junctional Tachycardia
   B. Ventricular Tachycardia
      (1) With Sinus Rhythm
      (2) With Atrial Fibrillation
      (3) With Atrial Flutter
      (4) With Atrial Tachycardia
      (5) With A-V Junctional Tachycardia
3. A-V Conduction Disturbances
   A. Complete (or Advanced) A-V Block
      (1) Sinus Rhythm with A-V Junctional or Ventricular Escape Rhythm
      (2) Atrial Fibrillation with A-V Junctional or Ventricular Escape Rhythm
      (3) Atrial Flutter with A-V Junctional or Ventricular Escape Rhythm
      (4) Atrial Tachycardia with A-V Junctional or Ventricular Escape Rhythm
      (5) A-V Junctional Tachycardia with A-V Junctional or Ventricular Escape Rhythm
   B. Artificial Pacemaker Induced Ventricular Rhythm
      (1) With Sinus Rhythm
      (2) With Atrial Fibrillation
      (3) With Atrial Flutter
      (4) With Atrial Tachycardia
      (5) With A-V Junctional Tachycardia

present. Wenckebach (Mobitz Type I) A-V block is characterized by a progressive lengthening of the P-R interval until a P wave is present without a QRS complex after it (Fig. 21-1). This pattern may then repeat itself. Thus the atrial to ventricular ratio becomes 3:2, 4:3, etc. Less common forms of second-degree A-V block, namely Mobitz Type II, also produce a 3:2, 4:3, etc. A-V block, which may resemble the Wenckebach type, but the P-R intervals remain constant except when a blocked (nonconducted) P wave occurs.

First-degree A-V block has a constant but prolonged (0.21 second or more) P-R interval. This relationship between atria and ventricles may occasionally be reversed; Wenckebach retrograde ventriculoatrial block may be the resulting abnormality.

2. *Absence of P wave*

When the P wave is not discernible, one should determine whether (1) the P wave is truly absent; or (2) the P wave is present but unobserved.

It is not uncommon to observe a P wave superimposed on a portion of the QRS complex, S-T segment, or T wave of the preceding or subsequent cycle. This occurs frequently during atrial tachycardia or A-V junctional tachycar-

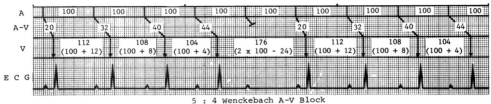

5 : 4 Wenckebach A-V Block

Fig. 21-1. This diagram illustrates Mobitz Type I (Wenckebach) A-V block. The numbers represent hundredths of a second. The numbers in the upper row represent the atrial cycle (P-P interval) with a rate of 60 per minute. The numbers within the oblique lines at A-V level indicate the A-V conduction time (P-R interval). The progressive lengthening of the P-R intervals is apparent until a blocked atrial impulse (dropped P wave) occurs. Following this blocked atrial impulse, the P-R interval shortens to its original value (0.20 second), and the sequence is repeated. The numbers in the lower row represent the duration of successive ventricular cycles. The progressive shortening of the ventricular cycle length (R-R interval) is due to the progressive increment of A-V conduction before the blocked atrial impulse, and the decrement immediately following the blocked P wave. The numbers in the parentheses in the lower row indicate the degree of increment or decrement in the ventricular cycle length.

dia and may occasionally be observed during sinus tachycardia. Various maneuvers, such as carotid sinus pressure or breath-holding, may enable us to delineate the P wave from other complexes by reducing the heart rate.

If after the above techniques the P wave is still not observed, the atrial mechanism must be determined. The most common cause of an absent P wave is atrial fibrillation; atrial flutter is less common. In these cases, an atrial fibrillation or flutter wave is present in place of the P wave. Untreated atrial fibrillation usually has a rapid ventricular rate (more than 120–160/min.), unless a significant A-V conduction defect is present. In untreated atrial flutter the ventricular rate is usually one-half that of the atrial. This block is not anatomic in nature and it is a physiologic phenomenon. Its presence is simply due to the fact that the A-V junction is unable to conduct the very rapid atrial rate. Thus, the ventricular rate is frequently around 150 to 175 per minute. In A-V junctional tachycardia or escape rhythm, the P wave may be totally superimposed on the QRS complex leading to absent P waves. This occurs when

atrial and ventricular depolarization occurs simultaneously. In rare circumstances, notably in severely diseased hearts, atrial activity may be completely absent because of atrial standstill.

DETERMINATION OF THE ORIGIN OF THE QRS COMPLEX WHEN ATRIAL ACTIVITIES ARE INDEPENDENT

When the atrial and ventricular activities are either temporarily or continuously independent, incomplete or complete A-V dissociation is said to exist (see list, causes of A-V Dissociation, above). When this occurs, either the atrial or ventricular mechanism may equally dominate. In other words, the atria may be controlled by the sinus node or any other atrial ectopic focus (atrial fibrillation, flutter or tachycardia), whereas the ventricles may be controlled by either the A-V junction or a ventricular ectopic focus.

When the QRS complex is unrelated to the P wave, the fundamental genesis of the impulse that activates the ventricles should be determined. It is essential to determine whether the QRS complex is produced by active or passive impulse formation. In addition, it should be determined whether the QRS complex originates from the A-V junction or the ventricle. If there is active impulse formation in the above examples, A-V junctional or ventricular tachycardia, respectively, will result. In contrast to this, passive impulse formation from the A-V junction and ventricle results in either A-V junctional or ventricular escape rhythm, respectively. The QRS complex that originates from the A-V junction is ordinarily of normal configuration, although it may be bizarre and wider than usual because of aberrant ventricular conduction. The QRS complex that originates in a ventricle is usually wide and has a bizarre configuration.

DETERMINATION OF THE NATURE AND ORIGIN OF BEATS OCCURRING PREMATURELY OR LATER THAN USUAL

Various fundamental mechanisms may produce a P wave or QRS complex that occurs prematurely. The most common example of this is the ordinary premature beat (extrasystole), which may originate from the atria, A-V junction, or ventricles. When a premature beat is found, one should determine its origin. The origin of a premature P wave is determined by the electrical axis and configuration of the P wave, and its relationship to the QRS complex. The configuration of the P wave of an atrial premature beat is usually slightly different in configuration from the sinus P wave. An atrial premature beat is ordinarily followed by a normal QRS complex. When a short coupling interval or Ashman's phenomenon is present, the QRS complex following an atrial premature beat may appear bizarre due to aberrant ventricular conduction. At times, a premature P wave may not be followed by a QRS complex, and this is termed a nonconducted or blocked atrial premature contraction. When the P wave is conducted in a retrograde fashion, it should be determined whether the P wave is related to the preceding QRS complex or to the QRS complex that followed or to both. The P wave of an A-V junctional premature beat may be preceded or followed by the QRS complex, depending upon whether the atria or ventricles were activated first. When a retrograde P wave is related to both the preceding and the following QRS complex and becomes placed between them, a reciprocal beat is usually present.

The QRS complex of A-V junctional premature or reciprocal beats may show a bizarre form because of aberrant ventricular conduction. The QRS complex of a ventricular premature beat is usually wide and bizarre. Rarely, as previously mentioned, a P wave may follow the QRS complex of a ventricular premature beat.

Recognition of an artificial pacemaker-induced ventricular rhythm is unmistakable because of the presence of the electrical artifact preceding each QRS complex.

Rare types of prematurely appearing P waves may be due to atrial or A-V junctional parasystole, atrial dissociation, or cardiac transplantation.

Ventricular parasystole produces prematurely appearing QRS complexes with varying coupling intervals.

In the presence of A-V dissociation, atrial or ventricular captured beats may produce prematurely appearing P waves or QRS complexes, respectively. Fusion beats, atrial or ventricular in origin, produce variations in the shape of the P waves and QRS complexes. Fusion beats are very common in parasystole. When a QRS complex appears later than usual in the basic rhythm, it is usually either an A-V junctional or ventricular escape beat. The QRS complex of A-V junctional escape beats is ordinarily normal in appearance, but not uncommonly it is wide and bizarre because of aberrant ventricular conduction. Ventricular escape (idioventricular) beats are always wide and bizarre. Escape beats, either A-V junctional or ventricular in origin, follow a long pause and are seen with various arrhythmias, including S-A block, sinus arrest, marked sinus bradycardia, sinus arrhythmia, second- or third-degree A-V block, and premature beats (extrasystoles).

DETERMINATION OF VENTRICULAR ABERRANCY VS. VENTRICULAR ECTOPY

It is extremely important yet often difficult to distinguish between supraventricular beats with aberrant ventricular conduction and ventricular ectopy, Aberrant ventricular conduction occurs when the supraventricular impulse is conducted to the ventricles during their partial refractory period. Ventricular aberrancy tends to occur when the coupling interval (the interval from abnormal beat to the preceding normal beat of the basic rhythm) is short or the ventricular cycle preceding the coupling interval is long (called *Ashman's phenomenon*). The diagnosis of ventricular aberrancy is supported by the following findings:

1. Short coupling interval
2. Ashman's phenomenon
3. Absence of a postectopic pause
4. Right bundle branch block pattern
5. Same initial vector between a normal and abnormal beat

If ventricular ectopy is diagnosed, needless to say, the above-mentioned ECG findings are absent.

CLASSIFICATION OF CARDIAC ARRHYTHMIAS

See the list on page 299 for detailed classification of cardiac arrhythmias.

REACHING FINAL CONCLUSIONS

After complete clinical and electrophysiological impressions are made, one should summarize all findings and ask himself the following questions.

1. What is the origin of the dominant rhythm?
   A. Is it normal sinus rhythm?
   B. Is it an ectopic rhythm?

2. What is the fundamental genesis of the arrhythmia?
   A. Is it abnormal impulse formation?
      (1) Is it active impulse formation?
      (2) Is it passive impulse formation?
      (3) Is it atrial, A-V junctional or ventricular in origin?
   B. Is it a conduction disturbance?
   C. Is it a combination of both?

3. Is the P wave present in the dominant rhythm?
   A. What is the origin of the P wave?
   B. What is the rate of the P wave?
   C. Is the P wave related to QRS complex?
      (1) If related, what is the mode of relationship between the P wave and the QRS complex?
      (2) If unrelated, what is the basic disorder producing A-V dissociation?

4. What is the atrial mechanism if the P wave is absent?
   A. Is the P wave truly absent, or superimposed on a portion of the QRS complex, S-T segment, T or U wave?
   B. Is the mechanism atrial fibrillation?
   C. Is it atrial flutter?
   D. Is it A-V junctional escape rhythm or tachycardia?
   E. Is it atrial standstill?

5. What is the origin and nature of the QRS complex if atrial and ventricular activities are independent?
   A. Is it active impulse formation in the A-V junction?
   B. Is it passive impulse formation in the A-V junction?
   C. Is it active impulse formation in the ventricles?
   D. Is it passive impulse formation in the ventricles?
   E. Is it artificial-pacemaker-induced ventricular rhythm?

6. What is the nature and origin of the beats that occur prematurely?
   A. Is it atrial, A-V junctional or ventricular, or perhaps sinus in origin?

B. Is it an ordinary premature beat (extrasystole)?

C. Is it sinus arrhythmia?

D. Is it parasystole?

E. Is it a reciprocal beat?

F. Is it a captured beat? (In the presence of A-V dissociation?)

G. Is the wide and bizarre QRS complex due to aberrant ventricular conduction of a supraventricular beat or is the beat of ventricular origin?

7. Is this a simple or complex, common or uncommon cardiac arrhythmia?

A. Are there any complex mechanisms, such as concealed conduction, unidirectional block, supernormal A-V conduction, involved?

B. Is the interpretation of the arrhythmia entirely satisfactory?

C. Are there any alternative interpretations?

8. What is the clinical significance of the arrhythmia?

A. Is treatment indicated?

B. What is the treatment of choice, if treatment is indicated?

DIAGNOSTIC CRITERIA

NORMAL SINUS RHYTHM

Normal sinus rhythm is diagnosed only when the following five criteria are present in the electrocardiogram:

1. P wave of sinus origin (normal mean axis of the P wave)

2. Constant and normal P-R interval (0.12-0.20 second)

3. Constant P wave configuration in each given lead

4. Rate between 60 and 100 beats per minute

5. Constant P-P (or R-R) cycle

DISTURBANCES OF SINUS IMPULSE FORMATION AND CONDUCTION

1. *Sinus bradycardia*

Sinus rhythm with a rate below 60 beats per minute is termed sinus bradycardia. The diagnostic criteria for sinus bradycardia are:

A. P wave of sinus origin (normal mean axis of the P wave)

B. Constant and normal P-R interval (0.12-0.20 second)

C. Constant P wave configuration in each given lead

D. Rate between 45 and 59 beats per minute (at times slower than 45 beats per minute)

E. Regular or slightly irregular P-P (or R-R) cycle

Sinus bradycardia often coexists with sinus arrhythmia.

2. *Sinus arrhythmia*

Sinus arrhythmia is diagnosed when the P-P cycles in sinus rhythm vary 0.16 second or more. The diagnostic criteria of sinus arrhythmia are as follows:

A. P wave of sinus origin (normal mean axis of the P wave)

B. Constant and normal P-R interval (0.12-0.20 second)

C. Constant P wave configuration in each given lead

D. Rate between 45 and 100 beats per minute (occasionally slower than 45 and faster than 100 beats per minute)

E. Irregular P-P cycle (variation of P-P interval 0.16 second or more)

Sinus arrhythmia is divided into 2 major types, namely respiratory and nonrespiratory.

A. In respiratory sinus arrhythmia, the sinus rate increases gradually with inspiration and slows with expiration.

B. Nonrespiratory sinus arrhythmia is the irregular sinus cycle not related to the respiratory cycle.

Sinus arrhythmia is often associated with wandering pacemaker in the sinus node and sinus bradycardia.

3. *Sinus tachycardia*

Sinus tachycardia is diagnosed when all of the 5 criteria for the diagnosis of normal sinus rhythm are present except for a rate faster than 100 beats per minute. The diagnostic criteria of sinus tachycardia include:

A. P wave of sinus origin (normal mean axis of the P wave)

B. Constant and normal P-R interval (0.12–0.20 second)

C. Constant P wave configuration in each given lead

D. Rate between 101 and 160 beats per minute (may be faster than 160 and may reach to 180–200 beats per minute during physical exercise in children and young adults)

E. Regular or slightly irregular P-P cycle

It is important to remember that the rate change in sinus tachycardia is usually gradual and it is *not* paroxysmal in nature.

4. *Wandering pacemaker in the sinus node*

A wandering pacemaker in the sinus node is frequently associated with sinus arrhythmia. Thus, a wandering pacemaker in the sinus node is considered by many investigators as a variant of sinus arrhythmia or an exaggerated form of sinus arrhythmia. The diagnostic criteria include:

A. P wave of sinus origin (normal mean axis of the P wave)

B. Varying P wave configuration in each given lead

C. Relatively constant P-R interval (may vary between 0.12 and 0.20 second)

D. Slightly irregular or regular P-P cycles

E. Rate between 45 and 100 beats per minute (rarely slower than 45 or faster than 100 beats per minute)

5. *Sinus arrest*

A. Sinus arrest (pause or standstill) is defined as a failure of impulse formation in the sinus node.

B. Sinus arrest is diagnosed by absence of the expected P wave.

C. The long P-P interval due to sinus arrest has no relationship to the basic P-P cycle.

D. One or more A-V junctional (less commonly ventricular) escape beats often occur in sinus arrest and may produce A-V dissociation.

E. Sinus arrest is frequently associated with sinus bradycardia and sinus arrhythmia.

F. Sinus arrest is commonly a manifestation of sick sinus syndrome.

6. *Sino-atrial (S-A) block*

S-A block may be classified into first, second, and third degree S-A block analogous to degrees of A-V block. However, only second degree S-A block can be diagnosed with certainty.

Second degree S-A block can be divided into 2 categories: (1) Mobitz Type I (Wenckebach) S-A block, which is comparable to Wenckebach A-V block (Fig. 21-1); and (2) Mobitz Type II S-A block, which is comparable to Mobitz Type II A-V block.

A. *Mobitz Type I (Wenckebach) S-A block*

Mobitz Type I S-A block is one of the most difficult arrhythmias to diagnose even by experienced cardiologist. One or more A-V junctional (less commonly ventricular) escape beats may occur in Wenckebach S-A block, and A-V dissociation also may be observed. The diagnostic criteria of Mobitz Type I (Wenckebach) S-A block are:

(1) Progressive shortening of the P-P cycles followed by a long pause (long P-P interval)

(2) The pause (the longest P-P cycle) is shorter than 2 shortest P-P cycles

(3) Regular irregularity of the P-P cycles when the conduction ratio is constant

B. *Mobitz Type II S-A block*

In this type of S-A block, there is an occasional absence of one or more expected sinus P waves. The QRS complex and T wave are also usually absent in S-A block. One or more A-V junctional (less commonly ventricular) escape beats may occur, and A-V dissociation is often produced in Mobitz Type II S-A block.

The diagnostic criteria of Mobitz Type II S-A block include:

(1) Constant P-P cycles (unless sinus arrhythmia is present) followed by an absence of the expected sinus P wave

(2) The long P-P interval due to S-A block shows a multiple of the basic P-P cycles

(3) Regular irregularity of the P-P cycles when the conduction ratio is constant

ATRIAL ARRHYTHMIAS

1. *Atrial premature contractions (extrasystoles)*

Atrial premature contractions (APCs) may originate from anywhere in the atria outside the sinus node. In most instances, atrial premature impulse activates the entire atria, including the sinus node. It is important to remember that frequent APCs may lead to atrial tachycardia, flutter, or fibrillation.

The diagnostic criteria of APC include:

A. Prematurely occurring P wave with constant coupling interval (interval from ectopic beat to the preceding beat of the basic rhythm)

B. Ectopic P wave configuration different from the sinus P waves

C. The ectopic P wave is usually upright in lead II and inverted in lead aVR (rarely APCs originating from left atrium may show inverted P waves in leads II, III, aVF and V_{5-6}, and upright in leads aVR and V_1).

D. APC followed by a non-full compensatory pause (the sinus P-P cycle containing APC is less than 2 basic sinus P-P cycles)

E. Ectopic P wave followed by a normal QRS complex in most cases (The QRS complex may be bizarre because of aberrant ventricular conduction)

F. APC that may be not followed by QRS complex (nonconducted or blocked APC) when the ectopic atrial impulse reaches the A-V junction during an absolute refractory period

G. P-R interval of the APC that is often longer than that of sinus beats in a given ECG tracing

2. *Atrial tachycardia*

Atrial tachycardia, like APCs, may originate from anywhere in the atria other than the sinus node. Since the onset of atrial tachycardia is commonly sudden, the term *paroxysmal atrial tachycardia* (so-called PAT) is frequently used to designate this entity.

By definition, 6 or more consecutive APCs are considered sufficient for the diagnosis of atrial tachycardia. The diagnostic criteria of atrial tachycardia include:

A. Regular tachycardia with upright P waves in leads II (often the P waves may not be easily recognized because of their superimposition to other portions of the ECG complexes)

B. A rate between 160 and 250 beats per minute

C. QRS complexes that are usually normal (unless there is aberrant ventricular conduction or bundle branch block)

D. An A-V ratio of 1:1 (unless there is coexisting A-V block)

E. Termination of atrial tachycardia or no response by carotid sinus stimulation (see Chap. 28)

F. Atrial tachycardia with varying degree A-V block (commonly Wenckebach A-V block) is nearly always due to digitalis toxicity (see Chap. 23).

3. *Multifocal atrial tachycardia*

Multifocal atrial tachycardia (MAT) has been called "chaotic atrial tachycardia or rhythm," "wandering pacemaker in the atria," and "malignant atrial tachycardia." MAT is most commonly found in chronic cor pulmonale. The diagnostic criteria of MAT include:

A. Two or more ectopic P waves with different configurations with 2 or more different ectopic P-P cycles

B. Atrial rate between 100 and 250 beats per minute (occasionally slower than 100 beats per minute)

C. Isoelectric line present between P-P intervals

D. Frequent occurrence of varying P-R intervals and A-V block of varying degree

E. Normal QRS complexes (unless there is aberrant ventricular conduction or bundle branch block)

4. *Atrial flutter*

Atrial flutter, like atrial tachycardia, may originate from anywhere in the atria outside of the sinus node. It should be noted that the ventricular rate around 150 beats per minute always raises a possibility of atrial flutter with 2:1 A-V conduction. The diagnostic criteria of atrial flutter include:

A. Atrial rate between 250 and 350 beats per minute

B. Sawtooth appearance of flutter waves

C. Most atrial flutter showing 2:1 A-V conduction

D. Usually regular atrial flutter cycles

E. QRS complex that is normal (unless there is aberrant ventricular conduction or bundle branch block)

5. *Atrial fibrillation*

Atrial fibrillation is the most common underlying ectopic rhythm that may originate from any portion of the atria other than sinus node. The diagnostic criteria of atrial fibrillation include:

A. Grossly irregular atrial as well as ventricular cycles

B. Atrial rate of usually more than 400 beats per minute, but it is often difficult to count

C. In many cases, fibrillation waves that are so small (fine) that no clear atrial activity is seen on the ECG

D. No P waves (fibrillation waves replace P waves)

E. Pure atrial fibrillation that often shows rapid (120–200 beats per minute) ventricular response

F. Normal QRS complex (unless there is aberrant ventricular conduction or bundle branch block)

6. *Atrial flutter-fibrillation*

The term *atrial flutter-fibrillation* is used when atrial flutter is mixed with atrial fibrillation. In this case, the flutter cycles often show irregularity and the atrial rate tends to be faster than 350 beats per minute.

7. *Atrial impure flutter*

The term *atrial impure flutter* is used when the atrial flutter rate is between 350 and 400 beats per minute, and other diagnostic criteria of the ordinary atrial flutter are present. The flutter cycles of the impure atrial flutter may be slightly irregular.

8. *Atrial standstill*

Atrial standstill is usually due to other primary cardiac rhythm disorders, such as marked sinus bradycardia, sinus arrest and sinoatrial block. The diagnostic criteria of atrial standstill include:

A. No atrial activity (either sinus or ectopic) in any lead of conventional (surface) or intracardiac electrocardiogram

B. No "a" wave in the neck veins or in the intra-atrial pressure tracing

C. Immobile atria on fluoroscopy and cineangiocardiography

D. A regular and slow ventricular rhythm without atrial activity

9. *Supraventricular tachycardia*

The term *supraventricular tachycardia* is frequently used whenever the ECG tracing shows a regular and rapid tachycardia with normal QRS complexes. The P waves are often indiscernible. However, *supraventricular tachycardia* is a broad term that actually refers to either atrial or A-V junctional tachycardia, or to reciprocating tachycardia. Therefore, the usage of the term *supraventricular tachycardia* should be avoided as much as possible, and a specific diagnosis of a given arrhythmia should be made.

A-V JUNCTIONAL ARRHYTHMIAS

In most instances, the impulse from the A-V junction activates the entire atria, including the sinus node, unless the underlying rhythm is atrial fibrillation or flutter. An ectopic impulse originating from the A-V junction is conducted in two directions simultaneously. Retrograde conduction activates the atria, whereas antegrade (forward) conduction activates the ventricles. Although the onset of retrograde and antegrade conduction is simultaneous, atrial and ventricular activation do not necessarily occur simultaneously. In fact, more often, atrial and ventricular activations are completed at different times. The retrograde P wave of the A-V junctional impulse may be preceded by or followed by the QRS complex, depending upon whether the atria or ventricles are activated first.

1. *A-V junctional premature contractions (extrasystoles)*

A-V junctional premature contraction (JPC) may originate from any location in the A-V junction. The diagnostic criteria of the A-V JPC include:

   A. Prematurely occurring retrograde P wave (inverted in leads II, III and aVF and upright in lead aVR), provided that the basic rhythm is sinus

   B. A premature retrograde P wave that may precede or follow a normal QRS complex (unless there is aberrant ventricular conduction or bundle branch block)

   C. A P-R interval of usually 0.12 second or less (unless there is a delayed antegrade conduction)

   D. An R-P interval between 0.10 and 0.20 second (unless there is a delayed retrograde conduction)

   E. Non-full compensatory pause following JPC in most instances

   F. Prematurely occurring normal QRS complex (unless there is aberrant ventricular conduction) in atrial fibrillation or flutter (this is difficult to diagnose with certainty)

2. *A-V junctional tachycardia*

A-V junctional tachycardia (A-V JT) is classified into 2 major forms. One form is paroxysmal A-V JT, which is comparable to paroxysmal atrial tachycardia. Another form is nonparoxysmal A-V JT.

   A. *Paroxysmal A-V junctional tachycardia*

Paroxysmal A-V JT may be found in apparently healthy individuals although it may occur in various cardiac diseases. It is interesting to note that paroxysmal A-V JT has *not* been reported in patients with digitalis intoxication. The diagnostic criteria of paroxysmal A-V JT are:

   (1) Regular tachycardia with a rate of 160 to 250 beats per minute

   (2) Normal QRS complex, unless there is aberrant ventricular conduction or bundle branch block

   (3) Retrograde P waves that may precede or follow QRS complexes (unless atrial fibrillation or flutter coexists)

   (4) A P-R interval of usually 0.12 second or less (unless atrial fibrillation or flutter coexists)

   (5) R-P interval between 0.10 and 0.20 second (unless atrial fibrillation or flutter coexists)

   (6) Usually paroxysmal onset and termination

   B. *Nonparoxysmal A-V junctional tachycardia*

Nonparoxysmal A-V JT is most commonly found in digitalis intoxication. The second common cause is acute diaphragmatic (inferior) myocardial infarction. Less commonly, nonparoxysmal A-V JT may be found in myocarditis, cardiomyopathy, and hypoxia due to various causes. The diagnostic criteria of nonparoxysmal A-V JT include:

(1) Regular tachycardia with a rate between 70 and 130 beats per minute

(2) Normal QRS complex, unless there is aberrant ventricular conduction or bundle branch block

(3) Retrograde P waves that may precede or follow QRS complexes (unless atrial fibrillation or flutter coexists)

(4) A P-R interval of 0.12 second or less (unless atrial fibrillation or flutter coexists)

(5) An R-P interval of 0.12 to 0.20 second (unless atrial fibrillation or flutter coexists)

(6) An underlying rhythm that is frequently atrial fibrillation to produce A-V dissociation

(7) Onset and termination that are *not* paroxysmal

3. *A-V junctional escape rhythm*

A-V junctional escape rhythm (JER) is due to a passive impulse formation in the A-V junction. A-V JER is usually produced by other primary rhythm disorders, such as complete A-V block, marked sinus bradycardia, sinus arrest, and sinoatrial block. A pure A-V JER is uncommon. The diagnostic criteria of A-V JER are:

A. Slow and regular rhythm with a rate between 40 and 60 beats per minute

B. Normal QRS complex, unless there is bundle branch block

C. Retrograde P waves that may precede or follow QRS complexes (in a pure form)

D. A P-R interval of 0.12 second or less, but an R-P interval of 0.12 to 0.20 second (in a pure form)

E. Complete A-V block is a common underlying cause for the development of A-V JER. Therefore, atrial and ventricular activities are independent (A-V dissociation)

F. Less commonly, A-V JER coexists with sinus bradycardia, sinus arrest and S-A block to produce A-V dissociation.

4. *Atrioventricular (A-V) dissociation*

By definition, A-V dissociation indicates that the atria and ventricles beat independently, so that P waves or atrial fibrillation or flutter waves, and the QRS complexes do not have any relationship. It should be emphasized that A-V dissociation is by no means a complete description of the cardiac arrhythmia because it is always a consequence of some other primary cardiac rhythm disorder. The various causes responsible for the development of A-V dissociation are summarized in the list on page 302.

5. *Reciprocating beats and reciprocating tachycardia*

A. Reciprocal beats and reciprocating tachycardia are considered to be due to a re-entry mechanism occurring in the A-V junction.

B. Reciprocal beat is diagnosed when a retrograde P wave is noted to be ''sandwiched'' between two closely spaced QRS complexes.

C. Reciprocal beat is often indistinguishable from a pure A-V junctional premature contraction.

D. Reciprocating tachycardia is actually a form of supraventricular tachycardia, and so called paroxysmal atrial or A-V junctional tachycardia often represents reciprocating tachycardia.

A-V BLOCK

A-V block is the most common conduction disturbance involving the A-V conduction system. A-V block can be classified into: (1) first degree; (2) second degree; (3) high degree (advanced); and (4) complete (third degree) A-V block (see list on p. 299).

1. *First degree A-V block*

First degree A-V block is very common in elderly persons without apparent heart disease. In addition, it is also common in mild digitalis toxicity, acute diaphragmatic myocardial infarction, and acute myocarditis, especially in acute rheumatic fever. The diagnostic criteria of first degree A-V block include:

A. Prolongation of the P-R interval, 0.21 second or more in adults

B. Prolongation of the P-R interval, 0.18 second or more in children

C. Constant P-R intervals

2. *Second degree A-V block*

There are two major forms of second degree A-V block, including (1) Mobitz Type I (Wenckebach) A-V block; and (2) Mobitz Type II A-V block.

A. *Mobitz Type I (Wenckebach) A-V block*

Mobitz Type I (Wenckebach) A-V block is the most common form of second degree A-V block. The site of a block is almost always A-V nodal block, which is very common in digitalis intoxication, acute diaphragmatic myocardial infarction, acute myocarditis. Wenckebach A-V block is often transient in nature and the A-V block is usually reversible. The diagnostic criteria of Mobitz Type I (Wenckebach) A-V block (Fig. 21-1) include:

(1) Progressive lengthening of the P-R intervals until blocked P wave (pause) occurs

(2) Progressive shortening of the R-R intervals until blocked P wave (pause) occurs

(3) The longest R-R interval (pause) containing a blocked P wave is less than 2 shortest R-R intervals

(4) Regular irregularity of the ventricular cycles when A-V conduction ratio is constant.

(5) Normal QRS complex (unless bundle branch block is present)

B. *Mobitz Type II A-V block*

Mobitz Type II A-V block is a very uncommon form of second degree A-V block. A block usually develops at the site of an infranodal block, which is considered to be a precursor of complete A-V block (complete bilateral bundle branch block). Therefore, Mobitz Type II A-V block is usually *not* reversible and the underlying process is considered to be a sclerotic-degenerative change in the Purkinje network. The diagnostic criteria of Mobitz Type II A-V block are:

(1) Constant P-R intervals in all conducted beats with occasional occurrence of a blocked P wave

(2) Constant R-R intervals until a blocked P wave occurs

(3) The longest R-R interval (pause) containing a blocked P wave is 2 times that of the basic P-P (or R-R) cycles

(4) Regular irregularity of the ventricular cycle when the A-V conduction ratio is constant

(5) A QRS complex that often shows bundle branch block

C. *2:1 A-V block*

A 2:1 A-V block is either a variant of Mobitz Type I (Wenckebach) or Type II A-V block. Therefore, 2:1 A-V block can not be specified unless a transitional change from or to Mobitz Type I or II A-V block is found in the same ECG tracing. For the same reason, a site of 2:1 A-V block can be at either an A-V nodal or an infranodal block. The diagnostic criteria of 2:1 A-V block include:

(1) Blocked P waves occurring on every other beat

(2) Constant P-R intervals in all conducted beats

(3) An R-R interval 2 times that of the P-P cycle

(4) A QRS complex that may be normal or that may show bundle branch block

3. *High degree (advanced) A-V block*

High degree (advanced) A-V block is the most advanced form of incomplete A-V block, and it is often a precursor of complete A-V block. High degree A-V block is diagnosed when the A-V conduction ratio is 3:1 or greater. The site of high degree A-V block is at an infranodal block in most cases. The diagnostic criteria of high degree A-V block include:

A. A-V conduction ratio of 3:1 or greater

B. An R-R interval representing a multiple of the P-P cycle

C. Constant P-R intervals in all conducted beats

D. A ventricular cycle that is regular when the A-V conduction ratio is constant

E. A QRS complex that often shows bundle branch block

F. Frequent occurrence of escape beats

4. *Complete (third degree) A-V block*

Complete A-V block is characterized by independent atrial and ventricular activities resulting from complete block at the A-V node, His bundle (common bundle), and bilateral bundle branches. Thus, complete A-V block may be either A-V nodal block or infranodal block.

It should be noted that complete A-V block is one of the most common causes of A-V dissociation (see list on p. 302).

A-V junctional or ventricular escape rhythm occurs to control the ventricular activity in complete A-V block.

The nature of complete A-V block depends on the site of the block. Complete A-V nodal block is usually reversible, and it is commonly due to digitalis intoxication, acute diaphragmatic myocardial infarction, and acute myocarditis. On the other hand, complete infranodal block is usually permanent; the acute form is frequently due to acute anterior myocardial infarction, whereas the chronic form is considered to be due to a degenerative-sclerotic change in the Purkinje network.

The diagnostic criteria of complete A-V block are as follows:

A. Independent atrial and ventricular activities

B. Regular ventricular cycle (A-V junctional or ventricular escape rhythm)

C. Ventricular rate between 30 and 60 beats per minute (may be <30 b.p.m.).

D. Atrial mechanism that may be sinus or ectopic

E. A QRS complex that may be normal (A-V nodal block) or broad (infranodal block)

F. Ventriculophasic sinus arrhythmia (The P-P interval containing a QRS complex is shorter than the P-P interval without QRS complex) in 30 per cent of the patients with complete A-V block.

VENTRICULAR ARRHYTHMIAS

Ventricular arrhythmias may be generated by an active or a passive impulse formation in the ventricles. The ectopic focus may be located anywhere in the ventricles. The QRS complex in ventricular arrhythmias as a rule, is bizarre and broad. Ventricular arrhythmias with normal (narrow) QRS complexes are considered to be originating from a fascicle of the bundle branch system.

1. *Ventricular premature contractions (extrasystoles)*

Ventricular premature contractions (VPCs) are the most common arrhythmia in human beings. They may occur in apparently healthy individuals, but they are common in digitalis toxicity (see Chap. 23) and coronary heart disease (see Chap. 2). The diagnostic criteria of VPCs include:

A. Prematurely occurring bizarre QRS complex with constant coupling interval

B. Full compensatory pause following a VPC in most cases (the P-P interval containing a VPC is twice the P-P cycles of the basic rhythm).

C. In occasional cases, an interpolated ectopic QRS complex (VPC is sandwiched between two QRS complexes of the basic rhythm)

D. A QRS interval of the ectopic beat that is almost always 0.12 second or more

E. A secondary T wave change (the

direction of the T wave is opposite to that of the QRS complex)

F. In occasional cases, a postectopic T wave change that follows the VPC

2. *Ventricular tachycardia*

The term *ventricular tachycardia* is used when 6 or more consecutive VPCs occur. Ventricular tachycardia, like isolated VPCs, may originate from any portion of the ventricles. There are two forms of ventricular tachycardia: paroxysmal and nonparoxysmal. Paroxysmal ventricular tachycardia is an ordinary ventricular tachycardia that is more common than nonparoxysmal ventricular tachycardia.

A. *Paroxysmal ventricular tachycardia*

Paroxysmal ventricular tachycardia, as the name indicates, has a paroxysmal nature, and its rate is usually rapid. This type of ventricular tachycardia is almost always encountered in serious heart disease, particularly acute myocardial infarction, and the arrhythmia should be treated immediately. The diagnostic criteria of paroxysmal ventricular tachycardia include:

(1) Regular tachycardia with bizarre QRS complexes (QRS interval: 0.12 second or more in most cases)

(2) A ventricular rate between 160 and 250 beats per minute

(3) QRS complexes not preceded by P waves (often there is A-V dissociation)

(4) Often abrupt onset and termination

(5) Long post-tachycardia pause upon termination

(6) Identical configuration between an isolated VPC and the QRS complexes during the tachycardia

(7) No response to carotid sinus stimulation (see Chap. 28)

B. *Nonparoxysmal ventricular tachycardia*

Nonparoxysmal ventricular tachycar-

dia has been termed *accelerated idioventricular rhythm,* and *idioventricular tachycardia.* This form of ventricular tachycardia is not as common as paroxysmal ventricular tachycardia. Nonparoxysmal ventricular tachycardia is most commonly observed during the first 72 hours of acute myocardial infarction, and the arrhythmia is usually self-limited. The diagnostic criteria of nonparoxysmal ventricular tachycardia are:

(1) Regular tachycardia with bizarre QRS complexes (QRS interval: 0.12 second or more)

(2) A ventricular rate between 70 and 130 beats per minute (often a similar rate to the rate of the basic rhythm)

(3) QRS complexes not preceded by P waves (often there is A-V dissociation)

(4) Onset and termination that are *not* abrupt

(5) No significant postectopic pause

(6) No response to carotid sinus stimulation

3. *Ventricular flutter*

Ventricular flutter has the same clinical significance as ventricular fibrillation. Therefore, direct current shock should be applied immediately (see Chap. 25). Otherwise, a fatal outcome is unavoidable. The diagnostic criteria of ventricular flutter include:

(1) Sawtooth appearance of the entire ECG complexes (a separation of QRS complex from S-T and T waves is impossible), so that the ECG complexes appear to be a continuous loop

(2) A rate between 160 and 250 beats per minute (at times slower than 160 beats per minute)

(3) Flutter cycles that may be regular or slightly irregular

4. *Ventricular fibrillation*

Ventricular fibrillation is the worst cardiac arrhythmia, which should be defibrillated immediately. The diagnostic criteria of ventricular fibrillation include:

A. Grossly irregular (chaotic) ventricular rhythm

B. No descernible P waves

C. A ventricular rate that is difficult to count, but usually more than 250 beats per minute

5. *Ventricular escape (idioventricular) rhythm*

Ventricular escape rhythm (VER) is a passive rhythm originating from any portion of the ventricles. Thus, VER is usually produced when there is complete A-V (infranodal) block. The diagnostic criteria of VER include:

A. Regular and slow ventricular rhythm with bizarre QRS complexes (QRS interval: 0.12 second or more)

B. A ventricular rate between 25 and 45 beats per minute (at times slower than 25 beats per minute)

C. A ventricular cycle that may be precisely regular, but that may be slightly irregular

D. Usually independent atrial and ventricular activities (A-V dissociation)

E. Atrial mechanism that may be sinus or ectopic

6. *Ventricular standstill (arrest)*

A. Ventricular standstill (arrest), like atrial standstill, is usually the consequence of some other cardiac arrhythmia.

B. The term *ventricular standstill* is used when no QRS complex is observed for a few seconds or longer.

C. Ventricular arrest may occur in the presence of any atrial activity, but both atrial as well as ventricular activity may be absent altogether (cardiac arrest or standstill).

D. Ventricular standstill results when a subsidiary pacemaker fails to produce an escape impulse during sinus arrest, S-A block, and complete A-V block.

E. Ventricular arrest may follow upon the termination of ectopic tachyarrhythmia.

F. Ventricular standstill may be observed during carotid sinus stimulation (see Chap. 28).

7. *Chaotic ventricular rhythm*

A. The term *chaotic ventricular rhythm* has been used to designate multifocal ventricular rhythms with extremely unstable mechanisms. It usually designates a terminal cardiac rhythm.

B. Chaotic ventricular rhythm often consists of a period of ventricular tachycardia, ventricular flutter or fibrillation, multifocal VPCs, high degree or complete A-V block, ventricular escape rhythm, and ventricular standstill.

8. *Artificial pacemaker induced ventricular rhythm*

Artificial pacemaker induced ventricular rhythm (APIVR) is readily recognized because each QRS complex is initiated by the artificial pacemaker spike. The diagnostic criteria of APIVR include:

A. Regular tachycardia with broad QRS complexes (QRS interval: 0.12 second or more) initiated by the artificial pacemaker spikes

B. A ventricular rate usually between 60 and 70 beats per minute.

C. Independent atrial and ventricular activities (A-V dissociation) in most cases

MISCELLANEOUS ARRHYTHMIAS

1. *Wolff-Parkinson-White syndrome: (ventricular pre-excitation syndrome)*

A. Wolff-Parkinson-White (WPW) syndrome was first recognized as a clinical entity by Wolff, Parkinson, and White in 1930.

B. The recognition of this syndrome is important because 50 to 75 per cent of the cases of WPW syndrome experience paroxysmal supraventricular tachyarrhythmias.

C. The diagnostic criteria of WPW syndrome consist of a short P-R interval and a broad QRS complex due to a delta wave (initial slurring of the upstroke of the QRS complex).

D. The mechanism responsible for the production of unique ECG findings in WPW syndrome is considered to be due to premature activation of a portion of the ventricles via an anomalous conduction.

E. The WPW syndrome is classified into two major types:

(1) *Type A:* Delta wave is directed anteriorly and to the right so that the delta wave is usually upright in leads V_{1-3} (often through leads V_{4-6}). Type A WPW syndrome resembles right bundle branch block.

(2) *Type B:* Delta wave is directed posteriorly and to the left so that the delta wave is upright in leads V_{4-6} and inverted in lead V_1 (often through leads V_{2-3}). Type B WPW syndrome closely resembles left bundle branch block.

F. WPW syndrome (both Types A and B) often produces pseudodiaphragmatic myocardial infarction pattern.

G. The most common tachyarrhythmia in WPW syndrome is reciprocating tachycardia (so-called paroxysmal atrial tachycardia). The next common arrhythmia is atrial fibrillation, and atrial flutter is rare.

H. Type A WPW syndrome is prone to atrial fibrillation and flutter, which are not uncommonly refractory to drug therapy.

I. The mechanism of tachyarrhythmias in WPW syndrome is considered to be a re-entry phenomenon involving an anomalous pathway and normal A-V conduction system.

J. Treatment of tachyarrhythmias in WPW syndrome is outlined in Chapter 24.

2. *Sick sinus syndrome*

A. The term *sick sinus syndrome* is commonly used to designate an abnormal function of the sinus node.

B. The sick sinus syndrome, therefore, may present as various electrocardiographic findings. Common ECG findings indicative of sick sinus syndrome may include:

(1) Marked sinus bradycardia

(2) Sinus arrest

(3) Sinoatrial block

(4) Ineffectiveness of atropine or isoproterenol for the above-mentioned arrhythmias

(5) Longer than expected postectopic pause (returning cycle) following an atrial premature beat (marked depression of the sinus node by the ectopic atrial impulse)

(6) Chronic atrial fibrillation

C. Many patients with sick sinus syndrome require a permanent artificial pacemaker (see Chap. 26).

3. *Brady-tachyarrhythmia syndrome*

A. The term *brady-tachyarrhythmia syndrome* is used when the ECG tracing shows areas of slow rhythms mixed with areas of rapid rhythms.

B. The slow rhythms may include marked sinus bradycardia, sinus arrest, S-A block, second degree or complete A-V block, and A-V junctional or ventricular escape rhythm.

C. The rapid rhythms may include any ectopic tachyarrhythmias, but frequently they are multifocal VPCs or short runs of ventricular tachycardia.

D. Drug therapy alone is not satisfactory for brady-tachyarrhythmia syndrome, and many patients require artificial pacemakers (see Chaps. 24 and 26).

4. *Parasystole*

A. *Definition*

Parasystole consists of simultaneous activity of two (rarely more) independent impulse-forming centers, one of which is "protected" from the other, each competing to activate the atria or ventricles or both.

B. *Ectopic focus*

The parasystolic pacemaker may be located anywhere in the heart but is commonly located in the ventricles, less commonly in the A-V junction and rarely in the atria.

C. *Rate*

The rate of parasystole may range

from 20 to 400 beats per minute, but most commonly it is between 40 and 50 beats per minute.

D. *Diagnostic criteria*

(1) Varying coupling intervals

(2) Constant shortest interectopic intervals

(3) Long interectopic intervals show a multiple of the shortest interectopic interval.

(4) Frequent occurrence of fusion beats

E. *Clinical significance*

(1) Parasystole closely resembles ordinary premature beats (extrasystoles)

(2) Parasystole is *not* a digitalis-induced arrhythmia

(3) Parasystole is often refractory to the commonly used antiarrhythmic agents (see Chap. 24).

(4) Parasystole is usually self-limited.

5. *Coronary sinus rhythm*

It should be noted that it is impossible to distinguish between coronary sinus rhythm and A-V junctional rhythm (or tachycardia) with delayed antegrade (forward) conduction. The diagnostic criteria of coronary sinus rhythm include:

A. Inverted P waves in leads II, III, and aVF and upright P wave in lead aVR

B. A P-R interval longer than 0.12 second

6. *Coronary nodal rhythm*

It should be noted that it is not uncommon to observe a short P-R interval in many healthy individuals with sinus rhythm. The diagnostic criteria of coronary nodal rhythm include:

A. Upright P waves in leads II, III, and aVF, and inverted P waves in lead aVR (the same direction of the P waves as the sinus rhythm)

B. A P-R interval of 0.10 second or less

7. *Lown-Ganong-Levine (LGL) syndrome*

The identical ECG findings as coronary nodal rhythm have also been called as Lown-Ganong-Levine (LGL) syndrome when the patient suffers from paroxysmal tachyarrhythmias. In a practical sense, the LGL syndrome is considered to be a variant of WPW syndrome, but the delta wave is not obvious in the former.

MANAGEMENT OF ARRHYTHMIAS

Guideline to the Management of Arrhythmias

1. The best therapeutic result only follows the correct diagnosis of a given arrhythmia.

2. Eliminate the underlying cause if present.

3. Serious considerations regarding indications and contraindications of various antiarrhythmic agents (see Chap. 24).

4. Choice of a proper drug and its dosage.

5. Careful considerations of interrelationship between various drugs (see Chap. 25).

6. Prevention of recurrent arrhythmias.

7. Proper use of direct current shock (see Chap. 25).

8. Proper use of artificial pacemakers (see Chap. 26).

9. Prevention of side effects and toxicity of various antiarrhythmic agents (see Chaps. 18, 23, and 24).

10. Detailed descriptions regarding management of various arrhythmias are found in Chapters 22, 24 to 26, and 28.

SUGGESTED READINGS

Chung, E. K.: Parasystole. Prog. Cardiovasc. Dis., *11*:64, 1968.

———: Principles of Cardiac Arrhythmias. Baltimore, Williams & Wilkins, 1971.

———: Electrocardiography: Practical Applications with Vectorial Principles. Hagerstown, Harper & Row, 1974.

————: Clinical Electrocardiography (Part 5): Differential Diagnosis (Slide Series). New York, Medcom, 1974.

Chung, E. K. and Chung, D. K.: ECG Diagnosis: Self Assessment. Hagerstown, Harper & Row, 1972.

Damato, A. N. and Lau, S. H.: Clinical value of the electrogram of the conduction system. Prog. Cardiovasc. Dis., *13*:119, 1970.

Kastor, J. A.: Current concepts: Atrioventricular block (Parts I and II). N. Engl. J. Med., *292*:462; 572, 1975.

Kistin, A. D.: Problems in the differentiation of ventricular arrhythmia from supraventricular arrhythmia with abnormal QRS. Prog. Cardiovasc. Dis., *9*:1, 1966.

Marriott, H. J. L. and Sandler, I. A.: Criteria, old and new, for differentiating between ectopic ventricular beats and aberrant ventricular conduction in the presence of atrial fibrillation. Prog. Cardiovasc. Dis., *9*:18, 1966.

Pick, A. and Langendorf, R.: Differentiation of supraventricular and ventricular tachycardias. Prog. Cardiovasc. Dis., *2*:391, 1960.

Winkle, R. A. et al.: Arrhythmias in patients with mitral valve prolapse. Circulation, *52*:73, 1975.

22. DIGITALIZATION

Edward K. Chung, M.D.

GENERAL CONSIDERATIONS

Digitalis is an indispensable drug in managing congestive heart failure and various cardiac arrhythmias, particularly those of supraventricular origin. From the time digitalis was introduced by a British physician, William Withering, into the practice of medicine in 1785, it has probably been the most valuable drug available for various cardiac as well as many noncardiac diseases. Unfortunately, there has been an increasing incidence of digitalis intoxication in recent years due to the utilization of newer and potent cardiac glycosides in conjunction with the potent diuretics. It has been shown that 1 out of 5 patients receiving cardiac glycosides in general hospitals have some degree of digitalis intoxication. The incidence of digitalis intoxication has been relatively high because the margin between therapeutic and toxic doses is narrow. This narrow margin becomes further reduced in elderly and seriously ill patients. The therapeutic dose is estimated to be approximately 60 per cent of the toxic dose.

Although digitalis is an essential drug in the treatment of congestive heart failure, the drug may cause or aggravate the congestive heart failure if the patient develops digitalis intoxication. Aggravation of congestive heart failure due to digitalis intoxication may be the first recognizable evidence of digitalis toxicity without any other manifestation. Congestive heart failure from digitalis intoxication may be much more common than is recognized, and this is particularly true in patients with refractory congestive heart failure.

Although such gastrointestinal symptoms as anorexia, nausea, and vomiting have been said to be the most common early symptoms, cardiac arrhythmias may be the only evidence of digitalis toxicity without such signs. The occurrence of cardiac arrhythmias is particularly common when using the purified glycosides. In fact, the occurrence of various arrhythmias in digitalis intoxication has been a more common manifestation than gastrointestinal symptoms, when purified glycosides have been used. In addition, cardiac arrhythmias are frequently the earliest sign of digitalis intoxication. Since the most serious and life-threatening manifestations of digitalis intoxication are cardiac arrhythmias, these arrhythmias must be immediately treated, for pre-existing congestive heart failure becomes rapidly worse under superimposed arrhythmias.

Most of the serious and unavoidable problems in the use of digitalis concerning toxicity result from inability of physicians to measure precisely the optimal therapeutic dosage of the drug. The determination of serum digoxin or digitoxin level is widely available at many institutions in order to assess the therapeutic and toxic doses of digitalis, but its clinical implication is still far from ideal. This is observed because there is a significant overlap between the therapeutic and toxic doses. Nevertheless, a markedly increased serum digitalis level certainly indicates digitalis toxicity, whereas a very small amount of digitalis in the serum usually indicates underdigitalization. Serum digitalis determination is extremely valuable when dealing with patients who suffer from intractable congestive heart failure and/or complex cardiac arrhythmias when little or no information regarding previous digitalization is available.

Patients may differ greatly in required dosage and tolerance to digitalis. Some may experience signs of toxicity with small amounts; while others may receive more than the usual quantity for digitalization without the development of toxicity. Toxic and therapeutic dosage may be almost the same in patients with severe congestive heart failure.

Other situations predisposing to toxicity, even with dosages usually nontoxic, include further deterioration of the underlying lesion, hypokalemia, myxedema, thyrotoxicosis, and advanced age. Therefore, any patients who are receiving a digitalis preparation may develop digitalis intoxication at any time during therapy. A search for digitalis intoxication should be a routine part of the management of patients with congestive heart failure, as an early recognition of digitalis toxicity simplifies therapy and minimizes morbidity and mortality. It is not uncommon to fail to recognize digitalis toxicity, even when it is severe enough to cause death, for digitalis intoxication does not produce pathognomonic evidence. In retrospect, an inadequate explanation of the cause of death in patients with refractory congestive heart failure can often be attributed to digitalis.

THE FUNDAMENTAL PRINCIPLES OF DIGITALIZATION

Before any physician attempts to administer digitalis to a patient, he should be fully aware of the following information regarding his patient and the cardiac glycoside he has chosen to use:

1. *Indications and contraindications for digitalization*

A. One should know whether or not digitalis is definitely indicated. One should know whether or not the patient is suffering from congestive heart failure and/or supraventricular tachyarrhythmias. Needless to say, two major

indications of digitalis include congestive heart failure and various supraventricular tachyarrhythmias, except those induced by digitalis.

B. In addition, one should be aware that there is no contraindication for digitalization except digitalis toxicity and idiopathic hypertrophic subaortic stenosis. The reason for this is that digitalis improves the contractile state of the left ventricular myocardium, which further reduces the left ventricular outflow tract. The clinical status of a patient with idiopathic hypertrophic subaortic stenosis deteriorates during digitalization but usually improves upon discontinuation of digitalis.

2. *Information on previous digitalization*

A. Physicians should try their best to obtain precise information as to previous digitalization, if possible. In particular, full information regarding past digitalization up to 3 to 4 weeks prior to present digitalization is important.

B. Not only the duration of digitalization, but also exact information concerning the preparation, dosage, and route of administration is indispensable.

C. If the clinical symptoms are rather mild and a history of previous digitalization is equivocal, it is preferable not to give any more digitalis until a definite indication for digitalization is established.

D. Serum digitalis determination by radioimmunoassay is extremely valuable when a history of previous digitalization is unclear.

3. *Electrocardiograms before and during digitalization*

A. It is essential to take a control electrocardiogram immediately before digitalization regardless of the clinical situation except in the case of the unusually acute patient in a critical state. The most important reason for this is to confirm a fundamental mechanism of the cardiac rhythm, so that it will be clearly evident if any new cardiac arrhythmia develops after digitalization.

B. Any form of a new cardiac arrhythmia that develops during or after digitalization strongly suggests digitalis intoxication, since almost every known type of rhythm disturbance may be induced by digitalis.

C. Another reason for the necessity of a control electrocardiogram is to know if there are any unexpected ECG abnormalities, such as acute myocardial infarction or hypokalemia, which directly influence the efficacy of digitalis and the incidence of digitalis toxicity.

D. In addition to the control electrocardiogram, frequent follow-up electrocardiographic tracings are needed until the patient becomes fully digitalized.

E. Electrocardiogram should be taken immediately, when there is any change in cardiac rhythm detected by physical examination, or digitalis toxicity is clinically suspected.

F. For the confirmation of the current cardiac mechanism, long rhythm strips of leads II and V_1 are adequate for the purpose.

4. *Choice of preparations and methods*

A. Choice of preparation and method of digitalization, directly and indirectly, influence the efficacy of digitalis and the development of digitalis intoxication.

B. For urgent situations, such as acute pulmonary edema, particularly associated with supraventricular tachyarrhythmias, a short-acting preparation, such as deslanoside (Cedilanid-D) or digoxin should be given intravenously.

C. If there are any modifying factors, short-acting preparations are always preferable.

D. If the clinical situation is not urgent, oral administration with slower method is advisable.

E. Every physician should be fully

familiar with the preparation chosen. Precise oral and parenteral dosages as well as various advantages and disadvantages of the particular preparations should be clearly understood.

F. By and large, every physician should be fully familiar with at least one preparation for intravenous use in order to obtain very rapid digitalization and one preparation for oral use for slow digitalization.

G. Digoxin has proven to be the most useful preparation that can be given in most clinical situations.

H. There is no point in changing from one preparation to another unless a definite advantage will be obtained or allergy to the former preparation is discovered.

5. *Factors modifying the efficacy of digitalis*

Various modifying factors, such as hypokalemia and various cardiac as well as noncardiac diseases, directly influence the efficacy and the development of digitalis toxicity. Therefore, these factors should be carefully considered (see Table 22-1).

6. *Determination of serum digitalis level*

In the past 10 years, various methods have been developed to determine serum digitalis level to assess an optimal therapeutic dosage and to diagnose digitalis toxicity with accuracy. Serum digitalis determination by radioimmunoassay method is extremely valuable when the values of serum digitalis levels are interpreted in conjunction with the total clinical picture and electrocardiographic findings. The usual therapeutic ranges of serum digoxin level are 1 to 2 ng./ml.

7. *Evaluation of refractory congestive heart failure*

A. Refractory congestive heart failure requires careful evaluation in order to determine whether the patient needs more digitalis or whether digitalis must be discontinued.

Table 22-1. Factors Modifying the Efficacy of Digitalis

Modifying factors		*Various conditions*
Age	Too young or too old	Advanced age, premature and newborn infant
Electrolyte imbalances	Potassium	Hypokalemia, hyperkalemia
	Calcium	Hypocalcemia, hypercalcemia
Various heart d.	Degree and diffuseness of heart d.	Advanced and generalized heart d.
	Primary myocardial d.	Idiopathic cardiomyopathy, Chagas' heart d., post-partum heart d., alcoholic cardio-myopathy
	Active heart d.	Acute myocarditis, pericarditis, endocar-ditis due to any cause
	Coronary heart d.	Acute M.I., severe coronary heart d.
	Mechanical obstruction	Mitral stenosis, constrictive pericarditis, cardiac tamponade or massive pericardial effusion, idiopathic hypertrophic subaortic stenosis
	Congenital and valvular heart d.	Any congenital and valvular heart d. with significant hemodynamic alteration
	Cardiac involvement from systemic d.	Amyloidosis, scleroderma, S.L.E., multiple myeloma, hemochromatosis, sarcoidosis, rheumatoid d.
	Tumors of heart	Primary or metastatic tumors
	Papillary muscle, ventricular or I-V septal rupture	Traumatic, post-M.I., or postendocarditis
	Right ventricular failure	Any cause
	Trauma of heart	Hemopericardium, I-V septal defect, myo-cardial rupture
	Idiopathic pulmonary hyper-tension	
Cardiac arrhythmias	A-V block and/or S-A block, ventricular arrhythmias, right or left bundle branch block, Wolff-Parkinson-White syndrome	
Noncardiac d.	Pulmonary d.	Pulmonary emphysema, bronchitis, pulmo-nary embolism and/or infarction
	Renal d. and related conditions	Renal failure due to any cause, peritoneal dialysis, nephrectomy
	Thyroid d.	Thyrotoxicosis, myxedema
	Other endocrine d.	Hyperaldosteronism, diabetic acidosis
	High output states	Anemias, beri-beri, A-V fistula, obesity, pregnancy
	Liver d.	Cirrhosis, liver involvement from systemic d. (amyloidosis, hemochromatosis, etc.), tumors of liver
	Psychoneurotic disorders	Hyperventilation syndrome, hysteria, cardi-ac neurosis, etc.
Concomitant other therapies	Diuretics	Thiazide preparations, mercurial diuretics, etc.
	Anti-hypertensive drugs	Reserpine, guanethidine, Aldomet, etc.
	Anti-arrhythmic drugs	Procaine amide, quinidine, etc.
	Beta-adrenergic blocking drugs	Pronethalol, propanolol
	Miscellaneous	Insulin, glucose, calcium salt, etc.
Miscellaneous conditions	Direct current shock, artificial pacemaker, cardiac catheterization, cardio-pulmonary bypass, general anesthesia, hypothermia, exercise (emotional and/or physical), carotid sinus stimulation, methods of digitalization, choice of digi-talis preparation, incorrect diagnosis of CHF and/or digitalis intoxication, misinterpretation of cardiac arrhythmias, prophylactic digitalization, cooper-ation of patients	

CHF, congestive heart failure; d., disease; M.I., myocardial infarction; I-V, interventricular; S.L.E., systemic lupus erythematosus. (From Chung, E. K.: Digitalis Intoxication. Amsterdam, Excerpta Medica, 1969.)

B. The presence of any modifying factors, (see Table 22-1) and the re-evaluation of the initial diagnosis are additional factors to be considered in treating refractory congestive heart failure.

C. It should be re-emphasized that digitalis intoxication is one of the important causes of refractory congestive heart failure.

8. *Evaluation of complex arrhythmias*

At times, digitalis-induced arrhythmias may be so complex that experienced electrocardiographers argue the mechanism of the cardiac rhythm. A given tracing may suggest a variety of mechanisms, and the cardiac rhythm may change quickly from one form to another every few seconds or minutes. It may be reasonable to state that an argument that ensues regarding the mechanism of the cardiac rhythm during digitalization is, in itself, often sufficient evidence to suspect digitalis intoxication.

INDICATIONS FOR DIGITALIZATION

Two major indications for digitalization include:

1. Congestive heart failure regardless of underlying heart disease (except when digitalis-induced)

2. Most supraventricular tachyarrhythmias (except when digitalis-induced)

A. Atrial fibrillation
B. Atrial flutter
C. Atrial tachycardia
D. Paroxysmal A-V junctional tachycardia
E. Reciprocating tachycardia

When the supraventricular tachyarrhythmias occur only transiently and when these arrhythmias last for a short duration, digitalis is not indicated.

It is also important to remember that the same tachyarrhythmia may be treated differently. Other antiarrhythmic agents can be used, or direct current shock may be used depending upon the clinical circumstance (see Chaps. 24 and 25).

CONTRAINDICATIONS FOR DIGITALIZATION

1. *Absolute contraindications*
A. Digitalis intoxication
B. Idiosyncrasy to digitalis
2. *Relative contraindications*
A. Idiopathic hypertrophic subaortic stenosis (IHSS)

Digitalis is relatively contraindicated in patients with IHSS because the drug improves the contractile state of the left ventricular outflow tract, leading to increased obstruction to left ventricular outflow, left ventricular systolic pressure, left ventricular-aortic pressure gradient, and a diminution of the effective orifice size of the left ventricular outflow tract. Deterioration in the clinical status by digitalization of this entity improves when digitalis is discontinued. However, if patients with idiopathic hypertrophic subaortic stenosis develop atrial tachyarrhythmias, particularly atrial fibrillation, digitalis may be required to reduce the heart rate.

B. Ventricular tachycardia

There is disagreement as to whether cardiac glycosides are indicated or contraindicated for treatment of ventricular tachycardia. If it is certain that ventricular tachycardia is a result of congestive heart failure or congestive heart failure is a result of ventricular tachycardia not due to digitalis, the drug is indicated and usually effective. Digitalis should be given with caution.

C. Complete A-V block

Although digitalis is not absolutely contraindicated in the presence of complete A-V block, if congestive heart failure is present, the effect of the drug is often not striking in this case. It is generally agreed that congestive heart failure with complete A-V block is often improved by increasing the heart rate with an artificial pacemaker. Digitalis should be continued even after artificial pacemaker implantation if congestive heart failure persists. However, in such emergency situations as acute pulmonary edema in patients with complete A-V block, a clinical trial of rapid digitalization may be necessary.

D. Acute myocardial infarction

During the first 72 hours of acute myocardial infarction, digitalization should be avoided if possible because often digitalis not only is ineffective but also may induce various life-threatening cardiac arrhythmias. When digitalis is considered to be definitely indicated, a smaller than usual dosage should be administered with caution.

METHODS OF DIGITALIZATION

Choice of the proper digitalis preparation and method of digitalization directly influence the therapeutic effect of digitalis and the incidence of digitalis intoxication. By and large, there are four ways to begin the administration of digitalis in most clinical situations:

1. Very rapid parenteral digitalization (within 12 hours)
2. Rapid oral digitalization (within 24 hours)
3. Moderately rapid oral digitalization (within 2 to 3 days)
4. Slow oral digitalization (within 5 to 8 days)

These may be carried out depending upon the degree of urgency, the nature of the underlying heart disease and/or the presence or absence of cardiac arrhythmias. Recently it has been shown that very slow digitalization can be carried out by giving a maintenance dosage for mild cases. In spite of the fact that there are marked variations in dosages in different individuals and even variations in the same individual, extensive clinical

experience enables us to set guidelines concerning average doses, usual ranges of dosages for full digitalization, and maintenance use. Methods of digitalization in adults are shown in Table 22-2.

Table 22-2. **Methods of Digitalization in Adults**

Drug	*Dosage and Regimen*
Very Rapid Parenteral Digitalization (within 12 hours)	
Digoxin	0.5–1 mg. I.V. initially and 0.25–0.5 mg. q̄ 2–4 hrs. as needed
Deslanoside (Cedilanid-D)	0.8–1.6 mg. I.V. initially and 0.4 mg. q̄ 2.–4 hrs. as needed
Ouabain	0.25–0.5 mg. I.V. initially and 0.1 mg. q̄ ½ hr. as needed
Rapid Oral Digitalization (within 24 hours)	
Digoxin	1–1.5 mg. initially and 0.5 mg. q̄ 6 hrs. until digitalized
Digitoxin	0.8 mg. initially and 0.2 mg. q̄ 6 hrs. until digitalized
Moderately Rapid Oral Digitalization (within 2–3 days)	
Digoxin	0.5 mg. t.i.d. for 2–3 days
Digitoxin	0.2 mg. t.i.d. for 2–3 days
Digitalis leaf	0.2 g. t.i.d. for 2–3 days
Slow Oral Digitalization (within 5–8 days)	
Digoxin	0.25 mg. t.i.d. for 5–8 days
Digitoxin	0.1 mg. t.i.d. for 5–8 days
Digitalis leaf	0.1 g. t.i.d. for 5 days

DIGITALIZATION (DIGOXIN) IN CHILDREN

1. Intravenous administration

A. Initial dosage is between ¼ and ½ of the estimated total digitalizing dose based upon the age and weight of the child.

(1) Under 2 years: 0.02 to 0.03 mg./lb.

(2) Over 2 years: 0.01 to 0.02 mg./lb.

B. Full digitalization dosage follows the initial dosage with ¼ of the estimated total digitalizing dose every 8 to 12 hours until the patient is digitalized.

2. Oral administration

A. Initial dosage is between ¼ and ½ of the estimated total digitalizing dose based upon the age and weight of the child.

(1) Under 2 years: 0.03 to 0.04 mg./lb.

(2) Over 2 years: 0.02 to 0.03 mg./lb.

B. Full digitalization dosage follows the initial dosage with ¼ of the estimated total digitalizing dose every 6 to 8 hours until the patient is digitalized.

C. Maintenance dosage is ¼ of the total digitalizing dosage.

MAINTENANCE DOSAGES

The usual daily maintenance dosages of commonly used digitalis preparations are as follows:

1. Digoxin: 0.125 to 0.75 mg. (average: 0.25 mg.)
2. Digitoxin: 0.05 to 0.2 mg. (average: 0.1 mg.)
3. Digitalis leaf: 0.05 to 0.2 g. (average: 0.1 g.)

SUGGESTED READINGS

Butler, V. P., Jr. and Lindenbaum, J.: Serum digitalis measurements in the assessment of digitalis resistance and sensitivity. Am. J. Med., 58:460, 1975.

Chung, E. K.: Digitalis Intoxication. Amsterdam, Excerpta Medica, 1969.

Cohn, J. N.: Indications for digitalis therapy. J.A.M.A., 229:1911, 1974.

Rahimtoola, S. H. and Gunnar, R. M.: Digitalis in acute myocardial infarction: Help or Hazard? Ann. Int. Med., 82:234, 1975.

Schick, D., and Scheuer, J.: Current concepts of therapy with digitalis glycosides. Part II. Am. Heart J., 87:391, 1974.

Smith, T. W.: Digitalis toxicity: epidemiology and clinical use of serum concentration measurements. Am. J. Med., 58:470, 1975.

Smith, T. W. and Haber, E.: Current techniques for serum or plasma digitalis assay and their potential clinical application. Am. J. Med. Sci., 259:30, 1970.

23. DIGITALIS INTOXICATION

Edward K. Chung, M.D.

GENERAL CONSIDERATIONS

Although cardiac glycoside is an indispensable drug in the treatment of heart failure and various supraventricular tachyarrhythmias, the drug is no longer beneficial to a patient when he develops toxic manifestations of digitalis. It is common experience that digitalis intoxication may develop with a relatively small dose that is either therapeutic or inadequate for other patients. This is especially true when there are various modifying factors, such as various electrolyte imbalances, advanced age, myxedema, and advancement of underlying heart diseases (see list below). Consequently, the digitalis requirement varies from patient to patient and within the same patient from time to time. Use of the standard dosage for digitalization without adjusting to the individual response is a common cause of digitalis toxicity. It is not uncommon to reach digitalis intoxication without having the desired therapeutic effect, especially in patients with intractable congestive heart failure. In retrospect, an inadequate explanation of the cause of death in patients with refractory congestive heart failure can often be completed by realizing that the death was due to digitalis intoxication.

Although digitalis is certainly one of the oldest and most commonly used drugs, it is not possible for physicians to determine precisely the optimal therapeutic dosage of the drug. The determination of serum digoxin or digitoxin value is widely utilized at many institutions in order to assess the therapeutic and toxic doses of digitalis. A markedly increased serum digitalis level usually indicates digitalis toxicity whereas a very small amount of digitalis in the serum often indicates underdigitalization. Serum digitalis determination is extremely valuable when dealing with patients who suffer from intractable congestive heart failure and/or complex cardiac arrhythmias when little or no information regarding previous digitalization is available.

The most common manifestations of digitalis intoxication are gastrointestinal disturbances, various cardiac arrhyth-

Manifestations of Digitalis Toxicity

Common	Uncommon
Gastrointestinal Symptoms	
Anorexia, nausea, vomiting	Abdominal pain, constipation, diarrhea, hemorrhage
Cardiac Symptoms	
Worsening of congestive heart failure, ventricular premature contractions, atrial tachycardia with A-V block, nonparoxysmal A-V junctional tachycardia, A-V block, sinus bradycardia	Atrial fibrillation, atrial flutter, ventricular tachycardia, ventricular fibrillation, sinus arrest, sinoatrial block, atrial premature contractions, junctional premature contractions
Visual Symptoms	
Color vision (green or yellow) with halos	Blurring or shimmering vision, scotoma, micropsia, or macropsia, amblyopia
Neurological Symptoms	
Fatigue, headache, insomnia, malaise, confusion, vertigo, depression	Neuralgia, convulsions, paresthesia, delirium, psychosis
Nonspecific Symptoms	
	Allergic reaction, idiosyncrasy, thrombocytopenia, gynecomastia

mias, aggravation of pre-existing congestive heart failure or the development of new congestive heart failure, neurological disturbances, and visual disturbances. Common and uncommon manifestations of digitalis intoxication are summarized in the list on page 326.

MANIFESTATIONS OF DIGITALIS INTOXICATION

1. *Gastrointestinal symptoms*
   A. Anorexia is often the earliest sign of digitalis toxicity.
   B. Anorexia is usually followed by nausea and vomiting within 2 to 3 days if digitalization is continued. Nausea and vomiting are considered to be central rather than gastric in origin.
   C. Diarrhea is rather uncommon manifestation of digitalis toxicity, and constipation or abdominal pain has been reported.
   D. Gastrointestinal symptoms are often not clearly evident in elderly patients, such symptoms probably being masked by the severity of the congestive heart failure and cerebral insufficiency.
   E. Most of the purified glycosides produce nausea and vomiting much less frequently than digitalis leaf.
   F. Digitalis-induced arrhythmias are frequently the earliest manifestation of digitalis toxicity from using these preparations.
   G. When nausea and vomiting develop, and the possibilities of over or underdigitalization are almost equal, digitalis should be discontinued immediately and these patients should be re-evaluated.

2. *Visual manifestations*
   A. Green or yellow color vision with colored halos has been considered to be a pathognomonic feature of digitalis toxicity for many years.
   B. Other visual disturbances may include scotoma, blurring, shimmering vision, and less commonly, micropsia,

and temporary or permanent amblyopias.
   C. Visual manifestations may easily be unrecognized unless the physician inquires specifically for its presence.

3. *Neurological manifestations*
   A. When toxicity develops, cardiac glycosides may produce various neurological symptoms, including headache, fatigue, lassitude, insomnia, malaise, depression, confusion, delirium, and vertigo, and less commonly convulsions and neuralgias, especially trigeminal nerve and paresthesia.
   B. Visual and neurological manifestations usually develop later than gastrointestinal symptoms or cardiac arrhythmias and most of the above-mentioned symptoms are less specific for digitalis toxicity.
   C. Neurological symptoms are often difficult to evaluate in elderly individuals because these manifestations may be due to many other conditions, such as cerebrovascular accidents and chronic brain syndrome.

4. *Rare manifestations*
   A. Allergic manifestations, such as urticaria and eosinophilia, and idiosyncrasy are *not* true manifestations of digitalis intoxication.
   B. Similarly, unilateral or bilateral gynecomastia that develops during digitalis therapy does *not* seem to be a manifestation of digitalis toxicity, although some investigators considered it as a toxic manifestation. Gynecomastia due to an estrogen-like activity of digitalis is most likely *not* a toxic manifestation. Digitalis-induced gynecomastia seems to be duration-dependent rather than dosage-dependent because the gynecomastia usually develops when patients have received cardiac glycosides for more than 2 years.
   C. A rare occurrence of digitoxin-induced thrombocytopenia was reported and it was considered to be a specific sensitivity reaction to digitoxin bound to

the gamma globulin fraction of the serum.

5. *Cardiac manifestations*

There are two major cardiac manifestations, which often occur simultaneously, induced by digitalis. These include: (1) alteration in contractility; and (2) digitalis-induced cardiac arrhythmias.

    A. *Alteration of contractility*

        (1) A worsening of pre-existing congestive heart failure or the development of new heart failure during digitalization is not an uncommon manifestation of digitalis toxicity.

        (2) Intractable or refractory congestive heart failure is frequently due to digitalis intoxication and this may be much more common than is recognized.

        (3) Regardless of the fundamental mechanism involved, all patients with intractable congestive heart failure should be carefully re-evaluated for possible digitalis toxicity.

    B. *Digitalis-induced cardiac arrhythmias (see list below)*

Recognition of digitalis-induced arrhythmias is extremely important because various cardiac arrhythmias may be not only the earliest but also the only sign of digitalis intoxication without any other clinical manifestation. This is observed more in recent years since the use of purified glycosides has become popular in our medical practice. Furthermore, hypokalemia induced by frequent use of potent diuretics predisposes a patient to the development of digitalis-induced cardiac arrhythmias.

It has been estimated that almost every known cardiac arrhythmia may occur in 80 to 90 per cent of the patients with digitalis intoxication. Various combinations of different cardiac arrhythmias are commonly observed in patients with advanced digitalis toxicity. It is not uncommon to observe that cardiac arrhythmias may change from one type to another in the same electrocardiographic tracing.

Digitalis-Induced Cardiac Arrhythmias

1. Digitalis-Induced Sinus Arrhythmias
   Sinus bradycardia
   Sinus arrhythmia
   Wandering atrial pacemaker
   Sinoatrial (S-A) block
   Sinus arrest
2. Digitalis-Induced Atrial Arrhythmias
   Atrial premature contractions
   Atrial Tachycardia with A-V block
     (P.A.T. with block)
   Atrial fibrillation
   Atrial flutter
   Atrial standstill (arrest)
3. Digitalis-Induced A-V Nodal (Junctional)
     Arrhythmias
   A-V nodal (junctional) premature contractions
   Nonparoxysmal A-V nodal (junctional)
     tachycardia
   A-V nodal (junctional) escape rhythm
   Multifocal A-V nodal (junctional) rhythms or
     tachycardias
   Reciprocal beats and reciprocating tachycardia
4. Digitalis-Induced A-V Conduction Disturbances
   First degree A-V block
   Second degree A-V block
       Wenckebach (Mobitz Type I) A-V block
       2:1 A-V block
   High degree (advanced) A-V block
   Complete (third degree) A-V block
5. Digitalis-Induced Ventricular Arrhythmias
   Ventricular premature contractions
   Ventricular tachycardia
   Ventricular flutter
   Ventricular fibrillation
   Ventricular standstill (pause)
6. Digitalis-Induced Arrhythmias in Artificial
     Pacemaker-Induced Ventricular Rhythm
     (A.P.I.V.R.)
   Sinus bradycardia
   Sinus arrest
   Sinoatrial block
   A-V nodal (junctional) tachycardia
   A-V nodal (junctional) escape rhythm
   Ventricular tachyarrhythmias

It should be emphasized that the classical digitalis effect (S-T, T-wave changes) in the electrocardiogram during digitalis therapy is completely independent of digitalis toxicity. This is observed because digitalis effect in the electrocardiogram may be absent in about ⅔ of the cases of digitalis toxicity. Furthermore, striking S-T, T-wave changes are frequently observed in the absence of any evidence of digitalis toxicity. By the same token, other electrocardiographic findings, such as a shortening of the Q-T interval, increased amplitude of the U waves, and peaking of the terminal portion of the T-waves during digitalis therapy, do not indicate digitalis toxicity.

Ventricular premature contractions are probably the most common digitalis-induced cardiac arrhythmia. An almost equally common one is A-V nodal (junctional) arrhythmia, especially in the presence of pre-existing atrial fibrillation.

Almost all types of cardiac arrhythmias may be induced by digitalis but certain arrhythmias do not seem to be related to cardiac glycosides. The term *non-digitalis-induced cardiac arrhythmias* may be used in later instances. *Non-digitalis-induced cardiac arrhythmias* may include Mobitz Type II A-V block, parasystole, hemiblocks, bilateral bundle branch block of varying degree (bifascicular and trifascicular block), sinus tachycardia, and paroxysmal A-V junctional tachycardia.

(1) *Disturbances of sinus impulse formation and conduction*

(a) Minor toxic effects of digitalis may induce sinus bradycardia, but it may lead to more serious arrhythmias, such as sinus arrest and sinoatrial (S-A) block, when digitalization continues.

(b) A sudden reduction of the heart rate below 50 beats per minute should raise the possibility of digitalis intoxication in all adult patients during digitalization. A slow pulse rate below 100 per minute in infancy has the same clinical significance.

(c) Sinoatrial block with or without Wenckebach phenomenon is not uncommon in digitalis intoxication, especially in children. Digitalis may be the most common cause of S-A block.

(2) *Atrial arrhythmias*

(a) Various atrial tachyarrhythmias may be produced by digitalis, although digitalis is often the drug of choice in the treatment of most atrial tachyarrhythmias.

(b) Atrial tachycardia is the commonest digitalis-induced atrial arrhythmia and it is frequently associated with varying degree A-V block (Fig. 23-1). In this circumstance, the term *PAT with block* has been used. Although the frequent occurrence of digitalis-induced PAT with block is emphasized repeatedly, its average incidence is only about 10 per cent of the total digitalis-induced cardiac arrhythmias. It has been said that carotid sinus stimulation frequently terminates PAT with block not due to digitalis toxicity but is ineffective when digitalis is the etiologic factor. However, it should be noted that applying carotid sinus stimulation to patients with suspected digitalis intoxication is

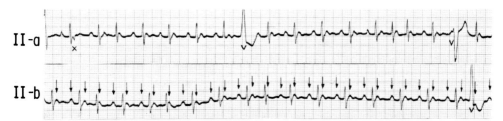

Fig. 23-1. Leads II-a and b are continuous. Arrows indicate P waves. The rhythm is atrial tachycardia (atrial rate: 190 beats per minute) with varying degree Wenckebach A-V block, occasional multifocal ventricular premature contractions (marked V) and one atrial echo beat (marked X).

dangerous. Some patients have expired from ventricular fibrillation or standstill during or after carotid sinus stimulation. Based on these observations, carotid sinus stimulation should be avoided as much as possible on patients who are taking even small amounts of digitalis.

(c) A combination of the depressive effect on the A-V conduction and the shortening effect on the atrial refractory period by digitalis results in atrial tachycardia with varying degree A-V block.

(d) Atrial fibrillation or flutter may be produced by digitalis, but its occurrence is very rare indeed. The exact reason why digitalis-induced atrial fibrillation or flutter is so rare, in comparison with atrial tachycardia, is uncertain.

(e) Although atrial premature contractions are not as common as ventricular ones, if the former occur the ectopic P waves are frequently not conducted to the ventricles (nonconducted or blocked atrial premature contractions) in spite of relatively long coupling intervals.

(3) *A-V nodal (junctional) arrhythmias*

(a) The incidence of various A-V nodal (junctional) arrhythmias in digitalis toxicity is probably as high as that of ventricular premature contractions.

(b) Digitalis induces various A-V nodal (junctional) arrhythmias, either due to passive impulse formation resulting in A-V junctional escape rhythm, or enhancement of A-V junctional impulse formation resulting in nonparoxysmal A-V nodal (junctional) tachycardia (Fig. 23-2) are frequently observed.

(c) In advanced digitalis intoxication, exit block of varying degree may develop around the A-V nodal (junctional) pacemaker so that the ventricular cycle may become slower and/or irregular. When the exit block is Wenckebach type, the ventricular cycle may show regular irregularity.

(d) In rare occasions, double A-V nodal (junctional) rhythm or tachycardia may be produced by digitalis, and this is a rare form of A-V dissociation (see Chap. 21).

(4) *A-V conduction disturbances*

(a) Digitalis may produce various degrees of A-V block resulting from both the direct and indirect actions of the drug. These actions are, needless to say, essential in the management of various

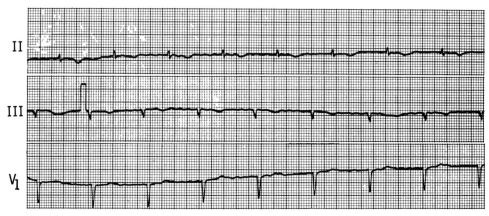

Fig. 23-2. Atrial fibrillation with nonparoxysmal A-V junctional tachycardia (rate: 70 beats per minute) producing complete A-V dissociation.

supraventricular tachyarrhythmias, especially atrial fibrillation.

(b) The degree of A-V block in digitalis intoxication depends largely upon the dosage of the drug, underlying heart disease, pre-existing A-V conduction disturbances, and the possible presence of electrolyte imbalances.

(c) First degree A-V block is one of the earliest manifestations of digitalis toxicity.

(d) Digitalis-induced second or higher degree A-V block is often followed by first degree A-V block when digitalis is stopped.

(e) The average incidence of second degree A-V block by different series is estimated to be 11 per cent.

(f) Among second degree A-V block, Wenckebach (Mobitz Type I) A-V block is more common than 2:1 A-V block.

(g) On the other hand, Mobitz Type II A-V block has not been reported as a manifestation of digitalis toxicity.

(h) It is common to observe that Wenckebach A-V block and 2:1 A-V block coexist in the same electrocardiographic tracing.

(i) High degree (advanced) or complete A-V block is very common in digitalis intoxication, when the underlying rhythm is atrial fibrillation (Fig. 23-3). It has been said that digitalis intoxication is the second most common cause of complete A-V block.

(5) *Ventricular arrhythmias*

(a) Ventricular premature contractions (VPCs) are the most common and often the earliest manifestation of digitalis toxicity in the adult population.

(b) The incidence of VPCs has been reported to be approximately 50 per cent of all digitalis-induced arrhythmias.

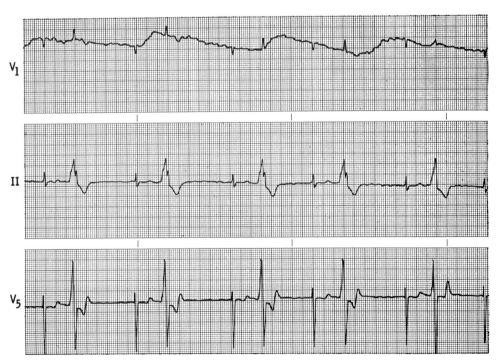

Fig. 23-3. Atrial fibrillation with advanced A-V block producing A-V junctional escape rhythm and ventricular bigeminy.

(c) Ventricular bigeminy (Fig. 23-3) is a hallmark of digitalis-induced arrhythmia.

(d) Diagnostic possibility of digitalis intoxication is 100 per cent when ventricular bigeminy coexists with non-paroxysmal A-V nodal (junctional) tachycardia or A-V block, especially in the presence of atrial fibrillation.

(e) In children, supraventricular arrhythmias and A-V conduction disturbances are a more common occurrence than VPCs in digitalis toxicity.

(f) VPCs may originate from a single focus or be multifocal. Multifocal VPCs are more pathognomonic for digitalis intoxication than unifocal ones.

(g) When VPCs, particularly multifocal or bidirectional ones, become frequent, ventricular tachycardia may develop, producing unidirectional or bidirectional tachycardia (Fig. 23-4) or even ventricular fibrillation.

(h) The average incidence of ventricular tachycardia has been estimated to be 10 per cent of all digitalis-induced arrhythmias.

(i) Bidirectional ventricular tachycardia is considered to be a more pathognomonic feature of digitalis toxicity than the unidirectional entity. This tachycardia is more common in advanced heart disease, and frequently the basic atrial mechanism is atrial fibrillation, flutter, or tachycardia (Fig. 23-4).

DETERMINATION OF SERUM DIGITALIS LEVEL BY RADIOIMMUNOASSAY METHODS

In the past 10 years, various methods for determining serum cardiac glycosides, in order to assess an optimal therapeutic dosage and to diagnose digitalis toxicity with accuracy, have been

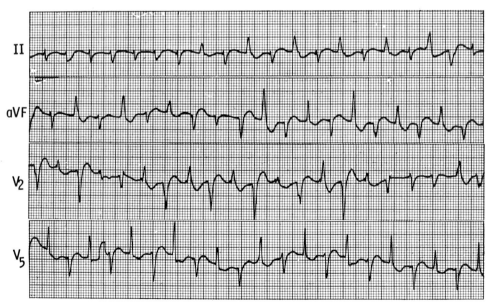

Fig. 23-4. Atrial fibrillation with bidirectional ventricular tachycardia producing complete A-V dissociation in a 70-year-old man with cor-pulmonale, thyrotoxicosis. Serum digoxin level, more than 10 ng./ml. is not compatible with life (the usual therapeutic range is below 2 ng./ml.).

developed. Radioimmunoassay method is the most popular (Fig. 23-5).

Clinical implications of serum cardiac glycosides levels are based upon the fact that there is reasonably close correlation between blood and tissue contents of digitalis so that the blood levels reflect total body and myocardial concentrations.

At present, it is generally agreed that patients with unequivocal digitalis intoxication have significantly higher serum or plasma levels of digoxin or digitoxin than nontoxic patients. Nevertheless, substantial overlap between toxic and nontoxic serum or plasma cardiac glycosides levels can not be avoided. This is particularly true when dealing with problem patients who suffer from intractable congestive heart failure and/or various complex arrhythmias. As repeatedly emphasized, the dosage of digitalis not only varies from patient to patient but also it may vary from time to time even in the same patient. Similarly, toxic and nontoxic serum or plasma digitalis levels may be different from patient to patient, depending largely upon vari-

ous modifying factors that include electrolyte imbalance, thyroid diseases, renal disease, acute or chronic lung disease, and particularly the nature and severity of underlying heart disease.

In general, serum digoxin levels of 2.0 ng./ml. or less, and serum digitoxin levels of 20 ng./ml. or less are considered to be nontoxic, although toxic patients may have serum levels below these values. Very low (digoxin levels below 0.4 ng./ml. or digitoxin levels below 10 ng./ml.) serum cardiac glycosides concentrations usually indicate under-digitalization. These low values are, as a rule, not observed among patients with digitalis intoxication.

The determination of serum digoxin or digitoxin levels by radioimmunoassay methods is extremely valuable when the values of serum cardiac glycoside levels are interpreted in conjunction with total clinical pictures and electrocardiographic findings. Serum digitalis level determination is very useful when little or no information is available as to previous digitalization. By knowing the serum digitalis level in a given patient in this

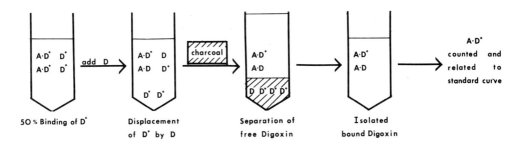

A - Antibody   D - Digoxin   * - Radioactivity   A·D - Antibody bound Digoxin

Fig. 23-5. Radioimmunoassay of digoxin. Tritiated digoxin (D*) and digoxin-specific antibody (A) are combined in fixed concentrations that result in the binding of 50 per cent of the digoxin to the antibody (A-D*). Nonradioactive digoxin (D) from serum or a standard preparation added to A-D* displaces bound D* in proportion to its own concentration. Dextranized charcoal added to the solution absorbs free D and D*. Amount of A-D* in supernatant fluid is then related to the standard curve to determine concentration of D originally added. Standard curve is prepared by displacing D* from A-D* by known amounts of D.

circumstance, an additional digitalis dosage may be determined much more accurately. On the other hand, the serum digitalis level may indicate digitalis intoxication. In addition, serum digitalis levels are valuable when dealing with patients who have various modifying factors (see list, Factors Modifying the Efficacy of Digitalis, p. 322), where daily regulation of digitalis dosage is indicated. Another role of serum digitalis level determination is to assess underdigitalization, which may be difficult or even impossible to ascertain clinically and/or electrocardiographically, especially in the presence of sinus rhythm.

It is hoped that these methods will enable many physicians to prescribe cardiac glycosides more effectively and properly so that digitalis intoxication can be minimized or even prevented.

DETERMINATION OF SALIVA ELECTROLYTES

Recently, it has been shown that electrolyte contents in the saliva have a close relationship to digitalis intoxication. It has been demonstrated that patients with digitalis intoxication have a disproportionately high concentration of potassium as well as calcium. Although mean values of saliva potassium and calcium were significantly higher in the group with digitalis toxicity this test also shows some overlapping between the groups. Further clinical evaluation will be needed to assess the value of the saliva test.

MANAGEMENT OF DIGITALIS INTOXICATION

Unfortunately, there is no known drug that has an antagonistic action to digitalis. Therefore, various agents have been tried in the treatment of digitalis intoxication with various success. Among many agents, diphenylhydantoin (Dilan-

tin) and potassium were proved to be the most effective in terminating various digitalis-induced tachyarrhythmias.

General Guidelines

1. The most important treatment of digitalis toxicity is, needless to say, the immediate withdrawal of the drug rather than reduction of the dosage. Most patients with mild digitalis intoxication, such as sinus bradycardia, first degree A-V block, and occasional ventricular premature contractions, can recover from digitalis toxicity by discontinuing the drug for several days only.

2. Generally, in patients with digitalis toxicity, emotional and physical activities should be restricted, and all factors that may aggravate the toxicity should be prevented and corrected.

3. Any patient with advanced digitalis intoxication, particularly serious cardiac arrhythmias, should be treated in a cardiac care unit or a room with similar facilities.

4. Various agents can be given orally, intramuscularly, or intravenously, depending upon the clinical situations.

Specific Treatment

1. Potassium

A. Potassium is probably one of the most effective agents in abolishing various atrial as well as ventricular tachyarrhythmias in digitalis intoxication.

B. The amount of potassium administration depends upon the severity of the toxicity, degree of suspected potassium deficiency in the myocardium and the response to potassium therapy.

C. Potassium is definitely contraindicated in the presence of renal failure and hyperkalemia.

D. Potassium is also relatively contraindicated in the presence of second degree or complete A-V block unless the serum potassium is proved to be very low.

E. Potassium in the form of potassium chloride may be administered orally in doses of 20 to 80 mEq/l. daily or by a slow intravenous infusion in doses of 40 to 60 mEq/l. over a 2- to 3-hour period initially. Intravenous administration is preferred because the exact amount received by the patient can be controlled and the drug may be discontinued at any time when indicated. Oral administration is widely used for milder cases with digitalis toxicity when hypokalemia is suspected or present.

F. During intravenous administration of potassium, continuous electrocardiographic monitoring is essential in order to prevent or avoid toxic signs of hyperkalemia or any cardiac arrhythmia.

G. Frequent determinations of serum potassium levels are also indicated.

2. Diphenylhydantoin (Dilantin)

A. Diphenylhydantoin (Dilantin) is probably the most effective agent in the treatment of digitalis-induced tachyarrhythmias, particularly, ventricular in origin.

B. Most patients respond within 3 seconds to 5 minutes to intravenous administration. The duration of response varies from 5 minutes to 4 to 6 hours.

C. The initial dose intravenously is between 125 and 250 mg. for 1 to 3 minutes under electrocardiographic monitoring. The same dose may be repeated every 5 to 10 minutes until the effect is established.

D. Toxic manifestations or side effects of diphenylhydantoin include respiratory arrest, skin reaction (urticaria, purpura), drowsiness, depression, nervousness, arthralgia, gingival hyperplasia, transient eosinophilia, and transient hypotension; but these manifestations are usually rare and not serious.

E. After conversion to sinus rhythm or the disappearance of digitalis-induced arrhythmias, oral maintenance doses (200–400 mg.) in divided doses are sufficient.

F. Diphenylhydantoin is of prophylactic value prior to direct current shock in a digitalized patient, since the drug is capable of preventing arrhythmias induced by cardioversion.

3. Beta adrenergic blocking agents

A. Propranolol (Inderal) is the only beta adrenergic blocking agent available in the United States at present.

B. The usual intravenous dose of propranolol is between 1 and 2 mg. under continuous electrocardiographic monitoring. The drug should be administered slowly, and the rate of administration should not exceed 1 mg. (1 ml.) per minute. Sufficient time should be allowed to enable a slow circulation to carry the drug to its site of action.

C. A second dose, if needed, may be repeated after 2 minutes. Additional medication should be withheld for at least 4 hours.

D. The oral route may be instituted as soon as cardiac arrhythmias are abolished or are markedly improved.

E. Intravenous atropine (0.5-1.0 mg.) may be needed if marked bradycardia occurs.

F. In nonurgent situations, atropine may be given in doses ranging between 10 and 30 mg. orally 3 to 4 times daily before meals and at bedtime. The same dosage schedule is also recommended for long-term use or for prophylactic purposes.

G. Propranolol is probably contraindicated for patients with bronchial asthma and allergic rhinitis (especially during the pollen season), marked sinus bradycardia, second or third degree A-V block, S-A block, sinus arrest, cardiogenic shock, and significant congestive heart failure. The drug is also contraindicated when patients are receiving any anesthetics, such as chloroform and ether, that produce myocardial depression. Patients receiving adrenergic-augmenting psychotropic drugs (including MAO inhibitors) should also not receive the drug. Propranolol may be given with caution after the 2-week withdrawal period from such drugs.

4. Procainamide (Pronestyl) and quinidine

A. Procainamide and quinidine may be effective in abolishing supraventricular and ventricular tachyarrhythmias induced by digitalis.

B. Procainamide may be used if potassium, diphenylhydantoin, and/or propranolol are ineffective or contraindicated.

C. Detailed descriptions of procainamide and quinidine are found in Chapter 24.

5. Xylocaine (Lidocaine)

A. Like procainamide, the antiarrhythmic mechanism of xylocaine is related to the drug's ability to raise the diastolic threshold of the ventricles to stimulation.

B. Xylocaine penetrates the tissue more rapidly than procaine or procainamide, but the action of the former is often transient.

C. Xylocaine may be effective for the treatment of digitalis-induced ventricular arrhythmias, but this drug is not the primary choice in most cases.

D. Detailed descriptions of Xylocaine are found in Chapter 24.

6. Chelating agents

A. Sodium EDTA (ethylenediamene tetra-acetic acid) is occasionally of value in the treatment of digitalis-induced ventricular arrhythmias and A-V block.

B. The chief advantage of this drug is its rapid onset of action, while its disadvantages include transient effect, occasional hypotension, and renal damage following large doses.

C. Chelating agents may be used when potassium and/or diphenylhydantoin are contraindicated or ineffective.

7. Magnesium

A. Recent clinical and experimental investigations have shown that hypo-magnesemia predisposes to digitalis intoxication.

B. Magnesium sulfate, therefore, should be administered when digitalis toxicity is associated with hypomagnesemia.

C. The drug may be given by slow (1 ml. per minute) intravenous infusion (20 ml. of 20% solution) under continuous electrocardiographic monitoring.

8. Direct current shock

A. Cardioversion should not be attempted on patients with suspected or proven digitalis-induced arrhythmias, because the procedure frequently induces more serious and irreversible arrhythmias such as ventricular tachycardia or fibrillation.

B. If cardioversion is definitely needed, prophylactic administration of diphenylhydantoin or potassium may prevent the occurrence of serious arrhythmias.

C. It is preferable to discontinue cardiac glycosides prior to the application of cardioversion. If a short-acting preparation has been given, the procedure should be postponed for at least 24 to 48 hours; if long-acting preparations have been used, the procedure should be delayed for at least 3 to 5 days.

D. In general, when treating the digitalis-induced arrhythmias, cardioversion may be attempted only as a last resort after all available measures have been exhausted.

9. Artificial pacemakers

A. Although digitalis intoxication is reported to be the second most common cause of complete A-V block, the Adams-Stokes syndrome as a manifestation of digitalis overdose has been found to be rare, since the ventricular rate in digitalis-induced complete A-V block tends to be faster than that in complete A-V block due to other causes. Therefore, a withdrawal of digitalis alone is often sufficient treatment.

B. If, however, the underlying

rhythm is atrial fibrillation, the incidence of Adams-Stokes seizures increases. When Adams-Stokes syndrome develops because of digitalis intoxication, a temporary "demand" (or "stand-by") pacemaker is quite suitable because the A-V block induced by digitalis is often transient and intermittent.

C. Permanent pacemaker implantation for the treatment of digitalis-induced A-V block is rarely called for unless other causes of A-V block co-exist.

SUGGESTED READINGS

Beller, G. A. et al.: Digitalis intoxication. A prospective clinical study with serum level correlations. N. Engl. J. Med., *284*:989, 1971.

Chung, E. K.: Digitalis Intoxication. Amsterdam, Excerpta Medica, 1969.

Doherty, J. E.: Digitalis glycosides. Pharmacokinetics and their clinical implications. Ann. Int. Med., *79*:229, 1973.

Doherty, J. E., Perkins, W. H., and Flanigan, W. J.: The distribution and concentration of tritiated digoxin in human tissues. Ann. Int. Med., *66*:116, 1967.

Harrison, D. C., Sprouse, J. H., and Morrow, A. G.: Antiarrhythmic properties of lidocaine and procaine amide: clinical and physiologic studies of their cardiovascular effects in man. Circulation, *28*:486, 1963.

Huffman, D. H. et al.: Association between clinical status, laboratory parameters, and digoxin usage. Am. Heart J., *91*:28, 1976.

Irons, G. V., Jr., Ginn, W. N., and Orgain, E. S.: Use of a beta adrenergic receptor blocking agent (Propranolol) in the treatment of cardiac arrhythmias. Am. J. Med., *43*:161, 1967.

Kim, Y. W., Andrews, C. E., and Ruth, W. E.: Serum magnesium and cardiac arrhythmias with special reference to digitalis intoxication. Am. J. Med. Sci., *242*:87, 1961.

Lyon, A. F. and DeGraff, A. C.: Reappraisal of digitalis. X. Treatment of digitalis toxicity. Am. Heart J., *73*:835, 1968.

Rosenbaum, J. L., Mason, D., and Seven, M. J.: The effect of disodium EDTA on digitalis intoxication. Am. J. Med. Sci., *240*:111, 1960.

Smith, T. W.: Digitalis toxicity: epidemiology and clinical use of serum concentration measurements. Am. J. Med., *58*:470, 1975.

Wotman, S. et al.: Cardiologists hear about rapid saliva tests for digitalis toxicity. J.A.M.A., *215*:1068, 1971.

24. ANTIARRHYTHMIC AGENTS

Edward K. Chung, M.D.

GENERAL CONSIDERATIONS

Since direct current cardioverters and artificial pacemakers have become readily available (see Chaps. 25 and 26), the therapeutic results of the management of various arrhythmias have improved markedly in the past decade. The best therapeutic results can be obtained when a precise diagnosis of the arrhythmia is entertained, because some drugs are more effective or even almost specific for certain arrhythmias. For instance, digitalis is usually the drug of choice for the treatment of various supraventricular tachyarrhythmias, especially atrial fibrillation with rapid ventricular response. Conversely, digitalis is ineffective or even contraindicated in the treatment of ventricular tachyarrhythmias (see Chap. 22).

It is essential to eliminate the cause if it is still present. For instance, the most important and the first step in treating digitalis-induced arrhythmias is immediate discontinuation of digitalis. In addition, underlying etiological factors also significantly influence the therapeutic result. For example, ventricular tachycardia associated with acute myocardial infarction is best treated with lidocaine (Xylocaine), whereas digitalis-induced ventricular tachycardia responds best to diphenylhydantoin (Dilantin) or potassium (see Chap. 23).

Prevention of the recurrence of tachyarrhythmias is another important aspect of management. For this reason, maintenance therapy with digitalis and many other antiarrhythmic drugs (see Table 24-1) is often necessary for long periods of time or even indefinitely.

Quinidine is known to be the best agent for the prevention of recurrence of atrial fibrillation or flutter, whereas procainamide (Pronestyl) is known to be the best agent for the prevention of ventricular tachyarrhythmias for long-term therapy. Propranolol (Inderal) is shown to be the most effective agent in the treatment of catecholamine-induced arrhythmias and arrhythmias related to Wolff-Parkinson-White syndrome. Bretylium tosylate (still under investigation) has been reported to be very effective in the treatment of refractory ventricular tachyarrhythmias.

Antibradyarrhythmic agents (see Table 24-2) have recently become much less frequently used because of the ready availability of artificial pacemakers (see Chap. 26). Commonly used antibradyarrhythmic agents include atropine and isoproterenol (Isuprel), especially during acute myocardial infarction (see Table 24-2).

It is not uncommon to use various antiarrhythmic drugs in conjunction with DC cardioverters and artificial pacemakers when dealing with refractory cardiac arrhythmias.

Since electrophysiologic studies have been carried out extensively, it is now possible to use a specific antiarrhythmic agent for a specific cardiac arrhythmia (see Table 24-3). For example, supraventricular (reciprocating) tachycardia with normal QRS complexes in WPW syndrome is best treated with either propranolol (Inderal) or digitalis because these drugs block the normal A-V conduction (see Table 24-3). On the other hand, lidocaine (Xylocaine) is found to be extremely effective in terminating atrial fibrillation with anomalous A-V conduction in WPW syndrome (see Table 24-4).

GUIDE TO THE ANTIARRHYTHMIC THERAPY

1. The purpose of the drug therapy for cardiac arrhythmias is for the prevention of various untoward sequelae of the arrhythmias.

2. The common untoward sequelae of arrhythmias include congestive heart failure, angina pectoris, fainting, dizziness, weakness, palpitations, skipped heart beats, convulsion, feeling of impending death, cerebral ischemia, and even actual death.

3. Correct diagnosis of a given arrhythmia is essential. There are 3 major categories (see Chap. 21):

A. Tachyarrhythmias, including premature contractions (extrasystoles) of various origins

B. Bradyarrhythmias

C. Bradytachyarrhythmias.

4. Careful considerations of indications and contraindications for various agents from electrophysiologic approaches (see Tables 24-3 and 24-4).

5. All physicians should be familiar with the recommended dosages of various antiarrhythmic agents (see Tables 24-1 and 24-2).

6. Prevention of side effects and toxicity of various agents is essential.

7. Eliminate the direct or indirect cause of a given arrhythmia if possible, before any antiarrhythmic agent is used.

8. Prevention of recurrent cardiac arrhythmia is another important aspect of antiarrhythmic therapy.

9. Refractory arrhythmias often require a combination of 2 or more antiarrhythmic agents.

10. Not uncommonly, some patients require direct current shocks and artificial pacemakers in addition to the antiarrhythmic agents.

MANAGEMENT OF PREMATURE CONTRACTIONS (EXTRASYSTOLES)

1. The first step of the management is to remove any possible cause for the development of premature contractions regardless of the origin of the ectopic impulses. For example, digitalis-induced premature contractions particularly ventricular in origin, are treated best by discontinuation of digitalis.

2. Sedation is another important method to eliminate premature beats, especially when dealing with high-strung or nervous individuals.

3. Premature contractions are often eliminated by stopping heavy smoking or excessive ingestion of coffee.

4. If the premature contractions are frequent (6 beats or more per minute) particularly in a diseased heart, such as in acute myocardial infarction, various antiarrhythmic agents may be required.

5. Supraventricular (atrial or A-V junctional) premature contractions are best treated with quinidine. Propranolol (Inderal) is almost equally effective in this situation.

6. Digitalis is particularly effective when premature contractions are associated with heart failure.

7. Lidocaine (Xylocaine) is the drug of choice for the treatment of ventricular premature contractions associated with acute myocardial infarction, or during catheterization and cardiac surgery.

8. In the following situations, treatment of ventricular premature contractions is indicated:

A. Frequent ventricular premature contractions (6 or more beats per minute)

B. R-on-T phenomenon (ventricular premature contraction superimposed on top of T wave of preceding beat)

C. Multifocal ventricular premature contractions

(Text continues on p. 344)

Table 24-1. Antitachyarrhythmic Agents, Including

Drugs	Full Dosage	Maintenance Dosage	Onset of Action	Maximum Effect
Digoxin (Lanoxin)	0.5–1 mg. I.V. initially. then 0.25–0.5 mg. q̄ 2 hrs. as needed (total: 1–2.5 mg.)	0.125–0.75 mg. (average: 0.25 mg.) daily (P.O.)	10–30 min.	2–3 hrs.
Deslanoside (Cedilanid-D)	0.8–1.6 mg. I.V. initially, then 0.4 mg. q̄ 2 hrs. as needed (total: 1.2–2 mg.)	——	10–30 min.	2–3 hrs.
Ouabain (G-Stro-phantin)	0.25–0.5 mg. I.V. initially, then 0.1 mg. q̄ ½ hr. as needed (total: 0.5–1.2 mg.)	——	3–10 min.	½–1 hr.
Lidocaine (Xylocaine)	75–100 mg. direct I.V. q̄ 10–20 min. as needed (total: 750 mg.) or 200–250 mg. I.M.	1–5 mg/min. I-V infusion	At once	At once
Procainamide (Pronestyl)	1–2 gm./200 ml. 5% D/W I.V. drip. 100 mg. q̄ 2–4 min. (1 gm. in ½–1 hr.) (total: 2 g.) or 1 g. p.o. initially, then 0.5 g. q̄ 2–3 hrs. (total: 3.5 g.)	0.25–0.5 g. q̄ 3 hrs. (P.O.)	At once / Rapid	Minutes / 1–2 hrs.
Quinidine Gluconate	0.8 g./200 ml. 5% D/W I.V. drip. 25 mg./min. or 0.4–0.6 g. I.M. initially then 0.4 g. q̄ 2–4 hrs. (total: 2.6 g.)		10–15 min. / 10–15 min.	Not im-mediate / 30–90 min.
Quinidine Sulfate	Oral route (see text)	0.3–0.4 g. q̄ 6 hrs. (P.O.)		2–3 hrs.
Diphenyl-hydantoin (Dilantin)	125–250 mg. I.V. q̄ 10–20 min. as needed (total: 750 mg./hr.)	100–200 mg. q̄ 6 hrs. (P.O.)	At once	Minutes
Propranolol (Inderal)	1–3 I.V. initially, then second dose may be repeated after 2 min. Additional medication should not be given less than 4 hrs. (total: 10 mg.)	10–30 mg. q̄ 6 hrs. (P.O.)	At once	Minutes

I.V.: intravenous injection; I.M.: intramuscular injection; q̄: every; D/W: dextrose in water; P.O.: orally; hrs.: hours; I-V block: intraventricular block; LE: lupus erythematosus; CHF: congestive heart failure; G-I: gastrointestinal; AF: atrial fibrillation; AFl: atrial flutter; AT: atrial tachycardia; A-V NT: A-V nodal tachycardia; S.V. tachyarrhythmias: supra-ventricular tachyarrhythmias; V. tachyarrhythmias: ventricular tachyarrhythmias. (From Chung, E.K.: Principles of Cardiac Arrhythmias. Baltimore, Williams and Wilkins, 1971.)

Dosage, Action, Indications, and Toxicity

Duration of Action	Indications	Toxicity	
		Dosage-dependent	Dosage-independent
3–6 days 3–6 days	S.V. tachyarrhythmias (AF, AFl, AT, A-V NT)	Almost every known arrhythmias, aggravation of CHF, anorexia, nausea, vomiting, color vision, blurring vision, headache, dizziness, confusion	Allergic manifestations (urticaria, eosinophilia), idiosyncracy, thrombocytopenia, G-I hemorrhage and necrosis
12 hrs.– 3 days			
Minutes	Primary: V. tachyarrhythmias Secondary: S. V. tachyarrhythmias	Dizziness, drowsiness, confusion, muscle twitching, disorientation, euphoria, cardiac and respiratory depression, convulsion, hypotension, A-V & I-V block	
6 hrs. 6–8 hrs.	Primary: V. tachyarrhythmias Secondary: S. V. tachyarrhythmias	A-V & I-V block, ventricular arrhythmias, LE, nausea, vomiting, lymphadenopathy, hypotension, convulsion	Allergic manifestations (eosinophilia, urticaria) agranulocytosis
6–8 hrs. 6–8 hrs. 6–8 hrs.	Primary: S. V. tachyarrhythmias Secondary: V. Tachyarrhythmias	A-V, I-V block, nausea, vomiting, photophobia, diplopia, headache. tinnitus, diarrhea, ventricular arrhythmias	Respiratory depression, hypotension, convulsion, rashes (macular or papular), thrombocytopenic purpura, thrombocytopenia, hemolytic anemia
4–8 hrs.	Primary: Digitalis-induced arrhythmias Secondary: Nondigitalis-induced arrhythmias (ventricular)	Cardiac depression, hypotension A-V, S-A block, sinus bradycardia, ataxia, tremor, gingival hyperplasia	Allergic manifestations (urticaria, purpura and eosinophilia)
3–6 hrs.	Various tachyarrhythmias	S-A, A-V block, CHF, nausea, vomiting, diarrhea, asthma, cardiogenic shock	Erythematous rashes, paresthesias of hands and fever

341

Table 24-2. Antibradyarrhythmic Agents, Including

Drugs	Dosage	Onset of Action	Maximum Effect
Atropine sulfate	0.3–2 mg. q̄ 4–6 hrs. I.V. inj. as needed or the same dose may be given by S.C. inj. (total: 4 mg.) or 0.4–0.8 mg. q̄ 4–6 hrs. P.O. for mild form	1–5 min.	Few minutes— 30 min.
Isoproterenol (Isuprel)	0.02–0.05 mg. (up to 0.1 mg.) I.C. or I.V. inj., or 0.1–0.4 mg. S.C. or I.M. inj. q̄ 2–6 hrs. as needed or 1 mg./200 cc. 5% D/W I.V. infusion, 1–4 μg./ min. initially and may increase to 5–10 μg./min. as needed. 10–30 mg. sublingually q̄ 1–6 hrs. (for mild cases)	At once Irregular	At once Irregular
Epinephrine hydrochloride (Adrenalin)	0.3–0.6 ml. of 1:1000 solution I.V., I.M., S.C., or I.C. inj., or 0.5–1 mg./250 ml. 5% D/W I.V. infusion, 1–4 μg./min. initially and may increase to 4–8 μg./min. as needed.	At once	At once
Ephedrine	30–60 mg. P.O. q̄ 2–4 hrs.	——	——
Corticosteroids	Hydrocortisone I.V. inj. 200–600 mg. for 24 hrs. or Solu-Medrol 80 mg. daily by I.M. inj. or Prednisone 40–60 mg. daily P.O.	——	——
Molar sodium lactate	5–7 ml./kg. I.V. infusion over periods of hours. If urgent 25–50 ml. rapid I.V. drip initially	——	——
Chlorothiazide	0.5–2 g. daily (P.O.) for 6–8 weeks	——	——

q̄: every; I.V.: intravenous; S.C.: subcutaneous; I.C.: intracardiac; I.M.: intramuscular; D-W: dextrose in water; P.O.: by mouth; min.: minute; hrs.: hours; A-S syndrome: Adams-Stokes syndrome; VPC: ventricular premature contraction; TB: tuberculosis; CHF: congestive heart failure. (From Chung, E.K.: Principles of Cardiac Arrhythmias. Baltimore, Williams and Wilkins, 1971.)

Dosage, Action, Indications, and Toxicity

Duration of Action	Indications	Side Effects and Toxicity
4–6 hrs.	Primary: Sinus brady-cardia, sinus arrest, S-A block Secondary: First degree & occasionally second degree A-V block	Dry mouth, urinary retention, exacerbation of glaucoma, hallucinations, hyperpyrexia, postural hypotension, sinus tachycardia, VPC, ventricular tachycardia
Minutes	Ventricular standstill, severe A-S syndrome Primary: High degree or complete A-V block Secondary: Sinus brady-cardia, sinus arrest & S-A block	Tremor, nausea, nervousness, sweating, weakness, dizziness, headache, palpitation, VPC, ventricular tachycardia & fibrillation, hypotension
Irregular		
Very short	High degree or complete A-V block & ventricu-lar standstill	Trembling, pallor, nervousness, hypertension, VPC, ventricu-lar tachycardia & fibrillation
——	High degree or complete A-V block	Urinary retention, nervousness, vertigo, insomnia, hyperten-sion, ventricular tachyar-rhythmias
——	Primary: A-V block with acute onset Secondary: Chronic A-V block	Prolonged steroid therapy may induce sodium retention, Cushing's syndrome, dissemi-nation of TB, aggravation of diabetes mellitus, glaucoma and psychosis
——	A-V block in the presence of acidosis or hyperkal-emia	Precipitation of CHF, alkalosis, hypokalemia, ventricular tachyarrhythmias
——	Sinus rhythm with inter-mittent A-V block	Hypokalemia, precipitation of gout, predispose to digitalis toxicity

Table 24-3. **Effects of Cardiac Drugs on Conduction Time**

Drugs	A-H Interval (A-V Nodal Conduction Time)	H-V Interval (His-Purkinje Conduction Time)
Digitalis	Increase (slowing)	No change
Propranolol (Inderal)	Increase (slowing)	No change
Quinidine	Decrease (accelerating)	Increase (slowing)
Procainamide (Pronestyl)	No change or increase (slowing)	Increase (slowing)
Diphenylhydantoin (Dilantin)	Decrease (accelerating) or no change	No change
Lidocaine* (Xylocaine)	No change	No change
Atropine	Decrease (accelerating)	No change
Isoproterenol (Isuprel)	Decrease (accelerating)	No change, or decrease (accelerating)

*Lidocaine prolongs or blocks the anomalous A-V conduction in WPW syndrome.

D. Grouped or paired ventricular premature contractions

E. Ventricular premature contractions after the termination of ventricular tachycardia or fibrillation.

9. For long-term therapy of the ventricular premature contractions, procainamide (Pronestyl) is the drug of choice.

10. Diphenylhydantoin (Dilantin) is probably the best agent for the treatment of digitalis-induced premature beats.

MANAGEMENT OF SUPRAVENTRICULAR TACHYARRHYTHMIAS

1. The first step of the management is elimination of the cause if present. For instance, atrial fibrillation associated with thyrotoxicosis can not be treated satisfactorily unless the thyroid function returns to euthyoid level.

2. Carotid sinus stimulation is often very effective in terminating paroxysmal atrial or A-V nodal (junctional) tachycardia (see Chap. 28).

3. Digitalis is usually the drug of choice in the treatment of various supraventricular tachyarrhythmias especially atrial fibrillation.

4. In digitalis-induced supraventricular tachyarrhythmias, digitalis must be discontinued immediately. In addition, diphenylhydantoin (Dilantin) or potassium is found to be very effective in ter-

Table 24-4. **Effect of Drugs on the Refractory Periods of the Normal A-V and Anomalous Pathways**

Drugs	Effective Refractory Period	
	A-V Node	Accessory Pathway
Propranolol (Inderal)	Lengthened	No change
Digitalis	Lengthened	Shortened
Lidocaine (Xylocaine)	No change	Lengthened
Quinidine	Shortened	Lengthened
Procainamide (Pronestyl)	No change	Lengthened
Diphenylhydantoin (Dilantin)	Shortened	Variable
Amiodarone*	Lengthened	Lengthened
Ajmaline*	No change	Lengthened
Verapamil*	Lengthened	Variable

*Not available for clinical use in the United States.

minating digitalis-induced supraventricular tachyarrhythmias (see Chap. 23).

5. Quinidine is the best agent to prevent the recurrence of atrial fibrillation or flutter.

6. Propranolol (Inderal) is shown to be most effective agent in the treatment of arrhythmias precipitated by exercise, emotional distress, or excessive sympathetic stimulation, and Wolff-Parkinson-White syndrome related supraventricular tachyarrhythmias.

7. Procainamide (Pronestyl) is less commonly used for the treatment of supraventricular tachyarrhythmias and lidocaine (Xylocaine) is rarely used in this situation except in the WPW syndrome.

8. Direct current (DC) shock is often very effective in terminating various acute supraventricular tachyarrhythmias. In addition, elective cardioversion is another important therapy of terminating chronic atrial fibrillation or flutter (see Chap. 25).

9. Artificial pacemakers (overdriving rate) are occasionally needed in the suppression of various supraventricular tachyarrhythmias that are refractory to various antiarrhythmic agents and/or DC shock (see Chap. 26).

10. Sedation is often beneficial for the treatment of supraventricular tachyarrhythmias in conjunction with other therapeutic measures.

MANAGEMENT OF VENTRICULAR TACHYARRHYTHMIAS

1. It is essential to eliminate any possible cause of ventricular tachyarrhythmias if present. Digitalis should be stopped immediately when ventricular tachyarrhythmias are due to digitalis toxicity.

2. Direct current shock is the most effective way of terminating ventricular tachycardia, flutter and fibrillation (see Chap. 25). Defibrillation should be carried out immediately for the treatment of ventricular fibrillation or flutter in addition to all necessary cardiopulmonary resuscitation as needed. However, DC shock should be avoided as much as possible if ventricular tachycardia is induced by digitalis. The reason for this is that DC shock often produces new cardiac arrhythmias, particularly ventricular fibrillation, in this situation.

3. Lidocaine (Xylocaine) is the drug of choice for the treatment of ventricular tachycardia associated with acute myocardial infarction, or during anesthesia and cardiac catheterization.

4. Procainamide (Pronestyl) is probably the next commonly used drug in this situation.

5. Quinidine or propranolol (Inderal) is less effective for the treatment of ventricular tachyarrhythmias.

6. Diphenylhydantoin (Dilantin) is the best drug for the treatment of digitalis-induced ventricular tachycardia (see Chap. 23).

7. Bretylium tosylate is an agent (still under investigation) which has been reported to be very effective in the treatment of refractory ventricular tachycardia.

8. When ventricular tachyarrhythmias are refractory to antiarrhythmic agents and/or DC shock, the use of an artificial pacemaker (over-driving pacing rate: 100 to 120 beats per minute) is often a life-saving measure (see Chap. 26).

MANAGEMENT OF SINUS BRADYCARDIA, SINUS ARREST AND S-A BLOCK

1. The therapeutic approaches vary markedly, depending upon the fundamental mechanism responsible for the production of bradyarrhythmias, the ventricular rate, and the underlying cause and degree of symptoms.

2. Sinus bradycardia of mild degree

(rate: 50–59 beats per minute) is not uncommon in healthy individuals, especially in young athletes and elderly persons. When the sinus rate is between 40 and 50 beats per minute, there may be some symptoms. Marked sinus bradycardia with a rate below 40 beats per minute often produces significant hemodynamic alterations, especially when it is associated with acute myocardial infarction.

3. The most common causes of sinus bradycardia include the therapeutic or toxic effects of various drugs including digitalis, propranolol, reserpine and guanethidine, methyldopa (Aldomet), and acute diaphragmatic myocardial infarction. Drug-induced sinus bradycardia, sinus arrest or S-A block is best treated by stopping that particular drug.

4. Active treatment is indicated when marked sinus bradycardia persists and becomes symptomatic, and especially when it is associated with acute myocardial infarction. The treatment of choice in this case is atropine and the next commonly used agent is isoproterenol (Isuprel).

5. Essentially the same therapeutic approach may be used in the treatment of symptomatic sinus arrest or S-A block.

6. In drug-resistant sinus bradycardia, sinus arrest or S-A block, a temporary or even a permanent artificial pacemaker is the treatment of choice. In most situations, only a temporary pacemaker is required (see Chap. 26).

MANAGEMENT OF A-V BLOCK

1. A-V block per se does not require treatment. Therapeutic indication for A-V block depends primarily on the degree and the etiology of the A-V block, the ventricular rate, and the presence or absence of symptoms.

2. First degree A-V block usually requires no particular treatment, except that the direct cause, such as digitalis intoxication, should be eliminated. It has been reported that atropine is effective in abolishing digitalis-induced first and second degree A-V block. Isoproterenol (Isuprel) may be effective in this circumstance, but the drug often produces untoward reactions, such as increasing ventricular irritability.

3. Wenckebach (Mobitz Type I) A-V block usually does not require active treatment unless significant symptoms are produced.

4. On the other hand, Mobitz Type II A-V block often requires an artificial pacemaker because Mobitz Type II A-V block is considered to be a precursor of bilateral bundle branch block.

5. In complete A-V block, the therapeutic approach depends upon the ventricular rate, the exact site of the block, and the degree of symptoms. Active treatment is usually not indicated when the ventricular rate is relatively rapid (40–60 per minute) in A-V nodal (junctional) escape rhythm due to complete A-V block, such as is seen in acute diaphragmatic myocardial infarction, unless symptomatic. On the other hand, a temporary or often a permanent artificial pacemaker is indicated when the ventricular rate is slow (slower than 40 per minute) in ventricular escape (idioventricular) rhythm due to complete A-V block such as seen in acute anterior myocardial infarction, or in elderly individuals with degenerative changes in the conduction system.

6. Bilateral bundle branch block of varying degrees often requires a permanent artificial pacemaker (see Chap. 26).

7. In urgent situations before the insertion of an artificial pacemaker, various agents such as isoproterenol (Isuprel) or epinephrine (Adrenalin) may be tried.

ANTITACHYARRHYTHMIC AGENTS

As emphasized previously, the best therapeutic results can be obtained when a precise diagnosis of the arrhythmia is entertained, because some drugs are more effective or even almost specific for certain arrhythmias. In addition, indications of various antitachyarrhythmic agents (see Table 24-1) vary markedly depending upon the underlying cause for the tachycardia. Most commonly used tachyarrhythmic agents include cardiac glycosides, quinidine, lidocaine (Xylocaine), procainamide (Pronestyl), diphenylhydantoin (Dilantin), and propranolol (Inderal).

1. *Quinidine*

Quinidine has been probably the most valuable antiarrhythmic agent available for more than 50 years. Quinidine has two major effects, namely, direct and indirect. The direct effect of the drug is on the cell membrane, whereas the indirect effect is anticholinergic. As a result of the net clinical effect of combined anticholinergic and direct actions, a marked prolongation of the refractory period in the atria and lesser degree of the prolongation of the ventricles are produced. In addition, a shortening of the refractory period in the A-V junction is induced by quinidine. The sinus rate tends to be slowed by the direct effect of quinidine but the indirect (vagolytic) effect tends to reverse this. As a result, the sinus rate may not be altered significantly by quinidine or it may even be accelerated.

A. *Indications*

(1) Quinidine has been an indispensable drug primarily to convert atrial fibrillation or flutter to sinus rhythm. Before DC cardioverters were available, large amounts of quinidine sulfate had to be used to restore sinus rhythm, but it is no longer necessary to do so except when a DC cardioverter is not available.

(2) At present, the role of quinidine is primarily to prevent the recurrence of atrial fibrillation or flutter following a restoration of sinus rhythm by either digitalization or DC shock.

(3) In addition, quinidine is also useful in the treatment of various acute supraventricular as well as ventricular tachyarrhythmias. In acute tachyarrhythmias, quinidine is found to be more effective for the treatment of supraventricular than ventricular ones.

(4) Quinidine is also useful for the suppression of premature beats, especially those of supraventricular origin.

(5) Quinidine is very effective in the treatment of supraventricular tachyarrhythmias with anomalous conduction in WPW syndrome.

B. *Full dosage*

(1) For the treatment of acute tachyarrhythmias, quinidine gluconate 0.8 g. diluted in 200 mg. of 5 per cent dextrose in water may be given intravenously at a rate of about 25 mg. per minute, under continuous electrocardiographic monitoring.

(2) Intramuscular administration of quinidine gluconate may be carried out by giving 0.4 to 0.6 g. initially and followed by 0.4 g. every 2 to 4 hours as needed. Total dosage by intramuscular route should not exceed 2 to 2.4 grams.

C. *Maintenance dosage*

The usual maintenance dosage of quinidine sulfate for the prevention of recurrence of various arrhythmias is 0.3 to 0.4 g. every 6 hours.

D. *Side effects and toxicity*

(1) Side effects or mild toxic manifestations include nausea, vomiting, diarrhea, tinnitus, slight impairment of hearing and vision, and slight widening of the QRS complex and/or Q-T interval.

(2) When quinidine toxicity is advanced, the above manifestations become more severe. Thus, the patient may develop blurring vision, disturbed

color perception, photophobia, diplopia, abdominal pain, headache, confusion, and ventricular tachyarrhythmias.

(3) When the patient has an unusual sensitivity or idiosyncracy to quinidine, he may develop respiratory depression, hypotension, convulsion, urticaria, macular or papular rashes, fever, thrombocytopenia, hemolytic anemia, and even sudden death.

(4) It has been shown that so-called quinidine syncope or sudden death from quinidine is attributed to the ventricular fibrillation as a result of R-on-T phenomenon.

2. *Lidocaine (Xylocaine)*

The discovery of antiarrhythmic properties of lidocaine is probably the most important addition to the therapeutic approach to cardiac arrhythmias. Lidocaine has a similar structure to quinidine or procainamide, but its electrophysiological properties are quite different. Since lidocaine has little effect on the atria, the drug is of little use in the treatment of atrial tachyarrhythmias. Lidocaine depresses diastolic depolarization and automaticity in the ventricles. It is of interest that lidocaine, in standard doses, has no effect on conduction velocity and generally shortens both the action potential and the refractory period. Approximately 90 per cent of an administered dose of the drug is metabolized in the liver, and the remaining 10 per cent is excreted unchanged via the kidneys. The action of lidocaine is more transient than that of procainamide and the former penetrates the cardiac tissues more rapidly than the latter drug.

A. *Indications*

(1) Lidocaine has been widely used, primarily for the treatment of ventricular tachyarrhythmias and ventricular premature contractions associated with acute myocardial infarction and cardiac surgery or cardiac catheterization.

(2) In the past decade, lidocaine has gradually replaced procainamide because the former is more effective and seldom produces hypotension when given properly.

(3) Lidocaine is found to be the drug of choice in the treatment of atrial fibrillation with anomalous conduction in WPW syndrome.

(4) The secondary indication of lidocaine may be for the treatment of various supraventricular tachyarrhythmias if other arrhythmic agents are ineffective.

B. *Administration*

(1) For the initiation of therapy, direct injection of 75 to 100 mg. of lidocaine (1-1.5 mg./kg.) is given slowly, and the second dose may be repeated 5 minutes later.

(2) In general, total doses should not exceed 750 mg., and it is advisable that no more than 300 mg. should be administered during a 1-hour period.

(3) When intravenous injection is not immediately feasible, alternatively, 200 to 300 mg. of lidocaine may be given intramuscularly into the deltoid muscle. An additional intramuscular injection may be carried out 60 to 90 minutes later as needed.

(4) It is recommended that lidocaine be administered under continuous electrocardiographic monitoring.

(5) Following the termination of ventricular tachyarrhythmia, continuous intravenous infusion with a rate of 1 to 5 mg. per min. is needed for 24 to 72 hours in most cases in order to prevent recurrence of the arrhythmia.

(6) When ventricular tachyarrhythmias do not recur, lidocaine may be replaced gradually with oral procainamide (oral use of lidocaine in clinical practice is not available).

C. *Side effects and toxicity*

(1) Toxicity of lidocaine is relatively uncommon.

(2) The drug may produce dizziness, drowsiness, confusion, muscle twitching, disorientation, euphoria, cardiac and respiratory depression, convulsion, and hypotension.

(3) Caution should be employed in the repeated use of lidocaine in patients with severe liver or renal disease because accumulation may lead to toxicity.

3. *Propranolol (Inderal)*

Propranolol is a beta-adrenergic receptor blocking agent that has been widely used for the management of various tachyarrhythmias, including those induced by digitalis and those resistant to digitalis. Antiarrhythmic actions of propranolol are produced by two effects, namely, inhibition of adrenergic stimulation of the heart and direct action on the electrophysiologic properties of cardiac tissue. The inhibition of adrenergic stimulation of the heart is needed for the treatment of catecholamine-induced arrhythmias. Direct membrane action on the electrophysiologic property is essential in the treatment of digitalis-induced arrhythmias. Thus, the overall effects of propranolol usually result in reduction of automaticity, including reduction of the sinus rate and prolongation of atrial and A-V conduction time.

A. *Indications*

(1) Tachyarrhythmias associated with WPW syndrome. Propranolol is considered to be the drug of choice in the treatment of regular supraventricular (reciprocating) tachycardia with normal QRS complexes.

(2) Catecholamine-induced tachyarrhythmias. Propranolol is very effective in the treatment of tachyarrhythmias (any origin) precipitated by physical exercise, emotional distress, or any other excessive sympathetic stimulation.

(3) Arrhythmias associated with mitral valve prolapse syndrome (Barlow's syndrome).

(4) Digitalis-induced tachyarrhythmias. Propranolol (Inderal) is used when potassium or diphenylhydantoin (Dilantin) is found to be ineffective or contraindicated.

(5) Atrial fibrillation or flutter. Propranolol is useful to reduce the ventricular rate in atrial fibrillation or flutter when the rapid ventricular response is difficult to control by digitalis.

(6) Miscellaneous indications. Propranolol is found to be effective in terminating some cases of multifocal atrial tachycardia. In addition, propranolol is useful when the arrhythmias are associated with idiopathic hypertrophic subaortic stenosis, angina pectoris, or anesthesia.

B. *Contraindications*

(1) Bradyarrhythmias: Marked sinus bradycardia, sinus arrest, S-A block, second or third degree A-V block, brady-tachyarrhythmia syndrome.

(2) Congestive heart failure

(3) Hypotension, cardiogenic shock

(4) Bronchial asthma, bronchitis, and other chronic lung diseases

(5) History of hypersensitive reaction to beta-blockers

C. *Administration and dosage*

(1) Intravenous injection. Propranolol (Inderal) should be administered slowly under the ECG monitoring. One to 2 mg. is the usual dosage and the second dose can be repeated 5 to 10 minutes later. Total dosage should not exceed 10 milligrams.

(2) Oral administration. In nonurgent situations, propranolol may be given orally in doses ranging between 10 and 40 mg., 3 to 4 times daily. The same dosage is recommended for long-term use or for prophylactic purposes.

D. *Side effects or toxicity*

Various side effects or toxicity of propranolol can be divided into 3 major categories: cardiovascular manifestations, respiratory manifestations, and miscellaneous manifestations.

(1) Cardiovascular manifestations

(a) Marked slowing of the heart rate, including sinus bradycardia, sinus arrest, S-A block, A-V junctional escape rhythm, ventricular escape rhythm, ventricular standstill. Note that atropine should be used to counteract for propranolol action.

(b) Development or worsening of congestive heart failure. Proper digitalization and diuretic therapy are essential.

(c) Development of hypotension. Isoproterenol (Isuprel) should be used.

(d) Development of acute myocardial infarction. Development of acute myocardial infarction has been reported upon sudden discontinuation of propranolol. Thus, gradual reduction of dosage is preferable whenever feasible.

(e) Difficulty of cardiac resuscitation. When the patient on propranolol therapy develops cardiac arrest, especially during cardiac surgery, it is often difficult to resuscitate him. Thus, it is recommended to discontinue propranolol for 24 to 48 hours before cardiac surgery if possible.

(2) Respiratory manifestations

The development of asthmatic attacks has been reported in susceptible individuals, particularly in patients with history of asthma or bronchitis. The reason for this is that Inderal increases the airway resistance.

(3) Miscellaneous manifestations

(a) Hypoglycemia has been reported in patients under insulin therapy or recovering from anesthesia and in pediatric age groups during periods of restricted food intake.

(b) Neurologic manifestations such as light-headedness, fatigue, lethargy, hallucination, mental depres-

sion, insomnia, and peripheral neuropathy

(c) Nonspecific or allergic manifestations include nausea, vomiting, diarrhea, constipation, fever, erythematous rashes, thrombocytopenia, granulocytosis, alopecia.

4. *Procainamide (Pronestyl)*

Procainamide had been the traditional drug of choice in the treatment of ventricular tachycardia until lidocaine was proven in the past decade to be a safer and more effective agent than the former drug. Large amounts of procainamide (Pronestyl) had often been used in the treatment of ventricular tachycardia, especially until DC cardioverters became readily available.

Procainamide has very similar electrophysiological effects to quinidine. Procainamide slows electrical conduction, increases the refractory period, and depresses diastolic depolarization and automaticity. It has an indirect vagolytic action, and A-V conduction may be facilitated when low doses are used. However, the direct effect of procainamide produces depression of A-V conduction when a higher dose is used. The therapeutic levels are easily achieved by oral administration, since this drug is almost completely absorbed from the gastrointestinal tract. This drug should be administered with caution to patients with significant renal disease, because the drug is excreted primarily by the kidneys in unchanged form.

A. *Indications*

(1) Although procainamide has very similar electrophysiological actions to quinidine, the former drug has been used primarily in the treatment of ventricular tachyarrhythmias.

(2) At present, the primary indication for procainamide is to prevent the recurrence of ventricular tachyarrhythmias following their termination by DC shock and/or intravenous lidocaine.

(3) Procainamide is also effective for the treatment of supraventricular tachyarrhythmias, although it is not the primary drug of choice. Procainamide has been used in place of quinidine when the patient is unable to take the latter drug.

(4) At present, large dosage of parenteral procainamide is only used when a DC cardioverter is not available and lidocaine is found to be ineffective.

(5) Procainamide is very effective for suppression of ventricular premature beats.

B. *Full dosage*

(1) Intravenous administration: When intravenous procainamide has to be used, 1 to 2 g. of the drug diluted in 200 ml. of 5 per cent dextrose in water are administered by continuous intravenous drip at a rate of 100 mg. every 2 to 4 minutes under continuous ECG monitor. A total intravenous dose should not exceed 2 grams.

(2) Oral administration: When the clinical situation is not urgent, procainamide may be given orally. Initially, 1 g. of procainamide may be given by mouth and followed by 0.5 g. every 2 to 3 hours as needed. A total oral dose should not exceed 3.5 grams.

C. *Maintenance dose*

The usual maintenance dose of procainamide is 0.25 to 0.5 g. every 3 hours by mouth.

D. *Side effects and toxicity*

(1) Side effects and toxic manifestations of procainamide include nausea, vomiting, fever, leukopenia, lymphadenopathy, lupus erythematosus-like syndrome, convulsions, A-V block and intraventricular block of varying degree, ventricular tachyarrhythmias and hypotension.

(2) In some patients who are sensitive to procainamide such allergic manifestations as eosinophilia, urticaria and agranulocytosis may be observed.

(3) The major disadvantageous aspect of procainamide is that the drug has to be given every 3 hours (by mouth) in order to maintain the therapeutic blood level.

5. *Diphenylhydantoin (Dilantin)*

The discovery of the antiarrhythmic properties of diphenylhydantoin (Dilantin) is another important addition to the management of various cardiac arrhythmias, particularly those induced by digitalis. Diphenylhydantoin has a similar structure to the barbiturates, but the electrophysiological properties are quite different from other antiarrhythmic agents. The conduction velocity in the atria is accelerated by diphenylhydantoin, resulting from a faster depolarization of the atria although the sinus rate is usually uninfluenced by this drug. Although the A-V conduction may not be influenced by this drug, diphenylhydantoin may accelerate it. Intraventricular conduction is not altered significantly by this drug as a rule. One of the most important actions of diphenylhydantoin is that the drug counteracts the depressant effect on the A-V conduction induced by digitalis or procainamide. In addition, diphenylhydantoin depresses diastolic depolarization and automaticity, and shortens the duration of the action potential and the effective refractory period.

A. *Indications*

(1) At present, diphenylhydantoin is considered to be the drug of choice in the treatment of various tachyarrhythmias induced by digitalis. This is especially true in the management of digitalis-induced ventricular tachycardia.

(2) For the secondary indications of diphenylhydantoin, the drug is also very useful in the place of procainamide or lidocaine when the latter drugs are found to be ineffective.

B. *Full dosage*

(1) Intravenous administration: The initial dose of diphenylhydantoin is between 125 and 250 mg. intravenously for 1 to 3 minutes under ECG monitoring. Most patients respond within 3 seconds to 5 minutes. The same dose may be repeated every 10 to 20 minutes as needed, but a total dose should not exceed 750 mg. per hour. Continuous intravenous drip of diphenylhydantoin is not practical because the drug easily precipitates with various commonly used intravenous solutions.

(2) Oral administration: When the situation is not urgent, 200 mg. of diphenylhydantoin may be given orally as an initial dose followed by 100 mg. every 4 to 6 hours as needed.

C. *Maintenance dosage*

Following the termination of the tachyarrhythmias, a maintenance dose of diphenylhydantoin 100 mg. 3 to 4 times daily is often needed for varying periods depending upon the clinical situation. Oral diphenylhydantoin is often useful in place of procainamide or quinidine for a long-term therapy.

D. *Side effects and toxicity*

Side effects and toxic manifestations of diphenylhydantoin (Dilantin) include respiratory and cardiac depression, such skin reactions as urticaria and purpura, eosinophilia, drowsiness, ataxia, tremor, depression, nervousness, arthralgia, gingival hyperplasia, hypotension, and A-V block of varying degree. Fortunately, these manifestations are usually rare.

ANTIBRADYARRHYTHMIC AGENTS

Because of ready availability of artificial pacemakers, various antibradyarrhythmic agents (see Table 24-2) have been much less commonly used in the past decade. Nevertheless, these agents are valuable for the management of such milder forms of slow rhythms as marked sinus bradycardia, sinoatrial block, etc. In addition, antibradyarrhythmic agents

are extremely useful for urgent situations, such as in Adams-Stokes syndrome, when artificial pacemakers are not immediately available. Atropine sulfate and isoproterenol are probably the most commonly used drugs.

1. *Atropine sulfate*

A. *Indications*

(1) Atropine is primarily used to accelerate the sinus rate by vagal inhibition. Thus, this is the drug of choice for marked symptomatic sinus bradycardia, sinus arrest, or sinoatrial block.

(2) Secondary indication of atropine is for first degree or Wenckebach A-V block due to digitalis toxicity or acute diaphragmatic myocardial infarction. However, in most cases, first degree or Wenckebach A-V block does not require treatment.

B. *Administration*

(1) Atropine is best administered intravenously in a dosage between 0.3 and 1 mg. (up to 2.0 mg.), and a similar dosage may be repeated every 4 to 6 hours as needed. The total dosage of atropine should not exceed 4 milligrams. The effect of the drug is usually prompt.

(2) Atropine may be given subcutaneously if the intravenous route is not feasible immediately.

(3) Oral administration of atropine has been used, but its effectiveness is less predictable.

C. *Side effects and toxicity*

(1) Serious toxic effects of atropine are uncommon, but ventricular premature contractions or ventricular tachyarrhythmias may be induced.

(2) Common side effects or mild toxicity include a dry mouth, urinary retention, exacerbation of glaucoma, hallucinations, hyperpyrexia, and marked sinus tachycardia.

2. *Isoproterenol (Isuprel)*

Before artificial pacemakers were available for clinical use, the treatment of choice for complete A-V block was the administration of isoproterenol. The drug is still very useful in the treatment of Adams-Stokes syndrome during an emergency, or temporarily until an artificial pacemaker can be inserted. Thus, isoproterenol is at present still the drug of choice in the treatment of Adams-Stokes syndrome due to bradyarrhythmias, primarily complete A-V block. Isoproterenol is capable of accelerating both the supraventricular and the ventricular pacemakers and of improving A-V conduction. The drug possesses a potent inotropic action leading to an increment in the stroke volume, the amplitude of myocardial contraction, and the coronary blood flow.

A. *Indications*

(1) Primary indication of isoproterenol is in the treatment of Adams-Stokes syndrome due to complete A-V block or ventricular standstill until an artificial pacemaker is inserted.

(2) For secondary indication, isoproterenol may be used, in place of atropine, in the treatment of symptomatic sinus bradycardia, sinus arrest, and S-A block.

B. *Administration*

(1) Isoproterenol can be given by direct intracardiac (I.C.), intravenous (I.V.), intramuscular (I.M.) or subcutaneous (S.C.) injection, or it may be given by intravenous infusion.

(2) In emergency situations, such as in severe Adams-Stokes syndrome or ventricular standstill, isoproterenol can be given by intracardiac or intravenous injection.

(3) The usual dosage is between 0.02 and 0.05 mg., but up to 0.1 mg. may be administered. Otherwise, the drug can be given subcutaneously or intramuscularly in a dosage of 0.1 to 0.4 mg. every 2 to 6 hours as needed.

(4) In addition, continuous intravenous infusion of isoproterenol is indicated in severe cases in order to maintain the ventricular rate around 50 to 60 beats per minute until an artificial pace-maker can be inserted. The usual method is to dilute 0.1 mg. of isoproterenol in 200 ml. of 5 per cent dextrose in water, and the initial infusion rate is 1 to 4 μg. per minute. The infusion rate may be increased to 5 to 10 μg. per minute, and, occasionally, up to 40 μg. per minute may be required to maintain an ideal ventricular rate.

(5) The most popular route for this drug is sublingually, and the usual dosage is 10 to 30 mg. every 1 to 6 hours. Occasionally, the drug can be given as often as every 30 minutes as needed.

C. *Side effects and toxicity*

(1) Side effects or mild toxicity of isoproterenol include tremor, nervousness, sweating, nausea, weakness, headache, dizziness, palpitation, and hypotension.

(2) A serious toxic effect is the production of ventricular tachyarrhythmias, which may occur equally with small or large doses.

3. *Epinephrine (Adrenalin)*

Epinephrine has been almost equally as popular as isoproterenol in the treatment of Adams-Stokes syndrome. However, epinephrine is considered to be definitely inferior to isoproterenol because the former drug produces significant hypertension and is prone to provoke ventricular irritability, particularly ventricular fibrillation.

Epinephrine is capable of accelerating the atrial rate as well as the ventricular rate. The degree of acceleration of the atrial rate has no relationship to the initial atrial rate, whereas the degree of the acceleration of the idioventricular rate is closely related to the initial ventricular rate. Namely, the degree of acceleration of the idioventricular rate is the greatest when the initial ventricular rate is very slow, while the enhancement of the ventricular rate is insignificant when the initial ventricular rate is relatively rapid.

A. *Indications*

(1) The primary indication for

epinephrine is in the treatment of ventricular standstill, particularly associated with acute myocardial infarction.

(2) The secondary indication for epinephrine is in the treatment of Adams-Stokes syndrome due to high degree or complete A-V block, until an artificial pacemaker is inserted.

B. *Administration*

(1) In urgent situations, as in ventricular standstill, epinephrine 0.3 to 0.6 ml. of 1:1000 solution may be given by intravenous (I.V.), intramuscular (I.M.), subcutaneous (S.C.) or even intracardiac (I.C.) injection. Slow injection over a period of several minutes is recommended under the ECG monitoring and the rate of injection should be regulated according to the patient's response.

(2) For long-term therapy, 0.5 to 1 mg., 1:1000 solution of epinephrine diluted in 250 ml. of 5 per cent dextrose in water can be given by a continuous intravenous infusion. The initial rate of the intravenous drip is usually 1 to 4 μg. per minute, and the rate may be increased to 4 to 8 μg. per minute according to the patient's response.

C. *Side effects and toxicity*

(1) Side effects or mild toxicity of epinephrine include nervousness, trembling, pallor, and hypertension.

(2) A serious toxic effect is the production of ventricular tachycardia and fibrillation.

MANAGEMENT OF TACHYARRHYTHMIAS ASSOCIATED WITH WOLFF-PARKINSON-WHITE SYNDROME

When tachyarrhythmias occur only transiently, with a short duration in the patient with Wolff-Parkinson-White (WPW) syndrome, treatment is usually not indicated. However, WPW syndrome characteristically produces recurrent supraventricular tachyarrhythmias in many patients. Therefore, every physician should be fully familiar with the diagnostic criteria (see Chap. 21) as well as the management of the WPW syndrome.

There are several ways to approach the management of WPW syndrome-related tachyarrhythmias (see list below and Table 24-4).

Therapeutic Approaches to Tachyarrhythmias in WPW Syndrome

1. Carotid sinus stimulation
2. Drug Therapy
   (1) Propranolol (Inderal)
   (2) Digitalis
   (3) Quinidine
   (4) Lidocaine (Xylocaine)
   (5) Procainamide (Pronestyl)
   (6) Sedatives
   (7) Other drugs:*
      (a) Amiodarone
      (b) Ajmaline
      (c) Verapamil
3. Direct current shock
4. Artificial pacemakers
5. Surgery

*Not available for clinical use in the United States.

1. The first step is to apply carotid sinus stimulation (CSS) when the diagnosis is established.

2. When CSS is ineffective, propranolol (Inderal) is the drug of choice in the treatment of regular supraventricular (reciprocating) tachycardia with narrow (normal) QRS complexes. The drug can be given either intravenously or orally, depending upon the clinical circumstance. Propranolol is extremely effective in young individuals.

3. Digitalis is equally effective for above-mentioned situation, but the drug seems to be more useful in older individuals.

4. Lidocaine (Xylocaine) is the drug of choice in the treatment of atrial fibrillation or flutter with anomalous conduction (resembles ventricular tachycardia) in WPW syndrome.

5. For regular supraventricular (reciprocating) tachycardia with anomalous conduction, lidocaine should be used first. Digitalis or propranolol may be occasionally effective in this case.

6. In extremely urgent situations, especially in atrial fibrillation or flutter with anomalous conduction and very rapid ventricular rate, direct current shock should be applied immediately.

7. At times, artificial pacemaker with overdriving pacing is indicated in refractory cases.

8. Various surgical approaches, such as ligation of anomalous pathways, have been tried in the treatment of refractory tachyarrhythmias associated with WPW syndrome but the surgical result is not always promising.

9. For prophylactic purposes, propranolol (small dosage) is most commonly used, and digitalis is almost equally effective, especially for regular supraventricular tachycardia.

10. For the prevention of atrial fibrillation or flutter, with anomalous A-V conduction, quinidine or Pronestyl alone, or combination of quinidine and Inderal or digitalis can be tried, but prevention of fibrillation or flutter is often difficult.

11. Sedatives or mild tranquilizers are often beneficial in many cases.

SUGGESTED READINGS

Bigger, J. T.: Pharmacologic and clinical control of antiarrhythmic drugs. Am. J. Med., 58:479, 1975.

Bissett, J. K. et al.: Electrophysiology of atropine. Cardiovasc. Res., 9:73, 1975.

Chung, E. K.: Drug therapy for cardiac arrhythmias. Postgrad. Med., 53:107, 1973.

———: Prophylactic use of antiarrhythmic drugs in acute myocardial infarction. Postgrad. Med., 54:197, 1973.

Collinsworth, K. A., Kalman, S. M. and Harrison, D. C.: The clinical pharmacology of lidocaine as an antiarrhythmic drug. Circulation, 50:1217, 1974.

Coltart, D. J. et al.: Investigation of the safe withdrawal period for propranolol in patients scheduled for open heart surgery. Br. Heart J., 37:1228, 1975.

Josephson, M. E. et al.: The electrophysiological effects of intramuscular quinidine on the atrioventricular conducting system in man. Am. Heart J., 87:55, 1974.

Josephson, M. E. et al.: Electrophysiologic properties of procainamide in man. Am. J. Cardiol., 33:596, 1974.

Josephson, M. E., Kastor, J. A. and Kitchen, J. G., III.: Lidocaine in Wolff-Parkinson-White syndrome with atrial fibrillation. Ann. Int. Med., 84:44, 1976.

Karlsson, E.: Procainamide and phenytoin. Comparative study of their antiarrhythmic effects at apparent therapeutic plasma levels. Br. Heart J., 37:731, 1975.

Koch-Weser, J. and Klein, S. W.: Procainamide dosage schedules, plasma concentrations, and clinical effects. J.A.M.A., 215:1454, 1971.

Luomanmäki, K., Heikkilä, J. and Härtel, G.: Bretylium tosylate. Arch. Int. Med., 135:515, 1975.

Miller, R. R. et al.: Propranolol-withdrawal rebound phenomenon. Exacerbation of coronary events after abrupt cessation of antianginal therapy. N. Engl. J. Med., 293:416, 1975.

Nies, A. S. and Shand, D. G.: Clinical pharmacology of propranolol. Circulation, 52:6, 1975.

Roos, J. C. and Dunning, A. J.: Effects of lidocaine on impulse formation and conduction defects in man. Am. Heart J., 89:686, 1975.

Rosen, K. M. et al.: Effects of lidocaine and propranolol on the normal and anomalous pathways in patients with preexcitation. Am. J. Cardiol., 30:801, 1972.

Scheinman, M. M., Thorburn, D., and Abbott, J. A.: Use of atropine in patients with acute myocardial infarction. Circulation, 52:627, 1975.

Seides, S. F. et al.: The electrophysiology of propranolol in man. Am. Heart J., 88:733, 1974.

Vargas, G., Akhtar, M. and Damato, A. N.: Electrophysiologic effects of isoproterenol on cardiac conduction system in man. Am. Heart J., 90:25, 1975.

Wellens, H. J. J.: Effect of drugs on Wolff-Parkinson-White syndrome. In Narula, O. S. (ed.): His Bundle Electrocardiography and Clinical Electrophysiology. Philadelphia, F. A. Davis, 1975.

———: The electrophysiologic properties of the accessory pathway in the Wolff-Parkinson-White syndrome. In Wellens, H. J. J., Lie, K. I., and Janse, M. J. (eds.): The Conduction System of The Heart. Philadelphia, Lea & Febiger, 1976.

25. DIRECT CURRENT SHOCK

Edward K. Chung, M.D.

GENERAL CONSIDERATIONS

Direct current (DC) shock has been widely used to terminate supraventricular as well as ventricular tachyarrhythmias due to various causes. DC shock is often a life-saving measure in terminating ventricular tachycardia or fibrillation. Because of the ready availability of DC cardioverters, the use of large dosages of various antiarrhythmic drugs (see Chap. 24), especially quinidine and procainamide, is no longer necessary in most clinical situations. It has been shown that about 90 per cent of the cases of atrial fibrillation are successfully converted to sinus rhythm, whereas 95 to 97 per cent of cases of ventricular tachycardia can be terminated by the procedure. It has also been shown that 90 out of 100 patients with atrial fibrillation refractory to large doses of quinidine could be converted to sinus rhythm by DC shock. Electrical cardioversion has been found to be much safer than various antiarrhythmic drugs, when the procedure is applied properly. For instance, when quinidine was used in order to convert chronic atrial fibrillation, a 30 per cent incidence of toxicity was observed along with a 1 to 2 per cent mortality. On the other hand, no fatalities nor episodes of ventricular fibrillation were observed when 500 consecutive cardioversions were performed by Lown et al.

For successful cardioversion, it is very important to apply the procedure properly, and all possible contraindications should be eliminated. It should be emphasized that DC shock may not only be ineffective for digitalis-induced tachyarrhythmias, but also may be fatal, since ventricular tachyarrhythmias or ventricular standstill may be induced. In general, when treating digitalis-induced tachyarrhythmias, DC shock may be attempted only as a last resort after all available measures have been exhausted. The reason for avoiding DC cardioversion is lowered fibrillatory threshold. This lowered threshold leads to ventricular arrhythmias. It is true that it may be aggravated by potassium loss during electrical countershock and tiia. this leads to relative digitalis intoxication, but the primary defect is the diminished fibrillatory threshold.

INDICATIONS FOR DIRECT CURRENT SHOCK

The use of the DC cardioverter may be divided into two major categories, namely (1) the treatment of acute tachyarrhythmias; and (2) elective cardioversion for chronic atrial fibrillation and flutter.

DC CARDIOVERSION FOR ACUTE TACHYARRHYTHMIAS

1. For the treatment of various supraventricular and ventricular tachyarrhythmias with acute onset, DC cardioversion is often a life-saving measure.

2. When a clinical situation is extremely urgent, such as in the treatment of life-threatening ventricular tachycardia or fibrillation, premedication for transient amnesia or anesthesia is not needed. Thus, 100 to 200 watt seconds of DC shock can be applied directly. If the arrhythmias persist, DC shock with increased energy (200–400 watt seconds)

should be applied immediately following the first shock.

3. On the other hand, if the clinical situation is not extremely urgent, small amounts of thiopental sodium (Pentothal) or diazepam (Valium) may be administered in order to induce a transient anesthesia or amnesia immediately before the application of DC shock.

4. Premedication may not be indicated when only a small energy discharge is required, particularly in the treatment of atrial flutter.

5. Following termination of ventricular tachyarrhythmias, continuous intravenous infusion of lidocaine (Xylocaine) (less commonly procainamide) is usually indicated and followed by oral maintenance therapy with procainamide (Pronestyl) (or diphenylhydantoin or quinidine).

6. When atrial flutter or fibrillation is terminated by DC shock, maintenance doses of oral quinidine, following digitalization, are needed in most instances.

CONTRAINDICATIONS OR NONINDICATIONS OF DIRECT CURRENT SHOCK

One of the most important aspects in considering the indications for DC cardioversion is the probability of restoration of sinus rhythm and of its maintenance for a reasonable period of time. In general, a heart that is difficult to convert to sinus rhythm is also difficult to maintain in sinus rhythm. It has been shown that the success of conversion is not directly influenced by the type of heart disease, prior resistance to quinidine therapy, age or sex of the patient, presence or absence of congestive heart failure, occurrence of thromboembolism, or degree of ventricular enlargement.

In the following situations, DC shock is either contraindicated or not indicated:

1. Digitalis toxicity and/or hypokalemia

2. Severe mitral insufficiency and/or marked left atrial hypertrophy

3. Atrial fibrillation or atrial flutter with complete A-V block

4. Chronic atrial fibrillation with duration of 5 years or longer

5. Imminent valvular surgery

6. Lone atrial fibrillation with slow ventricular rate

7. First degree A-V block before the onset of atrial fibrillation

8. Recurrence of atrial fibrillation or flutter during adequate digitalis and quinidine therapy

9. Sick sinus syndrome (*Sick sinus syndrome* is defined as a diseased sinus node that is incapable of producing adequate impulses, such as seen in marked sinus bradycardia, sinus arrest, or S-A block.)

10. Marked obesity (DC shock is often ineffective regardless of the type of cardiac arrhythmia.)

COMPLICATIONS OF DIRECT CURRENT SHOCK

Complications can be reduced to a minimum or even avoided in most instances when the patient is properly selected and the procedure is properly applied. In general, complications of DC cardioversion are directly related to technical errors during the procedure, severity of the atrial damage, and improper use or over-dosage of antiarrhythmic drugs. Technical errors in using a DC cardioverter include failure to synchronize the discharge, disregard for electrocardiographic artifacts that may trigger electrical discharge during the vulnerable period and lead to the development of ventricular fibrillation, and excessive energy settings. In addition, excessive dosage of digitalis and/or insufficient dosage of quinidine often produce postcardioversion arrhythmias or recurrence of atrial fibrillation or flutter.

1. DC shock may unmask digitalis-induced arrhythmias (Fig. 25-1).

2. Ventricular tachyarrhythmias may develop following DC shock, particularly during digitalis therapy (Fig. 25-1).

3. Pre-existing complete A-V block or ventricular standstill may occur following DC shock.

4. In 8 per cent of patients with chronic atrial fibrillation or flutter, stable sinus rhythm is not restored following termination of the former arrhythmia. In this case, A-V junctional or ventricular escape rhythm becomes the dominant rhythm with or without unstable sinus activity. In this circumstance, the term *sick sinus syndrome* is applied and is considered to be due to a failure of the sinus node to discharge an impulse (sinus arrest) or impaired conduction at the sinoatrial junction (S-A block) or in the atrial myocardium (intra-atrial block). Sick sinus syndrome may also be observed following the termination of other types of tachyarrhythmias (see Chap. 21).

5. DC cardioversion may induce new atrial tachyarrhythmias. This is considered to occur when the electric discharge is given during the atrial vulnerable period. Cardioversion-induced atrial tachyarrhythmias can be terminated by an additional DC shock in most cases.

6. Occurrence of thromboembolism, particularly cerebrovascular accidents in elderly individuals, within 24 to 48 hours following DC shock is not uncommon.

7. Intense and repeated DC shocks in dogs produce myocardial damage associated with increased serum MB creatine phosphokinase (CPK), but conventional DC shock does not cause such change in humans.

8. Superficial burn of the skin under the paddle may be induced by repetitive applications of direct current shock, especially when jelly is not sufficiently applied.

CARDIAC ARRHYTHMIAS RELATED TO DC SHOCK

Although DC shock is indispensable in terminating various supraventricular as well as ventricular tachyarrhythmias in many patients, certain cardiac arrhythmias may develop following the procedure. Some cardiac arrhythmias may be observed immediately following DC shock, even during ideal situations. Serious arrhythmias tend to develop from the procedure when there is digitalis intoxication or electrolyte imbalances (especially hypokalemia), when the patient is elderly with advanced heart disease and/or pre-existing conduction defect, and when the procedure is improperly performed.

1. It is very common to observe atrial or A-V junctional premature contractions following the termination of supraventricular tachyarrhythmias (atrial fibrillation, flutter or tachycardia and A-V junctional tachycardia), and in some cases, ventricular tachyarrhythmias.

2. Similarly, occasional appearances of A-V junctional escape beats or a period of A-V junctional escape rhythm with or without A-V dissociation are not uncommon during the first 1 to 3 seconds following cardioversion.

3. In addition, sinus bradycardia and sinus arrhythmia preceded by a short period of sinus arrest is also not infrequently encountered one or two seconds after the termination of a tachyarrhythmia. Irregular and slow sinus activity in this circumstance is simply due to the sinus node's requiring a warm-up period following a depression by a rapid ectopic impulse discharge. However, a failure of the sinus node to take over cardiac activity for a long period of time,

such as is seen in A-V junctional escape rhythm without discernible P waves, or with extremely slow and irregular sinus activity, indicates that the sinus node is diseased, and this is termed *sick sinus syndrome*.

4. When the heart is severely damaged and the sinus node as well as ectopic escape pacemakers are unable to produce impulses following cardioversion, atrial as well as ventricular standstill is produced.

5. Varying degrees of A-V block may be observed following DC shock when there is a pre-existing A-V conduction defect. First degree A-V block is extremely common following the termination of chronic atrial fibrillation or flutter. In this case, recurrence of the atrial fibrillation or flutter is very common and repeated cardioversion has little value.

6. It has been reported that cardioversion may change a pre-existing atrial fibrillation to atrial flutter or atrial tachycardia or vice versa instead of a sinus rhythm. The reason for the development of new atrial tachyarrhythmias following DC shock is probably the fact that the electrical discharge may fire during the vulnerable period of the atria. This is particularly true when the P-R intervals are long and the A-V conduction ratios vary. Cardioversion-induced atrial tachyarrhythmias can be terminated by an additional DC shock in most cases.

7. The appearance of occasional ventricular premature contractions immediately following DC shock is relatively common and is insignificant clinically.

8. However, frequent ventricular premature contractions and runs of ventricular tachycardia or fibrillation are serious problems.

9. The most common cause of ventricular fibrillation that develops immediately following DC shock is im-

proper synchronization, that is, the electrical discharge falls during the vulnerable period of the ventricles.

10. In addition, the development of ventricular tachyarrhythmias immediately after DC shock is often attributed to digitalis and/or quinidine intoxication, even in the presence of proper synchronization (Fig. 25-1).

11. Frequent ventricular premature contractions or even short runs of ventricular tachycardia may be provoked when DC shock is applied to a patient with hypoventilation during deep anesthesia.

12. In general, unnecessarily high energy discharges are prone to induce various cardiac arrhythmias.

ELECTIVE CARDIOVERSION

1. Elective cardioversion is indicated for the treatment of chronic tachyarrhythmias, primarily atrial fibrillation or flutter, when restoration of sinus rhythm is considered to be beneficial.

2. Less commonly, elective cardioversion is applied to terminate other tachyarrhythmias such as atrial or A-V nodal (junctional) tachycardia.

3. *Purpose of elective cardioversion*

Elective cardioversion is indicated when a restoration of sinus rhythm is considered to be beneficial. In general, cardioversion is expected to provide the following:

A. Increment of cardiac output leading to improvement of congestive heart failure and increase in exercise tolerance.

B. Better control of the ventricular rate.

C. Reduction of thromboembolic phenomenon.

4. *Preparation for elective cardioversion*

A. Before DC cardioversion is attempted, all possible contraindications

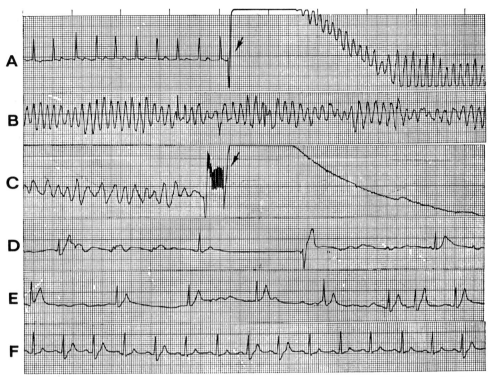

Fig. 25-1. Strips taken from a 43-year-old female with rheumatic heart disease who has been taking 0.25 mg. digoxin daily. Rhythm strips A-F are continuous. Her precardioversion arrhythmia is atrial fibrillation with rapid ventricular response. She developed ventricular fibrillation upon the application of DC shock, but fortunately ventricular fibrillation was terminated by the application of the second DC shock. Arrows indicate the applications of DC shocks. Note very unstable and slow rhythm (strips D and E) until sinus rhythm is restored.

and nonindications must be carefully avoided.

B. Every patient with chronic atrial flutter or fibrillation must be fully digitalized, and quinidinized 24 hours to 1 week prior to DC cardioversion. About 15 per cent of cases of chronic atrial fibrillation can be converted to sinus rhythm by quinidine (oral maintenance dose).

C. It is important to remember that short-acting digitalis preparations such as digoxin should be withheld for 24 to 48 hours immediately before DC shock is applied. If a long-acting digitalis prepara-

tion, such as digitoxin, has been used, the drug should be discontinued for 3 to 5 days prior to cardioversion.

D. The use of an anticoagulant 1 to 2 weeks before and after DC cardioversion has been emphasized by many investigators in order to prevent thromboembolism, but its practical value is uncertain. However, anticoagulation is recommended in patients with prior or recent systemic emboli.

E. Pentothal or diazepam (Valium) may be used prior to cardioversion especially when high energy discharge is required.

SUGGESTED READINGS

Chung, E. K.: Electrocardiography: Practical Applications with Vectorial Principles. Hagerstown, Harper & Row, 1974.

Ehsani, A., Ewy, G. A. and Sobel, B. E.: Effects of electrical countershock on serum creatine phosphokinase (CPK) isoenzyme activity. Am. J. Cardiol., *37*;12, 1976.

Gilbert, R. and Cuddy, R. P.: Digitalis intoxication following conversion to sinus rhythm. Circulation, *32*:58, 1965.

Hagemeijer, F. and Van Houwe, E.: Titrated energy cardioversion of patients on digitalis. Br. Heart J., *37*:1303, 1975.

Hurst, J.W. et al.: Management of patients with atrial fibrillation. Am. J. Med., *37*:728, 1964.

Jensen, J.B. et al.: Electroshock for atrial flutter and atrial fibrillation. J.A.M.A., *194*:1181, 1965.

Killip, T. and Yormak, S.: Short and long-term results from direct current conversion for atrial fibrillation and flutter. Circulation (supp. II), *31* and *32*:125, 1965.

Kleiger, R. and Lown, B.: Cardioversion and digitalis. II. Clinical studies. Circulation, *33*:878, 1966.

Lemberg, L. et al.: Arrhythmias related to cardioversion. Circulation, *30*:163, 1964.

Lindsay, J. Jr.: Quinidine and countershock: a reappraisal. Am. Heart J., *85*:141, 1973.

Lown, B.: "Cardioversion" of arrhythmias. I. Modern Conc. Cardiovasc. Dis., *33*:863, 1964.

———: "Cardioversion" of arrhythmias. II. Modern Conc. Cardiovasc. Dis., *33*:869, 1964.

———: Electrical reversion of atrial fibrillation.

Dreifus, L. S. and Likoff, W. (eds.): Mechanisms and Therapy of Cardiac Arrhythmias. New York, Grune & Stratton, 1966.

———: Electrical reversion of cardiac arrhythmias. Br. Heart J., *29*:469, 1967.

Lown, B., Kleiger, R. and Williams, J.: Cardioversion and digitalis drugs: Changes threshold to electric shock in digitalized animals. Circulation Res., *17*:519, 1965.

Morris, J. J. Jr. et al.: Experience with "Cardioversion" of atrial fibrillation and flutter. Am. J. Cardiol., *14*:94, 1964.

Oram, S. and Davies, J. P. H.: Further experience of electrical conversion of atrial fibrillation to sinus rhythm: Analysis of 100 patients. Lancet *1*:1294, 1964.

Rabbino, W., Likoff, W., and Dreifus, L. S.: Complications and limitations of direct current countershock. J.A.M.A., *190*:417, 1964.

Radford, M. D. and Evans, D. W.: Long-term results of DC reversion of atrial fibrillation. Br. Heart J., *30*:91, 1968.

Resnekov, L.: Electroversion of cardiac dysrhythmias. Am. Heart J., *79*:581, 1970.

———: Direct current shock. *In* Chung, E. K. (ed.): Cardiac Emergency Care. Philadelphia, Lea & Febiger, 1975.

Robinson, H. J. and Wagner, J. A.: DC cardioversion causing ventricular fibrillation. Am. J. Med. Sci., *249*:300, 1965.

Rokseth, R. and Storstein, O.: Quinidine therapy of chronic auricular fibrillation: Occurrence and mechanism of syncope. Arch. Int. Med., *3*:184, 1963.

Selzer, A. et al.: Immediate and long-term results of electrical conversion of arrhythmias. Prog. Cardiovasc. Dis., *9*:90, 1966.

26. ARTIFICIAL PACEMAKERS

Edward K. Chung, M.D.

GENERAL CONSIDERATIONS

At present, more than 30 different artificial pacemakers are available for internal or external use, temporary or permanent pacing. There are four major types of artificial pacemakers: the fixed rate pacemaker, the standby (demand) ventricular pacemaker, the atrial synchronized pacemaker, and the bifocal demand pacemaker.

The fundamental principles for the utilization of an artificial pacemaker were established as early as 1932, and external cardiac pacing was introduced into clinical medicine in 1952. In 1957, temporary direct myocardial stimulation in the treatment of complete A-V block was introduced and a transistorized, self-contained, implantable pacemaker for long-term correction of complete A-V block was established in 1960. Since then, artificial pacemakers have become indispensable and are the most reliable method for treating various bradyarrhythmias.

Initially, fixed-rate ventricular pacemakers were used, but demand ventricular pacemakers have been gradually replacing the former because of their various superior aspects. Atrial synchronized pacemakers have become popular recently, in view of the fact that it is a more physiologic form of pacing and the ventricular rate can be changed to correspond to the varying physiologic requirements. In addition, the atrial contribution to ventricular filling further improves the cardiac output. Very recently, the bifocal (sequential atrioventricular) demand pacemaker has been introduced. This pacemaker consists of two demand units; conventional QRS-inhibited ventricular pacemaker and a QRS-inhibited atrial pacemaker. The use of an artificial pacemaker in the treatment of various drug-resistant supraventricular as well as ventricular tachyarrhythmias is also an important aspect of management.

INDICATIONS FOR ARTIFICIAL PACEMAKERS

The precise criteria for the use of a temporary or a permanent pacemaker vary slightly from institution to institution, but the following conditions are generally accepted.

1. *Short-term pacing*

A. Symptomatic second degree or third degree A-V block, especially during acute myocardial infarction, requires temporary pacing. It should be noted that A-V block per se does not require artificial pacing.

B. Symptomatic and drug-resistant sinus arrhythmias including sinus bradycardia, sinus arrest, and sinoatrial (S-A) block

C. Left bundle branch block and bifascicular or trifascicular block associated with acute anterior myocardial infarction usually requires short-term pacing because these findings are often followed by a slow ventricular escape rhythm due to complete A-V block

D. Emergency treatment for Adams-Stokes syndrome and symptomatic bilateral bundle branch block

E. Before or during implantation of a permanent pacemaker

F. Therapeutic trial for intractable congestive heart failure, cardiogenic shock, cerebral or renal insufficiency

G. Prophylactic pacing during major surgery when Adams-Stokes syndrome is anticipated

H. Drug-resistant tachyarrhythmias by overdriving pacing rate

At present, the most commonly used pacemaker for a short-term pacing is the temporary transvenous type. In almost all situations, a demand unit is preferable to a fixed-rate unit. This is because normal A-V conduction may be present during the insertion of a pacemaker (especially when it is being used prophylactically) and because it is not uncommon to observe normal A-V conduction occurring intermittently following the development of complete A-V block. A bipolar or unipolar catheter electrode is inserted, via a jugular or arm vein, into the right ventricle, preferably in the apical region, under direct vision utilizing fluoroscopy with an image intensifier. Otherwise, the blind float technique may be used in certain circumstances. In this method, the catheter electrode is advanced gently into position as the location of the tip is monitored electrocardiographically. The usual pacing rate is between 60 and 70 beats per minute.

2. *Indications for long-term pacing (permanent pacing)*

The decision as to whether long-term pacing is indicated or not is very serious, because the patient must live with an artificial pacemaker all his life and must observe various necessary cautions and daily care. In addition, the battery should be changed every 18 to 30 months in most cases, depending upon the model. One of the most serious problems following permanent pacemaker implantation is malfunction of the unit, which may be fatal. At times, it is difficult to judge whether a permanent artificial pacemaker is definitely required. In general, in the following situations, long-term pacing is considered to be indicated.

A. Symptomatic, chronic second degree (usually Mobitz Type II) or third degree A-V block

B. Symptomatic, chronic and drug-resistant sinus arrhythmias including sinus bradycardia, sinus arrest and sinoatrial (S-A) block

C. Complete A-V block in acute myocardial infarction lasting more than 2 to 3 weeks

D. Symptomatic bilateral bundle branch block (see list below)

E. Recurrent Adams-Stokes syndrome

F. Intractable congestive heart failure, cerebral or renal insufficiency benefited by temporary pacing

G. Recurrent drug-resistant tachyarrhythmias benefited by temporary pacing

When the indication for a permanent pacemaker has been determined, the type of pacemaker suitable for the specific patient must be determined in view of the patient's age and general condition and the underlying disease process. Of the four major types of pacemakers available for a long-term pacing (fixed-rate and demand [standby] ventricular units, atrial synchronized and bifocal demand units), the two latter units are suitable for young and active individuals when a changing heart rate according to physiological demands is highly desirable. The older epicardial types have the disadvantage of requiring thoracotomy, which carries with it a significant surgical mortality and morbidity,

Diagnostic Criteria of Bilateral Bundle Branch Block

1. Right bundle branch block with left anterior hemiblock
2. Right bundle branch block with left posterior hemiblock
3. Alternating left and right bundle branch block
4. Left or right bundle branch block with first or second degree A-V block
5. Left bundle branch block on one occasion and right bundle branch block on another occasion
6. Any combination of above findings
7. Complete A-V block with ventricular escape rhythm

whereas the newer transvenous catheter types may cause right ventricular perforation and failure of ventricular capture due to movement of the catheter electrode. A fixed-rate ventricular pacemaker must be avoided when there is intermittent A-V block. Otherwise competition between the natural and artificial pacemaker rhythm (parasystole) will occur.

3. *Artificial pacemakers in acute myocardial infarction*

A special comment is in order regarding the use and abuse of artificial pacemakers in acute myocardial infarction (MI) because there is a significant controversy among physicians.

A. *Indications for pacing in acute myocardial infarction regardless of location*

(1) Symptomatic and drug resistant bradyarrhythmias of any origin or mechanism

(a) Sinus bradycardia, sinus arrest, S-A block

(b) A-V block (second degree, high degree and complete)

(c) Bilateral bundle branch block (see list on p. 363)

(2) Bradytachyarrhythmia syndrome

(3) Drug-resistant tachyarrhythmias

(4) Ventricular standstill

B. *Indications for pacing in acute diaphragmatic (inferior) myocardial infarction*

(1) Drug-resistant symptomatic, second degree, high degree, or complete A-V block, sinus bradycardia, sinus arrest, S-A block

(2) Extremely slow ventricular rate (below 45 beats per minute)

(3) Bradytachyarrhythmia syndrome

(4) Refractory tachyarrhythmias

(5) Ventricular standstill

C. *Indications for pacing in acute anterior myocardial infarction*

(1) Complete A-V block: Pacing (often permanent) is indicated in every case regardless of symptoms.

(2) Mobitz Type II or 2:1 A-V block

(3) Drug-resistant symptomatic sinus bradycardia, sinus arrest, S-A block, slow escape rhythm without A-V block

(4) Bradytachyarrhythmia syndrome

(5) Various forms of bilateral bundle branch block or left bundle branch block alone with acute onset

(6) Refractory tachyarrhythmias

(7) Ventricular standstill

D. *Equivocal or no indications for pacing in acute myocardial infarction*

(1) First degree A-V block

(2) Asymptomatic Wenckebach A-V block in diaphragmatic myocardial infarction

(3) Asymptomatic or transient sinus or A-V junctional bradyarrhythmias

(4) Right bundle branch block

(5) Left anterior hemiblock or left posterior hemiblock

(6) Transient bifascicular block

(7) Late development of bifascicular block

TYPES OF ARTIFICIAL PACEMAKERS

1. *Fixed-rate pacemakers*

A. The fixed-rate pacemaker is designed to function regardless of the patient's own natural rhythm (Fig. 26-1).

B. There are at least 24 different fixed-rate pacemakers available in the market.

C. A fixed-rate ventricular pacemaker can be used with relative safety in patients with established chronic complete A-V block when normal A-V conduction is unlikely to occur, even temporarily.

D. In addition, older patients using

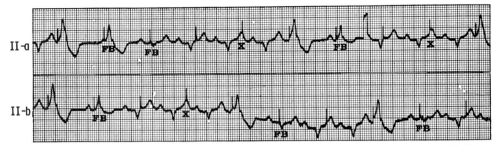

Fig. 26-1. Leads II-a and b are not continuous. The patient's own sinus rhythm with first degree A-V block competes with a fixed-rate pacemaker rhythm. Note frequent ventricular fusion beats (marked FB) and occasional areas showing the R-on-T phenomenon (marked X).

a fixed-rate pacemaker are able to carry out their ordinary activities quite adequately, since a maximum cardiac output is not important to sustain their limited physical requirements.

E. In approximately 25 per cent of patients who require permanent pacing for Adams-Stokes syndrome, normal A-V conduction (either normal sinus rhythm or second degree A-V block) may return either temporarily or even for long periods of time. In this case, the patient's own rhythm competes with the pacemaker rhythm so that the patient may develop ventricular fibrillation as a result of the R-on-T phenomenon (Fig. 26-1). Primarily because of this reason, a demand pacemaker is preferable in many patients in whom normal A-V conduction may return even momentarily (see no. 2 below).

F. A fixed-rate ventricular pacemaker is often used when overdriving pacing is indicated for the treatment of drug-resistant ectopic tachyarrhythmias.

2. *Demand (standby) pacemaker*

A. In the past several years, demand pacemakers have been gradually replacing fixed-rate pacemakers because a definite superiority in the former is that competition between the natural rhythm and artificial pacemaker rhythm can be avoided.

B. The demand pacemaker func-

tions only when the R-R intervals of the natural rhythm exceed a preset limit. Therefore, the demand pacemaker is particularly ideal for temporary pacing when bradyarrhythmias are transient or intermittent (Fig. 26-2).

C. There are two main types of demand units. The most commonly used demand pacemakers are the Medtronic, American Optical and Ventricor II (Cordis) units.

D. It is important to recognize "hysteresis" (the interval from the natural beat to the immediately following pacing beat is longer than the consecutively occurring pacing interval) in some models of demand units. Otherwise, the finding may be misdiagnosed as malfunction (Fig. 26-3).

E. Nonetheless, there are some disadvantages in using transvenous catheter electrodes, including perforation of the ventricles, failure of pacing due to migration or exit block, infection and fracture.

3. *Atrial synchronized pacemaker*

A. A more physiological type of artificial pacemaker is the atrial synchronized pacemaker (synchronous pacemaker, Nathan Pacemaker, atrial-triggered pacemaker).

B. In this type of pacemaker, the pulse generator is triggered by the natural P wave of atrial depolarization and

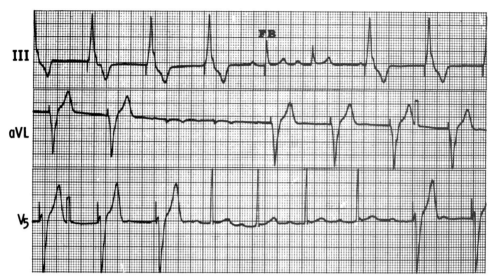

Fig. 26-2. Sinus rhythm with first degree A-V block and intermittent demand ventricular pacemaker rhythm with occasional ventricular fusion beats (marked FB). Note that there is no competition between the patient's own rhythm and the pacemaker rhythm.

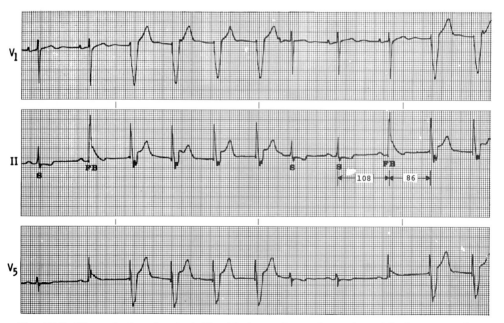

Fig. 26-3. Sinus rhythm (marked S) with intermittent demand ventricular pacemaker rhythm and occasional ventricular fusion beats (marked FB). Note that the R-R interval from the sinus beat to the immediately following pacemaker beat (1.08 seconds) is longer than the consecutively occurring pacing interval (0.86 second). This finding is called *hysteresis.* (The numbers represent hundredths of a second).

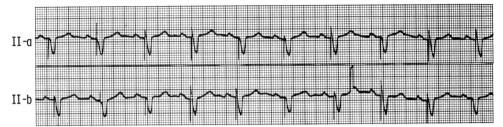

Fig. 26-4. Leads II-a and II-b are not continuous. The rhythm is sinus with atrial synchronized pacemaker rhythm.

ventricular stimulation follows after an optimal delay corresponding to the P-R interval (Fig. 26-4). In other words, an atrial synchronized pacemaker functions as an electronic bundle of His.

C. The major advantage of this type of pacemaker is its ability to provide maximum augmentation of the cardiac output at changing atrial rates in order to meet varying physiological requirements.

D. Another benefit is its utilization of the atrial contribution to ventricular filling to further augment the cardiac output.

E. Thus, the atrial synchronized pacemaker becomes extremely valuable in younger or more active patients.

F. When atrial tachycardia or flutter occurs, the pacemaker induces A-V block of varying degree so that an optimum ventricular rate is maintained.

G. Although the advantages of an atrial synchronized pacemaker are definitely known, electronic failure is frequent, and thoracotomy takes longer because of the complexity of the device.

H. An atrial synchronized pacemaker is contraindicated in atrial fibrillation, marked sinus bradycardia, unstable atrial activity such as S-A bloc', or sinus arrest, and atrial standstill.

4. *Bifocal demand pacemaker*

A. Bifocal (sequential atrioventricular) demand pacemaker consists of two demand units; a conventional QRS-inhibited ventricular pacemaker and a

QRS-inhibited atrial pacemaker (Fig. 26-5).

B. In this model, the escape interval of the atrial pacemaker is designed to be shorter than that of the ventricular pacemaker. Thus, the difference between these two escape intervals is a determining factor for the A-V sequential delay.

C. The bifocal demand pacemaker can stimulate both atria and ventricles in sequence, or it may stimulate the atria alone, or remain totally dormant. Thus, the pacemaker functions automatically according to the individual patient's needs.

D. In general, the bifocal demand pacemaker is considered to be indicated in the following situations:

(1) Sick sinus syndrome

(2) Significant atrial bradyarrhythmias associated with intermittent high degree or complete A-V block (symptomatic)

(3) High degree or complete A-V block (symptomatic), in that atrial contribution to the ventricular output is essential

E. The bifocal demand pacemaker does not compete with spontaneous ventricular contractions.

5. *Miscellaneous remarks*

Pacing site may be in the atria or coronary sinus region in order to utilize the atrial contribution and normal activation of the entire heart.

In coronary sinus pacemaker rhythm,

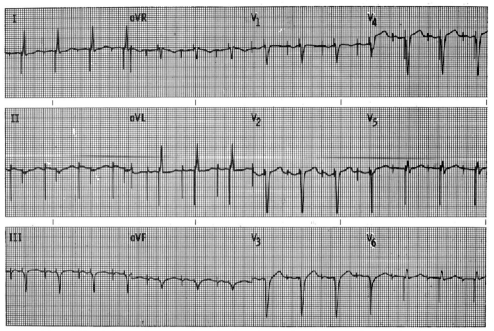

Fig. 26-5. Bifocal demand pacemaker rhythm. Note that there are 2 sets of artificial pacemaker spikes: one precedes the P waves and the other precedes the QRS complexes. There is evidence of anterior myocardial infarction and probable diaphragmatic (inferior) myocardial infarction.

the retrograde P wave is initiated by the pacing spike and followed by the optimal P-R interval and normal QRS complex (Fig. 26-6).

COMPLICATIONS OF ARTIFICIAL PACING

During the insertion or implantation of an artificial pacemaker, the danger of inducing ventricular fibrillation is always possible and, therefore, a cardioverter must be available immediately. In addition, various commonly used antiarrhythmic agents also should be available immediately. Common complications are as follows:

1. *Malfunctioning artificial pacemakers*

A malfunctioning unit may be manifested in the following ways:

A. *Acceleration of pacing rate (runaway pacemaker)*

(1) Runaway pacemaker is common when a fixed-rate pacemaker is used (Fig. 26-7).

(2) When the runaway pacemaker runs extremely fast, the preexisting bradyarrhythmia reappears (Fig. 26-8).

(3) In advanced cases of runaway pacemaker, ventricular fibrillation may occur. On the other hand, ventricular fibrillation can occur even in normally functioning pacemaker (Fig. 26-9).

(4) Runaway pacemaker is a medical emergency. In this case, the malfunctioning unit should be disconnected from the heart promptly. This can be done by cutting the electrode wires near their attachments to the pacemaker. Replacement with a temporary pacemaker

(Text continues on p. 371)

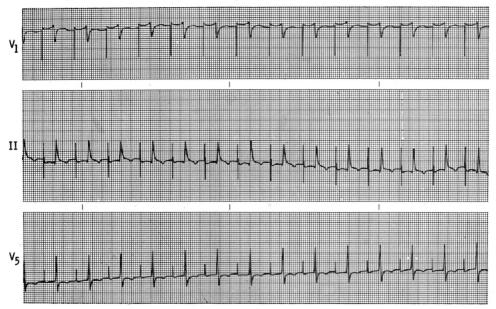

Fig. 26-6. Coronary sinus pacemaker rhythm. Note that all retrograde P waves are preceded by the pacemaker spikes and the P-R intervals are constant.

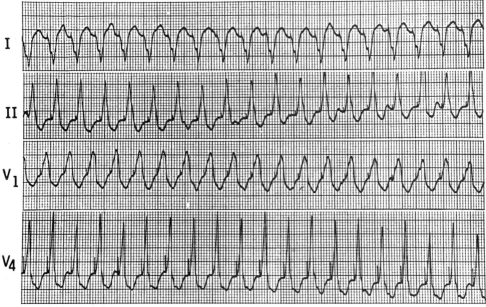

Fig. 26-7. Runaway pacemaker as a result of malfunctioning fixed-rate ventricular pacemaker (pacing rate: 167 beats/min.).

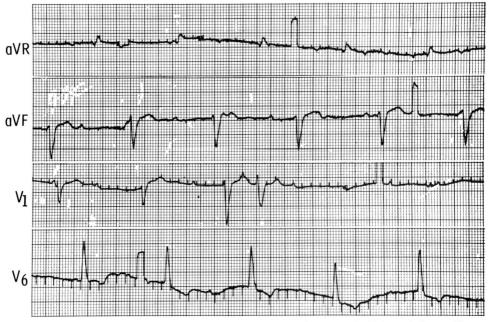

Fig. 26-8. Far-advanced runaway pacemaker with a pacing rate of 430 beats/minute. Note that none of the pacing spikes capture the ventricles, and the pre-existing complete A-V block is present with one ventricular premature beat (lead V_1).

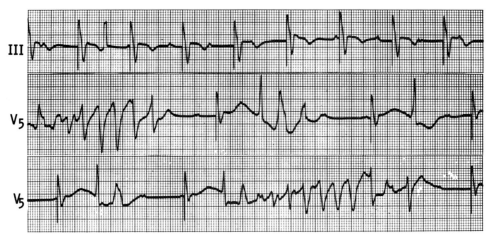

Fig. 26-9. A demand ventricular pacemaker rhythm with frequent ventricular premature contractions and paroxysmal ventricular fibrillation. Note that the artificial pacemaker functions normally.

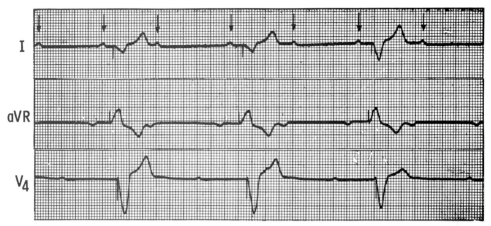

Fig. 26-10. Arrows indicate sinus P waves. A malfunctioning ventricular demand pacemaker produces a very slow pacemaker rhythm (pacing rate: 32 beats/min.). The preset pacing rate in this patient was 65 beats/minute.

connected to the bare electrode ends usually results in a prompt recovery in most patients.

(5) Antitachyarrhythmic agents are ineffective for the runaway pacemaker.

B. *Slowing of pacing rate*

(1) Slowing of pacing rate is a common form of malfunction when a demand unit is used (Fig. 26-10).

(2) Slowing of pacing may be associated with irregular pacing (Fig. 26-11).

C. *Irregular pacing*

(1) Irregular pacing is usually observed in advanced or late stage of malfunction (Fig. 26-11).

(2) Irregular pacing may be associated with slowing or acceleration of the pacing rate.

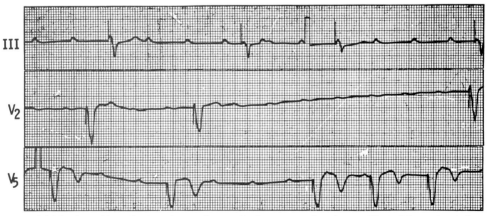

Fig. 26-11. A malfunctioning demand ventricular pacemaker is manifested by extremely slow and irregular pacemaker rhythm. Note a long ventricular pause in lead V_2.

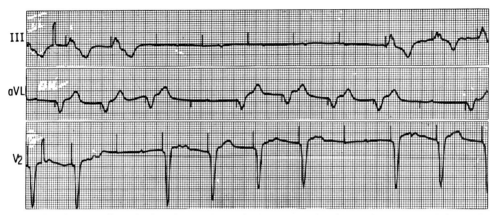

Fig. 26-12. A malfunctioning demand ventricular pacemaker is manifested by a failure of the ventricular capture in many areas. Note a long ventricular standstill in lead III.

D. *Failure of ventricular capture*

(1) Failure of ventricular capture is a very common problem (Fig. 26-12).

(2) Failure of ventricular capture may be associated with runaway pacemaker or slowing of pacing rate.

2. *Perforation of the ventricles*

A. Perforation of the ventricles can occur when a transverse catheter electrode is used.

B. Perforation of the ventricles may be suspected when the following findings occur unexpectedly:

(1) Right bundle branch block

(2) Recurrent diaphragmatic contractions

(3) Pericarditis or pericardial effusion

(4) A pansystolic murmur (due to rupture of the ventricular septum)

3. *Other findings*

(1) Electrode fracture

(2) Infection

(3) Thrombosis or embolism

(4) Knotting of the wire

(5) Various cardiac arrhythmias, which may be due to malfunction of the unit or which may simply coexist with the normally functioning pacemaker rhythm.

POSSIBLE INTERFERENCE WITH ARTIFICIAL PACEMAKER FUNCTION

The following may interfere with artificial pacemaker function:

1. Electric shavers
2. Automobile motors
3. Motorcycles
4. Malfunctioning TV sets
5. Direct contact with an ungrounded electrical appliance
6. Indirectly by proximity to equipment producing strong, rapidly fluctuating electromagnetic fields
7. Muscle stimulator for home use
8. Electric motors fitted with brushes and commutators
9. Motor-operated hospital beds
10. Electrosurgical and physical therapy equipment
11. Direct current shock

FACTORS MODIFYING PACEMAKER FUNCTION

There are various factors that may modify the artificial pacemaker function:

1. Sympathomimetic amines may increase myocardial irritability.

2. Hyperkalemia may cause failure of ventricular capture.

3. Fibrosis around pacemaker electrode may cause failure of ventricular capture.

4. Advancement of underlying heart disease may cause failure of ventricular capture.

AFTERCARE OF PATIENTS WITH ARTIFICIAL PACEMAKERS

1. *What the patient has to do*

A. Every patient with a permanent pacemaker should check the pulse 1 or 2 times daily in order to be certain that the pacemaker's preset rate remains constant.

B. In case of alteration of the pulse rate (either slowing or increasing), a physician should be notified immediately because this may be indicative of a malfunction of the pacemaker.

C. When any new symptoms or signs, such as chest pain, syncopal episode, dizziness, or wound infection occur, a physician should be notified immediately.

2. *What the physician has to do*

A. The patient should be fully instructed regarding the usual daily care, including common signs of malfunctioning pacemaker, following the pacemaker implantation before discharge.

B. The patient should be given an identification card indicating:

(1) Name of the patient

(2) Date of pacemaker implantation

(3) Name of the physician who performed the pacemaker implantation and/or a physician who will follow the pacemaker care after discharge.

(4) Name of the institution where the pacemaker implantation was performed.

(5) Type and model number of pacemaker and the manufacturer's name

(6) Medical summary, including medications (optional)

C. Pacemaker follow-up care

(1) First visit: 1 month after discharge

(a) Check surgical wound

(b) Detect gross evidence of malfunction

(c) Ask usual pulse rate and any complaint, such as chest pain or syncopal episode

(2) Routine visit: Every 3 to 6 months. Perform such procedures as ECG analysis

(3) Elective hospitalization: For battery change

(4) Emergency hospitalization: For replacing malfunctioning unit

D. Pacemaker follow-up procedure for each visit

(1) Complete check-up of the patient's cardiac status and status of pacemaker implantation site and the pacemaker function

(2) Long rhythm strips (leads II and V_2) to check the pacing rate to compare with the preset rate

(3) A 12 lead ECG (at least once or twice a year) to detect any unexpected or new ECG abnormality

(4) When the patient's own sinus rhythm returns following implantation of a demand pacemaker, certain maneuvers, such as reducing the patient's own heart rate by carotid sinus stimulation (see Chap. 28) or by edrophonium chloride (Tensilon) injection, or by accelerating the artificial pacemaker rate by using an induction coil, should enable one to check the function of the pacemaker.

(5) Ask about any unusual or new complaint, such as chest pain or fainting episodes.

(6) Arrange elective or emergency admission as needed.

E. ECG analysis of pacemaker function

(1) Long rhythm strip (lead II) and preferably 6 lead ECG at each visit.

(2) A 12 lead ECG:

(a) Every 12 months (routine check-up)

(b) When malfunction is suspected

(c) When the patient has unusual or new symptoms

(3) Measure pacing rate to compare with preset rate.

(4) Measure pacemaker artifact amplitude to compare with preset amplitude (often special equipment is needed).

(5) Detect cardiac arrhythmias.

F. Radiographic analysis of pacemaker function

(1) Chest radiographs (sometimes of abdomen) are taken

(a) Before discharge

(b) 6 to 9 months after discharge

(c) Yearly films thereafter

(d) Immediate radiographs when malfunction is suspected

(2) Check the position of the pacemaker and lead system. Malposition, twisting, angulation, rotation of electrode or pulse generator should be checked.

(3) Check the state of the mercury cell.

(a) Normal state: cell's outer core and its inner rings are radiopaque, and the electrolyte between is radiolucent.

(b) Mercury cell exhaustion: sharply delineated margins of rings become hazy as contained mercury compound moves into electrolyte zone.

SUGGESTED READINGS

Bacharach, B., Chung, E. K. and Morris, J., Jr.: Your Pacemaker Patient. Minneapolis, Medtronic, Inc., 1975.

Batchelder, J. E. and Zipes, D. P.: Treatment of tachyarrhythmias by pacing. Arch. Int. Med., *135*:1115, 1975.

Castellanos, A., Jr. and Lemberg, L.: Electrophysiology of Pacing and Cardioversion. New York, Appleton-Century-Crofts, 1969.

Chung, E. K.: Cardiac Arrhythmias: Management. Baltimore, Williams & Wilkins Co., 1973.

Furman, S. and Escher, D. J. W.: Principles and Techniques of Cardiac Pacing. Hagerstown, Harper & Row, 1970.

Krishnaswami, V. and Geraci, A. R.: Permanent pacing in disorders of sinus node function. Am. Heart J., *89*:579, 1975.

Lemberg, L. and Castellanos, A. Jr.: Artificial pacing. *In* Chung, E. K. (ed.): Cardiac Emergency Care. Philadelphia, Lea & Febiger, 1975.

Love, J. W. et al.: The Johns Hopkins rechargeable pacemaker. J.A.M.A., *234*:64, 1975.

Moss, A. J.: Therapeutic uses of permanent pervenous atrial pacemakers: A review. J. Electrocardiology, *8*:373, 1975.

Parsonnet, V., Furman, S. and Smyth, N. P. D.: Implantable cardiac pacemakers. Status reports and resource guideline. ICHD Report. Circulation, *50*:A21, 1974.

Schaldach, M. and Furman, S.: Pacemaker Technology. New York, Springer-Verlag, 1975.

Seremetis, M. G. et al.: Cardiac pacemakers. Am. Heart J., *85*:739, 1973.

Siddons, H. and Sowton, E.: Cardiac Pacemakers. Springfield, Charles C Thomas, 1967.

Spence, M. I. and Lemberg, L.: Cardiac pacemakers. IV. Complications of pacing. Heart & Lung, *4*:286, 1975.

Stoney, W. S. et al.: Cost of cardiac pacing. Am. J. Cardiol., *37*:23, 1976.

Vera, Z. et al.: Cardiac pacemakers: indications and complications. Heart & Lung, *4*:444, 1975.

27. CARDIOPULMONARY RESUSCITATION

Stephen C. Manus, M.D., *and Edward K. Chung,* M.D.

DEFINITIONS

1. Cardiopulmonary arrest is defined as the cessation of an effective cardiac output and functional ventilation.
2. Cardiopulmonary resuscitative measures are chemical and mechanical means attempted to restore an effective cardiac output and ventilatory function. Resuscitative measures include:
   A. Establishment of an airway
   B. Establishment of breathing for the patient
   C. Establishment of effective circulation

GENERAL CONSIDERATIONS

In the United States, more than 650,000 persons die annually because of ischemic heart disease. More than half of these, or approximately 350,000 persons, die outside of hospitals.[15] The acute onset of symptoms and sudden death frequently occur in the presence of relatives, friends, and medical personnel. In order to decrease this large number of deaths outside as well as inside the hospital setting, cardiopulmonary resuscitative measures should be learned by all physicians, nurses, police and firemen, rescue squads, hospital personnel, and the public.

ETIOLOGY

1. Syndromes of myocardial underperfusion:
   A. Atherosclerotic coronary heart disease (i.e., myocardial infarction)
   B. Shock due to various causes (see Chap. 20)

2. Electrolyte and acid-base imbalances. Extracellular or intracellular concentration changes of potassium, calcium, sodium or magnesium can cause cardiac arrhythmias and arrest.
3. Drugs
   A. Procainamide, diphenylhydantoin, and quinidine toxicity may be associated with ventricular tachycardia and fibrillation.
   B. Digitalis intoxication may produce ventricular tachycardia or fibrillation and ventricular standstill, in the setting of hypoxia, hypokalemia, and hypomagnesemia.
   C. Narcotic and sedative drug overdose with hypoventilation.
4. Electrocution
5. Hypoxemia and pulmonary embolism

PATHOPHYSIOLOGY

The pathophysiology of cardiac arrest is serious cardiac arrhythmias:
1. Ventricular tachycardia
2. Ventricular fibrillation
3. Idioventricular rhythm
4. Ventricular standstill (asystole)

SYMPTOMS AND SIGNS

1. *The absence of an effective cardiac output*
   A. The absence of an effective cardiac output is recognized by syncope, unconsciousness, seizures, or cyanosis.
   B. Physical examination may reveal the following:
      (1) Absent precordial pulsation
      (2) Absent heart sounds
      (3) Absent or markedly di-

minished central arterial pulses, such as carotid or femoral (The radial pulse should not be used.)

(4) Cool, moist, and cyanotic extremities and trunk

(5) The pupils may be dilated secondary to the inadequate cerebral perfusion. Pupil size can be used to estimate duration of cerebral anoxia and reveal any response to resuscitation measures. If dilated before resuscitation is begun, the prognosis is not as favorable as if constricted. If the pupils constrict during resuscitation, this indicates brain perfusion and oxygenation.

2. *The absence of functional ventilation*

The absence of functional ventilation may be recognized by:

A. The lack of abdominal or thoracic movement

B. The absence of breath sounds

C. The decrease or lack of air movements through the nose and mouth. Chest and abdominal movements without mouth or nose air motion is suggestive of upper airway obstruction.[15]

MANAGEMENT

1. *General measures*

Successful resuscitation requires speed and organization. The most experienced physician directs the team effort. This person monitors the electrocardiogram, orders the necessary cardiac drugs (see Chaps. 20, 22 and 24), and assigns team members to ventilation, external cardiac compression, securing an intravenous route, administering drugs, etc. Successful resuscitative effort is a team effort.

2. *Specific measures*

The purpose of cardiopulmonary resuscitation is to restore a cardiac rhythm that produces an effective cardiac output for tissue perfusion. Successful resuscitation also requires effective ventilation

for oxygenation as well as for correction of respiratory acidosis. The procedure followed during resuscitation depends on the specific cardiac arrhythmia encountered. Continuous ventilation and effective cardiac output must be maintained by any means.

A. *Chest thump*

(1) A quick blunt blow with the bottom of the closed fist to the midsternum should be immediately attempted.

(a) "Thump version" may revert ventricular tachycardia to normal sinus rhythm by depolarizing a portion of myocardium interrupting a re-entrant pathway responsible for ventricular tachycardia.[12]

(b) May terminate ventricular fibrillation[6]

(c) Has produced ectopic ventricular beats and ectopic automatic ventricular rhythms in patients with ventricular standstill.[13]

(2) The precordial thump should not be used when ventricular tachycardia provides adequate circulation.

(3) Precordial thump is not recommended for use in children.

(4) Time should not be wasted in repeated futile chest thumps.

B. *Defibrillation*

(1) If "thump version" does not immediately restore a cardiac rhythm with effective cardiac output, further therapy will require a DC defibrillation and/or the use of drugs (see Chaps. 24 and 25).

(2) While the defibrillator or drugs are being obtained, an effective cardiac output must be obtained by external cardiac compression, effective ventilation must be achieved, and an intravenous route must be found.

(3) In the critically ill patient, 200 to 400 watt-sec. with the DC defibrillator is recommended.[7] This will terminate ventricular tachycardia or fibrillation but will have no effect on asystole.

C. *Ventilation*

(1) Obtaining a patent airway

(a) The problem of upper airway obstruction should be recognized.[4]

(b) The mouth is examined for obstructive materials. Vomitus or foreign bodies should be removed by hand or forceps. The patient can also be turned laterally and struck forcibly between the scapula.

(c) In an unconscious patient:

(i) The jaw muscles supporting the tongue are relaxed, allowing the base of the tongue to rest on the posterior pharyngeal wall obstructing the air flow.

(ii) This obstruction can be relieved if the head is extended on the neck with the neck slightly flexed forward.

(iii) One hand is placed under the patient's neck, one on the forehead, elevating the neck while tilting the head backward.[14]

(iv) Care should be used in moving the neck if neck injury is suspected.

(v) The anterior portion of the lower jaw can also be pulled forward, pulling the base of the tongue with it and thereby opening the pharynx. This can also be done by pushing forward on the angles of the jaw.

(d) If these measures fail, emergency cricothyroid puncture with insertion of a small patent tube is required.

(e) Once the airway is patent, ventilation can be restored by using mouth to mouth resuscitation, tracheal intubation, or the use of the self-inflating bag.

(2) Methods of artificial ventilation

(a) Mouth to mouth technique

(i) The patient's nose is sealed with the thumb and forefinger.

(ii) A tight seal is produced between the resuscitator's mouth and the patient's mouth.

(iii) The mouths are separated during exhalation.

(iv) The initial ventilatory maneuver should be 4 full breaths into the patient without allowing time for lung deflation between breaths.

(v) After the initial respiratory maneuver, a respiratory cycle should be repeated every 5 seconds as long as respiratory difficulty persists (Fig. 27-1).

(b) Mouth to nose technique

(i) Adults

(A.) The patient's mouth is sealed with the rescuer's hand and the nose is sealed by the rescuer's mouth.

(B.) Because of a valve action by the soft palate, the victim's mouth may need to be opened to allow exhalation.

(C.) The respiratory cycle is repeated every five seconds.

(ii) Infants and children

(A.) The rescuer covers both the nose and mouth of the child with his mouth and uses smaller breaths with respiratory cycles every three seconds.

(B.) Overextension of the neck in children should be avoided.

(c) Self-inflating bag and mask

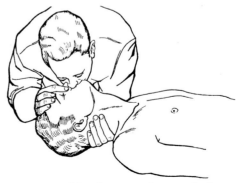

Fig. 27-1. Mouth-to-mouth resuscitation.

(i) An oral airway to depress the tongue is used.

(ii) The mask should form a tight seal over the patient's nose and mouth.

(iii) An oxygen-enriched air mixture should be used.

(iv) With the use of both the mouth to mouth technique or use of the self-inflating bag and mask, the chest should be observed in order to be certain of sufficient chest expansion and bilateral lung aeration.

(d) Endotracheal intubation

(i) If a trained person and equipment are available, endotracheal intubation with either an oral or nasotracheal tube can be done.

(ii) Prolonged attempts at intubation should not be done without intermittent ventilation by either mouth to mouth or bag and mask techniques.

(iii) Resuscitation efforts may be stopped momentarily for intubation but for no longer than 20 to 30 seconds. Prolonged attempts at unsuccessful intubation without interruption by other ventilatory techniques may lead to irreversible neurologic defects or intractable cardiac arrhythmias.

(iv) Auscultation should establish bilateral lung aeration.

(A.) The endotracheal tube may have to be pulled back if there is no aeration of the left lung due to slippage of the endotracheal tube down the right mainstem bronchus during insertion.

(B.) Bilateral lung aeration should be definitely established to insure that the esophagus and stomach have not been intubated, causing abortive successful resuscitation.

(v) A nasogastric tube may be inserted for gastric decompression.

(vi) All ventilation should be done with oxygen-enriched mixtures.

(vii) Pressure-cycled respirators should not be used during external cardiac compression because the chest pressure produced during compression causes early termination of inspiration.

(3) Coordination of ventilatory techniques with cardiac compression

(a) If only one person is performing resuscitation:

(i) Three or 4 breaths followed by 30 seconds of external cardiac compression should be performed.

(ii) This is followed by 2 quick lung inflations after each 15 chest compressions, which should be performed at an approximate rate of 80 compressions per minute.

(b) If two people are available:

(i) One performs external cardiac massage while the other performs ventilation.

(ii) There should be 4 or 5 external cardiac compressions for each ventilation effort.

(iii) External cardiac compression should not be interrupted to allow ventilation.

D. *External cardiac compression*

(1) An effective cardiac output and circulation must be restored for perfusion of the vital organs.

(2) This may necessitate the use of mechanical means when the restoration of the cardiac rhythm is unsuccessful.

(3) Both mechanical external cardiac compression and ventilatory efforts must be initiated simultaneously and immediately while treatment of the primary cardiac rhythm disturbance with drugs or by defibrillation is being initiated.

(4) Correctly applied external cardiac compression can produce systolic blood pressure of 100 mm. Hg. Cardiac output can be approximately 30 per cent of normal.[5] The palpated pulse wave is not necessarily indicative of adequate perfusion.[3]

(5) External cardiac compression

must be performed without interruption while one tries to obtain a cardiac rhythm capable of producing adequate cardiac output.

(6) External closed cardiac compression can be done by both mechanical and manual means[9] (Figs. 27-2 and 27-3).

(7) Manual techniques of compression for adults

(a) The patient should be supine on a firm surface, allowing compression to cause an effective decrease in the anterior-posterior diameter of the chest.

(b) The patient can be on a hard board, floor, or any available hard surface.

(c) The heel of one hand is placed over the lower third of the sternum superior to the xiphoid process.

(d) The heel of the second hand is placed over the dorsum of the heel of the lower hand.

(e) Only the heel of the lower hand should be in direct contact with the patient's chest. This application of sternal compression is important.

(f) The resuscitator should have his shoulders directly above the sternum.

(g) Compression should be carried out from force applied to the back and shoulders with the elbows fully extended so that downward force is transmitted from the shoulder through the forearm to the heel of the hands.

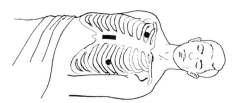

Fig. 27-2. The darkened rectangular area denotes where the heel of the hand is placed for closed-chest cardiac massage. The two darkened circular areas indicate where defibrillator electrodes should be placed.

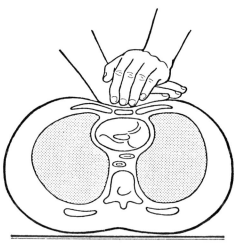

Fig. 27-3. External closed cardiac compression.

(h) Sufficient pressure is applied to move the sternum 3 or 4 cm. toward the vertebral column.

(i) At no time should the heel of the hand leave the sternum. The operator's fingers should always be extended off the chest wall of the victim to minimize the exertion of pressure anywhere except the proper place. This will prevent the fracture of ribs and possible lacerated viscera.

(j) Five external compressions are performed to one ventilation with no pause between the fifth and first compression.

(k) Firm pressure is applied approximately 60 times a minute.

(l) Massage is continued if the heart is not contracting, if a peripheral pulse (femoral or carotid) is weak, and if the cardiac output is inadequate to sustain life.

(m) The effectiveness of external compression can be judged by recognizing the strength of the carotid or femoral pulse. It can be judged also when the pupils begin to constrict from a dilated position.

(8) Manual techniques of compression for infants and young children

(a) For infants, 2 fingertips are applied to the midportion of the sternum, which is depressed 2.5 cm. at a rate of 100 to 120 compressions per minute.

(b) The older child's sternum may be depressed with the heel of only one hand.[5]

(9) Complications of compression

(a) Too vigorous compression may cause fractured ribs, or cardiac, lung, and other visceral damage.[11]

(b) Too high a compression over the sternum or too weak compression gives ineffective massage with inadequate cardiac output.

(c) There must be sufficient time for the heart to fill during mechanical diastole. A too-rapid compression rate can produce decreasing stroke volume and cardiac output.

E. *Route for administration of drugs*

(1) Intravenous route

(a) While ventilation and chest compression are being performed, an intravenous route should be found into a large vein of the arm.

(b) The femoral, jugular, or subclavian veins may be used.

(c) A cutdown is often indicated.

(d) All medications should be given either through the intravenous or intracardiac route because of inadequate or unpredictable absorption from other routes.

(e) A large-bore needle is used.

(f) The intravenous route is kept open with small quantities of 5 per cent dextrose in water.

(2) Intracardiac route

(a) A small-gauge spinal needle is passed through the fourth or fifth intercostal space 2 to 3 inches to the left of the sternum.

(b) External cardiac compression is stopped and artificial respiration halted temporarily so that the lingula of the left lower lobe of the lung is not punctured by the needle insertion.

(c) The intracardiac needle should be inserted with negative pressure until blood is obtained in the attached syringe. By doing so, it can be assessed that the needle is located in the ventricular cavity.

(d) Injection of drugs into the myocardium may result in intractable ventricular fibrillation.

(e) Disadvantages of the intracardiac route of drug administration include possible punctured coronary arteries, pericardial tamponade, pneumothorax, and interruption of cardiopulmonary resuscitation.

F. *Correction of acid-base abnormalities*

(1) Metabolic acidosis

(a) Cardiac arrest is associated with decreased cardiac output and poor tissue perfusion.

(b) Tissue underperfusion leads to anaerobic metabolism and lactic acid production.

(c) The metabolic acidosis subsequent to lactate accumulation has certain cardiovascular effects:

(i) Decreased myocardial contractility

(ii) Predisposition to cardiac arrhythmias

(iii) Decreased responsiveness of the heart and peripheral circulation to the effect of catecholamines[1]

(d) Treatment of metabolic acidosis is as follows:

(i) Sodium bicarbonate should be given to counteract the metabolic acidosis.

(ii) One or two ampules of sodium bicarbonate (44 mEq bicarbonate/ampule) are given immediately intravenously.

(iii) Arterial blood gases should be drawn to gauge further bicarbonate needs.

(iv) If no arterial blood gas measurements are available and an adequate circulation is not achieved, sodium bicarbonate at 1 mEq per kilogram can be repeated once after the initial bolus.[5]

(v) Acid-base balance is best achieved by frequent determinations of the arterial blood gases.

(vi) Sodium bicarbonate administration may cause serious problems if overused. Overzealous administration may result in the following:

(A.) Severe metabolic alkalosis

(B.) Hyperosmolality

(C.) Cerebral acidosis

(D.) Sodium and fluid overload causing pulmonary edema

(2) Respiratory acidosis

(a) Hypercapnia and respiratory acidosis play an important role in the acidosis of cardiac arrest.[1]

(b) The treatment of this acidosis is best achieved by improved ventilation instead of large doses of bicarbonate.

G. *Monitoring the patient*

(1) All patients should be placed in a monitored environment, such as intensive or cardiac care unit, as soon as possible.

(2) Treatment of the patient is determined by the specific cardiac arrhythmia responsible for the cardiac arrest (see Chaps. 21,24-26).

(3) The patient should be monitored continuously for adequate and appropriate control of cardiac arrhythmias.

H. *Use of the defibrillator*

(1) The use of the AC and DC defibrillators has saved many lives. The development of the defibrillator has been described.[8]

(2) DC countershock produces complete myocardial depolarization, allowing one of the spontaneously depolarizing areas to achieve pacemaker control of the heart, which then may produce effective cardiac output.

(3) The DC defibrillator must be used properly (see Chap. 25).

(a) Electrode paste is used between the paddles and the chest skin to allow proper electrical conduction to the heart.

(b) Saline-soaked gauze pads may be used.

(c) One electrode paddle is placed at the base of the heart at the right upper sternal border below the clavicle and the other is placed at the apex in the left anterior axillary line.

(d) Some DC defibrillators have one electrode paddle in the back, in the retrocardiac position, with the electrical shock delivered through an electrode in the anterior precordial area.

(e) The electrodes are held firmly against the patient's chest skin to allow good current flow. Insufficient chest wall contact has resulted in serious chest skin burns and infections.

(f) The operator of the defibrillator must not come into contact with the patient or the patient's bed when the electrical energy is discharged.

(g) With the defibrillator, various amounts of electrical energy may be delivered. In the seriously ill patient, 200 to 400 watt-sec. should be delivered.

(h) Failure of conversion by DC shock may be due to profound acidosis or hypoxemia.

I. *Treatment of various cardiac arrhythmias*

(1) Ventricular fibrillation

(a) Ventricular fibrillation is characterized by the chaotic spread of electrical activity. There is marked incoordination of muscle fiber contraction.[2]

(b) Ventricular fibrillation may be terminated by thump version.

(c) The most reliable and effective treatment of ventricular fibrillation is through use of DC countershock.

(d) There should be no delay.

(e) For patients that weigh over 50 kg., the full output of the defibrillator, usually 400 watt-sec. should be used.[16]

(f) Three hundred watt-sec. of energy may be inadequate to defibrillate 35 per cent or more of subjects weighing more than 50 kilograms. It has been suggested that the initial countershock for patients in ventricular fibrillation weighing less than 50 kg. be between 3.5 and 6.0 watt-sec. per kilogram of body weight.[16]

(g) A coarse ventricular fibrillation wave appears easier to convert than a fine fibrillatory wave.

(h) A fine fibrillation wave may be made coarser in an adult with an injection of epinephrine, 1:1,000 solution, 0.2–1.0 ml. given intravenously.[17] Epinephrine may also be given by intracardiac injection, 0.2 to 0.3 ml. in 1:1,000 solution (200-300 μg.).[18]

(i) Coarseness of fibrillation may also be induced by giving 3 to 10 ml. of 10 per cent solution of calcium chloride either intravenously or by intracardiac injection.

(j) Once a coarse fibrillatory pattern is achieved, DC shock is given immediately.

(k) External cardiac compression is continued and only temporarily interrupted by giving DC shock.

(l) Failure of the termination of ventricular fibrillation by DC shock may be due to profound acidosis and hypoxemia:

(i) The patient should be well ventilated and oxygenated.

(ii) Epinephrine is repeated.

(iii) A second bolus of bicarbonate is given.

(iv) A bolus of lidocaine (50–100 mg.) is given to inhibit ectopic foci.

(v) Countershock is then repeated.

(vi) The above steps may be repeated, substituting 100 mg. of procainamide for lidocaine if still unsuccessful.

(2) Ventricular tachycardia (see Chaps. 24–26).

(3) Ventricular standstill (asystole):

(a) If asystole has not responded to a vigorous blow to the chest, an intracardiac injection of epinephrine, 0.2 to 0.3 ml. of 1:1,000 solution (200–300 μg.) is given.

(i) Epinephrine may convert asystole to a sinus mechanism.

(ii) The rhythm may revert to a chaotic ventricular rhythm and proceed to ventricular fibrillation. The rhythm is then treated as ventricular fibrillation by DC shock.

(b) If epinephrine fails, one may give calcium chloride 5 to 10 ml. of 10 per cent solution by intracardiac injection.

(c) With failure of both epinephrine and calcium, isoproterenol (Isuprel) infusion, 1.0 to 4 μg. per min. is used.

(d) Artificial pacing may also be tried (see Chap. 26).

(i) A pacemaker may be inserted through a transthoracic needle into contact with the ventricular endocardium.

(ii) A pacemaker may also be inserted transvenously; however, more time is usually necessary for this route than for the transthoracic route.

(iii) Pacemaker electrical energy should be at the highest setting.

(4) Ventricular escape (idioventricular rhythm) and complete A-V block (see Chaps. 24 and 26).

(5) Sinus bradycardia (see Chaps. 24 and 26).

(6) Electrical mechanical dissociation

If the electrocardiogram shows an appropriate rhythm but there is no audible heart tone or peripheral pulse, electrical-mechanical dissociation is considered to be present.

(a) Epinephrine, 1:1000 solution, 0.2 to 0.3 ml. can be given by intracardiac injection; or an intravenous infusion of 1 to 4 μg. per min. may be used.

(b) Isoproternol (Isuprel) is an alternative therapy.

(c) Calcium chloride 0.5 g. or calcium gluconate 1.0 g. can be given. Caution should be observed with the use of calcium in digitalized patients because of synergistic effects of digitalis and calcium (see Chap. 23).

(d) Glucagon, 5 to 10 mg. intracardiac injection can be successful.

(e) Pericardial tamponade may result in electrical-mechanical dissociation. Withdrawal of as little as 50 to 100 ml. of pericardial fluid may restore good cardiac hemodynamics.

J. *Peripheral blood pressure (see Chap. 20)*

Hypotension causing decreased coronary perfusion may lead to refractory ventricular arrhythmias.

(1) Epinephrine as an intravenous infusion of 1 to 4 μg. per minute is used, and the dose may be increased to 4 to 8 μg. per minute.

(2) The infusion should be tapered or stopped if hypertension or frequent ectopic activity occurs.

(3) Isoproternol (Isuprel) is not useful when a vasopressor is required and if the heart rate is already accelerated.

(4) Levarterenol (Levophed), up to 32 μg. per minute, or metaraminol (Aramine), 200 mg. in 500 ml. 5 per cent solution of dextrose in water may be carefully titrated to appropriate blood pressure level.

(5) In a previously normotensive individual, the blood pressure should not be titrated to more than 90 to 100 mm. Hg systolic pressure.

(6) If the patient was previously hypertensive, the blood pressure should be maintained no higher than 40 mm. Hg systolic pressure below the pre-arrest pressure. Higher pressure increases peripheral resistance, increases myocardial oxygen demands, and may result in a decrease in cardiac output.

K. *Postresuscitation measures*

(1) Successfully resuscitated patients should be closely monitored in an intensive or cardiac care unit to insure aggressive therapy of arrhythmia and control of ventilation and blood pressure.

(2) One study has shown that 50 per cent of patients hospitalized for ventricular fibrillation developed ventricular fibrillation or ventricular tachycardia again within 24 hours of admission.[10]

(3) Ventricular premature contractions can be treated early by lidocaine, 50 to 100 mg. intravenous bolus followed by intravenous infusion of 1 to 5 mg. per minute.

(4) For long-term therapy for ventricular arrhythmias, procainamide, 0.25 to 5.0 g. every 3 to 6 hours or quinidine sulfate, 0.3 to 0.4 g. 4 times daily can be used orally.

(5) Second degree A-V block and complete A-V block may require artificial pacing (see Chap. 26).

(6) The intake and output and vital signs are frequently recorded.

(7) A diuretic therapy may be needed to excrete the excessive sodium and water given during resuscitation.

(8) A chest tube may be necessary if pneumothorax secondary to resuscitation maneuvers is present.

(9) A Swan-Ganz catheter measuring pulmonary artery and pulmonary capillary wedge pressure is helpful for medication and fluid therapy measuring second-to-second cardiac performance.

(10) Electrolytes and acid-base balance may need correction.

(11) Tracheal intubation, mechanical ventilation, and oxygen may be needed to correct hypoventilation and hypoxemia.

(12) The initiating factors causing the cardiac arrest must be identified and treated. Acute myocardial infarction must always be considered until the condition is proven to be otherwise.

L. *Termination of resuscitative efforts*

(1) Cardiopulmonary resuscita-

tion should be terminated if evidence of brain and/or cardiac death persists through 1 hour of cardiopulmonary resuscitation, or if it is definitely known that absence of circulation or respiration existed for 6 or more minutes before starting cardiopulmonary resuscitation.

(2) Cardiac death is manifested by persistent asystole, ventricular fibrillation, or slow agonal and chaotic rhythm unresponsive to all therapy.

(3) Brain death is manifested by dilated unresponsive pupils, no spontaneous movement or activity, and complete lack of responsiveness in the absence of hypothermia or drug intoxication.

REFERENCES

1. Chazan, J. A., Stenson, R. and Kurland, G. S.: The acidosis of cardiac arrest. N. Engl. J. Med., *278*:360, 1968.
2. Cranefield, P. F.: Ventricular fibrillation. N. Engl. J. Med., *289*:732, 1973.
3. DelGuerico, L. R. M., Coomaraswamy, R. P. and State, D.: Cardiac output and other hemodynamic variables during external cardiac massage in man. N. Engl. J. Med., *269*:1398, 1963.
4. Eller, W. C. and Haugen, R. K.: Current concepts: food asphyxiation-restaurant rescue. N. Engl. J. Med., *289*:81, 1973.
5. Goldberg, A. H.: Current concepts: cardiopulmonary arrest. N. Engl. J. Med., *290*:381, 1974.
6. Harwood-Nash, D. C. F.: Thumping of the praecordium in ventricular fibrillation. S. A. Medical J., *36*[Part I]:280, 1962.
7. Hurst, J. W. (ed.): The Heart, Arteries, and Veins, ed. 3. New York, McGraw-Hill, 1974.
8. Kouwenhoven, W. B.: The development of the defibrillator. Ann. Int. Med., *71*:449, 1969.
9. Kouwenhoven, W. B. et al.: Closed-chest cardiac massage. J.A.M.A., *173*:94, 1960.
10. Liberthson, R. R. et al.: Prehospital ventricular defibrillation: prognosis and follow-up. N. Engl. J. Med., *291*:317, 1974.
11. Lundberg, G. D. et al.: Hemorrhage from gastroesophageal lacerations following closed-chest cardiac massage. J.A.M.A., *202*:123, 1967.
12. Pennington, J. E., Taylor, J., and Lown, B.: Chest thump for reverting ventricular tachycardia. N. Engl. J. Med., *283*:1192, 1970.
13. Scherf, D. and Bornemann, C.: Thumping of the precordium in ventricular standstill. Am. J. Cardiol., *5*:30, 1960.
14. Shapter, R. K. et al.: Cardiopulmonary resuscitation: basic life support. Clinical Symposia, CIBA, *26*:12, 1974.
15. Standards for cardiopulmonary resuscitation (CPR) and emergency cardiac care (ECC). American Heart Association Committee on Cardiopulmonary Resuscitation and Emergency Cardiac Care. J.A.M.A., *227* [Supp.]:837, 1974.
16. Tacker, W. A., Jr. et al.: Energy dosage for trans-chest electrical ventricular defibrillation. N. Engl. J. Med., *290*:214, 1974.
17. Walinsky, P. and Chung, E. K.: Cardiopulmonary resuscitation. *In* Chung, E. K. (ed.): Cardiac Emergency Care. Philadelphia, Lea & Febiger, 1975.
18. Zoll, P. M.: Rational use of drugs for cardiac arrest and after cardiac resuscitation. Am. J. Cardiol., *27*:644, 1971.

28. CAROTID SINUS STIMULATION

Edward K. Chung, M.D., *and Lisa S. Chung,* M.D.

GENERAL CONSIDERATIONS

It has been known for many years that carotid sinus stimulation is very useful in differentiating various tachyarrhythmias, because the response to this procedure is different depending upon the origin and the nature of the arrhythmia. This is particularly true when dealing with regular ectopic tachycardia and wide QRS complex in which the differential diagnosis is often urgently needed. In addition, carotid sinus stimulation is extremely valuable in terminating supraventricular (atrial or A-V junctional) tachycardia. On the other hand, the danger of applying carotid sinus stimulation to patients with suspected digitalis intoxication is well known. The reason for this is that ventricular fibrillation may be induced during or after carotid sinus stimulation in this circumstance (see Chap. 23).

INDICATIONS OF CAROTID SINUS STIMULATION

Carotid sinus stimulation is indicated for 2 major purposes: therapeutic and diagnostic.

1. *Therapeutic*

A. Carotid sinus stimulation is extremely valuable in terminating paroxysmal atrial as well as A-V nodal (junctional) tachycardia.

B. In addition, regular and rapid (rate: 160–250 beats/min.) tachycardia is often terminated by carotid sinus stimulation even if the exact location of the ectopic focus is uncertain.

C. Carotid sinus stimulation may be effective whether the QRS complex is normal or wide.

2. *Diagnostic*

It has been known for many years that carotid sinus stimulation is extremely useful in differentiating various tachyarrhythmias. This is particularly true when dealing with regular ectopic tachycardia and wide QRS complex. Various responses to carotid sinus stimulation are described in Table 28-1. It should be emphasized that applying carotid sinus stimulation to patients with digitalis toxicity is dangerous and may induce ventricular fibrillation (see Chap. 23).

RESPONSES OF VARIOUS CONDITIONS TO CAROTID SINUS STIMULATION

1. *Sinus tachycardia*

In general it is not necessary to apply carotid sinus stimulation either diagnostically or therapeutically in cases of sinus tachycardia. However, the procedure is occasionally useful when the rate of sinus tachycardia is very rapid (around 150–160 beats per minute) and differentiation from atrial tachycardia is needed.

A. Sinus tachycardia slows only transiently in response to carotid sinus stimulation.

B. Less commonly, carotid sinus stimulation may produce varying degree A-V block transiently (Fig. 28-1).

2. *Atrial tachycardia*

Carotid sinus stimulation is extremely valuable in terminating paroxysmal atrial tachycardia (Fig. 28-2). The patient with atrial tachycardia may respond to carotid sinus stimulation in one of four ways:

A. Termination

B. No response

Table 28-1. **Various Responses to Carotid Sinus Stimulation**

Arrhythmias	*Responses*
Sinus tachycardia	1. Transient slowing of sinus (atrial) rate 2. Varying degree A-V block (less common)
Atrial tachycardia	1. Termination 2. No response 3. Slowing of ventricular rate due to increased A-V block (less common) 4. Increased atrial rate (less common)
Atrial fibrillation or flutter	Slowing of ventricular rate due to increased A-V block
A-V junctional tachycardia paroxysmal	1. Termination 2. No response
Nonparoxysmal	No response
Ventricular tachyarrhythmias	1. No response 2. Termination (extremely rare, see text)
W-P-W syndrome	Vary (see text)
Parasystole	Vary (see text)
Digitalis intoxication	Not recommended
Hypersensitive patients	Not recommended
Patients with demand pacemakers	Assessment of a demand ventricular pacemaker function (see text)

C. Slowing of ventricular rate due to increased A-V block

D. Increased atrial rate

When slowing of the ventricular rate occurs in atrial tachycardia because of increased A-V block, the underlying cause is usually digitalis toxicity (see Chap. 23).

3. *Atrial fibrillation or flutter*

A. When carotid sinus pressure is applied to patients with atrial fibrillation or flutter, the ventricular rate invariably slows because of the increased atrioventricular block (Fig. 28-3).

B. Occasionally a long ventricular standstill may result when carotid sinus pressure is applied to an elderly patient with atrial fibrillation or flutter.

4. *A-V nodal (junctional) tachycardia*

It is often difficult, and at times impossible, to distinguish between paroxysmal atrial tachycardia and paroxysmal atrioventricular junctional tachycardia when only conventional electrocardiograms are available. The P wave may be superimposed on the S-T segment, T wave, or QRS complex of the preceding or succeeding beat. Therefore, the term *supraventricular tachycardia* is often used in this circumstance. Reciprocating tachycardia also belongs to this category. Nevertheless, it is believed that the response to carotid sinus stimulation is similar in paroxysmal atrioventricular junctional tachycardia and paroxysmal atrial tachycardia.

A. Paroxysmal atrioventricular junctional tachycardia may convert to sinus rhythm or may not respond to the procedure.

B. Nonparoxysmal atrioventricular junctional tachycardia, on the other hand, is usually unresponsive to carotid sinus stimulation.

C. Ventricular fibrillation may ensue if the underlying cause is digitalis toxicity. Thus, carotid sinus stimulation is not recommended in the presence of nonparoxysmal atrioventricular junctional tachycardia, which is a common sign of digitalis toxicity.

5. *Ventricular tachyarrhythmias*

Carotid sinus stimulation is often used to differentiate ventricular tachycardia from supraventricular tachycardia, especially when the QRS complex is wide and bizarre.

A. In contrast to supraventricular tachyarrhythmias, as a rule, ventricular tachycardia does not respond to carotid sinus stimulation.

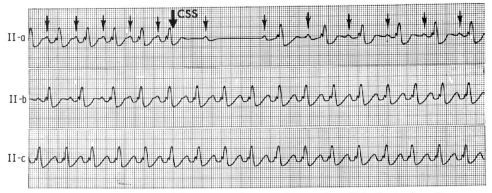

Fig. 28-1. Leads II-a, II-b, and II-c are continuous. Arrows (small) indicate sinus P waves. Note a transient slowing of the sinus rate associated with A-V block (first and second degree) by carotid sinus stimulation (marked CSS).

B. Therefore, any response to the procedure rules out ventricular tachycardia in most cases.

C. It should be noted, however, that in ventricular tachycardia due to a parasystolic mechanism, carotid sinus stimulation may slow or at times provoke a recurrence of the arrhythmia.

D. On extremely rare occasions, ventricular tachycardia may be terminated by carotid sinus stimulation (Fig. 28-4). This unusual phenomenon is considered to occur on the basis of a parasympathetic action in the ventricles.

6. *Wolff-Parkinson-White syndrome*

A. Carotid sinus pressure can abolish the ventricular preexcitation.

B. In occasional instances, the procedure may cause ventricular preexcitation to appear.

C. When carotid sinus pressure is applied in the presence of Wolff-Parkinson-White syndrome, it can produce an A-V junctional rhythm with a

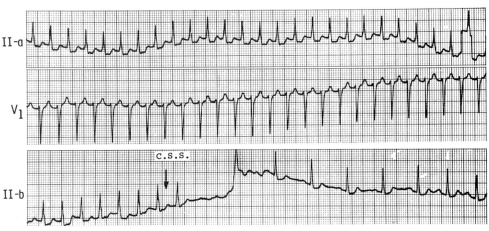

Fig. 28-2. Leads II-a and II-b are continuous. Supraventricular (probably atrial) tachycardia (rate: 188 beats/min.) is terminated by carotid sinus stimulation (marked C.S.S.) and sinus rhythm is restored.

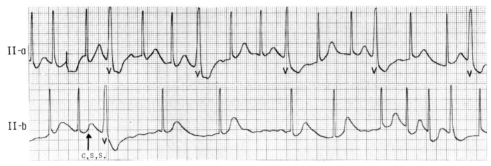

Fig. 28-3. Leads II-a and II-b are continuous. Note significant slowing of the ventricular rate due to increased A-V block by carotid sinus stimulation (marked C.S.S.). The basic rhythm is atrial fibrillation with frequent ventricular premature contractions (marked V).

normal QRS complex, since the vagal stimulation tends to prolong A-V conduction time or temporarily block the normal pathway and displace the pacemaker from the S-A node to the A-V junction.

D. Carotid sinus pressure is often effective in terminating supraventricular (atrial or reciprocating) tachycardia associated with Wolff-Parkinson-White syndrome.

7. *Parasystole*

A. The atrial or A-V junctional parasystolic rate may be decreased by the application of carotid sinus stimulation. This phenomenon never occurs in other forms of atrial or A-V junctional arrhythmias if the parasystolic mechanism is not present.

B. In ventricular parasystole, carotid sinus stimulation may slow or even provoke the recurrence of the arrhythmia.

C. The disappearance of ventricular parasystole due either to the appearance of exit block or the disappearance of the protection block due to the same mechanism has been reported.

D. The disappearance of atrial parasystole by carotid sinus stimulation has also been reported.

E. In certain cases, on the other hand, carotid sinus stimulation may not influence the arrhythmia.

8. *Digitalis intoxication (see Chap. 23)*

A. Some investigators observed that carotid sinus stimulation frequently

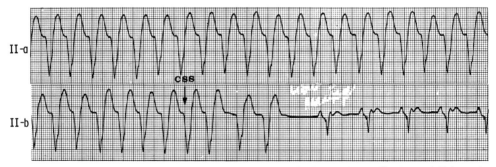

Fig. 28-4. Leads II-a and II-b are continuous. Ventricular tachycardia (rate: 148 beats/min.) is terminated by carotid sinus stimulation (indicated by arrow).

halts paroxysmal atrial tachycardia with A-V block not due to digitalis toxicity and is ineffective when digitalis is the etiologic factor.

B. On the other hand, a slowing of ventricular rate may result from increased A-V block by the procedure when underlying cause is digitalis toxicity.

C. However, the authors would like to emphasize the danger of applying carotid sinus stimulation to patients with suspected digitalis intoxication, because the patient may develop ventricular fibrillation or standstill during or after carotid sinus stimulation, which may result in a fatal outcome. Based on these observations, carotid sinus stimulation should be avoided as much as possible on patients who are taking even small amounts of digitalis.

9. *Hypersensitive patients*

A. Certain patients may be extremely sensitive to any pressure on the neck, including carotid sinus stimulation.

B. These hypersensitive patients may develop long ventricular standstill and/or fainting episodes simply by turning the head, a tight collar, or light carotid sinus stimulation (Fig. 28-5).

C. Obviously, carotid sinus stimulation should be avoided in these individuals, and some cases require permanent artificial pacemakers (see Chap. 26).

10. *Artificial pacemaker-induced rhythm*

A. Carotid sinus stimulation is a simple and useful procedure to assess the function of a demand ventricular pacemaker when there is only the patient's own sinus rhythm without any artificial pacemaker activity.

B. This is observed when the patient's natural rhythm is faster than the preset demand pacing rate.

C. When a slowing of the sinus rate

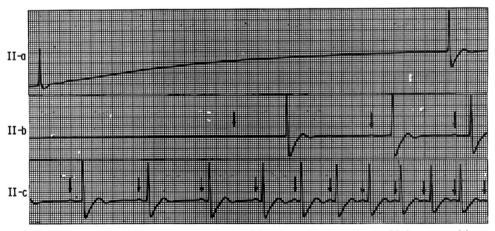

Fig. 28-5. These rhythm strips were obtained from an elderly patient with hypersensitive reaction to carotid sinus stimulation. Leads II-a, II-b and II-c are continuous. Arrows indicate sinus P waves. Note a long period of sinus arrest and ventricular standstill (complete cardiac arrest) associated with varying first degree A-V block by carotid sinus stimulation; this patient developed a brief period of unconsciousness. A permanent artificial pacemaker is implanted in this patient.

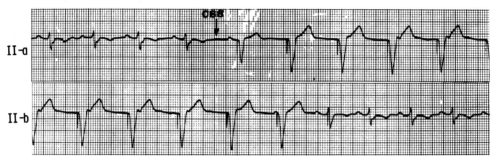

Fig. 28-6. Leads II-a and II-b are continuous. A demand ventricular pacemaker rhythm appears as a slowing of the sinus rate is produced by carotid sinus stimulation (marked CSS).

is produced by carotid sinus stimulation in this case, the rhythm of the demand pacemaker will appear to control the ventricular activity as the pacing rate exceeds the sinus rate (Fig. 28-6).

SUGGESTED READINGS

Alexander, S. and Ping, W. C.: Fatal ventricular fibrillation during carotid sinus stimulation. Am. J. Cardiol., *18*:289, 1966.

Chung, E. K.: Cardiac Arrhythmias: Management. Baltimore, Williams & Wilkins, 1973.

————: Digitalis Intoxication. Amsterdam, Excerpta Medica, 1969.

————: Parasystole. Prog. Cardiovasc. Dis., *11*:64, 1968.

Chung, E. K., Walsh, T. J. and Massie, E.: Wolff-Parkinson-White syndrome. Am. Heart J., *69*:116, 1965.

————:Ventricular parasystolic tachycardia. Br. Heart J., *27*:392, 1965.

Eliakim, M.: Atrial parasystole. Effect of carotid sinus stimulation, Valsalva maneuver and exercise. Am. J. Cardiol., *16*:457, 1965.

Golbey, M. et al.: Changes of ventricular impulse formation during carotid pressure in man. Circulation, *10*:735, 1954.

Hilal, H. and Massumi, R.: Fatal ventricular fibrillation after carotid sinus stimulation. N. Engl. J. Med., *275*:157, 1966.

Irons, G. V., Jr. and Orgain, E. S.: Digitalis-induced arrhythmias and their management. Prog. Cardiovasc. Dis., *8*:539, 1966.

Lorentzen, D.: Pacemaker-induced ventricular tachycardia. Reversion to normal sinus rhythm by carotid sinus massage. J.A.M.A., *235*:282, 1976.

Scherf, D., Bornemann, C., and Yildiz, M.: A-V nodal parasystole. Am. Heart J., *60*:179, 1960.

Scherf, D. et al.: Parasystole. Am. J. Cardiol., *12*:527, 1963.

29. CARDIAC CATHETERIZATION AND CORONARY ARTERIOGRAPHY

Martial A. Demany, M.D., *and Henry A. Zimmerman,* M.D.

DEFINITIONS AND GENERAL CONSIDERATIONS

1. Cardiac catheterization[8] is the study of the heart by means of catheters (from a Greek word meaning "tube"). The study of the great vessels leading to or from the heart constitutes an integral part of cardiac catheterization.

A. With right heart catheterization, the following structures can be studied: superior and inferior venae cavae, right auricle and ventricle, tricuspid and pulmonic valves, and the main pulmonary artery and its branches. By wedging the tip of the catheter into a pulmonary vein, it is possible to obtain a good approximation of the left atrial pressure.

B. With left heart catheterization, the following structures can be evaluated: left auricle and ventricle, mitral and aortic valves, and the ascending aorta. It is sometimes possible to advance the catheter in a retrograde fashion into one or more pulmonary veins.

C. Complete evaluation of the patient with heart disease as a rule requires right and left cardiac catheterization combined in a single procedure with coronary arteriography.

2. Coronary arteriography is the visualization of the coronary arteries by means of a contrast agent injected into their respective openings. Documentation is accomplished with cine films or with cut films.

A. With the advent of coronary artery bypass, the bypassed artery can be visualized (if the graft remains patent) when dye is injected into the ostium of the saphenous graft and/or the internal mammary artery.

3. The cardiac laboratory is composed of one or more rooms specifically equipped for performing cardiac catheterization and coronary arteriography.

4. The cardiovascular team consists of:

A. A cardiologist with special training in the techniques of cardiac catheterization and coronary arteriography.

B. A registered nurse with additional training in the field of cardiovascular nursing.

C. A technician capable of monitoring ECGs and vascular pressures.

NOTE: Each member of the team must be thoroughly familiar with the method of cardiopulmonary resuscitation.

EQUIPMENT

1. X-ray tube: a high-vacuum tube in which a stream of electrons is accelerated and focused upon a tungsten target to produce a beam of x-radiation.

2. Image intensifier: an electronic device to convert the spatial x-ray image into light in such a form that a highly intensified image can be viewed by a TV camera or photographed by a cine camera.

3. Fluoroscopic table: a cradle-like structure in which the patient may lie comfortably with the arm supported. Rotation of the table around the head-to-foot axis provides both lateral and longitudinal motion for scanning the field of study.

4. Monitoring equipment: an electronic device that allows the continuous display of ECG and intravascular/intracardiac pressures through a

cathode-ray tube and provides for graphic recording of the parameters monitored.

5. Oximeter densitometer: an optical device for a direct and rapid read-out of the O_2 saturation of blood samples taken from different sites in the cardiovascular system.

6. Cardiac output computer: an electronic apparatus that receives a signal from a densitometer through which blood and later a mixture of blood and dye are passed at a constant speed. The computer will analyze the variations in density and display directly the cardiac output in liters per minute on the basis of the dye dilution curve.

7. Pressure injector: a power-driven injection apparatus capable of delivering the contrast agent at a rate and in a quantity suitable for the examination desired.

8. Direct current defibrillator: an electrical device by means of which a charge, stored in a capacitor, may be delivered to the heart through paddle electrodes applied to the chest wall.

9. Catheters:

A. Composition: Catheters are made of such synthetic materials as radiopaque polyethylene, teflon, dacron, polyurethane, and polyvinyl chloride.

B. Sizes: 4F to 8F are most commonly used.

C. Length: 80, 100, or 125 centimeters.

D. Tips differ by presence or absence of a tapered portion; absence or presence (and numbers) of side holes; straight or hook-tail configuration. The type of catheter used depends upon the kind of information desired; for instance:

(1) The Cournand catheter, with only one end hole, is ideal for obtaining a good wedge pressure but should not be used for angiography because of excessive recoil.

(2) The Sones catheter, with its long tapered tip and four side holes, is ideal for coronary arteriography because

of the lesser risk of coronary artery occlusion.

(3) The hook-tail catheter is ideal for angiography because of quick delivery of a large amount of dye through multiple side holes with practically no recoil.

10. Guidewires: steel wires made of an inner core surrounded by a closely wound outer layer. The straight inner wire is either freely movable or fixed 3 cm. short of the distal tip of the sheath; the sheath thus has a soft, flexible spring tip. Some guides have a flexible tip of 6 to 8 inches in length ("floppy" wire). When a safety J guide is introduced to catheterize tortuous vessels, the inner wire may be withdrawn enough to allow a fairly long segment of the guide to become flexible and to form an intravascular loop which may be advanced in the vessel with much less risk of trauma.

11. The Seldinger needle: a needle consisting of:

A. An inner obturator

B. An inner needle with a short, sharp point with fixed stylet

C. An external cannula with a blunt, tapered tip

12. Sheath: the Mylar right sheath, introduced to allow the use of a closed-end catheter with the percutaneous technique. In procedures calling for several changes of catheter, it has been found to be of great value because of a much smaller incidence of complications.

13. Contrast agents: substances containing iodine, which makes them opaque to x-rays. Their injection in a cardiac chamber or a vessel will allow visualization of that structure. The final salification products appear to be responsible for the widely divergent degrees of myocardial toxicity of contrast agents; the methylglucamine salts are much less toxic than the sodium salts of the same iodine radicals.

14. Catheterization tray: a tray containing the following items: drapes,

syringes, needles, knife, towel clamps, straight and curved hemostats, umbilical tape, straight and curved pick-ups, needle holder, sutures, scissors, three-way stopcock, manifold, and xylocaine. Cardiac catheterization requires the same sterile technique as any surgical or invasive procedure. Everything on the tray must have been thoroughly sterilized beforehand and must be kept sterile during the procedure.

INDICATIONS

1. Cardiac catheterization is first a diagnostic procedure; its immediate goal is to secure a maximum amount of data that will allow as accurate an assessment as possible of congenital and/or acquired heart disease.

2. Cardiac catheterization is very valuable in the following situations:

A. Evaluation of the surgical treatment of congenital and/or acquired heart disease.

B. Management of the patient with acute myocardial infarction

C. Management of the patient immediately after cardiac surgery

D. Evaluation of the action of pharmacological agents on the cardiovascular system

E. Evaluation of the effects of pacing on cardiac performance

F. Evaluation of hemodynamic disturbances during cardiac arrhythmias

G. Study of the cardiovascular system (as a research tool)

TECHNIQUES OF CARDIAC CATHETERIZATION

1. Surgical exposure of vein/artery[3,20]

A. The basilic (or brachial) vein and the brachial artery are by far the most commonly used; when they are too small, however, the femoral vein and artery are exposed by cutdown, but their depth makes this a more difficult procedure, particularly when expert surgical help is not available.

B. The elbow and surrounding area are surgically scrubbed and draped with sterile towels. The skin is infiltrated with a 2 per cent solution of lidocaine and a transverse incision of approximately 20 cm. is made just above the flexor crease over the point of maximum pulsation of the artery.

C. The vessels are isolated by gentle, blunt dissection. Two lengths of umbilical tape are passed under each vessel to control bleeding around the catheter at its point of introduction.

D. The venous catheter is introduced through a small phlebotomy; after it reaches the axilla, further advancement is done under fluoroscopy. Through the superior vena cava the catheter enters the right auricle; after forming a J loop in this chamber, the tip of the catheter is rotated toward the tricuspid valve, introduced into the right ventricle and further advanced into the pulmonary artery. Finally, the catheter is wedged in a pulmonary vein; this position is confirmed by the display of an atrial-type pressure curve (the so-called reflexion of the left atrial pressure).

E. From each cavity and large vessel, blood samples can be withdrawn; through the catheters, pressures are recorded and studies with gas inhalation or drugs performed.

F. To prevent clotting, 3,000 units of heparin are injected into the distal segment of the artery, and the arterial catheter is then introduced through a small arteriotomy.

G. When the tip of the catheter reaches the axilla, further advancement is under fluoroscopic surveillance. The ascending aorta is reached through the subclavian and innominate arteries (when entry is made by way of the right arm) and the aortic arch. By making a J loop against the wall of the aorta, the tip of the catheter readily crosses the aortic valve to fall into the left ventricle (except in the presence of calcific aortic stenosis). A few premature ventricular beats occur commonly upon entrance of the catheter into a ventricle; they disappear if the tip of the catheter is readjusted away from the ventricular wall. The appearance of ventricular tachycardia or fibrillation calls for immediate withdrawal from the ventricle and rapid DC countershock.

H. Occasionally, when the J loop formed by the tip of the catheter finds the mitral valve open, it is possible for the catheter to enter the left atrium. Use of a special catheter, designed by Shirey, facilitates this last maneuver.

I. From each chamber and from the ascending aorta, blood samples can be withdrawn; through the catheter pressures can be recorded.

J. With one catheter in the venous circulation and another in the arterial circuit, it is possible to perform cardiac output determination and dye dilution studies.

K. Cineangiography performed after the hemodynamic studies have been completed avoids the changes produced by the contrast agent on ventricular performance.

L. Different parts of the study may call for the use of different catheters; replacement catheters are advanced as described above.

M. When the study has been completed, the catheters are withdrawn and care is taken to ascertain the patency of the vessels, particularly of the artery. The arteriotomy and phlebotomy are closed with 6-0 Ethiflex and the skin with 4-0 Ethilon.

N. Surgical exposure of the femoral vessels is done in a manner similar to that of the brachial vessels and the catheters are introduced in the same way. The venous catheter reaches the right auricle through the iliac vein and

inferior vena cava while the arterial catheter travels the length of the abdominal and thoracic aorta and follows the aortic arch to reach the ascending aorta. The remainder of the manipulation is as described above and the vessels are closed in the same way.

2. Percutaneous puncture of vein or artery for cardiac catheterization

The femoral vessels are by far the most commonly used; a few, however, have advocated the puncture of the brachial or axillary artery.

A. Seldinger technique[17]

(1) The basic principle is that of the replacement of the needle by a catheter advanced over a guidewire.

(2) The inguinal area is surgically scrubbed and draped with sterile towels. The skin and tissues overlying the vessels are infiltrated with 2 per cent solution of lidocaine.

(3) With the tip of a sharp blade a 2- to 3-mm. incision is made through the anesthetized skin and the needle is then advanced into the vessel.

(4) The obturator is removed; adequate intravenous position is confirmed by the appearance of dark blood.

(5) The internal needle is removed and the flexible tip of the guidewire is introduced through the external cannula, then advanced 10 to 15 cm. beyond it.

(6) The outer cannula is withdrawn over the whole length of the guidewire while manual pressure is applied over the puncture site.

(7) Once the guidewire is felt to advance freely, the catheter is slipped over the guidewire and when it reaches the skin, guide and catheter are pushed together through the vascular wall.

(8) Under fluoroscopy, guide and catheter are advanced until they reach the right auricle; the guidewire is withdrawn and the catheter connected to the pressure gauge. Right heart catheteriza-

tion is then performed as described earlier.

(9) Percutaneous puncture of the femoral artery is performed in a manner similar to that described for the femoral vein; adequate intra-arterial position is confirmed by the appearance of a brisk jet of bright red blood.

(10) Under fluoroscopy, guide and catheter are advanced along the iliac artery into the abdominal and thoracic descending aorta; letting the guidewire protrude beyond the tip of the catheter by 1 or 2 in. will make passage along the aortic arch much easier.

(11) Crossing the aortic valve is achieved with about 2 in. of the guide protruding beyond the tip of the catheter, advancing guide and catheter together will result in the tip of the guide forming a loop or a bend against the wall of the sinus of Valsalva. With slight to and fro motion this loop will pass between the aortic cusps and fall into the left ventricle; the guide is withdrawn and the catheter connected to the pressure gauge. Left cardiac catheterization is then performed as described earlier.

(12) If the catheter has to be replaced, the guidewire must be reinserted and advanced 10 to 15 cm. beyond the tip of the catheter. The catheter is then pulled out and another is slipped over the guide and advanced as previously described.

(13) Upon completion of the procedure, the catheter is pulled out and hemostasis is obtained by manual pressure over the puncture sites. When no further bleeding is evident, a sandbag is placed over the groin for about 5 hours to prevent the formation of a hematoma.

B. Percutaneous "sheath" catheterization

(1) Percutaneous catheterization of the femoral vessels can be done in children with a great deal of success; because of the smaller size of the vessels, however, the rate of failures and the in-

cidence of complications increase markedly in children weighing less than 10 kilograms.

(2) Netches and collaborators[11] have recommended a technique that is a compilation of the Seldinger method and of its modification by Desilets and Hoffman.[6]

(3) The femoral vein or artery is punctured as described previously and the guidewire advanced into the inferior vena cava or abdominal aorta.

(4) The needle is removed and a small straight hemostat is inserted into the tract along the guidewire. Opening the jaws of the hemostat slowly will widen the needle tract.

(5) The sheath and the Teflon dilator unit are advanced over the wire; the Teflon dilator is passed through the skin and with a rotary motion is advanced into the vessel; the sheath is advanced over the dilator and into the vessel.

(6) The Teflon (venous) sheath can be advanced and rotated in a manner similar to that used for the dilator.

(7) The thin-walled polypropylene (arterial) sheath should be grasped tightly between the thumb and index finger and with only a slight twisting motion advanced over the guidewire together with the dilator.

(8) The dilator and guidewire are removed; the sheath is left in the vessel lumen where it remains for the duration of the procedure.

(9) Any type of catheter can now be inserted through the sheath into the vessel.

(10) Excessive bleeding or air aspiration must be avoided; therefore the orifice of the sheath should always be occluded during catheter changes.

3. Bedside catheterization

Recognition in the past few years of the importance of hemodynamic alterations in patients with acute myocardial infarction has led to the use of cardiovascular catheterization in the cardiac or coronary care unit (i.e., outside the cardiac laboratory). In the absence of bedside fluoroscopy, new methods have been devised to catheterize the right side of the heart, the pulmonary artery, and the left ventricle.

A. Bedside catheterization of right cardiac chambers and pulmonary artery

(1) Swan, Ganz, et al.[19] have designed a catheter made of extruded polyvinyl chloride and so constructed that a small lumen exists in the wall and parallels the major lumen. A latex balloon is fastened approximately 1 mm. from the catheter tip and connected to the minor lumen via a side hole in the shaft.

(2) The catheter is inserted into the antecubital vein by cutdown, and, under pressure monitoring, advanced into the right atrium. (When the catheter is within the thorax, a cough produces deflections of 50 mm. Hg or more in the pressure tracing).

(3) The balloon is inflated with 0.8 ml. of air and, under continuous pressure and electrocardiographic monitoring, is advanced through the right ventricle into the pulmonary artery until "wedge" pressure is recorded.

(4) If more than 15 cm. of catheter are advanced into the right ventricle without producing a pulmonary artery pressure curve, the catheter is probably doubling up in the ventricle; it should be withdrawn into the atrium and passage should be attempted again.

(5) On withdrawal, the balloon should be partially deflated to prevent damage to the valves and supporting structures.

(6) Inflation of the balloon is associated with a feeling of resistance, so that on release of pressure the barrel slips back. If no resistance is encountered, the integrity of the balloon should be suspected and inflation discontinued at once.

(7) Before each inflation of the balloon to obtain wedge pressure, the syringe should be disconnected from the adaptor and reconnected to assume neutral position of the balloon before inflation.

B. Bedside catheterization of the left ventricle[2]

(1) To catheterize the left ventricle with only ECG monitoring, Cohn et al. use a catheter made of standard wall Kifa radiopaque polyethylene (available from United States Catheters and Instruments, Boston, Mass.).

(2) The catheter is immersed in water at 194° F and a terminal curve of 2 cm. in diameter is formed.

(3) The catheter is introduced into the femoral artery by percutaneous technique as described above; it is then advanced 20 cm. beyond the point of entry; the guidewire is withdrawn until it is estimated that its tip lies just beyond the terminal curve of the catheter. Entry into the left ventricle is usually heralded by a few ectopic ventricular beats that disappear after the catheter has been withdrawn for 1 or 2 centimeters.

(4) Tortuosity of the iliac vessels is the greatest obstacle to success with this method.

4. Use of a "flow directed" catheter[16] for cardiac catheterization and selective angiography in infants

A. Near the end of one lumen of the 5F 50-cm. catheter are six side holes. A second (inflation) lumen communicates via a side hole in its shaft with a latex balloon located 1 mm. proximal to catheter tip.

B. Carbon dioxide is used for balloon inflation to prevent air embolism.

C. The catheter is inserted into the femoral vein through a 6F sheath (percutaneous technique) or through a phlebotomy (surgical exposure).

D. Right cardiac catheterization is carried on as described previously.

E. In the great majority of infants, anatomic patency of the foramen ovale gives easy access to the left atrium. When access to the left atrium has been achieved, the balloon is inflated and the catheter quickly enters the left ventricle.

F. In positioning for left ventriculography, the balloon is inflated maximally (1 mm.) to insure that the tip of the catheter is retracted within the circumference of the balloon. The balloon is then wedged into the left ventricular apex in contact with the endocardium, without disturbing the cardiac rhythm. The inflated balloon keeps the side holes away from the endocardium.

G. Antegrade catheterization of the aorta (pulmonary artery in transposition of the great vessels) is achieved by the formation of a catheter loop in the left atrium. The loop and balloon are backed into the left ventricle. Once the loop has cleared the mitral valve, inflation of the balloon propels the catheter into the left ventricular outflow tract and the aorta.

5. Transseptal cardiac catheterization

A. J. Ross, Jr.[14] has demonstrated that the interatrial septum can be successfully punctured by means of a retractable needle passed through a cardiac catheter introduced into the right atrium via the saphenous vein, with its tip positioned against the fossa ovalis.

B. The original transseptal technique was later modified by Brockenbrough[1] (percutaneous introduction of the catheter into the femoral vein; modifications of the needle and catheter to allow left ventricular catheterization and angiography). Ross himself[13] introduced further modifications in equipment and technique to increase safety.

C. The catheter is introduced by percutaneous puncture into the right femoral vein and advanced into the right atrium.

D. The site for the puncture is decided upon after location of: (a) the tricuspid valve (by right heart catheterization); and (b) the aortic valve and ascending aorta (by placement of an arterial catheter, its tip lying at the bottom of the posterior sinus of Valsalva).

E. The needle is inserted in the catheter to the point where its tip lies just within the distal end.

F. The tip of the catheter is positioned at the junction of the lower and middle third of the atrial septum and directed posteriorly to the left at an angle of 45° from the horizontal plane. During the septal puncture by the needle, there is a sudden decrease in resistance, indicating that penetration has occurred; if no resistance is encountered, and the catheter can be easily advanced without the needle, a patent foramen ovale is present.

G. The needle should be connected to a pressure transducer to provide for constant monitoring prior to, during, and after puncture of the atrial septum. If the needle has entered the left atrium, a somewhat higher atrial pressure curve will be displayed, depending upon the severity of the mitral valve disease or of the decompensation of the left ventricle.

H. After septal puncture, the catheter tip is advanced into the left atrium and the needle withdrawn. A blood sample is drawn for O_2 saturation determinations; the value should be in the arterial range. The atrial pressure is recorded and a left atriogram is taken. After indicator dye has been injected into the left ventricle, the catheter may also be used for detecting and quantifying mitral regurgitation.

I. Further manipulation of the transseptal catheter may result in its passage across the mitral valve into the left ventricle, but most of the time it is necessary to use a catheter tip occluder with a specially made bend that will curve the tip of the catheter in the direction of the mitral valve. After withdrawal of the catheter tip occluder, the left ventricular pressure is recorded and left ventriculography is carried out. After indicator dye has been injected into the aortic root, the catheter may also be used for detecting and quantifying aortic regurgitation.

J. The transseptal technique has been particularly useful in the study of mitral and aortic stenosis, since it precludes the necessity of crossing the stenotic valve in a retrograde manner, usually a difficult maneuver. The pressure gradient in mitral stenosis is obtained by placement of a transseptal catheter proximal to the mitral valve and an arterial catheter in the left ventricle across the aortic valve, and by a simultaneous recording of both pressures. The gradient across the stenotic aortic valve is obtained by the advancement of the transseptal catheter into the left ventricle while the arterial catheter remains in the ascending aorta, and by a simultaneous recording of both pressures.

6. Percutaneous left ventricular puncture[12]

A. The advent of the transseptal method for catheterization of the left ventricle has considerably reduced the need for left ventricular puncture. It is still used in conjunction with the transseptal technique (catheter tip in the left atrium) and retrograde aortic catheterization to record the left ventricular systolic and end-diastolic pressures in patients with prosthetic mitral and aortic disc valves. It is also used for left ventricular pressure recording and angiography when other methods have failed.

B. With the patient in supine position, the anterior chest wall is surgically scrubbed and draped. The point of maximum apical impulse and the second right costochondral junction are located and marked on the skin. The skin and subcutaneous tissues are infiltrated with lidocaine until the pericardium is encountered.

C. The needle is inserted through a small incision and advanced along an axis going from the apex to the second costochondral junction, backward at 30°

from the anterior surface of the chest in order that it may enter the left ventricular cavity along the longest axis.

D. If the puncture is done with the needle connected to a syringe, rapid filling of the syringe with bright red blood will confirm entry into the left ventricle; if the needle is connected to a pressure transducer, a left ventricular pressure curve will be displayed.

E. After pressure recordings have been taken, contrast agents may be injected for ventriculography or indicator dye for detection of shunts and/or valvular regurgitation.

F. It is also possible to perform left ventricular puncture by a technique identical to that of Seldinger for percutaneous puncture of the femoral artery, with subsequent replacement of the needle by a catheter that has been advanced over a guidewire.

COMPLICATIONS OF CARDIAC CATHETERIZATION

1. *Trauma, dissection and/or perforation of the arterial wall by the guidewire and/or catheter*

   A. *Causes*
     (1) Faulty arterial puncture
     (2) Faulty catheter manipulation
     (3) Lifting of an arteriosclerotic plaque
     (4) Faulty injection of dye
   B. *Prevention*
     (1) Do not introduce guidewire until puncture has yielded brisk, jet-like bleeding.
     (2) Do not thread the catheter over the guidewire until the latter moves freely and painlessly.
     (3) Keep the tip of the guidewire at least 1 in. ahead of the tip of the catheter.
     (4) Use a J guide for tortuous vessels.
     (5) Stop pushing when resistance is met; withdraw the catheter for a short

distance and make a small injection of dye by hand to visualize the tortuous segment.

C. *Treatment*

Call for vascular surgeon if vascular dissection or perforation has taken place.

2. *Knotting of the catheter*

A. *Cause:* Catheter too soft

B. *Prevention:* Check catheter for excessive softness prior to insertion.

C. *Treatment*

(1) Pull the knotted catheter as far back peripherally as possible.

(2) Call for vascular surgeon for removal of knotted catheter.

3. *Clotting of the catheter*

A. *Detection*

(1) Progressive damping of arterial or ventricular pressure curve.

(2) Impossibility of withdrawing blood through catheter.

B. *Prevention*

(1) Flush catheter with a heparinized solution of glucose or saline every 3 to 5 minutes throughout the procedure.

(2) After a few minutes of manipulation of a catheter with guidewire, remove the latter. Aspirate the catheter of its content, and fill it with a heparinized solution of glucose or saline prior to reinsertion of the guidewire.

C. *Treatment* Withdraw clotted catheter and replace with a new one.

4. *Arterial/venous spasm*

Spasm may occur rather frequently, particularly in children and in adults with small vessels; it may preclude any further manipulation and lead to thrombus formation in situ.

A. *Causes*

(1) Inadequate sedation

(2) Inadequate local/perivascular anesthesia

(3) Small size of vessels

(4) Catheter too large for the size of the vessel

(5) Forceful and traumatic advancement of the guidewire and/or catheter despite resistance and/or pain

B. *Prevention*

(1) Give adequate sedation to allay patient's anxiety.

(2) Provide generous local anesthesia.

(3) Try to match the size of the catheter with that of the vessel.

(4) Do not manipulate guidewire and/or catheter forcefully against resistance.

C. *Treatment*

(1) Increase sedation if it is inadequate.

(2) Increase local infiltration with lidocaine if necessary.

(3) Step down to a smaller size catheter if necessary.

(4) If spasm persists or develops after the procedure is over, administer papaverine 30 to 50 mg. I.V. every 4 hours four times, and alternate with phentolamine, 15 mg. in 100 ml. of a 5 per cent solution of dextrose in water to run in one hour, also every four hours.

(5) If the above measures are unsuccessful, do a brachial or lumbar plexus block.

5. *Arterial thrombosis*

A. Predisposing factors

(1) Previous history of thrombosis

(2) Advanced age

(3) Diffuse atheromatous disease

(4) Conditions with decreased cardiac output

(5) Diabetes mellitus

(6) Polycythemia

(7) Prolonged arterial spasm

(8) Long and difficult catheter manipulation

(9) Small size of vessel catheterized

(10) Catheter too large for vessel catheterized

(11) Trauma to the posterior wall of the artery at the level of the arteriotomy

(12) Inadequate repair of the arteriotomy

(13) Excessive pressure over the puncture site to stop bleeding

(14) Surface clotting over the catheter with stripping of the clot upon withdrawal of the catheter

B. *Prevention*

(1) See all four points mentioned above to prevent arterial spasm.

(2) See all five points mentioned previously to prevent trauma to the arterial wall.

(3) Avoid percutaneous puncture of arteries with diminished pulsation.

(4) Avoid prolonged manual pressure over the puncture site.

(5) Inject 3,000 units of heparin immediately distal to the site of the arteriotomy.

(6) Consider systemic heparinization.

(7) Check patency of proximal and distal arterial segments prior to repair of the arteriotomy.

(8) Repair the arteriotomy with the most meticulous care.[5]

C. *Treatment*

Thrombectomy with Fogarty catheter within 24 hours after catheterization.[7]

(1) After reopening the arteriotomy, advance a 4F Fogarty embolectomy catheter as far as the subclavian artery.

(2) Inflate the balloon at the tip with a small amount of heparinized glucose solution (0.5–0.75 ml. will usually suffice).

(3) Withdraw the catheter slowly with the balloon inflated; in this way the clot may be brought out through the arteriotomy.

(4) Follow the same procedure in the distal arterial segment, advancing the catheter approximately to the level of the wrist.

(5) To help prevent further thrombosis, inject heparin directly in each arterial segment through a 4F Fogarty irrigation catheter (3,000 units in each site).

(6) Repair the arteriotomy as usual.

(7) Keep the patient on heparin I.V. for another 24 hours (5,000 units every 6 hours).

6. *Arterial emboli*

A. *Causes*

(1) Dislodgement of fragments of atherosclerotic plaques or of calcium by the catheter or guidewire.

(2) Air embolus resulting from injection of air bubbles mixed with dye.

B. *Prevention*

(1) Manipulate the catheter and guidewire gently.

(2) Use transseptal catheterization for patients with calcific aortic stenosis instead of attempting to cross the valve.

(3) Check the dye-containing syringe for presence of air prior to injection; if present, air should be expelled immediately.

C. *Treatment*

(1) Use vasodilators and anticoagulants or regional block for an extremity exhibiting a decrease in temperature and/or change in color.

(2) Employ embolectomy with a Fogarty catheter and anticoagulants for larger emboli, which produce the same clinical picture as arterial thrombosis.

7. *Hematoma at site of arterial puncture or arteriotomy*

A. *Causes*

(1) Inadequate occluding pressure over the puncture site

(2) Pressure applied for too short a period of time (adequate time is 15 minutes)

(3) Inadequate suture of the arteriotomy

(4) Small subcutaneous arterioles (cut or torn during the procedure) left unsutured

(5) Puncture needles and catheters of large size

(6) Excessive heparinization

(7) Blood dyscrasias

(8) Anticoagulant therapy

B. *Prevention*

(1) Apply adequate manual pressure over the puncture site until bleeding stops.

(2) Repair the arteriotomy with the most meticulous care.

(3) Insure excellent hemostasis before closing the incision.

(4) Avoid excessive heparinization.

(5) Avoid, if at all possible, catheterization of patients with blood dyscrasias.

(6) For patients on oral anticoagulants, omit the dose on the day of the catheterization if the prothrombin time is below 30 per cent of normal activity and resume in the evening after the procedure; do not catheterize if prothrombin time is below 25 per cent of normal activity.

C. *Treatment*

(1) Evacuate large hematomas; inspect the repair of the arteriotomy and suture all bleeding points (inspect the whole cutdown area for eventual bleeders).

(2) If, after 30 min. of adequate manual pressure, bleeding at the puncture site continues, surgically explore the area; a tear in the vessel is likely to be found and its surgical repair is mandatory.

8. *Arteriovenous fistula*

A. Fistula occurs very rarely.

B. A continuous murmur or thrill may be detected.

C. Surgical repair is necessary.

9. *False aneurysm*

A. Aneurysm may occur after multiple punctures weaken the arterial wall.

B. Treatment is surgical.

10. *Intramural injection of dye*

A. *Cause*: Unrecognized misplacement of the catheter tip

B. *Prevention*

(1) Check the contour of the pressure curve for "damping" prior to injection of dye.

(2) Double-check the free position of the catheter tip by first making a small injection of dye by hand; if necessary, reposition the catheter tip away from the wall.

(3) Use a hook-tail catheter whenever possible to avoid recoil during injections under high pressure.

C. *Treatment*

(1) Perforation of the left ventricular wall with extravasation of dye in the precordial sac may result in rapid development of tamponade. Emergency pericardiotomy under general anesthesia may be needed.

(2) Dissection of the aortic root should be watched extremely closely, particularly if it involves the sinuses of Valsalva, from which the coronary arteries originate. A cardiac surgical team should be alerted for eventual repair under cardiopulmonary bypass.

11. *Arrhythmias*

A. *Cause*: ventricular arrhythmias occur most commonly in the following.

(1) Overdigitalization and/or hypokalemia

(2) Aortic calcific valvular stenosis

(3) Severe congestive cardiac failure

B. *Prevention*

(1) Check amount of digitalis taken; omit digitalis dose on morning of the procedure.

(2) Check serum potassium level; if level is too low, give I.V. potassium chloride and/or triamterene orally depending upon time available before the procedure.

(3) Use the transseptal technique rather than attempting to cross a severely stenotic and calcified aortic valve.

(4) Treat congestive failure before the procedure if at all possible.

C. *Treatment*

(1) Ventricular tachycardia calls for immediate I.V. administration of one or more antiarrhythmic agents. If patient loses consciousness, give immediate DC countershock.

(2) Ventricular fibrillation is treated with immediate DC countershock, followed by I.V. administration of antiarrhythmic agents if ventricular irritability persists.

(3) Nasal O_2 and I.V. sodium bicarbonate should be given to increase arterial O_2 saturation and to combat metabolic acidosis.

12. *Complete atrioventricular block*

A. *Cause*: In patients with preexistent bundle branch block, catheterization of the ventricle opposite that which is already the site of the bundle branch block may result in complete atrioventricular block and in sudden asystole if an idioventricular rhythm fails to take over.

B. *Prevention*: Manipulate catheter with the greatest care in the ventricle opposite that which is already the site of a bundle branch block.

C. *Treatment*

(1) Prophylactic insertion of a catheter pacer in the right auricle, ready for immediate advancement into the right ventricle and for pacing in case asystole develops

(2) Cardiopulmonary resuscitation while a temporary pacer is inserted as fast as possible

(3) I.V. administration of steroids to reduce the extent and duration of the irritation caused by the catheter

(4) I.V. drip of isoproterenol

13. *Allergic reaction to dye*

A. *Cause*: Sensitivity to iodine.

B. *Prevention*

(1) Perform skin sensitivity test prior to injection.

(2) If test is positive, do not inject dye in the venous side of the circulation.

(3) Inject dye in the left ventricle, aorta, and/or coronary arteries after giving 25 mg. diphenhydramine (Benadryl) I.M. and an I.V. bolus of methylprednisone (125 mg.).

C. *Treatment*

(1) Diphenhydramine (Benadryl) I.M. for rash or hives (50 mg. stat., then every 4 to 6 hours for 1 or 2 days)

(2) I.V. bolus of methylprednisone for swelling of face and eyelids (125 mg. stat., then every 4 to 6 hours until swelling subsides)

(3) Possible tracheal intubation in case of angioneurotic edema

COMPLICATIONS PERTAINING TO THE TRANSSEPTAL TECHNIQUE

1. *Injury to the atrial septum*

A. *Causes*

(1) A permanent atrial septal defect resulting from the needle puncture and passage of the catheter (rare)

(2) Forceful injection through the side holes of the catheter when its tip has not been advanced sufficiently into the left auricle

B. *Prevention*: Check position of catheter with small hand injection of dye prior to injection with pressure apparatus.

2. *Cardiac tamponade*

A. *Causes*

(1) Puncture of the aortic root by the catheter or by a large size transseptal needle

(2) Perforation of the left atrial appendage

(3) Puncture of the posterior left atrial wall

B. *Prevention*

(1) Advance a catheter in the posterior aortic sinus of Valsalva and visualize the configuration of the ascending aorta with small hand injections of dye.

(2) Use a small-size transseptal needle.

(3) Check the position of the needle tip by watching the position of its curve indicator before puncturing the atrial septum.

(4) Monitor pressure constantly to pick up immediately the high aortic pressure as soon as the tip of the needle has entered the aortic root.

NOTE: An experienced thoracic surgeon should be immediately available when a transseptal puncture is performed.

C. *Treatment*

(1) If the catheter or a large-size needle has entered the aortic root, it should be left in place and taped over the groin to avoid dislodgement.

(2) If tamponade develops, pericardiocentesis will buy some time while surgical help is obtained.

(3) Perform pericardiostomy and drainage under general anesthesia.

(4) Surgically repair the puncture hole.

3. *Hemopericardium*

Accumulation of serosanguineous fluid in the pericardial sac in an amount too small to cause cardiac tamponade may result from puncture of the aortic root or atrial wall with a small-size needle.

A. *Prevention*: Same as for tamponade.

B. *Treatment*

(1) Short term observation in intensive care unit for frequent recording of vital signs.

(2) Chest x-ray for cardiac size immediately after the procedure and again at 12- and 24-hour intervals.

4. *Systemic embolization*

A. *Causes*

(1) Dislodgement of a thrombus loosely adherent to the left atrial wall (risk much greater in patients with atrial fibrillation)

(2) Dislodgement of fragments of an atrial myxoma

B. *Treatment*: As described earlier in complications of cardiac catheterization.

5. *Breakage of the tip of the transseptal needle*

A. Such breakage has occurred very rarely.

B. No untoward effects were reported.

6. *Atrial arrhythmias* occur rather infrequently; their treatment is routine.

COMPLICATIONS OF LEFT VENTRICULAR PUNCTURE

1. *Pneumothorax*

A. Pneumothorax occurs commonly in varying degrees.

B. If it is large, treat with aspiration or closed drainage.

2. *Pleural effusion*

A. Pleural effusion is usually small.

B. If it is large, aspirate.

3. *Postpericardiotomy syndrome*

A. Occurs rarely.

B. Treat with steroids.

4. *Cardiac tamponade and/or hemopericardium*

A. Both may occur if the needle damages a branch of a coronary artery.

B. For treatment, see Complications of Transseptal Catheterization, page 402.

5. *Faulty dye injection*

A. *Cause*: Unrecognized misplacement of tip of needle or catheter.

B. *Prevention and Treatment*: See Complications of Cardiac Catheterization, page 398.

HEMODYNAMIC STUDIES

GOALS

1. To establish or confirm the presence of shunts between the left and the right side of the heart, between the great vessels, or between the coronary arteries and the cardiac chambers

2. To measure the magnitude of the shunts and their effect upon the pulmonary vascular resistance

3. To confirm the presence of supravalvular, valvular and/or subvalvular stenosis, and/or valvular incompetence, and to measure its severity

4. To arrive at an accurate preoperative diagnosis of complex congenital cardiac malformations

5. To assess the performance of the left ventricle in conditions that impose a greater burden upon this chamber (i.e., coronary artery disease, aortic and/or mitral disease, myocardiopathies).

Detection and Measurement of Shunts

1. *Oxymetry* is the determination of oxygen content and/or saturation of blood samples withdrawn in rapid succession from areas proximal and distal to the site of the shunt by Van Slyke manometric technique (very cumbersome) or by cuvette oxymeter.

A. A left to right shunt of sufficient size results in a step-up in the oxygen saturation/content of the venous blood at the level of the shunt and distal to it.

B. A right to left shunt results in a step-down in the oxygen saturation/content of the arterial blood at the level of the shunt and distal to it.

C. A bidirectional shunt will be a combination of A and B.

D. The application of the Fick principle gives the magnitude of the shunt, which is equal to the difference between systemic and pulmonary blood flow.

artery and blood withdrawn from the aorta is passed through a cuvette densitometer; the optical density of the dye is transcribed as a curve by means of a connection to DC input of a multichannel oscillograph.

B. In case of a left to right shunt between the cardiac chambers or the great vessels, a hump due to early recirculation of dye appears on the downslope of the curve.

C. In the presence of a right to left shunt, a hump appears on the upstroke of the curve if the dye is injected proximal to or at the level of the shunt. When the dye is injected distal to a right to left shunt, this early hump will not appear; thus serial dye curves will aid in the localization of the shunt.

D. In patent ductus arteriosus with reversal of flow that is a right to left shunt, the tip of the sampling catheter must be located in the descending aorta.

NOTE: (1) The dye dilution curve is more sensitive than oxymetry for the detection of small shunts.

(2) Because the dye dilution curve entails the withdrawal of a considerable amount of blood, when several curves are mandatory it is not indicated in infants and children.

3. *Ascorbate curves*

$$\text{Cardiac Output (ml. per min.)} = \frac{O_2 \text{ consumption (cc/min.)} \times 100}{\text{arterial} - \text{venous } O_2 \text{ content (cc./l. blood)}}$$

$$\text{Systemic Blood Flow} = \frac{O_2 \text{ consumption}}{\text{arterial} - \text{venous } O_2 \text{ content (at level immediately proximal to shunt)}}$$

$$\text{Pulmonary Blood Flow} = \frac{O_2 \text{ consumption}}{\text{arterial} - \text{pulmonary artery } O_2 \text{ content}}$$

NOTE: (1) Small shunts are not easily detected by oxymetry.

(2) Fiber-optic catheters are very valuable for use in infants and small children from whom only a limited amount of blood can safely be withdrawn.

2. *Dye dilution curves*

A. Indocyanine green (Cardiogreen) dye is injected in the pulmonary

A. Their shape is almost identical to those obtained with indocyanine green (Cardiogreen) dye.

B. A few ml. of ascorbate are injected in the same way as indocyanine green (Cardiogreen) dye; detection is done by a catheter with a platinum tip electrode.

C. Left to right and right to left

shunts can be detected by the ascorbate method.

NOTE: (1) The ascorbate method is very safe.

(2) It can be used in infants and small children, as there is no withdrawal of blood.

4. *Krypton-85*

A. Krypton-85 is absorbed into the circulation by inhalation for the detection of left to right shunts by a sampling catheter advanced at various levels in the right side of the heart.

B. Two blood samples must be counted, a venous and an arterial one; the ratio of the number of counts of the former to that of the latter is used in determining the presence or absence of a shunt.

NOTE: (1) Radiation hazards limit the number of krypton curves.

(2) Krypton technique is time-consuming and cumbersome.

5. *Hydrogen*

side is indicative of the presence of a right to left shunt, barring interference with the electrode due to a fall in pH of the blood.

NOTE: (1) The hazards of storing and handling hydrogen gas, an explosive indicator, represent a serious drawback to its use.

(2) The quantitative analysis of the hydrogen curves is difficult.

6. *Passage of the catheter through the abnormal communication* between a right and a left cardiac chamber or between the pulmonary artery and the aorta, coupled with the finding of a high O_2 saturation, confirms the passage from the venous into the arterial circulation. This passage occurs in the presence of a shunt, except when a patent foramen ovale exists, as is the case in a large proportion of infants.

7. *Pulmonary vascular resistance*

A. Pulmonary vascular resistance is calculated by the following formula:

$$P.V.R. = \frac{\text{pulmonary artery mean pressure (mm. Hg)} - \text{left atrial mean pressure (mm. Hg)} \times 1.332 \text{ dynes}}{\text{pulmonary blood flow (cm.}^3/\text{sec.)}} \text{ cm.}^2$$

A. For the detection of left to right shunts, a breath of hydrogen gas is inhaled; in the presence of such a shunt, blood containing hydrogen gas appears in the right side of the heart, the potentiometric electrode mounted at the tip of the catheter shows a potential difference

Mean pulmonary capillary wedge may be substituted for left atrial mean pressure.

Normal values range from 100 to 250 dynes sec./cm.$^{-5}$

B. Pulmonary vascular resistance can also be expressed in units as follows:

$$P.V.R. = \frac{\text{pulmonary artery mean pressure (mm. Hg)} - \text{left atrial mean pressure (mm. Hg)}}{\text{pulmonary blood flow (l./min.)}}$$

with respect to the neutral electrode. By means of suitable recording equipment, the presence of hydrogen gas in the blood can be continuously monitored from several sites in the circulation.

B. Since in its first passage through the lungs a hydrogen-saturated saline solution is completely cleared of hydrogen, the presence of detectable gaseous hydrogen in the arterial blood following injection of such a solution on the venous

Normal values are between 1 and 3 units; one unit is equivalent to 80 dynes sec./cm.$^{-5}$

C. In some cases of left to right shunt, the pulmonary vascular resistance increases progressively as the patient grows older, and the shunt may become bidirectional.

D. As surgical repair is contraindicated in the presence of a high pulmonary vascular resistance, the importance of resistance measurement cannot be overemphasized.

E. Of even greater importance is the differentiation between cases with "fixed" high pulmonary vascular resistance, due to irreversible changes in the pulmonary arterioles, and those in which a major part of the increase in pulmonary vascular resistance is due to increased pulmonary arteriolar tone. In the latter, a high-oxygen breathing mixture may produce a significant reduction of a markedly elevated pulmonary artery pressure. Infusion of acetylcholine into the pulmonary artery in amounts that are effective in dilating pulmonary arterioles has been used for the same purpose and with the same results as the inhalation of 100 per cent oxygen.

If the O_2 (or acetylcholine) causes an appreciable fall in pulmonary arterial pressure, it can be assumed that a major part of the increased pulmonary resistance was due to increased pulmonary arteriolar tone; a decrease in pulmonary resistance may then be anticipated after closure of the defect. On the other hand, if the O_2 (or acetylcholine) has little or no effect, it can be assumed that increased pulmonary arteriolar resistance is fixed; in such a case closure of the defect might be of no benefit.

Detection and Evaluation of Valvular Stenosis and/or Incompetence

Pressure recordings in the cardiac chamber and great vessels constitute an important parameter in the evaluation of valvular malfunction. Their value is greatly enhanced by the addition of other hemodynamic studies: determination of cardiac output, stroke volume, and regurgitant fraction.

1. *Pressure gradient*

A. The difference in pressure between the sides of a valve or between two segments of a vessel during the period of the cardiac cycle when there should be no difference or only a very small one (1 mm. Hg or less across the mitral and tricuspid valves; 10 mm. Hg or less across the aortic or pulmonic valves).

B. Diastolic atrioventricular gradients are found across the stenotic mitral or tricuspid valves.

C. Systolic left ventricular-aortic and right ventricular-pulmonic gradients are recorded across the stenotic aortic or pulmonic valves.

D. The gradient increases as the square of the blood flow; when the cardiac output and stroke volume are normal, the higher the gradient, the more severe the stenosis; on the other hand, when the cardiac output and stroke volume are smaller, even a small gradient is most impressive.

E. The exact location of the pressure gradient obtained by a continuous recording is of the greatest importance in the differentiation between valvular stenosis and stenosis located proximal to the valve (subvalvular stenosis) or distal to it (supravalvular stenosis).

F. *Sequential* or *combined* pressure gradients can be found in some conditions. Some cases of tetralogy of Fallot have both infundibular (or subvalvular) pulmonic stenosis with a systolic gradient between the right ventricular chamber and the right ventricular outflow tract and valvular pulmonic stenosis with a second systolic gradient between the right ventricular outflow tract and the pulmonary artery. Some cases of valvular aortic stenosis are complicated by such a degree of subvalvular hypertrophy that a double systolic gradient is recorded during pullback of the catheter from the left ventricular cavity through the left ventricular outflow tract and across the aortic valve.

2. *Pressure curve analysis*: Examination of the different segments of the atrial, ventricular, or arterial pressure

curves may yield some useful diagnostic information.

A. The A wave in the right atrial pulse tracing is increased in the presence of tricuspid stenosis.

B. The A wave in the left atrial pressure curve (or a satisfactory pulmonary capillary wedge recording) is also higher than normal in mitral stenosis when sinus rhythm is present. The A wave is accompanied by a slow descent of the V wave (= slow Y descent), due to slow atrial emptying, and by a continuing fall in pressure throughout diastole (instead of the normal rise in pressure during diastasis).

C. In the presence of severe aortic stenosis, the A wave of the left atrial pressure curve is higher than its V wave.

D. In some cases of pure mitral regurgitation, the left atrial pressure curve shows a gradually rising, peaked V wave of great amplitude in systole and a rapid Y descent of the V wave beginning at the end of systole; when regurgitation is severe, the X descent becomes virtually obliterated. At times the V wave becomes so tall that its configuration resembles that of the left ventricular pressure contour; this effect is called *ventricularization* of the atrial pressure curve.

E. In cases of tricuspid regurgitation, identical changes appear in the right atrial pressure curve.

F. In cor triatriatum, the pulmonary capillary wedge pressure is elevated while a simultaneously recorded left atrial pressure is normal (= pressure gradient between pulmonary capillary and left atrium).

G. Intraventricular systolic pressure gradients in tracings obtained by continuous pullback are diagnostic for infundibular pulmonic stenosis (right ventricle) or subvalvular aortic stenosis (left ventricle).

H. An early diastolic dip suddenly terminating early rapid diastolic ven-tricular filling, followed by a diastolic plateau, is characteristic of disease that impairs ventricular distensibility, such as constrictive pericarditis, endocardial fibroelastosis, or cardiac amyloidosis.

I. In pure pulmonic regurgitation, the pulmonary artery systolic pressure is normal or elevated, but the pulmonary diastolic pressure is lower and identical to the right ventricular diastolic pressure.

J. In pure mitral regurgitation, the pulmonary artery pulse pressure is wide; the systolic peak of the left atrial V wave corresponds to the elevated pulmonary systolic pressure and the low diastolic Y point in the left atrium corresponds to the low diastolic pulmonary artery pressure.

K. In valvular aortic stenosis, the aortic pressure curve usually reveals a slow rise to the summit and a delay from the onset to the incisura on the downstroke. A prominent anacrotic notch or shoulder is commonly found on the ascending limb, and the greater the stenosis, the lower the position of the notch. The upstroke time is a good index of the severity of valvular aortic stenosis.

L. In idiopathic subvalvular hypertrophic aortic stenosis, the aortic pressure curve shows a rapidly rising upstroke with a high peak; there may be a sharp cutoff in midsystole followed by a second lower peak.

M. In cases of supravalvular aortic stenosis, the continuous pressure recording reveals no difference in pressure across the aortic valve, but a pressure gradient is seen between the aortic root and the area of the ascending aorta distal to the obstruction.

N. In coarctation of the aorta, a systolic pressure gradient is found between the aortic arch and the descending aorta.

O. In patients with aortic regurgitation, the aortic pulse pressure is characterized by a rapid rise, a rapid fall, and a low dicrotic notch with the systolic pressure often higher and the diastolic pressure lower than normal.

3. *Cardiac output (C.O.) determination* (by dye dilution technique with indocyanine green or by thermodilution) helps greatly in the evaluation of the gradient found across a stenotic valve.

A. Cardiac output equals the amount of blood pumped by the heart, expressed in liters per minute.

B. Cardiac index (C.I.), which is a more accurate measure of the gradient than the cardiac output because it is related to the surface area of the patient, equals:

$$\frac{\text{cardiac output}}{\text{body surface area (m.}^2)}$$

C. Stroke volume (S.V.) equals the number of ml. of blood per beat, and it equals:

$$\frac{\text{cardiac output}}{\text{heart rate}}$$

Stroke volume is particularly important in the evaluation of the systolic gradient in patients with aortic stenosis.

D. Stroke volume index (S.V.I.) equals:

$$\frac{\text{stroke volume}}{\text{body surface area}}$$

Thus S.V.I. relates the stroke volume to the individual size of the patient.

4. *Regurgitant volume:* Quantitative assessment of valvular incompetence is possible by dye dilution technique.

A. In the presence of aortic regurgitation, indocyanine green dye is injected 1 cm. above the valve; simultaneous blood sampling from the left ventricle and the femoral artery follows.

B. To quantify mitral insufficiency, the dye is injected in the left ventricle; simultaneous sampling in the left atrium and femoral artery follows.

C. The more severe the aortic regurgitation, the more dye will be forced back into the left ventricle and the greater will be the ratio of the ventricular curve area to the femoral curve area. Aortic regurgitant fraction (Fa) equals:

$$\frac{\text{ventricular curve area}}{\text{femoral curve area}}$$

Aortic regurgitant volume equals:

$$\frac{\text{Fa} \times \text{cardiac output (l./min.)}}{1 - \text{Fa}}$$

D. In mitral incompetence also, the worse the mitral leak, the greater the ratio between the atrial curve area and the femoral curve area. Mitral regurgitant fraction (Fm) equals:

$$\frac{\text{atrial curve area}}{\text{femoral curve area}}$$

Mitral volume equals:

$$\frac{\text{Fm}}{1 - \text{Fm}} \times \text{cardiac output (l./min.)}$$

5. *Calculation of valvular area:* is done by the Gorlin formula.

A. Mitral valve area equals:

$$\frac{\text{mitral valve flow}}{31\sqrt{\text{left atrial pressure} - \text{diastolic l.v. pressure}}}$$

where mitral valve flow equals:

$$\frac{\text{cardiac output (l./min.)}}{\text{diastolic filling period (sec./min.)}}$$

The normal mitral valve area is about 4.5 cm.^{2} Mitral stenosis is symptomatic at areas less than 1.0 cm.^{2}

B. Aortic valve area equals:

$$\frac{\text{aortic valve flow}}{k\sqrt{\text{systolic l.v. pressure} - \text{systolic aortic pressure}}}$$

where aortic valve flow equals:

$$\frac{\text{cardiac output (l./min.)}}{\text{systolic ejection period (sec./min.)}}$$

The normal aortic valve area is about 4.0 cm.² Significant stenosis occurs when the orifice is less than 1.0 cm.²

Hemodynamic Studies in the Diagnosis of Complex Congenital Malformations

1. Complex congenital cardiovascular malformations are due to the coexistence of several anomalies in the heart and great vessels: septal defect with shunts, valvular atresia, stenosis, regurgitation or displacement, transposition of the great vessels, double outlet right ventricle, or common arterial trunk.

stenosis where the rise has been explained by a decrease in left ventricular compliance during the diastolic relaxation phase.

2. *Cardiac index and stroke volume index*: In the presence of failure, the stroke volume index (S.V.I.) falls below normal. Sinus tachycardia may be able to maintain the cardiac index in the lower normal range for a while, but as the left ventricular performance deteriorates further, the cardiac index too will fall below normal.

3. *Left ventricular stroke work index* is calculated by the following formula:

$$L.V.S.W.I. = S.V.I. \times (\text{systolic mean arterial pressure} - \text{l.v. filling pressure}) \times \frac{1.36}{100}$$

2. Accurate diagnosis of malformations depends to a great extent upon the evaluation of their multiple components by the different types of hemodynamic studies described above and by the abnormal course taken by the catheter passing through abnormal communications between right and left cardiac chambers, between great vessels, or between a cardiac chamber and the abnormally located origin of the great vessels.

Hemodynamic Studies for the Evaluation of Left Ventricular Performance in Diseases Affecting the Left Ventricle

The left ventricle performs the major part of the cardiac work. It is thus very important to evaluate as accurately as possible its functional status in patients suffering from mitral incompetence, aortic stenosis and/or regurgitation, coronary artery disease, hypertensive cardiovascular disease and myocardiopathies. The following hemodynamic studies are helpful in this regard:

1. *Left ventricular end diastolic pressure*: Elevation of pressure is almost always evidence of myocardial failure except in cases of severe, pure aortic

Stroke work index is an excellent index of left ventricular function because it takes into account the preload, the afterload, the contractility and the heart rate; it has been found to have an excellent prognostic value in patients with acute myocardial infarction.

4. *Systolic time intervals*: These can be obtained without cardiac catheterization but if such a procedure is performed, they may be integrated with other parameters of left ventricular function.

A. *Total electromechanical systole or Q-S2 interval* is the time between the onset of the QRS complex and the onset of the second heart sound; this interval spans the entire period of systole from the onset of electrical activation to the closure of the aortic valve.

Pre-ejection phase (PEP) is the time between the onset of ventricular depolarization and the actual beginning of ejection; this interval is obtained by subtracting the left ventricular ejection time from the total electromechanical systole.

C. *Left ventricular ejection time (LVET)* is the period during which the left ventricle actually ejects blood into the aorta; it is the time between the onset of the rapid rise in the aortic pressure and the incisura, which corresponds to the closure of the aortic valve.

NOTE: (1) These measurements should be corrected for the patient's heart rate and sex.

(2) Decreased left ventricular function lengthens the PEP and shortens the LVET while the total Q-S2 remains unchanged. The ratio of PEP to LVET offers a quick and easy way to express alterations in the systolic time intervals (normal PEP/LVET ratio is 0.35 with standard deviation of 0.04).

Other Indications for Hemodynamic Studies

1. *Evaluation of surgical treatment of congenital heart disease*

A. Oxymetry, dye dilution curves, and gas inhalation demonstrates the correction of a shunt or its persistence.

B. Intracardiac pressure recordings afford a more thorough evaluation of valvotomy for valvular stenosis and of valvuloplasty or artificial valve insertion for valvular incompetence; dye dilution studies also detect post surgical valvular regurgitation.

2. *Evaluation of surgical treatment of acquired valvular disease*

A. A thorough evaluation of mitral commissurotomy and of mitral, aortic and/or tricuspid prostheses can be obtained by pressure recordings with gradient measurement and determinations of cardiac output at rest and during exercise.

B. Mitral regurgitation following mitral commissurotomy and regurgitation after mitral and/or aortic prostheses insertion can be detected by dye dilution studies.

3. *Evaluation of myocardial revascularization* (venous graft bypass and/or internal mammary artery anastomosis to a coronary artery)

Hemodynamic studies for the evaluation of left ventricular performance form an important part of the evaluation of the postoperative results.

4. *Evaluation of hemodynamic disturbances secondary to cardiac arrhythmias*

Alterations on intracardiac pressure, cardiac output and stroke volume resulting from disturbances in the cardiac rhythm have been better defined due to cardiac catheterization.

5. *Evaluation of pacing on cardiac performance*

Comparison between hemodynamic studies performed prior to pacing and during pacing at different heart rates is required for evaluation of pacing.

6. *Evaluation of cardiovascular drugs*

Hemodynamic studies, particularly those pertaining to the performance of the left ventricle, are essential to a judgment of the value of pharmocological agents.

7. *Management of patients with acute myocardial infarction or in cardiogenic shock*

Monitoring of the left ventricular end diastolic filling pressure, either directly or indirectly by using the Swan-Ganz catheter, and for repeated determinations of cardiac output, preferably by the thermodilution method (to avoid the withdrawal of too large an amount of blood) is required.

CINEANGIOGRAPHIC STUDIES

1. Cineangiography is the visualization of one or more cardiac chambers and/or great vessels by the injection of a contrast agent under relatively high pressure with high-speed recording on motion picture film (16 or 35 mm.) by a camera exposing 30 or 60 frames per second.

2. Those projections are selected which best reveal the defect or structure under investigation.

3. Filming can also be done by biplanar rapid film changer with conven-

tionally sized x-ray film providing 2 to 6 plates per second.

4. *Right atriogram* reveals the presence of a right to left shunt at the atrial level or an intracavitary tumor (myxoma).

5. *Right ventriculogram* confirms the presence of tricuspid regurgitation and outlines the right ventricular outflow tract (of particular importance in tetralogy of Fallot); it also visualizes a right to left shunt at the ventricular level.

6. *Pulmonary arteriogram* confirms the presence of pulmonary valvular incompetence, supravalvular pulmonic stenosis (single, in the main trunk, or multiple, in the branches) and pulmonary emboli.

7. A dye injection in the right side of the heart or in the pulmonary artery can be used to visualize the left cardiac chambers and the ascending aorta; however, left-sided cardioangiography or aortography gives better results and should be used when possible.

8. *Left atriogram* is of great importance in mitral valve disease to evaluate the size of this chamber, its rate of emptying, and the motion of the mitral leaflets, and to ascertain the presence of mural thrombi. Left atriography is used to visualize an atrial septal defect with left to right shunt and to confirm the presence of a myxoma.

9. *Left ventriculogram* visualizes mitral valvular regurgitation and mitral leaflet prolapse; it delineates obstruction to outflow of blood in patients with idiopathic hypertrophic subaortic stenosis; in patients with aortic valve disease, coronary artery disease and myocardiopathies, it shows the size of the left ventricular cavity, the disturbance in contractility involving different segments of the left ventricular wall (from hypokinetic areas to frank paradoxical aneurysms) and, in some cases, the presence of mural thrombi; when repeated after the administration of a quick

acting vasodilator, it shows the improvement (or lack of improvement) in contractility of the involved segments.

10. *Aortography* confirms the presence of aortic regurgitation; it shows the motion of the aortic cusps and the configuration of the aortic root; it also visualizes a patent ductus arteriosus and localizes exactly the site and delineates configuration of supravalvular aortic stenosis or aortic coarctation. Finally, it outlines an aortic aneurysm, with or without dissection.

CORONARY ARTERIOGRAPHY

Indications

1. "Mapping" of coronary artery disease: number, location and severity of lesions and/or aneurysms; presence and extent of coronary circulation.

2. To establish the presence or absence of coronary artery disease in patients with atypical angina or with chest pain of obscure origin.

3. Selection of candidates for myocardial revascularization.

4. To confirm the presence of coronary arterial spasm and the effectiveness of vasodilators.

5. Visualization of congenital malformations of the coronary arterial system, particularly of the fistulae between a coronary artery and a right cardiac chamber and the anomalous origin of the left coronary artery from the main pulmonary artery.

6. Opacification of venous grafts and/or internal mammary artery anastomoses to the coronary arteries plays an important role in the evaluation of myocardial revascularization.

Techniques

1. *Sones technique*[18]

A. Following surgical exposure of a brachial artery, usually the right, a Sones catheter (usually a #7 or 8F, rarely 6F for patients with a small brachial artery) is introduced through a small arteriotomy and advanced into the ascending aorta.

B. Small amounts of dye are injected by hand into the sinuses of Valsalva to locate the ostium of each coronary artery.

C. The tip of the catheter is then manipulated gently into the coronary ostium and the vessel opacified with a small hand injection (approximately 5 ml.) of contrast agent.

D. Each vessel is opacified in several projections to obtain better visualization of different segments of the coronary arterial tree.

E. Sublingual nitrates are given for relief of coronary arterial spasm or of chest pain in patients with coronary artery disease.

F. Left ventriculography is always done after coronary arteriography; it can be done with the Sones catheter, but better opacification with less recoil is obtained with the Judkins pigtail catheter.

G. At the end of the procedure, the catheter is withdrawn and the arteriotomy is sutured in order to maintain adequate flow while preventing bleeding.

H. *Advantages*

(1) In 95 per cent of the cases, both coronary arteries can be opacified with the same catheter.

(2) The long, soft, tapered tip of the Sones catheter reduces considerably the risk of trauma to the intima of the coronary artery.

2. *Judkins technique*[10]

A. Following percutaneous puncture of a femoral artery, usually the right, the needle is replaced by a guidewire; the catheter is then threaded over the guidewire as described above in the Seldinger technique.

B. When the catheter-guide assembly has reached the ascending aorta, the guidewire is withdrawn and the catheter connected to the manifold.

C. The coronary artery ostium is located by small hand injections of dye.

D. The catheter tip is then advanced into the entrance of the vessel which is opacified with a small hand injection (approximately 5 ml.) of contrast agent.

E. Each vessel is opacified in several projections.

F. *Advantages:* There is no need for surgical exposure of the artery used for entrance of the catheter.

G. *Disadvantages*

(1) Two different catheters made of polyurethane are required, one with a curve designed for entry into the left coronary ostium and the other with a different curve molded for catheterization of the right coronary artery.

(2) Left ventriculography requires a third catheter, preferably a Judkins pigtail catheter.

3. *Schoonmaker-King technique*[15] (multipurpose catheter)

A. The multipurpose catheter, made of polyurethane, is introduced percutaneously into the femoral artery by the Seldinger technique.

B. It is advanced over a 0.35 Teflon coated guidewire with floppy tip into the abdominal aorta only.

C. The guidewire is removed at this point and the catheter is flushed vigorously with a heparinized solution of glucose or saline.

D. Because of the gentle 45° bend near its tip, the catheter may be advanced around the aortic arch into the ascending aorta without guidewire.

E. Each coronary artery ostium is located by a small hand injection of dye and each vessel selectively opacified in different projections.

F. Left ventriculography is done at the end of the procedure.

G. *Advantages*

(1) There is no need for surgical cutdown to expose the vessel used for entrance of the catheter.

(2) There is no need for multiple catheter and guidewire changes.

4. *Visualization of vein grafts to coronary arteries*

The Sones catheter and the multipurpose catheter are particularly well suited for this task. These techniques have been described.

5. *Visualization of internal mammary artery anastomoses to coronary arteries*

A. Each internal mammary artery can be selectively catheterized by a catheter introduced through the brachial artery on the same side.

B. After surgical exposure of the brachial artery, a Viamonte catheter, made of polyurethane, is introduced through a small arteriotomy and advanced into the subclavian artery.

C. Small hand injections of dye in the proximal portion of the subclavian artery help locate the ostium of the internal mammary artery.

D. The tip of the catheter is then manipulated gently into the ostium of the internal mammary artery and the vessel opacified with a small hand injection (approximately 5 ml.) of contrast agent.

E. When an internal mammary artery has been anastomosed to a coronary artery, its catheterization should be undertaken with the same care as that of a coronary artery.

Complications

1. Sinus bradycardia, junctional escape rhythm, cardiac standstill.

A. *Causes*

(1) Vasovagal reaction, as at the beginning of any medical procedure.

(2) Injection of dye in a coronary artery (usually the dominant one) or in a saphenous vein graft or in an internal mammary artery connected to a coronary artery.

B. *Prevention*

(1) Make a "test" injection of 2 ml. of dye to outline the size of the artery to be studied and to show the presence of branches to the sinoatrial and/or atrioventricular nodes. If significant cardiac slowing follows this small injection, give 0.4 mg. atropine I.V. before proceeding further.

(2) Instruct patient to cough immediately and vigorously upon command (= self-induced cardiac massage).

C. *Treatment*

(1) Order the patient to cough immediately and vigorously.

(2) Give a blow on the precordium.

(3) Give closed chest cardiac massage.

(4) Give atropine 0.8 mg. I.V. push.

(5) Give I.V. drip of isoproterenol.

NOTE: Some cardiologists routinely insert a catheter pacer in the right auricle prior to coronary arteriography and turn it on if standstill develops.

2. *Ventricular fibrillation*

A. *Cause*

The frequency of ventricular fibrillation is directly related to the sodium concentration of the dye injected; it is exceedingly rare with diatrizoate methylglucamine.[4,9]

B. *Prevention*: Use a dye with low sodium concentration.

C. *Treatment*

(1) Immediate direct current countershock

(2) Sodium bicarbonate I.V. if more than 30 seconds have elapsed between the onset and the termination of the arrhythmia.

(3) Propanolol (1.0 mg.), I.V., procainamide (250 mg.), and/or lidocaine (50 mg.) to decrease ventricular irritability

3. *Acute coronary insufficiency*

A. *Cause*: Pre-existent coronary artery disease, usually severe

B. *Treatment*

(1) Administer sublingual quick acting nitrate.

(2) Wait till the pain has been relieved before resuming dye injection.

4. *Acute left ventricular failure*

A. *Cause*: Borderline left ventricular function prior to the procedure

B. *Treatment*

Sitting position, nasal O_2; morphine sulfate; I.V. digitalis and furosemide; sublingual vasodilator

5. *Coronary artery occlusion*

A. *Causes*

(1) Catheter advanced too far into the vessel

(2) Lifting of an arteriosclerotic plaque by the tip of the catheter

(3) Dissection of the intima by the tip of the catheter; the forward flow progressively enlarges the tear that was initially small, and the lumen is narrowed, then occluded, by the loosened intima. Dissection of the intima in the proximal right coronary artery has occurred mostly with the Judkins right coronary catheter. This catheter must be watched carefully for possible whipping that may result in a too forceful entrance into the vessel.

(4) Dislodgement of a clot from the catheter tip. Dislodgement has occurred mostly with the Judkins left coronary catheter; when it results in complete occlusion of the left coronary artery main trunk, it is invariably fatal.

B. *Prevention*

(1) Extreme vigilance in pressure monitoring will avoid the consequences from too deep a penetration into a coronary artery.[4] The technician in charge of monitoring will report immediately any sudden pressure drop. Withdrawal of the catheter from the coronary artery within a few seconds will avoid any serious consequences of this occlusion of very short duration. On the other hand, when the drop in pressure is not noticed or reported, the catheter may be left too long

in an occluded artery or may even be forcefully wedged further down; then acute myocardial infarction, ventricular fibrillation, cardiac standstill and/or death may result.

(2) Gentle manipulation of the catheter (preferably soft-tipped) and use of a first-rate image intensifier greatly reduces the risk of lifting an arteriosclerotic plaque.[4]

(3) A small injection of dye in the sinus of Valsalva prior to catheterization outlines the proximal segment of the coronary artery and signals the presence of plaques in that area.

(4) When the Judkins technique is used, after removal of the guidewire from the catheter, brisk bleeding from the catheter's proximal end is essential before any dye injection is made.

C. *Treatment*

(1) Withdraw catheter immediately into ascending aorta.

(2) Flood the sinus of Valsalva with dye to locate the occlusion.

(3) When a myocardial infarction has occurred because a coronary artery was occluded for too long a period of time, its treatment is the same as that of a spontaneously occurring myocardial infarction.

(4) When coronary occlusion is the result of plaque lifting, intimal dissection or clot injection, supportive measures should be started while preparations are being made for emergency coronary artery bypass. The chances of success are reasonably good when the right coronary artery has been occluded, but they are practically nil following occlusion of the left coronary artery main trunk because death occurs before emergency bypass can be done.

6. The following are complications of the Sones technique for coronary arteriography:

A. Brachial artery spasm

B. Brachial artery thrombosis

C. Bleeding and hematoma, arteriovenous fistula at the site of the arteriotomy

D. Dissection of the subclavian or innominate artery by the lifting of an arteriosclerotic plaque

NOTE: Prevention and treatment of the above complications have been outlined in the section dealing with the complications of cardiac catheterization.

7. The following are complications of the Judkins technique for coronary arteriography:

A. Trauma, dissection and/or perforation of the arterial wall by the guidewire and/or catheter

B. Breakage of the flexible tip of the guidewire

C. Breakage of the catheter tip during its insertion

D. Femoral artery spasm

E. Femoral artery thrombosis

F. Bleeding and hematoma, arteriovenous fistula, false aneurysm at the site of the arterial puncture.

NOTE: Prevention and treatment of the above complications have been outlined in the section dealing with the complications of cardiac catheterization.

8. Complications related to dye sensitivity and toxicity are the same as those encountered with cineangiography. Their prevention and treatment have been outlined in the section dealing with the complications of cineangiography.

REFERENCES

1. Brockenbrough, E. C. and Braunwald, E.: A new technique of left ventricular angiocardiography and transseptal left heart catheterization. Am. J. Cardiol., 6:1062, 1960.
2. Cohn, J. N., Khatri, I. M. and Hamosh, P.: Bedside catheterization of the left ventricle. Am. J. Cardiol., 25:66, 1970.
3. Cournand, A. and Ranges, H. A.: Catheterization of the right auricle in man. Proc. Soc. Exper. Bio. and Mod., 46:462, 1941.
4. Demany, M. A., Tambe, A. A. and Zimmerman, H. A.: Coronary cine arteriography: a safe diagnostic procedure. Am. J. Cardiol., 26:436, 1970.
5. Demany, M. A., Tambe, A. A. and Zimmerman, H. A.: Meticulous repair of the arteriotomy in prevention of thrombosis following left cardiac catherization and coronary arteriography. Vasc. Surg., 5:102, 1971.
6. Desilets, D. T. and Hoffman, R. B.: A new method of percutaneous catheterization. Radiology, 85:147, 1965.
7. Fogarty, T. J. et al.: A method for extraction of arterial emboli and thrombi. Surg. Gyn. Obst., 116:241, 1963.
8. Forssmann, W.: Die Sondierung. des rechten Herzens. Klin. Wschr., 8:2085, 1929.
9. Gensini, G. G. and DiGiorgi, S.: Myocardial toxicity of contrast agents used in angiography. Radiology, 82:24, 1964.
10. Judkins, M. P.: Selective coronary arteriography, part 1: a percutaneous transfemoral technique. Radiology, 89:815, 1967.
11. Neches, W. H. et al.: Percutaneous sheath cardiac catheterization. Am. J. Cardiol., 30:378, 1972.
12. Ponsdomenech, E. R. and Nunez, V. B.: Heart puncture in man for diodrast visualization of the ventricular chambers and great arteries. Am. Heart J., 41:643, 1951.
13. Ross, J. Jr.: Considerations regarding the technique for transseptal left heart catheterization. Circulation, 34:391, 1966.
14. Ross, J. Jr., Braunwald, E. and Morrow, A. G.: Left heart catheterization by the transseptal route. A description of the technique and its applications. Circulation, 22:927, 1960.
15. Schoonmaker, F. W. and King, S. B.: Coronary arteriography by the single catheter percutaneous femoral technique. Circulation, 50:735, 1974.
16. Schwartz, D. C. and Kaplan, S.: Cardiac catheterization and selective angiography in infants with a new flow-directed catheter. Catheterization and Cardiovascular Diagnosis, 1:7, 1975.
17. Seldinger, S. I.: Catheter replacement of the needle in percutaneous arteriography, a new technique. Acta. Radiol., 39:368, 1953.
18. Sones, F. M., Jr., and Shirey, E. K.: Cine coronary arteriography. Mod. Concepts Cardiovasc. Dis., 31:735, 1962.
19. Swan, H. J. C. et al.: Catheterization of the heart in man with use of a flow-directed balloon-tipped catheter. N. Engl. J. Med., 283:447, 1970.
20. Zimmerman, H. A., Scott, R. W. and Becker, N. O.: Catheterizatin of the left side of the heart in man. Circulation, 1:357, 1950.

30. POSTOPERATIVE CARE FOLLOWING CARDIOVASCULAR SURGERY

Donal M. Billig, M.D.

GENERAL CONSIDERATIONS

Cardiovascular surgical procedures, especially operations performed upon the heart or major intrathoracic vessels, are almost always performed upon patients having pre-existing physiologic disturbances of cardiac function. These disturbances may be mild and totally reversible, as in the child with an atrial septal defect of the ostium secundum type (see Chap. 10). They may be severe and only partially reversible, as in many patients with severe valvular heart disease, coronary atherosclerosis, or both. In some patients these abnormalities are not treated in any way by the surgical procedure but pose potential problems in the postoperative period. An example of this is the frequent association of arterial hypertension, coronary atherosclerosis and cerebral vascular disease in patients undergoing surgery for aneurysms of the thoracic aorta and aneurysms or occlusive disease of the abdominal aorta, its branches, and the peripheral arteries (see Chaps. 14–16).

The surgical procedure itself imposes further pathophysiologic disturbances by increasing metabolic demands and imposing increases in the necessity for oxygen consumption and cardiac output. At the same time, a depression of ventricular function often occurs following cardiac surgery. This is usually reversible but may be permanent, as in the case of perioperative myocardial infarction. The extent of the depression in cardiac function is variable in degree and duration, and depends upon many factors such as the pre-existing hemodynamic state, the completeness of the repair, the amount of surgical trauma, and other factors.

Changes in blood and extracellular fluid volumes impose another physiologic variable that is closely related to changes in cardiac performance. The filling pressures required to maintain an adequate cardiac output in the postoperative period may be different from the preoperative values, adding still another unknown.

Serum electrolyte abnormalities are frequent (see Chap. 31). Hyponatremia and hypokalemia usually occur following the use of hemodilution primes for open intracardiac operations. These cations are also reduced by water retention secondary to inappropriate antidiuretic hormone secretion, and altered by abnormal gastrointestinal fluid losses.

Respiratory gas exchange may be altered by retained secretions, changes in alveolar ventilation relative to pulmonary capillary perfusion, acid-base imbalances, and red blood cell enzyme deficits. Most of these changes are temporary, but may require ventilatory assistance, adjustments in acid-base abnormalities, and (in some instances) transfusion of whole fresh blood to maintain homeostasis.

Abnormalities of cardiac rhythm may occur in the postoperative patient, further compromise cardiac performance, and require prompt recognition and treatment (see Chaps. 21–28).

The foregoing brief remarks indicate the number and complexity of the physiologic adjustments that occur in the postoperative period. Many or most of the abnormalities (e.g., congestive heart failure, arrhythmias, cardiogenic shock) are discussed in other sections, and their management differs little in the postoperative patient. The extreme complexity of the adjustments however, requires not only careful attention to clinical signs but also a continuous correlation of these with intracardiac and intra-arterial pressure measurements, blood gas determinations, amount of chest drainage, urine output, cardiac output measurements, radiographic examinations, and other measurements.

The most important ingredient in adequate postoperative care is knowledge of the preexisting pathophysiology, of how it is likely to be altered by surgical treatment, and therefore an awareness of the potential problems in each individual patient.

Postoperative Clinical Radiographic, Hemodynamic and Laboratory Observations

Clinical observations
  Skin: temperature, moisture, color
  Conjunctivae: prominence and color of vessels
  Sensorium: alertness, restlessness, appropriateness of responses
  Motor functions: appropriate extremity motions and strength
  Urine: hourly volume, specific gravity or osmolality
  Chest drainage: amount and character
  Chest: breath sounds, heart sounds, sternal stability, excursions of chest wall, respiratory rate, character and amount of secretions
  Abdomen: distention, bowel sounds, flank ecchymosis or fullness
  Extremities: character of pulses
Radiographic observations
  Routine chest film immediately postoperatively, and daily thereafter until chest tubes removed. More often as required.
Physiologic monitoring
  Electrocardiogram
  Left and right atrial pressure cannulae
  Pulmonary artery pressure (direct or transvenous Swan-Ganz catheter)
  Systemic artery pressure cannula
  Cardiac output (Indocyanine green or thermodilution)
  Skin and core temperature (mostly in infants)
Laboratory observations
  Hemoglobin, hematocrit
  BUN, creatinine, Na, K, CO_2, Cl
  Arterial blood bases, pH and base excess
  Clotting profile, platelet count
  Serum lactate

Potential Postoperative Complications

Hemorrhage
  Hypovolemia
  Cardiac and mediastinal tamponade
  Hemothorax
Low cardiac output
  Cardiogenic shock
  Congestive heart failure
Cardiac arrhythmias
Respiratory abnormalities
Peripheral vascular complications
Central nervous system complications

The majority of surgical patients have a relatively simple and uncomplicated postoperative course, make their own circulatory adjustments, and require such intensive monitoring for only short periods.

POSTOPERATIVE HEMORRHAGE

1. *Definition*

Excessive hemorrhage may be defined as bleeding of more than 600 ml. per square meter of body surface in the first 24 hours following surgery, or bleeding of an amount to produce hypovolemia, shock, cardiac tamponade, or hemothorax of one-third or more the volume of one hemithorax.[5,13]

2. *General features*

A. There is inevitably some blood loss into the chest, mediastinum, retroperitoneal space, or leg (depending on the site of surgery) following all operations on the heart or major vessels.

B. The majority of the blood loss occurs in the first 2 to 3 hours following surgery.[13]

C. During this early period it is not uncommon for chest drainage after cardiac surgery to approximate 90 ml. per square meter of body surface (150 ml. per hour) in the average adult patient.

D. Should this rate of blood loss continue and/or signs of hypovolemia, cardiac tamponade or both ensue, then hemorrhage is clearly causing physiologic impairment and therapeutic measures to correct coagulation deficits, reoperation, or both become mandatory.

E. The effects of hypovolemia and of cardiac-mediastinal tamponade may act in tandem and are often present together.

F. Certain operations and lesions, such as aortic valve replacement, repair of tetralogy of Fallot, and operations in cyanotic and polycythemic patients, are more likely to result in significant postoperative hemorrhage.[13]

G. Hemothorax may produce varying degrees of pulmonary dysfunction and may account for significant blood loss, which may be unappreciated unless repeated chest examinations and roentgenograms are carried out.

H. The physiologic alterations of hypovolemia, cardiac tamponade, and respiratory insufficiency secondary to hemothorax or shock, have many features in common, and often occur together. Their manifestations will be considered separately below to avoid confusion.

3. *Etiology*

A. Excessive bleeding is most often due to lack of perfect surgical hemostasis.

B. The type of surgery influences this, with aortic valve replacement and repair of tetralogy of Fallot with an outflow patch having the highest incidence of bleeding.

C. The duration of cardiopulmonary bypass, the presence of cyanosis and polycythemia and the presence of preoperative coagulation deficits also influence this by causing abnormalities of coagulation, as does massive transfusion of banked blood.[2,13,18]

4. *Diagnosis*

A. In patients undergoing cardiothoracic operations, the diagnosis of excessive hemorrhage is usually simple, and predicated upon excessive chest tube drainage or the presence of symptoms, signs, roentgenographic, labora-

tory, and hemodynamic manifestations of hypovolemia, tamponade or hemothorax, to be described below.

B. In abdominal or peripheral vascular surgery, the diagnosis is predicated upon the manifestations of hypovolemia (see below), bleeding through the incisions, swelling of the neck, abdomen, or leg as the case may be, and flank ecchymosis or fullness (or both, in the case of retroperitoneal hemorrhage).

5. *Management*

A. It is imperative to ascertain whether or not a coagulation deficit exists.

B. An immediate hematologic consultation with performance of a complete coagulation profile is mandatory.

C. Fresh frozen plasma or fresh whole blood transfusions usually remedy most of these deficits.

D. If heparin has been used, additional protamine may be required. If disseminated intravascular coagulation is present, small doses of heparin may be appropriate therapy.

E. On rare occasions, platelet transfusions and special concentrates of fibrinogen or other plasma factors may be necessary but this is unusual.

F. The cornerstones of therapy remain adequate transfusion to prevent hypovolemia, utilizing fresh frozen plasma and whole fresh blood if available, and early reoperation if hemorrhage continues or tamponade develops, providing the clotting mechanism is near normal or adequately corrected.[2,13,18]

6. *Prognosis*

A. The prognosis of patients having excessive postoperative bleeding is significantly poorer than that of patients with adequate postoperative hemostasis.

B. This varies, depending upon:

(1) The cause of the bleeding

(2) The presence of such other complications as low cardiac output, central nervous system abnormalities, respiratory problems, or others.

Hypovolemia

1. *General features*

A. The requirements for circulating blood volume in the postoperative patient depend upon the balance between cardiac performance, the degree of compensatory vasoconstriction, the changeable metabolic and cardiac output requirements, and other variables.

B. That volume which allows the patient to maintain adequate hemostasis is the one appropriate for his clinical condition.

C. Careful clinical and hemodynamic assessment on a continuous basis in the early postoperative period are mandatory, to assess the changing requirements for blood volume imposed by these variables.[6—8,10,14,15]

2. *Definition*

In the postoperative patient, hypovolemia can only be defined as a circulating blood volume not large enough to maintain adequate cardiac filling pressures, cardiac output, and clinical circulatory hemostasis.

3. *Etiology*

A. Inadequate blood volume may result from undertransfusion at the time of surgery or from preoperative reduction in blood and extracellular fluid volume, as in aortic stenosis or intestinal malfunction in patients with mesenteric artery lesions or duodenal obstruction secondary to a large abdominal aneurysm.[6,7]

B. Excessive postoperative blood loss, inadequately replaced gastric suction volume, or sequestration of "third space" fluid may also account for hypovolemia.

C. Blood volume requirements may be increased, as in many postoperative septic patients and in some patients having an immediate fall in blood pressure following renal artery revascularization or repair of aortic coarctation, and this may cause relative hypovolemia.

4. *Pathophysiology*

A. Atrial filling pressures and cardiac output are reduced.

B. Skin, renal, and splanchnic vasoconstriction occur to compensate for this, and for a time serve to maintain arterial blood pressure, though pulse pressure is usually narrowed.

C. Renal blood flow and glomerular filtration are reduced, as is skin and splanchnic flow.

D. As these compensatory alterations that serve to decrease the size of the vascular compartment fail to compensate for increasing reductions in blood volume arterial blood pressure falls, effective renal flood flow may be close to zero, coronary and cerebral blood flow begin to fail reducing cardiac performance and resulting in central nervous system symptoms.

E. Inadequate organ blood flow results in inadequate tissue oxygenation and anaerobic glycolysis ensues, causing lactic acidemia.[20]

5. *Symptoms and signs*

A. The skin is cool, damp, pale, or mottled, and there is often peripheral cyanosis.

B. The conjuctival vessels are constricted, and pale or cyanotic.

C. Restlessness, disorientation, and occasionally frank seizures, or abnormal extraocular muscle signs appear.

D. In the final stages, coma may ensue.

E. Urine volume is diminished.

F. Pulse volume is sharply reduced to palpation.

G. Ileus is frequent.

H. Respiratory rate is increased, and there may also be hyperpnea as a compensatory mechanism against metabolic acidosis.

I. Nostril flaring and sternal retractions are often present, more frequently in children.

J. The liver edge, which prior to surgery may have been palpable below the costal margin, especially in children with preoperative congestive heart failure, may no longer be palpable.

6. *Laboratory findings*

A. *Roentgenographs*

(1) When the hypovolemic state is due to excessive postoperative hemorrhage, there is often mediastinal widening, increase in the cardiac-pericardial silhouette and often varying degrees of opacification of a hemithorax, especially if a pleural space has been entered during the operative procedure.

(2) If another etiologic agent is responsible, or if the blood has been well drained by mediastinal tubes, the cardiac silhouette is smaller than prior to surgery. This is often an early sign of hypovolemia, and one should not gain a false sense of security from an early and immediate decrease in cardiac size.

(3) The lung fields often appear underperfused.

(4) Abdominal films following abdominal aortic operations are rarely of help in ascertaining retroperitoneal bleeding. Obliteration of the psoas shadows is so frequently present following these procedures that it has no diagnostic value.

(5) When hypovolemia is due to extracellular fluid loss as a result of postoperative ileus or intestinal obstruction, distended loops of small bowel, with an empty colon (small bowel obstruction), or loops of small bowel plus colon gas to the sigmoid area (usually following resection of ruptured abdominal aortic aneurysm), with air fluid levels, are usually present.[6]

B. *Hemodynamic findings*

(1) There is almost always a reduction in left and right atrial pressures or central venous pressure.

(2) When cardiac performance has been affected adversely either by operation or by reduction in coronary flow with severe hypovolemia, atrial pressures may be somewhat above normal.[20]

(3) Cardiac index is always re-duced, usually below 2.0 liters per square meter per minute.[1,6,20]

(4) Pulmonary artery pressures and pulmonary wedge pressures, when measured, reflect changes in left atrial pressure. Peripheral and pulmonary vascular resistance is elevated.

(5) All of these changes must be interpreted within the context of the preoperative and surgically altered pathophysiology. Serial measurements are much more valuable than a single set of determinations.[3,5]

(6) Arterial pressure as measured via an indwelling cannula evidences a narrowed pulse pressure, damped peaks, and due to peripheral vasoconstriction may show only sine-wave fluctuations as if a mean pressure were being recorded.

(7) Simultaneous recording of skin and core temperature (esophageal or high rectal) show a widening, with skin temperature becoming progressively lower than core temperature. Differences of more than 3 degrees centigrade, and increasing differences, are ominous and early signs of impending circulatory collapse and often precede other hemodynamic or laboratory abnormalities.*

C. *Other laboratory findings*

(1) Hemoglobin and hematocrit may not be an accurate index of blood loss early in acute bleeding situations. In open cardiac operations where hemodilution priming solutions are used, they may be low even when circulating volume is normal. When there is sequestration of third space fluid, these values may be high in the face of a low blood volume, and the same is true when intestinal fluid loss is not adequately replaced.[6,15]

(2) BUN, and later creatinine, will rise as renal blood flow, glomerular filtration, and urine output fall.[6]

(3) Arterial blood gas determinations are variable, but in general arterial

---

*Deverall, P. B.: Personal communication.

hypoxemia develops as pulmonary blood flow falls and pulmonary vasoconstriction and shunting begin.[14]

(4) Hypocarbia is often present early, as hyperventilation ensues as a compensation for metabolic acidosis. Later, as gas exchange deteriorates further, hypercarbia and respiratory acidosis may result.

(5) Arterial blood pH is often well maintained because of the balance produced by metabolic acidosis and respiratory alkalosis, but this is easily detectable as abnormal, since the arterial pCO_2 is too low and the base deficit too high for the pH.[21]

(6) Serum lactate levels are elevated if cardiac output is too low to meet the tissue demands for oxygen, so that anaerobic glycolysis is therefore taking place. There is always associated metabolic acidosis.[20]

7. *Diagnosis*

A. The assessment of the clinical picture, laboratory, x-ray, and hemodynamic data will usually allow prompt recognition of the hypovolemic state.

B. As will be seen, there are only subtle differences to distinguish cardiogenic shock and tamponade, and they may be present together.

C. In general, inadequate circulating blood volume is the most frequent etiology of inadequate circulatory status in the postsurgical patient.

8. *Management*

A. Treatment consists of transfusion of appropriate solutions: Whole blood is usual, but the alternatives are packed red blood cells when there is associated cardiac failure, fresh frozen plasma when a hemostatic deficit exists, and balanced electrolyte solutions when the losses are intestinal fluid rather than blood.

B. Occasionally, if hematocrit is low, diuretics in conjunction with packed red blood cells are appropriate, especially if cardiac failure is present.

C. The aim of therapy is to restore appropriate cardiac filling pressures (left atrial and right atrial) and thus improve cardiac output.

D. Raising the left atrial pressure above 14 to 16 mm. Hg does not seem to improve cardiac output further, and this value should only rarely be exceeded by additional transfusion.[1,15]

9. *Prognosis*

A. If treated promptly before serious metabolic, renal, central nervous system and cardiac complications arise, and the underlying cause for hypovolemia is corrected, the prognosis should be good.

B. Once renal, cardiac, and central nervous system complications arise, the prognosis is much poorer.[13]

Cardiac and Mediastinal Tamponade

Cardiac and mediastinal tamponade may occur whether or not the pericardium is closed following cardiac surgery. Since the subject is discussed in Chapter 8 in detail, only features unique to the postoperative period will be covered here.

1. *Symptoms and signs*

A. Since in the postoperative patient tamponade is almost always a phenomenon of the first 24 to 48 hours and is almost invariably secondary to excessive bleeding, an early abnormal amount of chest tube drainage is most often present.

B. The symptoms and hemodynamic abnormalities of hypovolemia and of reduced ventricular function are often superimposed.

C. The restlessness, sweating, pallor, and other symptoms and signs of circulatory failure described under hypovolemia are all present in this condition, the consequences of an inadequate cardiac output.

D. As a rule there is also distention of neck veins. On inspiration these veins fill, as opposed to their complete inspiratory emptying when hypovolemia is unaccompanied by tamponade.[12]

2. *Laboratory findings*

A. *Roentgenographs*

The hallmark is a widened mediastinal shadow and obliteration of the aortic and cardiac silhouette. Hemothorax is frequently associated.

B. *Hemodynamics*

(1) Filling pressures (left and right atrial) are both elevated, and tend to be almost equal.

(2) Cardiac output is reduced, usually below 2.0 liters per square meter per minute.

(3) If pulmonary artery pressure is measured, it usually is low.

(4) Systemic arterial pressure is low with a low pulse pressure and the damped arterial pressure curve characteristic of low cardiac output in the postoperative patient.

(5) In general, the more severe the degree of tamponade, the more nearly equal pressures in all cardiac chambers and arterial systems become.

C. *Other laboratory findings* are identical to those described under Hypovolemia.

3. *Diagnosis*

A. This is predicated on the clinical and laboratory signs of circulatory failure as described above under hypovolemia, the characteristic roentgenographic and hemodynamic features, usually accompanied by excessive blood loss.

B. It is best to err on the side of making the diagnosis more frequently.

C. Temporizing while the patient's condition is still fair may result in a catastrophic episode within the next few hours, should even a small additional amount of bleeding occur.

D. Moreover, in the late hospital period, as clot liquifies and becomes hygroscopic, additional fluid may accumulate and cause acute circulatory embarrassment with catastrophic results when the patient is out of the intensive care unit and under less continuous observation.

4. *Management*

A. The tamponading material is almost always clot.

B. As in all postoperative bleeding, coagulation studies are indicated but are usually near normal.

C. Fluid loading to maintain cardiac filling pressures serves to temporarily increase cardiac output. This is one of the few instances where left atrial pressures should be elevated as high as 20 mm. Hg in a postoperative patient. Whole blood or fresh frozen plasma are the preferred solutions.

D. "Milking" the mediastinal tubes, removal of a few lower sutures and probing the mediastinum to evacuate some clot are temporizing measures that may serve to temporarily improve the circulation until the operating room can be readied.

E. The mainstay and the only safe therapy is reoperation, removal of all clot, and surgical control of bleeding.

5. *Prognosis*

A. If early recognition, application of measures to temporarily relieve the situation, and prompt reoperation are carried out, the results are usually excellent.

B. Very few patients will bleed again and require further intervention.

C. Improvement in circulatory status is usually immediate upon reopening the chest and relieving the pressure.

Hemothorax

1. Hemothorax is seldom a serious problem.

2. While it may cause some respiratory impairment, even this is usually not marked, and is usually only an adjunctive problem to tamponade and hypovolemia.

3. Amounts of blood one-third or less the hemithoracic volume by x-ray examination can be evacuated by thoracentesis or an additional intercostal tube, and nothing further is necessary, even if the evacuation is incomplete.

4. Larger amounts should be evacuated, but reoperation for this as an isolated complication can easily be delayed for 10 to 14 days unless there are severe respiratory problems.

5. If by 14 days the blood cannot be evacuated, thoracotomy is advisable.

6. Fibrothorax and late sequelae are thus avoided.

LOW CARDIAC OUTPUT

Cardiogenic Shock

This subject has been well covered in Chapter 20. There are subtle differences in cardiogenic shock occurring in the early postoperative period, the most important of which is its temporary nature in many patients.[1,8,9,15] Only special postsurgical considerations will be discussed in this section.

1. *Etiology*

A. After cardiac operations there is almost always a decrease in ventricular function, which is usually temporary and improves within 48 to 72 hours.

B. The severity and reversibility of this depends upon:

(1) The underlying myocardial pathology

(2) The operative procedure performed

(3) The duration of intraoperative myocardial ischemia

(4) The method of myocardial preservation

(5) The completeness of the repair

(6) The cardiac rhythm

(7) Other factors[1,8,9,15,16]

C. In most instances the surgical team has a grasp of the factors in each particular patient and can thus be prepared to deal with them.

2. *Differential diagnosis*

As has already been stated, the manifestations of hypovolemia, tamponade, and decreased ventricular function may be present in the same patient, and the surgeon must often estimate which (or all) to treat by assessing hemodynamic changes as treatment ensues.[3,8,9,15]

3. *Management*

A. The initial steps consist of *increasing fluid load*

(1) The appropriate intravenous solution is determined by the assessment of such considerations as whether or not hypovolemia is also a factor, or hemorrhage is ongoing.

(2) Blood, fresh frozen plasma, salt-free albumin, or crystalloids may be used as the situation demands.

(3) Dextran is rarely indicated.

(4) Infusion may be rapid when left atrial or pulmonary wedge pressures and cardiac output are being measured, since one has instant appreciation of when one is approaching unsafe levels of infusion.

(5) Raising left atrial pressure above 15 mm. Hg by intravenous infusion will not increase cardiac output further, may decrease it by overloading the circulation, and is to be avoided.[8,15,16]

(6) When left ventricular compliance is extremely low, as in aortic stenosis and severe left ventricular hypertrophy, one may need to raise filling pressure (left atrial) to as high as 20 mm. Hg to achieve a satisfactory cardiac output.

B. *Inotropic drugs* are the next line of defense.

(1) Digitalis is always the preferable agent[8,15] in our experience, although it is less rapidly acting and less actively metabolized than some of the others.

(2) Dilute solutions of epinephrine (no more concentrated than 0.4 μg./ml.) are best in our experience.

(3) The end point is not only elevation of arterial systolic blood pressure to 90 mm. Hg but with it an improved renal, cerebral, skin, and muscle flow as evidenced by increased urine output, diminution of cerebral signs, warmer and dryer skin, decreases in serum lactate, and correction of metabolic acidosis.

(4) Isoproterenol in the same

concentrations can also be used, but in our experience it causes more tachycardia and has a more adverse effect on myocardial work and oxygen consumption.

(5) Norepinephrine is a poor drug for the postoperative patient and should only be used when all else fails.

(6) Dopamine HCl is a useful drug in these situations but is less reliable in accomplishing hemodynamic improvement, in our experience.

C. *Intra-aortic balloon counter pulsation*

(1) Should all these measures fail, intra-aortic balloon counter pulsation should be undertaken, and in the opinion of some, it is the modality of choice, though it is not without its own inherent complications.

(2) There is no question that use of the measure decreases cardiac work and oxygen consumption, increases cardiac output, and increases diastolic blood pressure and coronary perfusion.[9]

4. *Prognosis*

A. This is dependent upon:

(1) The disease treated

(2) The preoperative degree of cardiac impairment

(3) The severity and duration of the diminished ventricular function

(4) The reversibility of such associated or etiologic problems as hemorrhage, perioperative infarction, reoperation to repair incomplete corrections, valve or graft malfunctions when present.

B. For example, the overall surgical mortality for total correction of the tetralogy of Fallot is approximately 3 per cent in our hands and others.[4,8,15] Twenty-five per cent of patients having total correction require inotropic assistance in the early postoperative period. The mortality is almost entirely in this group, at about 12 per cent. But within this group, it is higher for patients requiring extensive muscle resection, outflow reconstruction with patch, or having in-

complete hemodynamic repair or marked augmentation of bronchial circulation. It approximates the same 3 per cent for patients with excellent postoperative repair and hemodynamics who have temporary edema due to right ventriculotomy and cardiac manipulation.

C. Each disease, preoperative and postoperative hemodynamics, and all other factors make the chances for survival different in each patient.

Congestive Heart Failure

Again, this entire subject is well reviewed in Chapter 19, and aside from a few special considerations need not be reiterated here.

1. *Etiology*

A. The (usually) temporary decrease in ventricular function is an additional surgical etiologic factor.

B. Important etiologic factors peculiar to surgical intervention include:

(1) Graft or valve malfunctions

(2) Incomplete repairs of congenital heart lesions

(3) The effects of ventriculotomy

(4) Ischemic intraoperative cardiac arrest with or without cooling

(5) Intraoperative coronary perfusion

2. *Management*

A. Management differs little in surgical patients, with a few exceptions.

B. Body temperature must be kept near normal to avoid marked increase in metabolic and cardiac output requirements. This is especially true in children. Shivering is to be avoided for the same reason.

C. Ventilatory assistance should be maintained to reduce the work of breathing, since this makes up a large proportion of the body's metabolic requirements in the early postoperative period.[10]

3. *Prognosis*

A. This depends upon the identical factors outlined under cardiogenic shock, and is variable in each situation.

B. In general, early and favorable responses to aggressive therapy imply a favorable outcome.

CARDIAC ARRHYTHMIAS

This topic has been dealt with at length in Chapter 21, and only factors of special surgical significance will be considered here.

1. *Etiology*

A. Certain surgical procedures have an expected higher incidence of cardiac arrhythmias because of the nature of the underlying pathology and the proximity of the surgical manipulation to the conducting system.

B. For example, repair of partial or complete A-V canal, ventricular septal defect, tetralogy of Fallot, transposition of the great vessels, and some other surgical procedures predispose to injury to the conducting system and atrioventricular dissociation.

C. Resection of atrial septum as in the Blalock-Hanlon and Mustard procedures for transposition of the great vessels may interrupt internodal pathways or traumatize them and cause a variety of supraventricular arrhythmias as well.

D. Ventricular premature beats are not infrequent following any cardiac surgical trauma and are by far the most frequent postsurgical arrhythmia.

E. Patients with mitral valve disease, coronary atherosclerosis, and to a lesser degree aortic valve pathology frequently develop atrial fibrillation spontaneously, and this tendency is heightened in the postoperative period.

F. Nonparoxysmal A-V junctional tachycardia with or without A-V dissociation is mostly produced by inflammation, ischemia, and digitalis, the former two of which are caused by all cardiac surgery. The heart is somewhat more prone to digitalis toxicity early after surgery, another factor predisposing to this arrhythmia. This particular rhythm itself is usually self-limited.

2. *Pathophysiology*

Arrhythmias often are less well tolerated in the early postoperative period for a variety of reasons, but largely because myocardial function is diminished, cardiac compliance is lower, and rapid or slow rates or loss of sequential atrioventricular conduction interfere more with cardiac performance.

3. *Management (see Chaps. 23–28)*

A. The differences in management for the surgical patient are few.

B. Pacing wires are left routinely by some surgeons in all patients.

C. Others tend to be more selective, utilizing them in patients whose procedures or pathology predispose them to serious arrhythmias, such as complete A-V block.

D. Corticosteroids can be used to attempt to reduce edema around the conduction system when complete A-V block occurs. However, this is rarely of benefit.

RESPIRATORY ABNORMALITIES

1. *General features*

A. Respiratory dysfunction is present to a degree in all patients undergoing anesthesia and surgery.[7,17]

B. Underlying pulmonary disease and abnormalities of pulmonary blood flow and distribution in the cardiovascular surgical patient augment these abnormalities, as do retained secretions, atelectasis, and infection.

C. Not all cardiovascular surgical patients require intensive respiratory care, mechanical ventilation, or other supports, but many do, and careful attention to respiratory status is mandatory in the first few days following cardiovascular surgery.

2. *Etiology*

A. Underlying chronic obstructive pulmonary disease is a frequent problem.

B. Other causes may be such congenital abnormalities of the lung as: (1)

congenital lobar emphysema, (2) sequestration, (3) absence of one pulmonary artery, or (4) hypoplasia or absence of one lung, especially in children with congenital heart defects.

C. Cardiac disease itself produces pulmonary congestion, active (left to right shunting) or passive (left heart failure), and in either case may result in progressive vascular changes.[17]

D. Chest and abdominal pain may result in retained secretions because of poor cough, and result in atelectasis and parenchymal infection.[7,19,22]

E. In infants, the chest wall may be too weak to accomplish the augmented work of breathing secondary to reduced pulmonary compliance and increased airway resistance.[11]

3. *Pathophysiology*

This has been extensively reviewed.[17] All of the etiologic factors mentioned above lead to abnormalities in the relationship of alveolar ventilation to pulmonary capillary perfusion, augment intrapulmonary shunting, and lead to arterial hypoxemia and ultimately to alveolar hypoventilation, hypercarbia, and respiratory acidosis. Hypoxia and acidosis have severe effects on all organ systems, as described in other sections.

4. *Symptoms and signs*

A. During early stages, there may be:

    (1) Tachypnea
    (2) Retractions
    (3) Nostril flare
    (4) Cyanosis
    (5) Restlessness
    (6) Tachycardia

B. Peripheral vasoconstriction and pallor ensue as the condition worsens.

C. Bradycardia and circulatory collapse are the end results.

D. Examination of the chest reveals:

    (1) Rhonchi
    (2) Rales
    (3) Uneven ventilatory excursions

    (4) Absent breath sounds, or
    (5) Other signs of poor ventilation in one or both lungs.

5. *Laboratory findings*

    A. *Roentgenographs*

    (1) Atelectasis of segments, lobes, an entire lung or its equivalent may be present.

    (2) Fluffy infiltrates, frank pulmonary edema, or combinations of these are present.

    (3) In some patients, the films are surprisingly unremarkable, though this is unusual.

    B. *Other laboratory findings*

    (1) Arterial oxygen tension is always below 50 mm. Hg.

    (2) Intrapulmonary shunting is usually above 25 per cent of pulmonary flow.[19]

    (3) Pulmonary compliance is decreased, dead space ventilation (V_D) is increased, tidal volume (V_T) decreased and V_D/V_T ratio is increased, usually at or above 50 per cent.[17]

    (4) In later stages, arterial hypercarbia and respiratory acidosis are present.

    (5) As circulatory collapse ensues, in the final stages, metabolic acidosis and lactic acidemia appear as well.

6. *Diagnosis*

    A. The above clinical laboratory and x-ray findings leave little doubt as to the diagnosis of respiratory difficulty.

    B. The underlying cause is usually apparent from the preoperative findings and clinical course.

7. *Management*

    A. Retained secretions are managed by the following:

    (1) Aggressive chest physiotherapy
    (2) Encouragement to cough
    (3) Ultrasonic nebulization
    (4) ''Blow'' bottles
    (5) Positive pressure nebulization of saline or bronchodilators
    (6) Early mobilization

(7) Nasotracheal suction

B. Bronchoscopy is useful if these fail.

C. Oral or nasotracheal intubation is necessary if these measures fail and repeat bronchoscopy is required.

D. Tracheostomy is also an alternative, but we prefer to reserve this for patients who require endotracheal intubation for more than 5 days.

E. In infants, we try to avoid tracheostomy and will leave nasotracheal tubes in place for extended periods if necessary.

F. Positive pressure ventilation may be necessary to provide adequate ventilation. Volume respirators are preferable. The content of inspired oxygen is reduced as arterial blood gases improve.

G. Continuous positive airway pressure (CPAP) or positive end expiratory pressure (PEEP) is useful in some patients and improves ventilation/perfusion abnormalities and blood gas contents. Careful attention to cardiac performance is necessary while this modality is being used.

H. Weaning from ventilatory assistance is predicated on trials of spontaneous ventilation while the patient is still intubated and the results of arterial blood gas determinations. Intermittent mandatory ventilation (IMV) is useful in the weaning process, especially in children.[11]

I. Other measures to treat the underlying cause of the problem, such as intensive treatment of congestive heart failure, management of infection, volume loading when shock is present, and drainage of sepsis must be individualized to clinical needs.[17,22]

8. *Prognosis* depends upon the following, and must be individualized for every case.

A. The reversibility of the underlying cause

B. The promptness of treatment

C. Degree of response to treatment

D. The patient's general condition

PROBLEMS IN PERIPHERAL VASCULAR RECONSTRUCTION

1. Aside from the potential problems already covered, such as hemorrhage, hypovolemia, cardiac failure, and arrhythmias, the problem specific to reconstruction of peripheral arteries is whether or not vascularity has been restored or improved.

2. In reconstructions involving the lower extremities, the presence and character of pulses, warmth and color of the extremity, ability to move the leg, presence of feeling in the leg, absence of pain in the foot, are all to be carefully checked at frequent intervals.

3. Early failure of graft function is almost always heralded by adverse findings in several of these modalities, and rearteriography or reoperation without arteriography must be strongly considered.

4. Following carotid surgery, no narcotics should be used, since they mask pupillary and sensorial changes. Careful check of motor and sensory functions, awareness, ability to count, and pupil reactions give early information as to the success of the procedure.

CENTRAL NERVOUS SYSTEM COMPLICATIONS

These are not infrequent in open heart operations. Most are reversible and transitory, some leave permanent disability. Their etiologies are multiple.

1. *Etiology*

Possible etiologic factors include:

A. Air embolism

B. Poor cardiopulmonary perfusion

C. Particulate embolism from calcified valves

D. Thrombotic emboli from prosthetic valves

E. Problems relative to pre-existing cerebral vascular disease or malformations

F. Hypoxemia

G. Low cardiac output

2. *Management*

A. Reduction of any potential brain swelling is carried out by use of:

(1) Urea solutions

(2) Mannitol

(3) Corticosteroids

B. Seizures must be controlled with curarelike drugs, and, when coma or seizures are present, mechanical ventilatory support via an endotracheal airway is mandatory.

C. Less catastrophic problems can be managed by physiotherapy, good nursing, and supportive care.

REFERENCES

1. Appelbaum, A. et al.: Early risks of open heart surgery for mitral valve disease. Am. J. Cardiol., *37*:201, 1976.
2. Bachmann, F. et al.: The hemostatic mechanism after open heart surgery I. Studies on plasma coagulation factors and fibrinolysis in 512 patients after extracorporeal circulation. J. Thorac. Cardiovasc. Surg., *70*:76, 1975.
3. Berger, R. L. et al.: Cardiac output measurement by thermodilution during cardiac operations. Ann. Thorac. Surg., *21*:43, 1976.
4. Billig, D. M.: Current review: Current considerations in the management of tetralogy of Fallot. Chest, *64*:79, 1973.
5. ———: Management of thoracic trauma. *In* Matsumoto, T. (ed.): Current Management of Trauma in Surgery and General Practice. Springfield, Charles C Thomas, 1975.
6. Billig, D. M. and Jordan, P. H. Jr.: Hemodynamic abnormalities secondary to extracellular fluid depletion in intestinal obstruction. Surg. Gynec. Obstet., *128*:1274, 1969.
7. ———: Hemodynamic and respiratory alterations following abdominal surgery. Am. J. Surg., *117*:582, 1969.
8. Billig, D. M. and Kreidberg, M. B.: Physiologic parameters in intra- and postoperative management. *In* Billig, D. M. and Kreidberg, M. B. (eds.): The Management of Neonates and Infants with Congenital Heart Disease. New York, Grune & Stratton, 1973.
9. Cleveland, J. C. et al.: The role of intra-aortic balloon counterpulsation in patients undergoing cardiac operations. Ann. Thorac. Surg., *20*:652, 1975.
10. Clowes, G. H., Jr., DelGuercio, L. R. M. and Barwinsky, J.: The cardiac output in response to surgical trauma. Arch. Surg., *81*:212, 1960.
11. Downes, J. J. and Raphaely, R. C.: Pediatric intensive care. Anesthesiology, *43*:238, 1975.
12. Ebert, P. A.: The pericardium. *In* Gibbon, J. H., Jr., Sabiston, D. C., Jr. and Spencer, F. C. (eds.): Surgery of the Chest. Philadelphia, W. B. Saunders, 1969.
13. Gomes, M. R. and McGoon, D. C.: Bleeding patterns after open heart surgery, J. Thorac. Cardiovasc. Surg., *60*:87, 1970.
14. Kinney, J. M.: Ventilatory problems in shock and trauma. *In* Matsumoto, T. (ed.): Current Management of Trauma in Surgery and General Practice. Springfield, Ill., Charles C Thomas, 1975.
15. Kirklin, J. W. and Karp, R.: Treatment during the post-operative period. *In* Kirklin, J. W. and Karp, R. (eds.): The Tetralogy of Fallot From a Surgical Viewpoint. p. 97. Philadelphia, W. B. Saunders, 1970.
16. Kirklin, J. W. and Theye, R. A.: Cardiac performance after open intracardiac surgery. Circulation, *28*:1061, 1968.
17. Laver, M. B., Hallowell, P. and Goldblatt, A.: Pulmonary dysfunction secondary to heart disease: Aspects relevant to anesthesia and surgery. Anesthesiology, *33*:161, 1970.
18. McKenna, R. et al.: The hemostatic mechanism after open heart surgery. II Frequency of abnormal platelet functions during and after extracorporeal circulation. J. Thorac. Cardiovasc. Surg., *70*:298, 1975.
19. Matsumoto, T. and Levy, B. A.: Management of pulmonary failure in surgical patients. *In* Matsumoto, T., (ed.):Current Management of Trauma in Surgery and General Practice. Springfield, Ill., Charles C Thomas, 1975.
20. Motsay, G. J. and Lillehei, R. C.: Hypovolemic shock. *In* Matsumoto, T., (ed.): Current Management of Trauma in Surgery and General Practice. Springfield, Ill., Charles C Thomas, 1975.
21. Siggard-Anderson, O. and Engel, K.: A new acid base nomogram. An improved method for the calculation of the relevant blood acid-base data. Scand. J. Clin. and Lab. Invest., *12*:172, 1960.
22. Solliday, N. H., Shapiro, B. A. and Grecey, D. R.: Adult respiratory distress syndrome. Chest, *69*:207, 1976.

31. VARIOUS CARDIAC SYNDROMES AND RELATED PROBLEMS

Stuart M. Deglin, M.D., and Edward K. Chung, M.D.

GENERAL CONSIDERATIONS

Chest pain, fatigue, shortness of breath, lightheadedness, fainting, edema, and various electrocardiographic changes are findings commonly encountered in various clinical entities. Some of these findings may be a part of a given syndrome that does not reflect significant heart disease, whereas other findings may indicate clinically significant organic heart disease. Differentiation is often difficult. For example, chest pain due to noncardiac disorders, such as Tietze's syndrome or hyperventilation syndrome, may closely resemble coronary heart disease. A variety of cardiac syndromes and related subjects that are considered to be clinically significant will be briefly reviewed in this chapter to assist in the differential diagnosis and management.

POST-MYOCARDIAL-INFARCTION SYNDROME (DRESSLER'S SYNDROME)

1. *Definition*

Pleuropericarditis secondary to myocardial infarction, generally occurring 2 to 11 weeks after the acute episode, is termed the post-myocardial-infarction syndrome.[1]

2. *Etiology*

An autoimmune etiology is suspected because of:

A. The latent period before pericarditis develops

B. The response to steroids

C. The frequent demonstration of antimyocardial antibodies in the patients[2]

3. *Symptoms and signs*

A. Symptoms

(1) The patient may experience a recurrence of chest pain weeks to months after the acute episode of a myocardial infarction.

(2) The chest discomfort is sharp in character.

(3) It is usually precordial but may radiate to the shoulder or into the neck.

(4) It is aggravated by deep respiratory movements and by recumbency.

B. Physical findings.

(1) A pericardial friction rub is the most important physical diagnostic feature.

(2) There may be associated low grade fever, tachycardia, and evidence of pleural or pericardial effusion.

(3) Rales may be heard in the chest.

4. *Diagnosis*

A. There are no specific laboratory findings.

B. Radiologic studies may reveal pulmonary infiltrates or pleural effusion.

C. A globular-shaped heart may be seen only if there is a large pericardial effusion.

D. The electrocardiogram classically demonstrates diffuse S-T segment elevation without reciprocal changes in addition to pre-existing myocardial infarction.

E. Diagnosis is made on the basis of recurrent chest pain after an appropriate interval following acute myocardial infarction and on the basis of physical findings as described above.

5. *Differential diagnosis*

The differential diagnosis includes extension of myocardial infarction and pulmonary embolism or infarction.

A. Extension of myocardial infarction is accompanied by the more typical retrosternal discomfort of ischemic cardiac pain and by the development of new Q waves on the ECG.

B. The presence of a pericardial friction rub most frequently differentiates the post-myocardial-infarction syndrome from pulmonary infarction.

C. Pulmonary embolic phenomena are likely to produce more discrete infiltrates than those seen in Dressler's syndrome.

6. *Complications*

A. Supraventricular tachyarrhythmias occur commonly in this syndrome.

B. Hemorrhagic pericardial effusions and pericardial tamponade are known complications, particularly if anticoagulants are administered in the presence of pericarditis.

7. *Management*

A. Aspirin may relieve pain in some instances, although protracted or severe discomfort may call for the use of corticosteroids.

B. Prednisone may be started at a dose of 40 to 60 mg. daily, often resulting in dramatic relief of symptoms. The dose is slowly decreased over a 4-week period.

C. Symptoms often recur when lower dosage levels have been reached or the drug has been withdrawn, necessitating reinstitution of steroids, sometimes for prolonged periods of time.

8. *Prognosis*

A. Good in most cases

B. The post-myocardial-infarction syndrome has not been shown to alter the prognosis of the underlying coronary heart disease.

POSTCARDIOTOMY SYNDROME

1. *Definition*

The postcardiotomy syndrome is a febrile illness with pericardial and sometimes pleuropulmonary reaction that follows pericardiotomy by 2 weeks to 3 months.[3] It occurs after approximately 30 per cent of pericardiotomies.

2. *Etiology*

Postcardiotomy syndrome may be due to various causes.[3,4] They may include:

A. Cardiac surgery (common)

B. Penetrating trauma to the chest (common)

C. Blunt trauma to the chest (less common)

D. Artificial pacemaker implantation (rare)[4]

3. *Pathophysiology*

The exact pathophysiology of this syndrome remains controversial. Prominent theories include:

A. Infectious agents

B. Hypersensitivity to blood in the pericardium

C. Autoimmunity to damaged myocardial or pericardial tissue.[3]

4. *Symptoms and signs*

A. As in other forms of pericarditis, there is chest pain that is intensified by inspiration and recumbency.

B. There may be cough and dyspnea.

C. Unexplained prolongation of postoperative fever or reappearance of fever weeks after surgery are typical.

D. Pericardial and/or pleural effusions may be present.

E. A pericardial friction rub is commonly heard.

5. *Laboratory findings*

Radiologic and electrocardiographic findings, if present, are identical to those described in Dressler's syndrome except for the absence of a myocardial infarction pattern.

6. *Complications*

A. The course is generally benign.

B. Cardiac tamponade may rarely occur.

C. Cardiac arrhythmias, particularly supraventricular, are common.

7. *Management*

A. Corticosteroid therapy induces

prompt defervescence and alleviation of symptoms although relapses are common when therapy is withdrawn.

B. Salicylates may be helpful when symptoms are less severe.

8. *Prognosis* is good in most cases.

Q-T INTERVAL SYNDROME

1. *Definition*
These syndromes are familial disorders characterized by prolongation of the Q-T interval associated with cardiac arrhythmias and syncope or even sudden death.

2. *Classification*
A. Families have been reported with deaf-mutism, an autosomal recessive pattern of inheritance, and sometimes iron deficiency anemia.[5]

B. Other families have demonstrated autosomal dominant inheritance of Q-T prolongation with normal hearing.[6]

3. *Pathophysiology*
A. The cause of the Q-T prolongation is not certain.

B. The episodes of syncope generally occur during physical exercise.

C. Syncope and even sudden death are considered to occur because of ventricular fibrillation as a result of the R-on-T phenomenon (see Chap. 21).

4. *Treatment*
A. Prophylactic antiarrhythmic (procainamide, quinidine, propranolol or diphenylhydantoin) therapy is most important. Antiarrhythmic therapy is discussed in detail in Chapter 24.

B. Avoid strenuous physical activities.

C. Electrocardiographic screening of family members of the patient is necessary to prevent a possible syncopal episode or even sudden death.

5. *Prognosis*
A. Unpredictable
B. Sudden death is always a possibility.

BRADYTACHYARRHYTHMIA SYNDROME

1. *Definition*[7]
A. The bradytachyarrhythmia syndrome is characterized by components of bradyarrhythmias due to any mechanism and components of tachyarrhythmias due to any mechanism.

B. The underlying rhythm is usually bradyarrhythmias, and tachyarrhythmias occur intermittently.

C. Bradyarrhythmias may be marked sinus bradycardia, sinus arrest, S-A block, A-V junctional or ventricular escape rhythm and second degree, high degree, or complete A-V block.

D. Tachyarrhythmias may be atrial tachycardia, flutter or fibrillation and A-V junctional tachycardia, more commonly ventricular tachyarrhythmias.

E. Adams-Stokes syndrome is common.

2. *Etiology and pathophysiology*
A. Disease of the sinus node
B. Disease of the A-V node
C. Disease in the S-A junction and A-V junction
D. Disease in the Purkinje network
E. Disease process often involves 2 or more sites simultaneously.
F. The histopathology may vary but is commonly fibrosis, fatty infiltration, or arteriosclerosis.

3. *Signs and symptoms*
A. Lightheadedness or fainting (Adams-Stokes syndrome)
B. Irregular pulse, palpitations, and skipped heartbeats
C. Hypotension, and congestive heart failure may occur.
D. Signs and symptoms of underlying heart disease

4. *Diagnosis*
A. The diagnosis is made by demonstration of underlying bradyarrhythmias of various origins and mechanisms associated with intermittent tachyarrhythmias of various origins and mechanisms.

B. The underlying bradyarrhythmias are commonly unstable with slow sinus bradycardia and high degree or complete A-V block.

C. Tachyarrhythmia components are commonly multifocal ventricular premature contractions, ventricular group beats, and short runs of ventricular tachycardia.

D. Continuous monitoring system, such as Holter monitor ECG, is often required to confirm the diagnosis of bradytachyarrhythmia syndrome.

5. *Treatment*

A. Drug therapy alone is usually unsatisfactory because of the following reasons:

(1) Antiarrhythmic medications used to suppress the tachyarrhythmias may interfere with impulse formation in the sinus and may depress escape mechanisms.

(2) Adrenergic stimulation of the sinus or A-V node, for example with isoproterenol, may have the adverse effect of precipitating tachyarrhythmias.

B. Artificial pacing with slight overdriving pacing rate (80–120 beats per minute) alone is often effective (see Chap. 26).

C. Antiarrhythmic therapy in conjunction with the use of artificial pacemaker is necessary in some cases (see Chaps. 24 and 26). This therapeutic approach provides:

(1) Suppression of tachyarrhythmias

(2) Prevention of asystolic periods

6. *Prognosis*

A. Guarded

B. Many patients require permanent pacemakers.

SICK SINUS SYNDROME

1. *Definition*

A. The term *sick sinus syndrome* is used when the sinus node is unable to produce sufficient impulses.

B. Broad use of this term often includes the impairment of the sinus impulse conduction at the sino-atrial junction (S-A block).

C. Disease of the A-V node and other conduction systems often coexists with the sick sinus syndrome.

D. Sick sinus syndrome is commonly present as a part of bradytachyarrhythmia syndrome (see above).

E. Some investigators use the terms *sick sinus syndrome* and *bradytachyarrhythmia syndrome* interchangeably, but they are *not* identical.

2. *Etiology and pathophysiology*

A. Acute form

(1) Digitalis intoxication (see Chap. 23)

(2) Quinidine toxicity

(3) Atrial myocardial infarction

(4) Surgical (cardiac) trauma

(5) Chest injury

(6) Endocarditis

B. Chronic form

(1) Degenerative-sclerotic change in the sinus node and sinoatrial junction

(2) Cardiomyopathies

(3) The same disease process often involves the A-V node and other conduction system.

3. *Signs and symptoms*

A. May be asymptomatic in mild cases

B. Slow and irregular pulse

C. Lightheadedness or fainting (Adams-Stokes syndrome)

D. Palpitations (when bradytachyarrhythmia syndrome is present)

E. Congestive heart failure or shock may occur.

F. Signs or symptoms of underlying disorders

4. *Diagnosis*

Sick sinus syndrome may be manifested by the following findings:

A. Marked sinus bradycardia, sinus arrest and S-A block

B. Drug-resistant (atropine and/or isoproterenol) sinus bradyarrhythmias

C. Longer than usual pause following an atrial premature contraction

D. Long sinus node recovery time by atrial pacing (longer than 1500 msec.)

E. Atrial fibrillation:

(1) Often slow ventricular rate

(2) Often preceded by sinus bradycardia or first degree A-V block

F. Chronic first degree A-V block with intermittent atrial fibrillation

G. A-V junctional escape rhythm

H. Bradytachyarrhythmia

5. *Treatment*

A. Eliminate the cause if possible (acute form)

B. No therapy in asymptomatic patients

C. Artificial pacemaker in symptomatic patients (see Chap. 26)

D. Antiarrhythmic therapy is ineffective.

6. *Prognosis*

A. Guarded

B. Many patients require permanent artificial pacemakers.

HYPERKINETIC HEART SYNDROME

1. *Definition*

A. The hyperkinetic heart syndrome is characterized by an increased rate of ventricular ejection.

B. This results in bounding peripheral pulses, systolic ejection murmurs, and (commonly) ejection clicks.

C. Patients with this syndrome generally but not always have an increased cardiac output.[8]

2. *Clinical and laboratory findings*

A. Most patients described have been young or middle-aged.

B. Most patients with this syndrome are hyperactive in their daily activities.

C. Electrocardiograms may show left ventricular hypertrophy, but commonly it shows just high left ventricular voltage (voltage criteria of left ventricular hypertrophy).

D. Congestive heart failure has occurred during follow-up period in some cases.

3. *Treatment*

A. Beta-adrenergic blockage has been utilized in some patients.

B. The use of beta-adrenergic blocking agents in asymptomatic patients has not been advocated.[9]

4. *Prognosis* is good.

SHOULDER-HAND SYNDROME

1. *Definition*

A. The shoulder-hand syndrome is a periarthritis of the shoulder occurring during recovery from acute myocardial infarction.

B. The syndrome is primarily considered to be due to a long-standing disuse of the arms and shoulders as a result of acute myocardial infarction.

2. *Etiology*

A. The pain in the shoulders probably represents reflex spasm of the shoulder girdle muscle due to referred cardiac pain impulses.[10]

B. Structural damage to the hand has been attributed to hypoxia due to local reflex vasoconstriction.

C. The contributory role of protective disuse is suggested by the decreasing incidence of this complication as patients are more promptly mobilized when acute phase of myocardial infarction is over.

3. *Symptoms and signs*

A. Pain, stiffness, and limitation of motion of the shoulders and arms, generally on the left side, are characteristic.

B. The skin of the hands may become swollen and discolored.

C. Dupuytren's contracture of the palmar fascia may occur.

4. *Management*

A. Treatment consists of a program of physical therapy.

B. Corticosteroids either systemically or by injection into local trigger zones are effective in more refractory cases.

C. Reassurance is the most important therapeutic approach.

5. *Prognosis* is good.

TIETZE'S SYNDROME (COSTOCHONDRAL JUNCTION SYNDROME)

1. *Definition*

A. Tietze's syndrome is characterized by painful swelling at the costochondral junctions.

B. It most commonly occurs in young adults and during middle age.

C. The syndrome seems to be more common in females than males.

2. *Etiology*

A. The etiology is unknown.

B. Biopsy of the involved areas reveals normal cartilage.

3. *Symptoms and signs*

A. Tietze's syndrome often resembles acute myocardial infarction or acute pericarditis.

B. Pain and swelling usually develop at a single articulation, although multiple points may be involved.

C. The syndrome usually involves one side only and bilateral involvement is uncommon.

D. Examination reveals firm swelling with tenderness but no fluctuation or erythema.

E. There is no evidence of cardiovascular disorders.

F. There are no systemic manifestations.

4. *Laboratory findings*: There are no associated laboratory abnormalities.

5. *Differential diagnosis*

A. The anterior chest wall pain must be differentiated from angina pectoris or acute myocardial infarction and acute pericarditis.

B. Points in favor of the costochondral junction syndrome are:

(1) The markedly localized area of discomfort and local tenderness often associated with swelling.

(2) An electrocardiogram, during pain, which does not show findings of myocardial ischemia, injury, or infarction.

(3) Immediate relief by infiltration with local anesthetics.

6. *Management*

A. Reassurance of the absence of organic heart disease.

B. Mild analgesics.

C. In case of severe discomfort, nerve block or infiltration with corticosteroids.

7. *Prognosis*

A. The disorder is self-limited.

B. Episodes may last up to several months.

C. The syndrome is occasionally recurrent.

HYPERVENTILATION SYNDROME

1. *Definition*

A. This term refers to a syndrome of recurrent attacks of dyspnea associated with palpitations, tachycardia, atypical chest pain, lightheadedness, fatigue, and pararesthesias.

B. It is often associated with functional disorders of other organs systems including the gastrointestinal and musculoskeletal systems.

C. It is frequently seen in soldiers during the stress of war, but is more common in female civilians.[11]

2. *Etiology*

A. The syndrome is a manifestation of an underlying neuropsychiatric disorder, generally an anxiety neurosis.

B. It is commonly precipitated by environmental stress.

C. Most of the clinical features directly result from the underlying anxiety state.

D. Paresthesias and even frank tetany may be secondary to hyperventi-

lation and subsequent respiratory alkalosis.

3. *Symptoms and signs*

A. There is no objective evidence
of organic heart disease.

B. Dyspnea and chest pain commonly occur at rest.

C. The pain is often sharp in
character, does not radiate, and may be
associated with precordial tenderness.

4. *Diagnosis*

Differential diagnosis between functional chest pain and coronary chest pain
is described in Tables 31-1 and 31-2. The
diagnosis of hyperventilation is made by:

A. Recognition of the symptom
complex

B. Exclusion of organic heart disease

C. Uncovering a past or current history of neuropsychiatric disorder.

5. *Treatment*

A. Reassurance of the absence of
organic heart disease

Table 31-1. **Differential Diagnosis Between Coronary and Functional Chest Pain**

	Coronary	*Functional*
Age	Older persons (age above 45)	Young (age: 20–40)
Sex	Common in male	Common in female
Etiology	Coronary artery disease (atherosclerosis)	Psychologic insecurity and maladjustment
Precipitating factors	Exercise (eating, working), excitement, stress	Spontaneous or emotional
Hereditary	Family history of coronary heart disease and/or hypertension	Family history of psychoneurotic disorder
Initial symptom	Chest-pain, pressure sensation, tightness in the chest	Anxiety, dyspnea, hyperventilation
Feeling of palpitation	Often present, and may be associated with tachyarrhythmias	May be present without true cardiac arrhythmias
Objective signs of heart disease	Present	Absent
Fever	May be present (up to 102°F.)	May be present but rarely exceeds 100.5°F.
Fainting	Often present	May be present but transient
Shock	Often present in acute myocardial infarction	Absent
Heart failure	Often present	Absent
Chest x-ray	Often shows cardiomegaly or signs of congestive heart failure	Normal
Resting ECG	Often abnormal (myocardial infarction, ischemia or injury)	Normal
ECG during attack	Usually abnormal	Almost always normal
Cardiac arrhythmias	Common (almost every known type)	Rarely present (may show sinus tachycardia and extrasystoles)
Exercise ECG test	Often positive	Negative
Serum enzymes	Usually elevated in acute myocardial infarction	Normal
Commonly associated disorders	Hypertension diabetes mellitus, hyperlipidemia, obesity	Various psychoneurotic disorders

Table 31-2. **Characteristics of Coronary vs. Functional Chest Pain**

	Coronary	*Functional*
Location	Mostly substernal but anywhere in the chest	Cardiac apex and around the nipple
Area	Diffuse	More localized
Quality	Squeezing, burning, pressure, tightness, heavy feeling	Dull-aching or knife-like, sharp, stabbing
Radiation	Both shoulders, arms, fingers, neck, cheeks, teeth, interscapular region	Left hemithorax, left shoulder or back
Duration	Often less than 5 minutes in angina pectoris	Often more than 10 minutes or continuous
Local tenderness	Usually absent	Often present
Rest	Pain often disappears or improves	Pain unchanged or becomes worse
Response to antianginal drugs	Good	No effect or doubtful
Response to morphine	Good	Doubtful or unchanged
Factors aggravating chest pain	Exercise, excitement, and other similar stress, cold weather, after meals, sexual intercourse	Emotional stress, anxiety, complete rest

B. Judicious use of sedatives or mood elevators

C. Most importantly, guidance through stressful life situations by the physician or by referral to someone experienced in this area

ELECTROLYTE DISTURBANCES

General Features

Various electrolyte abnormalities may alter myocardial function from both mechanical and electrophysiologic standpoints. There are classic electrocardiographic abnormalities associated with each disturbance (described below). It must be realized that various underlying heart diseases, use of cardioactive drugs, and combined electrolyte disturbances frequently make the clinical problems more complex.

1. *Hyperkalemia*

A. Hyperkalemia may result from renal insufficiency, acidosis, and over-administration of potassium, especially in conjunction with potassium-sparing diuretics.

B. The common electrocardiographic changes during mild hyperkalemia (serum K: up to 7.5 mEq/L.) are:

(1) A tall and peaked T wave with a narrow base (Fig. 31-1).

(2) T waves that had been inverted for other reasons, such as left ventricular hypertrophy, may become upright in the face of hyperkalemia (Fig. 31-1).

C. With marked elevations of potassium (greater than 7.5 mEq/l.) there may be:

(1) Flattening, widening, and eventually disappearance of the P wave (atrial standstill)

(2) Prolongation of the P-R interval (first degree A-V block) followed by second degree or complete A-V block.

(3) Intraventricular block including diffuse and nonspecific intraventricular block, hemiblocks, bifas-

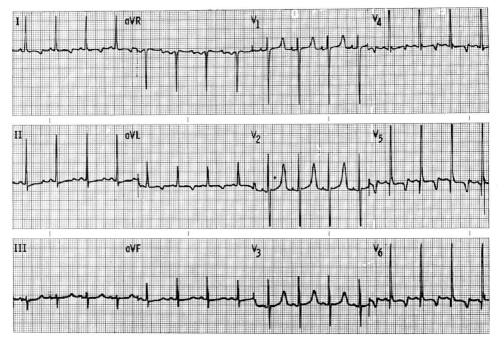

Fig. 31-1. This tracing was obtained from a patient with chronic renal failure. The rhythm is sinus with a rate of 95 beats per minute. Abnormalities include peaked and tall T waves due to hyperkalemia and prolonged Q-T interval (lengthening of the S-T segment) as a result of hypocalcemia. Note also an evidence of left ventricular hypertrophy.

cicular block, (Fig. 31-2) and trifascicular block.

D. In advanced hyperkalemia (more than 8.5 mEq./l.):

(1) A-V junctional or ventricular escape rhythm may occur without any atrial activity.

(2) In severe cases, ventricular standstill, tachycardia, or fibrillation (Fig. 31-2) can be observed.

(3) Advanced hyperkalemia often causes death.

2. *Hypokalemia*

A. Hypokalemia may be caused by inadequate dietary intake, gastrointestinal loss, salt-losing nephritis, use of corticosteroids or diuretics, aldosteronism, insulin administration, or alkalosis of any cause.

B. The most common electrocardiographic finding is that of a prominent U wave (Fig. 31-3).

C. In addition, S-T segment depression, T wave inversion, and prominence of the P wave may be seen.

D. Various cardiac arrhythmias may occur with hypokalemia alone.

E. The most important fact we should be aware of is that hypokalemia frequently predisposes to digitalis intoxication.

3. *Hypercalcemia*

A. Hypercalcemia may occur with hyperparathyroidism, vitamin D intoxication, malignant neoplasms (especially when osseous metastases have occurred), milk alkali syndrome, sarcoidosis, immobilization, overadminis-

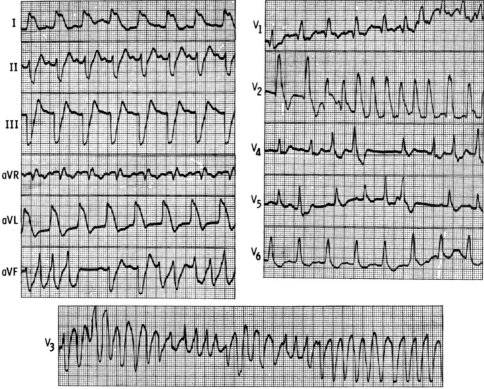

Fig. 31-2. Advanced hyperkalemia is manifested by bifascicular block (a combination of right bundle branch block and left anterior hemiblock) and short runs of ventricular tachycardia with paroxysmal ventricular fibrillation.

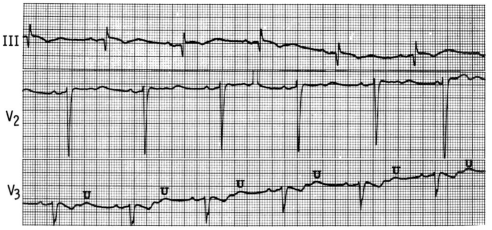

Fig. 31-3. Sinus bradycardia (rate: 50 beats per minute) with diaphragmatic (inferior) myocardial infarction. Note prominent U waves (marked U) indicative of hypokalemia.

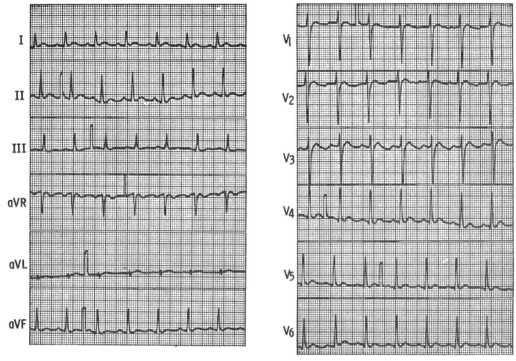

Fig. 31-4. The rhythm is sinus tachycardia with a rate of 105 beats per minute. Hypercalcemia is manifested by a shortening (actual absence of the S-T segment) of the Q-T interval.

tration of calcium, Paget's disease of bone, multiple myeloma, and hyperthyroidism.

B. The common ECG finding is shortening of the Q-T interval (Fig. 31-4).

C. Occasionally there may be prolongation of the P-R interval and QRS duration.

D. Ventricular premature contractions and ventricular tachycardia have been reported in severe cases although arrhythmias are relatively uncommon with this disturbance.

4. *Hypocalcemia*

A. Hypocalcemia may occur in chronic renal failure, essential hypercalcuria, renal tubular acidosis, vitamin D deficiency, hypoparathyroidism, and alkalosis.

B. The common ECG abnormality is prolongation of the Q-T interval, primarily due to lengthening of the S-T segment (Fig. 31-5).

C. Hypocalcemia and hyperkalemia often coexist, especially in chronic renal failure (Fig. 31-6).

D. Significant cardiac arrhythmias on the basis of hypocalcemia alone are rare.

5. *Hypomagnesemia*

A. Hypomagnesemia may predispose to digitalis toxicity.

B. It may result in cardiac arrhythmias in the absence of digitalis, and hypomagnesemia-induced ventricular fibrillation has been reported.

C. Hypomagnesemia and hypokalemia often coexist, and both conditions predispose to digitalis toxicity.

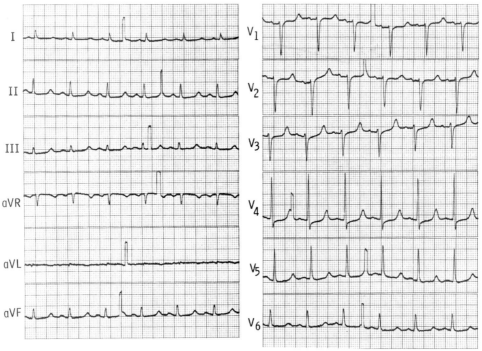

Fig. 31-5. The rhythm is sinus with a rate of 85 beats per minute. The striking abnormality is a prolongation of the Q-T interval (lengthening of the S-T segment) due to hypocalcemia.

6. *Hypermagnesemia*

Hypermagnesemia may result in ECG abnormalities similar to those seen in hyperkalemia.[11]

PREGNANCY AND HEART DISEASE

Pregnancy imposes a stress on the heart due to the metabolic requirements of the embryo. While the circulatory alterations that occur are normal adaptive mechanisms, the diseased heart may be unable to accommodate them, with heart failure being the result.

1. *Etiology*

Rheumatic (particularly mitral stenosis) and congenital cardiac disorders are the usual underlying problems.

2. *Pathophysiology*

A. Oxygen consumption may increase by up to 25 per cent.

B. Blood volume increases by 30 per cent at about the 32nd week.

C. Cardiac output increases by 30 to 50 per cent.

D. Because of the time sequence of circulatory overload, heart failure, if it occurs, is most common in the eighth month.[10]

3. *Symptoms and diagnosis*

A. The diagnosis of heart disease must be made with caution in the pregnant patient since edema, palpitations, systolic flow murmurs, and a third heart sound may all occur in the absence of cardiac abnormalities.

B. The elevated diaphragm may even give the false impression of cardiomegaly.

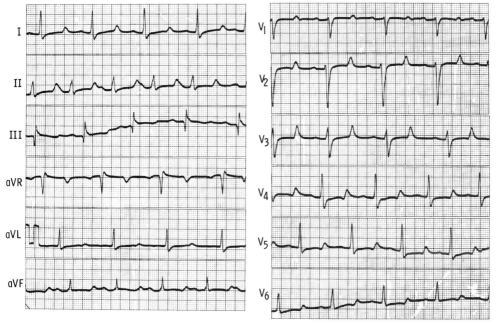

Fig. 31-6. This tracing was obtained from a patient with a far-advanced renal failure. Marked hyperkalemia is manifested by a flattening of the P waves, first degree A-V block, peaking T waves and diffuse intraventricular block. In addition, the Q-T interval is markedly prolonged because of a coexisting hypocalcemia.

C. A history of previous known heart disease and the presence of diastolic or continuous murmurs usually indicate organic heart disease.

D. Sinus tachycardia is very common during pregnancy without heart disease.

E. Ventricular premature contractions are relatively common during late pregnancy and in puerperal period in the absence of heart disease.

4. *Management*

A. Control of heart failure is the major problem in management of pregnant patient with heart disease.

(1) Frequent visits to the physician are mandatory.

(2) Overexertion, excessive sodium intake, and anemia should be avoided.

(3) If heart failure should occur, bed rest, marked sodium restriction, digitalis, and diuretics are instituted.

B. Cardiac arrhythmias may require various antiarrhythmic agents.

C. In severe cases with organic heart disease, pregnancy may have to be terminated.

5. *Prognosis*

A. The prognosis of cardiac patients during pregnancy parallels their functional status at the onset of pregnancy.

(1) There is no significant rise in morbidity in well compensated patients.

(2) The risk increases proportionately with severity of organic heart disease.

B. Fetal mortality has been estimated as being up to four times normal in patients with congestive heart failure during pregnancy.[10]

OBESITY

1. The presence of obesity is correlated with the coronary risk factors including hypertension and hypertriglyceridemia. Both of these abnormalities may improve to some extent by simple weight reduction.

2. In severe obesity, there may be marked cardiomegaly and heart failure with no other demonstrable cause.[12]

3. Cardiac disease may be simulated by obesity in the following fashions:

A. The dyspnea of obese patients is generally due to poor conditioning.

B. Dependent edema may be due to local factors.

C. The appearance of cardiomegaly on chest roentgenogram is often second-ary to elevated diaphragms and a large pericardial fat pad.

D. Frequent occurrence of sinus tachycardia in obesity may mimic organic heart disease.

CHEST DEFORMITY

Abnormalities of the thoracic skeleton can have significant effects upon the heart. The chest deformity may produce the ECG abnormality that may mimic myocardial infarction (Fig. 31-7).

1. *Kyphoscoliosis*

A. Kyphoscoliosis results in atelectasis, loss of lung compliance, and ventilation-perfusion abnormalities with subsequent arterial hypoxemia and hypercapnia.

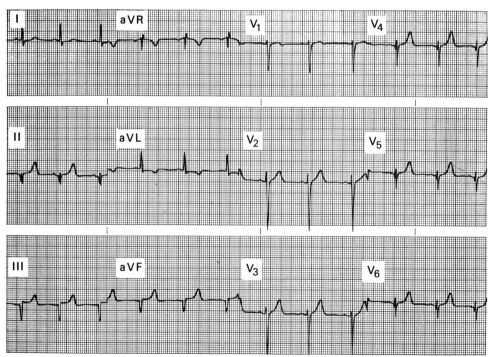

Fig. 31-7. This tracing was taken on a patient (23-year-old female) with marked chest deformity. Diaphragmatic-lateral myocardial infarction is closely simulated. This patient was found to have no heart disease.

B. Cor pulmonale is known to be a clinical consequence of kyphoscoliosis, and studies have demonstrated right ventricular hypertrophy and dilitation in 50 to 75 per cent of cases.[10]

2. *Pectus excavatum*

A. Pectus excavatum is a congenital abnormality with inward concavity of the lower end of the sterum. Because of the reduced anteroposterior diameter of the chest, compression of the heart may occur.

B. Physical examination reveals lateral displacement of the apical impulse, sometimes a left parasternal impulse, and a functional systolic murmur, most commonly in the pulmonic area.

C. The radiologic appearance is that of leftward displacement and the appearance of cardiac enlargement in posteroanterior views. However, in the lateral view, the sternal depression and narrowed anteroposterior diameter of the heart is seen.

D. The deformity is of significance only because its physical and radiological findings are so frequently misinterpreted as representing organic heart disease. In actuality, it rarely results in significant cardiopulmonary dysfunction.

3. *The straight back syndrome*

A. The straight back syndrome describes loss of the normal curvature of the thoracic spine with resultant reduction in anteroposterior diameter of the chest and compression of the heart.

B. The physical findings are similar to those in pectus excavatum, and radiologically the characteristic compressed cardiac shadow and straight thoracic spine are seen on lateral view.

C. The deformity results in no significant cardiovascular consequences.

REFERENCES

1. Chung, E. K.: Principles of Cardiac Arrhythmias. Baltimore, Williams & Wilkins, 1971.
2. Dressler, W.: Management of pericarditis secondary to myocardial infarction. Prog. Cardiovasc. Dis., *3*:13, 1960.
3. Engle, M. E. et al.: Postpericardiotomy syndrome. A new look at an old condition. Mod. Concepts Cardiovasc. Dis., *44*:59, 1975.
4. Friedberg, C. K.: Diseases of the Heart. ed. 3, Philadelphia, W. B. Saunders, 1966.
5. Frohlich, E. D., Dustan, H. P. and Page, I. H.: Hyperdynamic beta-adrenergic circulatory state. Ann. Int. Med., *117*:614, 1966.
6. Glock, G. and Braunwald, E.: Cardiac tumors and other unusual forms of heart disease. *In* Harrison, T.: Principles of Internal Medicine. New York, McGraw-Hill, 1974.
7. Hurst, J. W. (ed.): The Heart, Arteries and Veins, ed 3. New York, McGraw-Hill, 1974.
8. Kaplan, M. and Frengbry, J. D.: Autoimmunity to the heart in cardiac disease. Am. J. Cardiol., *24*:459, 1969.
9. Kaplan B. M. et al.: Tachycardia-Bradycardia syndrome (so called, "Sick Sinus Syndrome"). Am. J. Cardiol., *31*:497, 1973.
10. Kaye, D., Frankl, W. and Arditi, L. I.: Probable postcardiotomy syndrome following implantation of a transvenous pacemaker: Report of the first case. Am. Heart J., *90*:627, 1975.
11. Langslet, A. and Sorland, S. J.: Surdocardiac syndrome of Jervell and Lange-Nielsen, with prolonged Q-T interval present at birth and severe anemia and syncopal attacks in childhood. Br. Heart J., *37*:830, 1975.
12. Schwartz, P. J., Periti, M., Mulliani, A.: The long Q-T syndrome. Am. Heart J., *89*:378, 1975.

INDEX

Page numbers in *italics* refer to graphic, tabular and illustrative material. The term *passim* indicates scattered references to a subject within the noted sequence of pages.